1999 YEAR BOOK OF DIAGNOSTIC RADIOLOGY®

Statement of Purpose

The YEAR BOOK Service

The YEAR BOOK series was devised in 1901 by practicing health professionals who observed that the literature of medicine and related disciplines had become so voluminous that no one individual could read and place in perspective every potential advance in a major specialty. In the final decade of the 20th century, this recognition is more acutely true than it was in 1901.

More than merely a series of books, YEAR BOOK volumes are the tangible results of a unique service designed to accomplish the following:

- to *survey* a wide range of journals of proven value
- to *select* from those journals papers representing significant advances and statements of important clinical principles
- to provide *abstracts* of those articles that are readable, convenient summaries of their key points
- to provide *commentary* about those articles to place them in perspective

These publications grow out of a unique process that calls on the talents of outstanding authorities in clinical and fundamental disciplines, trained literature specialists, and professional writers, all supported by the resources of Mosby, the world's preeminent publisher for the health professions.

The Literature Base

Mosby and its editors survey approximately 500 journals published worldwide, covering the full range of the health professions. On an annual basis, the publisher examines usage patterns and polls its expert authorities to add new journals to the literature base and to delete journals that are no longer useful as potential YEAR BOOK sources.

The Literature Survey

The publisher's team of literature specialists, all of whom are trained and experienced health professionals, examines every original, peer-reviewed article in each journal issue. More than 250,000 articles per year are scanned systematically, including title, text, illustrations, tables, and references. Each scan is compared, article by article, to the search strategies that the publisher has developed in consultation with the 270 outside experts who form the pool of YEAR BOOK editors. A given article may be reviewed by any number of editors, from one to a dozen or more, regardless of the discipline for which the paper was originally published. In turn, each editor who receives the article reviews it to determine whether the article should be included in the YEAR BOOK. This decision is based on the article's inherent quality, its probable usefulness to readers of that YEAR BOOK, and the editor's goal to represent a balanced picture of a given field in each volume of the YEAR BOOK. In addition, the editor indicates when to include figures and tables from the article to help the YEAR BOOK reader better understand the information.

Of the quarter million articles scanned each year, only 5% are selected for detailed analysis within the YEAR BOOK series, thereby assuring readers of the high value of every selection.

The Abstract

The publisher's abstracting staff is headed by a seasoned medical professional and includes individuals with training in the life sciences, medicine, and other areas, plus extensive experience in writing for the health professions and related industries. Each selected article is assigned to a specific writer on this abstracting staff. The abstracter, guided in many cases by notations supplied by the expert editor, writes a structured, condensed summary designed so that the reader can rapidly acquire the essential information contained in the article.

The Commentary

The YEAR BOOK editorial boards, sometimes assisted by guest commentators, write comments that place each article in perspective for the reader. This provides the reader with the equivalent of a personal consultation with a leading international authority—an opportunity to better understand the value of the article and to benefit from the authority's thought processes in assessing the article.

Additional Editorial Features

The editorial boards of each YEAR BOOK organize the abstracts and comments to provide a logical and satisfying sequence of information. To enhance the organization, editors also provide introductions to sections or individual chapters, comments linking a number of abstracts, citations to additional literature, and other features.

The published YEAR BOOK contains enhanced bibliographic citations for each selected article, including extended listings of multiple authors and identification of author affiliations. Each YEAR BOOK contains a Table of Contents specific to that year's volume. From year to year, the Table of Contents for a given YEAR BOOK will vary depending on developments within the field.

Every YEAR BOOK contains a list of the journals from which papers have been selected. This list represents a subset of approximately 500 journals surveyed by the publisher and occasionally reflects a particularly pertinent article from a journal that is not surveyed on a routine basis.

Finally, each volume contains a comprehensive subject index and an index to authors of each selected paper.

The 1999 Year Book Series

Year Book of Allergy, Asthma, and Clinical Immunology: Drs. Rosenwasser, Boguniewicz, Borish, Routes, Spahn, and Weber

Year Book of Anesthesiology and Pain Management®: Drs. Tinker, Abram, Chestnut, Roizen, Rothenberg, and Wood

Year Book of Cardiology®: Drs. Schlant, Collins, Gersh, Graham, Kaplan, and Waldo

Year Book of Chiropractic®: Dr. Lawrence

Year Book of Critical Care Medicine®: Drs. Parrillo, Balk, Calvin, Franklin, and Shapiro

Year Book of Dentistry®: Drs. Meskin, Berry, Jeffcoat, Leinfelder, Roser, Summitt, and Zakariasen

Year Book of Dermatology and Dermatologic Surgery™: Drs. Thiers and Lang

Year Book of Diagnostic Radiology®: Drs. Osborn, Birdwell, Dalinka, Groskin, Maynard, Pentecost, Ros, Smirniotopoulos, and Young

Year Book of Emergency Medicine®: Drs. Wagner, Dronen, Davidson, King, Niemann, and Hamilton

Year Book of Endocrinology®: Drs. Bagdade, Braverman, Fitzpatrick, Horton, Kannan, Landsberg, Molitch, Morley, Odell, Poehlman, and Rogol

Year Book of Family Practice®: Drs. Berg, Bowman, Davidson, Dexter, and Scherger

Year Book of Gastroenterology: Drs. Aliperti and Fleshman

Year Book of Hand Surgery®: Drs. Amadio and Hentz

Year Book of Medicine®: Drs. Klahr, Frishman, Malawista, Mandell, Jett, Young, Barkin, and Bagdade

Year Book of Neonatal and Perinatal Medicine®: Drs. Fanaroff, Maisels, and Stevenson

Year Book of Nephrology, Hypertension, and Mineral Metabolism: Drs. Schwab, Bennett, Emmett, Hostetter, and Moe

Year Book of Neurology and Neurosurgery®: Drs. Bradley and Gibbs

Year Book of Nuclear Medicine®: Drs. Gottschalk, Blaufox, Coleman, Strauss, and Zubal

Year Book of Obstetrics, Gynecology, and Women's Health®: Drs. Mishell, Herbst, and Kirschbaum

Year Book of Oncology®: Drs. Ozols, Eisenberg, Glatstein, Loehrer, and Urba

Year Book of Ophthalmology®: Drs. Wilson, Augsburger, Cohen, Eagle, Grossman, Laibson, Maguire, Nelson, Penne, Rapuano, Sergott, Spaeth, Tipperman, Ms. Gosfield, and Ms. Salmon

Year Book of Orthopedics®: Drs. Morrey, Beauchamp, Currier, Tolo, Trigg, and Swiontkowski

Year Book of Otolaryngology–Head and Neck Surgery®: Drs. Paparella, Holt, and Otto

Year Book of Pathology and Laboratory Medicine®: Drs. Raab, Cohen, Dabbs, Olson, and Stanley

Year Book of Pediatrics®: Dr. Stockman

Year Book of Plastic, Reconstructive, and Aesthetic Surgery®: Drs. Miller, Bartlett, Garner, McKinney, Ruberg, Salisbury, and Smith

Year Book of Psychiatry and Applied Mental Health®: Drs. Talbott, Ballenger, Frances, Lydiard, Meltzer, Jensen, and Tasman

Year Book of Pulmonary Disease®: Drs. Jett, Castro, Maurer, Peters, Phillips, and Ryu

Year Book of Rheumatology, Arthritis, and Musculoskeletal Disease™: Drs. Panush, Hadler, Hellmann, LeRoy, Pisetsky, and Simon

Year Book of Sports Medicine®: Drs. Shephard, Drinkwater, Eichner, Torg, Alexander, and Mr. George

Year Book of Surgery®: Drs. Copeland, Bland, Deitch, Eberlein, Howard, Luce, Seeger, Souba, and Sugarbaker

Year Book of Urology®: Drs. Andriole and Coplen

Year Book of Vascular Surgery®: Dr. Porter

1999

The Year Book of DIAGNOSTIC RADIOLOGY®

Editor in Chief

Anne G. Osborn, M.D.

Professor, Department of Radiology, University of Utah School of Medicine, Salt Lake City; Nycomed Visiting Professor in Diagnostic Imaging, Armed Forces Institute of Pathology, Washington, D.C.

Mosby

St. Louis Baltimore Boston Carlsbad Naples New York Philadelphia Portland London Madrid Mexico City Singapore Sydney Tokyo Toronto Wiesbaden

Mosby
Dedicated to Publishing Excellence

Publisher: Cheryl A. Smart
Associate Publisher: Terrie Du Hadway
Senior Developmental Editor: Laura C. Berendson
Manager, Periodical Editing: Kirk Swearingen
Production Editor: Pat Costigan
Project Supervisor, Production: Joy Moore
Production Assistant: Karie House
Manager, Literature Services: Idelle L. Winer
Illustrations and Permissions Specialist: Steve Ramay

1999 EDITION

Printed in the United States of America
Composition by Reed Technology and Information Services, Inc.
Printing/binding by Maple-Vail

Editorial Office:
Mosby, Inc.
11830 Westline Industrial Drive
St. Louis, MO 63146

International Standard Serial Number: 0098–1672
International Standard Book Number: 0–8151–9617-2

Table of Contents

Associate Editors

Robyn L. Birdwell, M.D.

Assistant Professor of Radiology, Department of Radiology, Stanford University Medical Center, Stanford, California

Murray K. Dalinka, M.D.

Chief, Musculoskeletal Radiology, Hospital of the University of Pennsylvania; Professor of Radiology, University of Pennsylvania Medical Center, Philadelphia

Stuart A. Groskin, M.D.

Associate Professor, Department of Radiology, State University of New York; Health Science Center at Syracuse, College of Medicine, Syracuse, New York

C. Douglas Maynard, M.D.

Director, Division of Radiologic Sciences, Professor and Chairman, Department of Radiology, Wake Forest University School of Medicine, Bowman Gray Campus, Winston-Salem, North Carolina

Michael J. Pentecost, M.D.

Professor and Chairman, Department of Radiology, Georgetown University, Washington, D.C.

Pablo R. Ros, M.D., M.P.H.

Executive Vice Chairman and Associate Radiologist-in-Chief, Department of Radiology, Brigham and Women's Hospital; Professor of Radiology, Harvard Medical School, Boston, Massachusetts

James G. Smirniotopoulos, M.D.

Chairman, Department of Radiology/Nuclear Medicine; Professor of Radiology and Neurology, Uniformed Services University of the Health Sciences, Bethesda, Maryland, and Department of Radiologic-Pathology, Armed Forces Institute of Pathology, Washington, D.C.

Lionel W. Young, M.D.

Professor and Director, Division of Pediatric Radiology, Loma Linda University Medical Center and Children's Hospital, Loma Linda, California

Douglas L. Brown, M.D.

Associate Professor, Department of Radiology, Harvard Medical School; Staff Radiologist, Ultrasound Section, Brigham and Women's Hospital, Boston, Massachusetts

Contributors

Alan E. Oestreich, M.D.

Professor of Radiology and Pediatrics, University of Cincinnati College of Medicine; Radiologist, Cincinnati Children's Hospital Medical Center, Cincinnati, Ohio

Tina Young Poussaint, M.D.

Assistant Professor of Radiology, Harvard Medical School; Staff Neuroradiologist, Department of Radiology, Children's Hospital, Boston, Massachusetts

Journals Represented

Mosby and its editors survey approximately 500 journals for its abstract and commentary publications. From these journals, the Editors select the articles to be abstracted. Journals represented in this YEAR BOOK are listed below.

Abdominal Imaging
Academic Radiology
Acta Neurochirurgica
American Journal of Emergency Medicine
American Journal of Gastroenterology
American Journal of Kidney Diseases
American Journal of Neuroradiology
American Journal of Otolaryngology
American Journal of Respiratory and Critical Care Medicine
American Journal of Roentgenology
American Journal of Sports Medicine
Annals of Emergency Medicine
Annals of Internal Medicine
Annals of Thoracic Surgery
Archives of Neurology
Archives of Surgery
Arthroscopy
Australasian Radiology
Blood
Brain Pathology
British Journal of Obstetrics and Gynaecology
British Journal of Radiology
British Journal of Surgery
British Medical Journal
Canadian Association of Radiologists Journal
Chest
Circulation
Clinical Orthopaedics and Related Research
Clinical Radiology
Developmental Medicine and Child Neurology
Digestive Diseases and Sciences
Epilepsia
European Respiratory Journal
Gut
Hepatology
Human Pathology
International Journal of Neuroradiology
Investigative Radiology
Journal of Bone and Joint Surgery (American Volume)
Journal of Bone and Joint Surgery (British Volume)
Journal of Computer Assisted Tomography
Journal of Digital Imaging
Journal of Gastrointestinal Surgery
Journal of Laryngology and Otology
Journal of Medical Genetics
Journal of Neurosurgery

Journal of Nuclear Medicine
Journal of Pediatric Gastroenterology and Nutrition
Journal of Pediatric Orthopaedics
Journal of Pediatric Surgery
Journal of Radiosurgery
Journal of Rheumatology
Journal of Spinal Disorders
Journal of Surgical Research
Journal of Thoracic and Cardiovascular Surgery
Journal of Ultrasound in Medicine
Journal of Urology
Journal of Vascular Surgery
Journal of Vascular and Interventional Radiology
Journal of the American College of Cardiology
Journal of the American Medical Association
Journal of the National Cancer Institute
Journal of the Neurological Sciences
Lancet
Mayo Clinic Proceedings
Neuroradiology
Neurosurgery
New England Journal of Medicine
New Zealand Medical Journal
Pediatric Neurology
Pediatric Pulmonology
Pediatric Radiology
Pediatrics
Plastic and Reconstructive Surgery
Radiology
Rivista di Neuroradiologia
Skeletal Radiology
Southern Medical Journal
Spine
Stroke
Surgical Neurology
Transplantation
Ultrasound in Obstetrics and Gynecology
Urology
World Journal of Surgery

Standard Abbreviations

The following terms are abbreviated in this edition: acquired immunodeficiency syndrome (AIDS), cardiopulmonary resuscitation (CPR), central nervous system (CNS), cerebrospinal fluid (CSF), computed tomography (CT), deoxyribonucleic acid (DNA), electrocardiography (ECG), health maintenance organization (HMO), human immunodeficiency virus (HIV), intensive care unit (ICU), intramuscular (IM), intravenous (IV), magnetic resonance (MR) imaging (MRI), ultrasound (US), and ribonucleic acid (RNA).

Note

The Year Book of Diagnostic Radiology® is a literature survey service providing abstracts of articles published in the professional literature. Every effort is made to assure the accuracy of the information presented in these pages. Neither the editors nor the publisher of the Year Book of Diagnostic Radiology® can be responsible for errors in the original materials. The editors' comments are their own opinions. Mention of specific products within this publication does not constitute endorsement.

To facilitate the use of the Year Book of Diagnostic Radiology® as a reference tool, all illustrations and tables included in this publication are now identified as they appear in the original article. This change is meant to help the reader recognize that any illustration or table appearing in the Year Book of Diagnostic Radiology® may be only one of many in the original article. For this reason, figure and table numbers will often appear to be out of sequence within the Year Book of Diagnostic Radiology®.

Introduction

The 1999 YEAR BOOK OF DIAGNOSTIC RADIOLOGY, the second volume produced with our new team of coeditors, proves once again that radiology is a burgeoning and exciting field of medicine. Doug Maynard takes us into the twenty-first century with his selections that illustrate how radiology as a discipline will "weather" the coming millennium. His selections address other hot topics of concern to both academic and private practice departments. Does "filmless" radiology deserve all the hype? How go the turf wars? What is the role of research? Dr. Maynard, never at a loss for turning a neat phrase, says that "research by radiologists may well determine our success at guaranteeing radiology by radiologists in the future" (see Chapter Five, introduction).

In Chapter One, Stuart Groskin revisits some old friends (tuberculosis, HIV infection, aortic rupture) and acquaints us with some new ones (eg, CT fluoroscopy and "virtual" bronchoscopy). Dr. Young, our pediatric radiology coeditor, focuses on new techniques such as MR lymphangiography and voiding US with echo enhancement for vesicoureteric reflux. Of the latter technique he says "this may be the ideal nonionizing radiation method that has been sought for many years" (see Chapter Four, introduction).

Michael Pentecost's prescience in dubbing uterine fibroid embolization one of 1998's hottest topics in interventional radiology has been further fortified this year. Outcomes research for issues such as treating patients with claudication and chronic venous insufficiency is emphasized in Chapter Six.

In Chapter Three, Murray Dalinka once again treats us to the complex (combined ligament injuries) and the simple (the "Ottawa Ankle Rules"). Jim Smirniotopoulos and I have selected a bunch of super neuroradiology articles that demonstrate the broadened applications of new imaging techniques for old diseases. Really hot this year is the issue of screening for intracranial aneurysms, especially in at-risk patients (eg, first-order relatives). And what should be done if a lesion is discovered?

Lionel Young, our pediatric radiologist, welcomes Drs. Alan Oestreich and Tina Young Poussaint as contributors to Chapter Four. The team chose abstracts that identify a number of hot topics, including predicting outcomes in perinatal asphyxia based on MR findings, MR lymphangiography for vascular anomalies, voiding US with echo enhancement for vesicoureteric reflex, and enhanced MR imaging for childhood pyelonephritis.

Pablo Ros, our coeditor of the gastrointestinal/genitourinary section welcomes Dr. Douglas Brown who served this year, and will continue to serve next year as associate editor for the section on abdominal US (Chapter 7). Pablo and Doug point out that there is a definite trend toward increasing the use of cross-sectional imaging in areas that were long considered the domain of conventional radiology (ie, small bowel series, barium enema, excretory urography). Also selected for review this year are new applications of nuclear medicine in abdominal imaging (eg, the use of colonic scintigraphy for transit time and PET for abdominal malignancies).

Finally, we welcome a new coeditor, Dr. Robyn Birdwell, to Chapter Two on breast imaging. Dr. Birdwell focuses on a number of important issues, including that of sentinel lymph node (SLN) identification. Her selections and commentaries are terrific. We think you'll really enjoy her fresh perspective.

To all of our readers, welcome to the 1999 YEAR BOOK OF DIAGNOSTIC RADIOLOGY. Here are more than 300 articles and stimulating commentaries to keep you updated, off the street, and out of mischief! Enjoy.

Anne G. Osborn, M.D.

1 Thoracic Imaging

Introduction

In this year's YEAR BOOK OF DIAGNOSTIC RADIOLOGY, I revisit some old friends (the section titled "something old" covers tuberculosis, HIV infection, and aortic rupture) and make some new acquaintances (the section titled "something new" includes articles on CT fluoroscopy, the use of computers in detecting interstitial lung disease and on virtual bronchoscopy). I have borrowed the perspective of a clinician (in the "something borrowed" section) and looked at the practical applications and implications of the studies we perform and of our interpretations of those studies. I take a look at new approaches to imaging diseases of the airways ("something blew") and I am impressed with what I see.

In the category "something completely different," I include a potpourri of interesting cases, from the carcinomatous to the leguminous.

I hope that you will find these selections both entertaining and educational.

Stuart A. Groskin, M.D.

Something Old

Detection of Pulmonary Tuberculosis in Patients With a Normal Chest Radiograph

Marciniuk DD, McNab BD, Martin WT, et al (Univ of Saskatchewan, Saskatoon, Canada)
Chest 115:445-452, 1999 1–1

Introduction.—Pulmonary tuberculosis (TB) in the presence of a normal chest radiograph (CXR) has been reported earlier, even in patients with primary disease. The clinical features and the method of detecting pulmonary TB in the absence of radiographic findings has not been well delineated. Early symptoms of pulmonary TB in 25 patients with culture-positive pulmonary TB and normal CXRs are described.

Methods.—Patients were identified from a review of 518 consecutive patients between Jan. 1, 1988, and March 31, 1997. Patients with abnormal CXRs at diagnosis were excluded. Data were gathered regarding anthropometric data, symptoms, previous antibiotic therapy, method of detection, cultures, Mantoux skin tests, and other associated medical conditions.

Results.—Twenty-three of the 25 patients (92%) had symptoms at the time their TB was diagnosed. The most common symptom, cough/sputum, was reported in 76% of the patients. Eleven patients were identified because of exposure to persons with infectious pulmonary TB. The other 14 patients were identified because they had symptoms. Twenty-four patients (96%) had 1 or more symptoms: cough for more than 1 month, fever for more than 1 week, or skin-test conversion after contact with infectious TB. Only 1 patient had a positive sputum smear. Of 2 patients who were pregnant at the time of diagnosis, 1 was HIV-positive and 1 had isoniazid-resistant organisms. Five patients had primary TB associated with Mantoux skin-test conversion. The rate of culture-positive TB associated with normal CXR was less than 1% between 1988 and 1989 and steadily rose to 10% in the period from 1996 to 1997.

Conclusion.—Culture-positive pulmonary TB with a normal CXR is not an uncommon finding, and its incidence is increasing. These patients usually have symptoms, or are identified by contact tracing to individuals with infectious pulmonary TB. It is recommended that patients seen with a cough that has persisted for more than 1 month, with a fever for more than 1 week in duration, or with documented skin-test conversion less than 2 years after known exposure to infectious TB should submit sputum for a *Mycobacterium tuberculosis* smear and culture, even in the presence of a normal CXR.

► After an alarming increase in incidence from the mid-1980s to the early 1990s, TB appears to once again be on the wane. But don't be fooled! This remarkably resilient disease has been with us since prehistoric times and will likely accompany us to the end of the next millenium and beyond.

Leung's state-of-the-art review[1] is the most comprehensive discussion of the microbiological, epidemiologic, clinical, and radiologic features of *M. tuberculosis* infection that I have come across. It should be required reading for all radiologists and clinicians, regardless of their area of specialization, and it should also be recommended to medical students and house officers.

The article by Marciniuk et al deals with a particularly worrisome problem, the patient with active pulmonary TB who has a normal CXR. According to the authors, this problem is best dealt with by physicians being aware that patients with active pulmonary TB can have a normal CXR and by physicians maintaining a high index of suspicion when evaluating patients who have the following warning signs: (1) an unexplained cough for more than 1 month, (2) an unexplained fever for more than 1 week, (2) a ppd that has converted to positive within the past 2 years, or (3) a history of close contact with a patient with active TB.

The article by Marciniuk et al forced me to also think about a broader, less defined problem: How should we describe findings on CXRs that might be related to tuberculosis? More specifically, how should we indicate the likelihood that these abnormalities signify the presence of viable organisms and the possibility of active pulmonary disease? A large apical cavity poses no problem, but what should you say when you see apical fibrocystic changes with evidence of associated volume loss on a routine preoperative CXR? How valuable are old films, since reactivation tuberculosis can occur after years of radiographic stability, implying that viable organisms were present all along despite the lack of radiographic change? What do the phrases *old tuberculosis* and *no radiographic evidence of active pulmonary tuberculosis* mean to radiologists and to clinicians? What should they mean? Bottom line, how can we make our dictations both clear and clinically helpful? I don't have any pat answers to these questions, but I encourage you to think about them and, if possible, to discuss them with your clinical colleagues.

S.A. Groskin, M.D.

Reference

1. Leung AN: Pulmonary tuberculosis: The essentials. *Radiology* 210:307-322, 1999.

Cold Abscess of the Chest Wall: A Surgical Entity?

Faure E, Souilamas R, Riquet M, et al (Hôpital Laennec, Paris)
Ann Thorac Surg 66:1174-1178, 1998 1–2

Introduction.—Tuberculosis (TB) has reappeared as a significant public health problem in western countries. Skeletal localizations are infrequent.

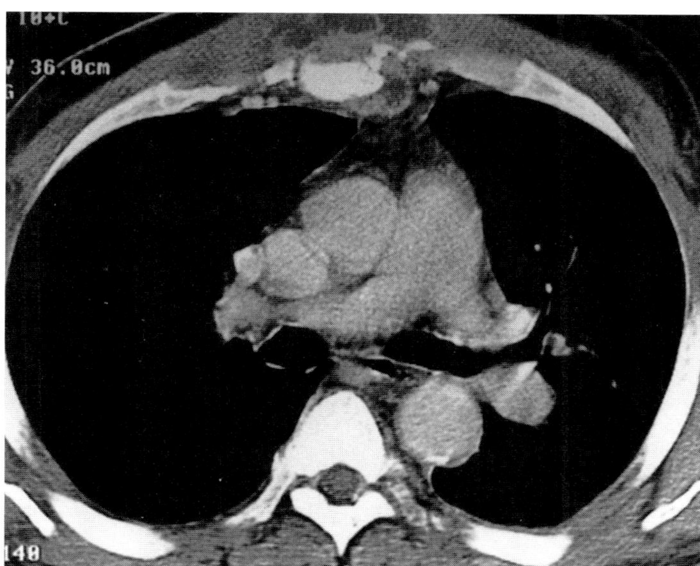

FIGURE 1.—CT scan showing a soft-tissue lesion destroying the sternum and extending anteriorly and posteriorly. The parasternal mass with low attenuation center and rim enhancement probably corresponds to a necrosis of an internal mammary lymph node. (Reprinted with permission from the Society of Thoracic Surgeons from Faure E, Souilamas R, Riquet M: Cold abscesses of the chest wall: A surgical entity? *Ann Thorac Surg* 66:1174-1178, 1998.)

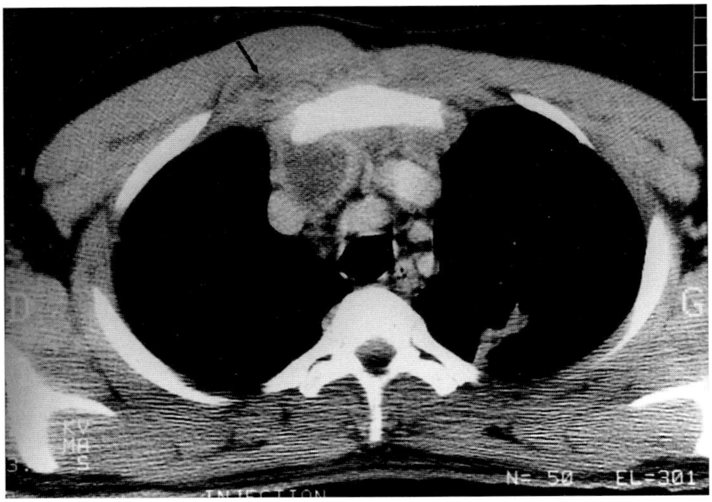

FIGURE 2.—CT scan showing a parasternal cold abscess (*arrow*) clearly resulting from a necrosis of the internal mammary lymph nodes. (Reprinted with permission from the Society of Thoracic Surgeons from Faure E, Souilamas R, Riquet M: Cold abscesses of the chest wall: A surgical entity? *Ann Thorac Surg* 66:1174-1178, 1998.)

The most common manifestations are lesions of the vertebrae, hips, and knees. Rib involvement is uncommon; yet it is necessary to update this pathologic condition of the chest wall. The role of surgical treatment of cold abscesses of the chest wall in patients with TB was evaluated.

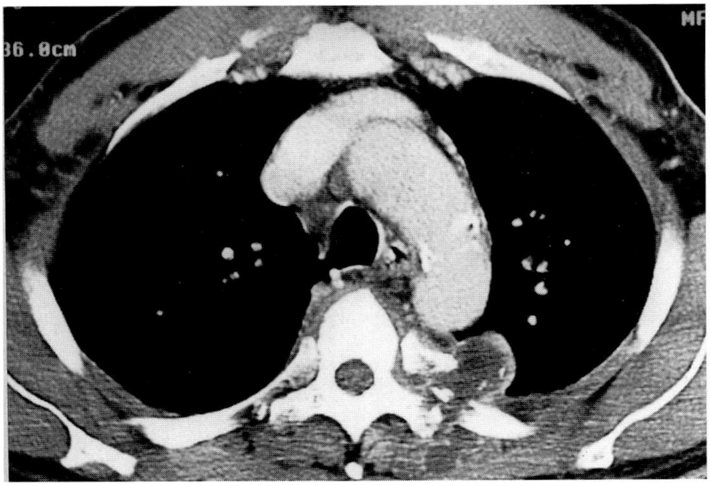

FIGURE 3.—CT scan showing a costovertebral cold abscess with destruction of the rib and the transverse process. (Reprinted with permission from the Society of Thoracic Surgeons from Faure E, Souilamas R, Riquet M: Cold abscesses of the chest wall: A surgical entity? *Ann Thorac Surg* 66:1174-1178, 1998.)

Methods.—Medical records of 18 patients with 1 or more cold abscesses of the ribs managed between 1980 and 1996 were reviewed retrospectively for data regarding epidemiologic characteristics, primary indications for surgery, methods and results of surgery, and pathogenesis of the abscesses.

Results.—The mean age of the 16 men and 2 women was 45 (range, 20-76 years). Sixteen patients were immigrants, and 1 had a history of intravenous drug use and was infected with human immunodeficiency virus. Nine patients had a history of TB (7 pulmonary and 2 mediastinal). Sixteen patients had a single chest wall lesion, 1 patient had 2 abscesses, and the remaining patient had 3 abscesses. Twelve patients had a clinically palpable mass. There were 21 lesion locations. Of these, 1 was located over a fractured sternum (Fig 1), 4 were parasternal (Fig 2) at the level of the lateral thoracic nodes, 12 were located in the rib shaft, and 4 were in the costovertebral joint (Fig 3). Chest wall images with low-density central area and ring enhancement were observed in 11 patients who underwent CT of the chest (Figs 1-3). Before surgery, needle aspiration or biopsy of the abscess gave a definitive diagnosis in only 4 of 11 patients. These 4 patients underwent antituberculous treatment before surgery. Four additional patients with associated active primary TB also received chemotherapy. The other 10 patients did not have a definitive diagnosis of TB at the time of operation. Operative management consisted of excision of the cold abscesses and required a costal or chondral resection in 15 patients. There was only 1 patient who did not undergo surgery after a favorable response to medical treatment. Eleven of 17 patients who underwent surgery were available for follow-up. One patient required a second operation because of recurrence at the same location. This patient had refused antituberculous therapy after the first operation. Locations of abscesses, CT scan results, and histologic examinations were in favor of a lymph-borne dissemination of tubercle bacilli.

Conclusion.—Since fine-needle aspiration is an inaccurate diagnostic tool and antituberculous medical treatment is not always efficacious, tubercular cold abscesses of the chest wall continue to be a surgical entity in most patients.

► As this article appeared in a surgical journal (*Annals of Thoracic Surgery*), what do you think is the answer to the question posed in the title? I selected this article not because I was particularly interested in whether or not tuberculous cold abscesses are surgical entities but because the resurgence of TB in the mid-1980s and early 1990s has made it mandatory that we recognize not only the common but also the uncommon manifestations of TB.

When I think of soft-tissue infections of the thorax, I think first of blastomycosis and actinomycosis, not TB. Musculoskeletal TB is not common, but it does occur, and when it does, it can be difficult to diagnose. One problem is our lack of awareness. Another problem is that musculoskeletal tuberculosis often occurs in patients who have no radiographic evidence of pulmonary tuberculosis. Because the clinical and imaging findings of musculoskeletal tuberculosis are nonspecific and microbiologic studies of aspirated material are often negative, surgery may be necessary for both diagnosis and treatment.

The authors don't address the question of what role percutaneous abscess drainage plays in treating these patients, but I wonder how effective it might be?

I recommend this article for its timeliness and for its surprisingly good illustrations.

S.A. Groskin, M.D.

Preliminary Results of Collapse Therapy With Plombage for Pulmonary Disease Caused by Multidrug-resistant Mycobacteria

Jouveshomme S, Dautzenberg B, Bakdach H, et al (Hôpital Pitié-Salpétrière, Paris; Centre Médico Chirurgical du Val d'Or, St Cloud, France)

Am J Respir Crit Care Med 157:1609-1615, 1998 1–3

Objective.—Although excisional surgery is recommended for patients with pulmonary diseases resulting from multidrug-resistant mycobacteria, two thirds of patients are high risk and therefore not eligible. As many as half of the remainder experience postoperative complications. Collapse therapy with plombage (filling of the intercostal extraperiostal space with lucite spheres) has been reported to cure 75% of these patients, but it was abandoned after several years. Results in a series of high-risk patients treated with collapse therapy with plombage are presented.

Methods.—Between September 1992 and March 1996, 7 patients (1 woman), aged 26 to 68 years, who had multidrug-resistant strains of mycobacteria and extensive bilateral cavitary disease were treated with collapse therapy. Six patients had active disease. The ribs over the disease area were denuded. The cavitary portion of the lungs was collapsed and the intercostal extra periostal space was filled with 5 to 18 polystyrene spheres that were 4 cm in diameter. Plombage was removed, if possible, when the periosteum had regenerated in the collapsed position (Fig 2).

Results.—Hospital stays averaged 12 days. After surgery, parenchymal cavities collapsed completely (Fig 1). In patients with active disease at surgery, sputum cultures remained negative for mycobacteria for 8 to 58 months. One patient infected with *M. xenopi* died at 4 months with culture-positive sputum. Plombage was removed from 4 patients at 3, 8, 11, and 25 months later. One patient with MAC infection died suddenly of unknown causes 8 months after collapse therapy and 5 months after plombage removal.

Conclusion.—Collapse therapy is an effective treatment for high-risk patients with pulmonary disease caused by multidrug-resistant mycobacteria.

► *Everything old is new again*—Barenaked Ladies.

Is there anyone who doesn't remember being shown a chest radiograph when he or she was a medical student or brand-new resident that showed multiple, remarkably similar, extremely symmetric pulmonary cavities?

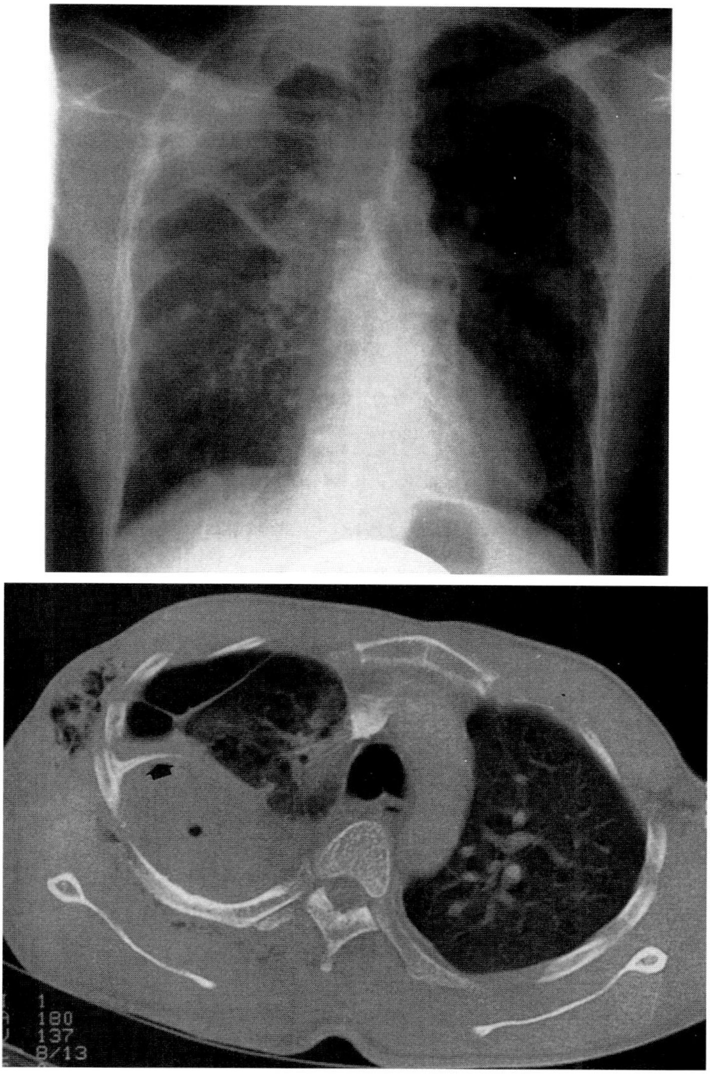

FIGURE 2.—Chest radiograph (**top**) and lung CT scan (**bottom**) of Patient 1 after withdrawal of the plombage. *Arrow*, calcifications of the periosteum that has regenerated in the collapsed position. The extrapleural space has filled spontaneously. (Courtesy of Jouveshomme S, Dautzenberg B, Bakdach H, et al: Preliminary results of collapse therapy with plombage for pulmonary disease caused by multidrug-resistant mycobacteria. *Am J Respir Crit Care Med* 157:1609-1615, 1998. Official Journal of the American Thoracic Society. Copyright American Lung Association.)

"Okay, hot shot, what's the differential?" asks the senior student/senior resident/junior attending.

"Cavitary mets."

"No."

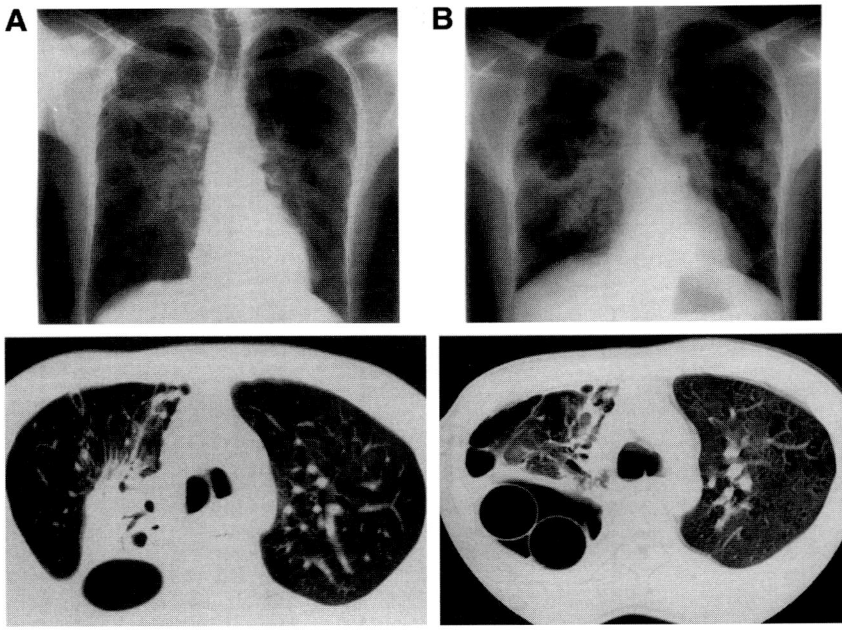

FIGURE 1.—Preoperative (**A**) and postoperative (**B**) chest radiographs and CT lung scans at the level of the carina of Patient 1. The previous cavity of the right upper lung is no longer demonstrable after collapse therapy. (Courtesy of Jouveshomme S, Dautzenberg B, Bakdach H, et al: Preliminary results of collapse therapy with plombage for pulmonary disease caused by multidrug-resistant mycobacteria. *Am J Respir Crit Care Med* 157:1609-1615, 1998. Official Journal of the American Thoracic Society. Copyright American Lung Association.)

"Abscesses, multiloculated empyema."

"No."

"Wegener's granulomatosis."

"No."

"I give up."

"You can't give up—is that what you're going to tell your patient?"

Last week, the candy stripers got this diagnosis in 13 seconds. They recognized ping-pong balls when they saw them, and they didn't have the dubious benefit of your medical education. It's called plombage, mister!"

And so yet another physician is done in by tuberculosis, the master of disguise.

The diagnosis and treatment of tuberculosis have literally and figuratively plagued us since prehistoric times. Although we seemed to gain the upper hand in the late 1940s and early 1950s (with the development of effective antimycobacterial drugs), the recent emergence of multidrug-resistant strains of tuberculosis and the increasing incidence of atypical mycobacterial infections have done a great deal to reverse those successes. Jouveshomme et al. describe remarkably good results of treating patients with refractory drug-resistant mycobacterial infections with the antique technique of plombage. The authors placed polystyrene spheres in surgically created subperiosteal, extrapleural pockets adjacent to large mycobacterial lung cavities. The bulky spheres caused the adjacent cavities to collapse, inhibiting mycobacterial growth. The results of this study made the authors happy and undoubtedly also pleased the patients. The results also made me happy, because I can now rest assured that future generations of medical students and radiology residents will also be shown chest radiographs that demonstrate multiple, remarkably similar, extremely symmetric pulmonary cavities.

S.A. Groskin, M.D.

Human Immunodeficiency Virus Infection and Pulmonary Hypertension: Two New Cases and a Review of 86 Reported Cases

Mesa RA, Edell ES, Dunn WF, et al (Mayo Clinic, Rochester, Minn)

Mayo Clin Proc 73:37-45, 1998 1–4

Introduction.—A myriad of pulmonary diseases have been associated with HIV and AIDS. As a result of longer survival and better prophylaxis, noninfectious complications are becoming more prominent. Lymphocytic or nonspecific interstitial pneumonia, bronchiolitis obliterans organizing pneumonia, diffuse infiltrative CD8 lymphocytis, bullous lung disease, pneumothorax, Kaposi's sarcoma, non-Hodgkin's lymphoma, and pulmonary hypertension are some of the noninfectious complications of HIV infection. HIV-related pulmonary hypertension was described.

Patients.—There were 88 patients, 61% of whom were male, with pulmonary hypertension and HIV infection. The usual initial symptom was dyspnea. Systolic pressure ranged from 49 to 118 mm Hg in the 74 patients who had their pulmonary artery pressure recorded. Lung tissue showed the plexogenic variant of pulmonary arterial hypertension in 85% of the 33 patients who had lung tissue evaluated microscopically. Three of 5 patients examined histologically had thrombotic pulmonary arteriopathy. In 1 case, it was caused by recurrent thromboembolism, and the other 2 patients had in situ thrombosis. Two patients had pulmonary veno-occlusive disease. One patient's chest x-ray study showed prominent pulmonary arteries and a patchy infiltrate in the left lower lobe of the lung (Fig 3).

Results.—The development of pulmonary hypertension was not associated with CD4 counts or a history of pulmonary infections. Confounding factors for hypertensive pulmonary vascular disease were present in 17% of the 88 patients, including coexisting liver disease and coagulation abnormalities. The chronic HIV infection seems to have been related to the development of pulmonary hypertension in 83% of the patients. Patients with HIV or AIDS had more rapidly progressive pulmonary hypertension than patients with primary pulmonary hypertension. In the patients with HIV or AIDS, there was an interval of 6 months between onset of symptoms and diagnosis. In the non-HIV and non-AIDS patients, there was an interval of 30 months.

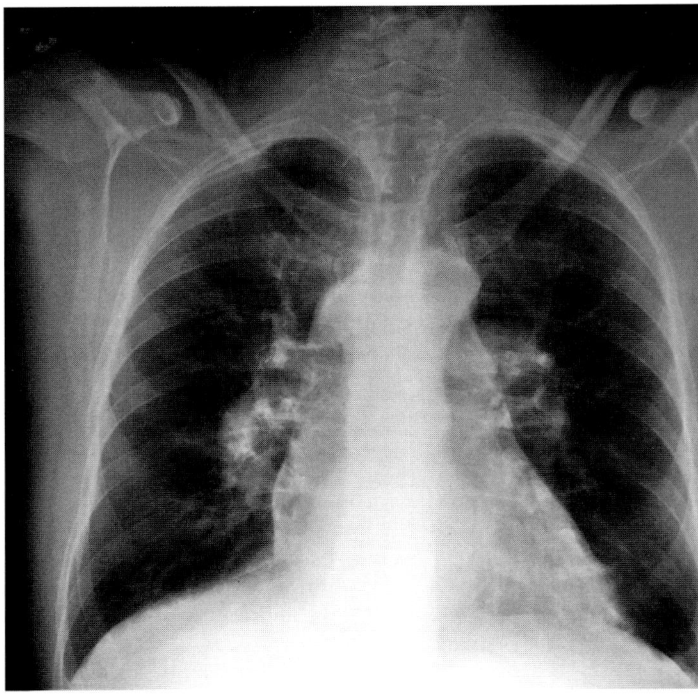

FIGURE 3.—Chest roentgenogram, showing prominent pulmonary arteries indicative of hypertensive pulmonary vascular disease. (Courtesy of Mesa RA, Edell ES, Dunn WF, et al: Human immunodeficiency virus infection and pulmonary hypertension: Two new cases and a review of 86 reported cases. *Mayo Clin Proc* 73:37–45, 1998.)

Conclusion.—For patients with HIV and pulmonary hypertension, the 1-year survival rate was 51%, compared with a 1-year survival rate of 68% for patients with primary pulmonary hypertension. In 29 of the 38 fatalities (76%), death was considered a direct consequence of pulmonary hypertension.

► I am sure that something profoundly philosophical could be said about the increasing frequency with which we now encounter noninfectious complications of AIDS. Maybe it is simply that our patients have become the victims of our success. In the beginning, most patients with AIDS died of opportunistic infections. As we have become more sophisticated in our prophylaxis and treatment of these infections, we have witnessed the emergence of whole new classes of complicating diseases that now challenge and confound us and kill our patients. It is interesting that many of these newly prominent diseases are thought to represent the direct result of HIV infection and not a complication of the immune suppression associated with systemic HIV infection.

Pulmonary arterial hypertension occurs with significantly increased frequency in patients with AIDS. Although some patients with AIDS have independent risk factors for pulmonary arterial hypertension (IV drug abuse, cirrhosis with portal venous hypertension), most do not, suggesting that this disorder may be the direct result of HIV infection. From a radiologic perspective, it is important to remember that enlarged hilar shadows in HIV-positive patients may represent distended pulmonary arteries caused by underlying AIDS-related pulmonary arterial hypertension, not lymphadenopathy caused by underlying infection or tumor.

S.A. Groskin, M.D.

Transbronchial Needle Aspiration (TBNA) in Patients Infected With HIV

Harkin TJ, Ciotoli C, Addrizzo-Harris DJ, et al (New York Univ; Bellevue Hosp, New York)

Am J Respir Crit Care Med 157:1913-1918, 1998 1–5

Objective.—Transbronchial needle aspiration (TBNA) of intrathoracic lymph nodes is useful in the diagnosis and staging of primary lung cancer and has demonstrated its value in the diagnosis of benign diseases. Results of the first 44 TBNA procedures using a histology needle in patients with HIV infection and intrathoracic adenopathy are presented.

Methods.—A total of 44 lymph node sampling procedures were performed in 41 patients with mediastinal or hilar adenopathy identified on chest radiographs or CTs. When undiagnosed intrathoracic adenopathy or parenchymal abnormalities were present, bronchoscopy was also performed.

Results.—Adequate lymph node sampling was performed in 35 procedures (80%) and sufficient diagnostic specimens were obtained in 23 procedures (52%). Transbronchial needle aspiration was the only diagnostic method used in 13 patients (32%). It was diagnostic of mycobacterial disease in 20 of 23 patients (87%), providing the sole diagnosis in 11 (48%). Transbronchial needle aspiration was diagnostic of *Mycobacterium tuberculosis* in 12 of 15 procedures (80%) and sarcoidosis in 2 of 4 patients (50%), providing the sole diagnosis in 1. It was diagnostic in 1 of 2 patients with non–small-cell lung cancer and was the sole diagnostic method used. The use of a histologic needle enhances the ability to diagnose nonmalignant diseases, including granulomatous disorders. In the HIV-infected population, intrathoracic adenopathy unrelated to lung cancer is primarily caused by tuberculosis. Transbronchial needle aspiration diagnosed intrathoracic adenopathy resulting from mycobacterial infection in 87% of the 50% of patients in this study, yielding a rapid diagnosis in 75% of the patients and the sole diagnosis in 50%. Thirteen negative bronchoscopic specimens and sputum smears and cultures were diagnosed by TBNA. It provided the sole diagnosis in 5 of 15 patients (33%) with *M. tuberculosis*, 6 of 8 (75%) with nontuberculous mycobacteria, 1 of 2 (50%) with bronchogenic carcinoma, and 1 of 4 (25%) with sarcoidosis.

Conclusion.—Transbronchial needle aspiration is a safe and effective—and sometimes the sole—technique for diagnosing the cause of intrathoracic adenopathy in HIV-positive patients.

Virtual Bronchoscopy for Directing Transbronchial Needle Aspiration of Hilar and Mediastinal Lymph Nodes: A Pilot Study

McAdams HP, Goodman PC, Kussin P (Duke Univ, Durham, NC)

AJR 170:1361-1364, 1998 1–6

Introduction.—Virtual bronchoscopy is a 3-dimensional, computer-generated procedure that uses helical CT data sets to generate simulated endobronchial images. Its potential uses include evaluation of endobronchial cancer or airway stenoses and guided bronchoscopy. Transbronchial needle aspiration (TBNA) is used to acquire a biopsy specimen of enlarged hilar or mediastinal lymph nodes during fiberoptic bronchoscopy. Reported is a preliminary investigation of virtual bronchoscopy as a guide for TBNA of hilar or mediastinal lymph nodes to determine the usefulness of this technique.

Methods.—Seventeen patients with a mean age of 65 (range, 43 to 80) underwent CT for examination of suspected adenopathy seen on chest radiographs. Primary cancer in 8 patients included 4 breast lesions, 2 renal cell lesions, 1 esophageal lesion, and 1 melanoma. To plan TBNA, enlarged nodes were manually traced on every third axial slice to create lymph node models. The models were embedded in the data set and displayed in green. Contrast material was injected into blood vessels and highlighted by means of a voxel seeding routine and displayed in red. Fiberoptic bronchoscopy and TBNA were performed with 22-gauge, 1- to 3-cm cytology needles. The mean number of needle passes was 3 (range, 2 to 10).

Results.—Eighteen nodes with a mean short-axis dimension of 1.9 cm (range, 1.0-5.0 cm) were aspirated in 17 patients. Locations were 7 paratracheal, 6 right hilar, 2 left hilar, 2 subcarinal, and 1 posterior tracheal. Findings were positive for cancer in 14 aspirates and negative for cancer in 4 aspirates. Of these, 2 aspirates had false negative findings. One patient had nodular sclerosing Hodgkin's disease that was diagnosed during open thoracotomy. The other patient had melanoma and a 1.8-cm right paratracheal node. Sensitivity of TBNA for cancer was 88% on a per node basis in this patient series. Time required to perform virtual bronchoscopy diminished over time.

Conclusion.—Virtual bronchoscopic images obtained from routine helical CT scans were useful in directing transbronchial needle aspiration. Bronchoscopy may have improved the yield of transbronchial needle aspiration with 22-gauge needles.

▶ Patients with AIDS who have mediastinal or hilar lymphadenopathy pose a perplexing but not uncommon problem in differential diagnosis. Enlarged intrathoracic lymph nodes in patients who have AIDS are usually caused not by the HIV infection but by either tuberculosis or tumor (lymphoma, Kaposi's sarcoma). Obtaining diagnostic material has been a challenge, and many patients undergo thoracotomy or mediastinoscopy.

TBNA of mediastinal and hilar lymph nodes has been successfully performed for a number of years.[1] Although it can be a very effective diagnostic tool, percutaneous needle biopsy does carry a significant risk of pneumothorax. Transbronchial needle biopsy has also been successfully performed for a number of years (since 1949 with a rigid bronchoscope and since 1978 with a flexible bronchoscope). The major problems with TBNA are knowing where to obtain a biopsy specimen (since the operator can't see through the airway wall, knowing where to puncture to hit a node and to avoid adjacent vessels can be a tricky business) and what size needle to use (bigger needles give better specimens, but they can also damage bronchoscopes). Harkin et al. describe their experience with a 19-gauge needle to perform TBNA biopsy of enlarged intrathoracic lymph nodes in patients with HIV. Their technique proved to be an effective diagnostic tool and produced no complications. Although all of their patients underwent CT scanning before biopsy, Harkin et al. never specified exactly how they used the information from the CT scans to plan and perform their biopsies. I am not an advocate of "virtual" anything, including virtual bronchoscopy (which seems to be largely visual sleight of hand and without real substance), but I wonder whether the results achieved by Harkin et al. might have been even better if they had used virtual bronchoscopy, as suggested by McAdams et al. Also, I wonder whether virtual bronchoscopy might have allowed Harkin et al. to use smaller biopsy needles, decreasing the risk of damage to their bronchoscopes.

S.A. Groskin, M.D.

Reference

1. Protopapas Z, Westcott JL: Transthoracic needle biopsy of mediastinal lymph nodes for staging lung and other cancers. *Radiology* 199:489-496, 1996.

Imaging of Acute Thoracic Aortic Injury Due to Blunt Trauma: A Review

Patel NH, Stephens KE Jr, Mirvis SE, et al (Univ of Washington, Seattle; Univ of Maryland, Baltimore)
Radiology 209:335-348, 1998 1–7

Introduction.—Up to 20% of fatalities in high-speed deceleration accidents are caused by acute thoracic aortic injury. The standard of care is prompt diagnosis and surgical management for successful surgical repair. Favorable results have been found with the use of CT and transesophageal echocardiography to screen for and facilitate the diagnosis of acute thoracic aortic injury in the patient with blunt chest trauma, and some have suggested that these imaging modalities could replace the thoracic aorto-

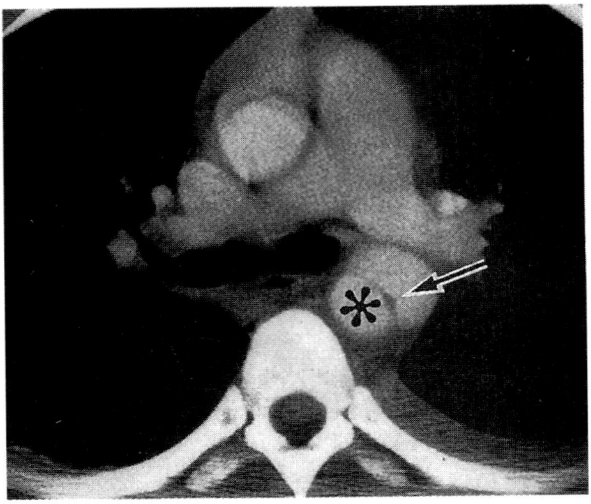

FIGURE 6.—Axial contrast-enhanced CT image at the level of the proximal descending thoracic aorta shows an intimal flap (*arrow*) separating the true lumen of the aorta from a pseudoaneurysm (*asterisk*). (Courtesy of Patel NH, Stephens KE Jr, Mirvis SE, et al: Imaging of acute thoracic aortic injury due to blunt trauma: A review. *Radiology* 209: 335-348, 1998. Radiological Society of North America.)

gram. The current status of the individual imaging modalities in use were summarized.

Computed Tomography.—Polyploid (clot) or linear (intimal flap) intraluminal areas of low attenuation, pseudoaneurysm, irregularity of the aortic wall or contour, pseudocoarctation, intramural hematoma, and dissection are the direct signs of acute thoracic aortic injury on CT. Figure

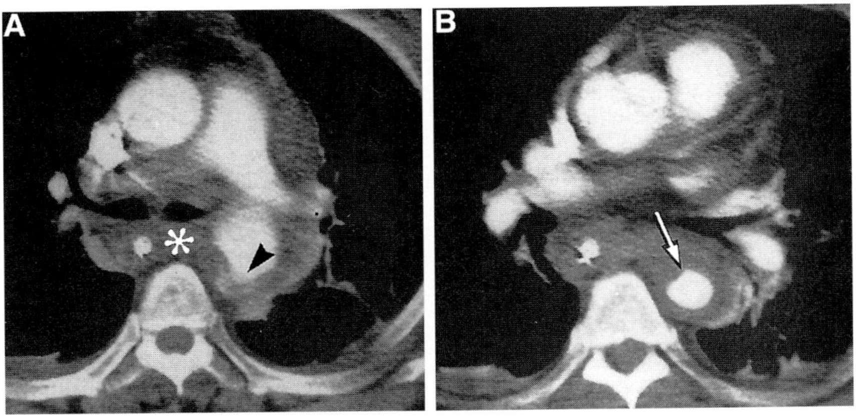

FIGURE 7.—**A**, Axial contrast-enhanced CT image at the level of the proximal descending thoracic aorta shows a contour abnormality (*arrowhead*) and a large periaortic hematoma (*asterisk*). **B**, A more caudal contrast-enhanced CT image obtained in the same patient shows that the caliber of the distal descending aorta (*arrow*) is narrowed (pseudocoarctation). (Courtesy of Patel NH, Stephens KE Jr, Mirvis SE, et al: Imaging of acute thoracic aortic injury due to blunt trauma: A review. *Radiology* 209: 335-348, 1998. Radiological Society of North America.)

6 shows an intimal flap separating the true lumen of the aorta from a pseudoaneurysm. Figure 7 shows a contour abnormality and a large periaortic hematoma, as well as pseudocoarctation. For depicting aortic lacerations longer than 16 mm, CT aortography is technically adequate. CT abnormalities that are not 100% diagnostic of acute thoracic aortic injury should be checked with transcatheter aortography.

Transesophageal Echocardiography.—Detailed, real-time images of cardiac anatomy are possible with transesophageal echocardiography; however, it cannot be used to reliably image the thoracic aorta. Intimal flap, intraluminal thick stripes, pseudoaneurysm, aortic occlusion, fusiform aneurysms, and aortic wall hematoma are direct transesophageal echocardiography signs of acute thoracic aortic injury. The extent of the injury is not reliably shown and may not depict the entire circumference of the aorta in up to 60% of patients.

Conclusion.—Thoracic aortography remains the standard of reference for demonstrating acute thoracic aortic injury, as it is the only imaging modality that allows complete evaluation of the thoracic aorta from the aortic root to the diaphragmatic hiatus and the brachiocephalic arteries and their branches. Timely diagnosis of acute thoracic aortic injury remains a challenge. To document the true sensitivity and negative predictive value of each modality, a comparative study of aortography, CT, and transesophageal echocardiography is needed.

▶ This is quite simply the best article about the imaging of suspected aortic trauma that I have read. It should be required reading for all radiologists, cardiologists, trauma physicians, and thoracic surgeons. Read it! The rest is silence.

S.A. Groskin, M.D.

Periaortic Hematoma on Helical CT of the Chest: A Criterion for Predicting Blunt Traumatic Aortic Rupture

Wong Y-C, Wang L-J, Lim K-E, et al (Chang Gung Mem Hosp, Taoyuan Hsien, Taiwan)

AJR 170:1523-1525, 1998 1–8

Introduction.—Helical CT, which provides less artifact than conventional CT does and decreases the number of equivocal or uninterpretable scans, is recommended for emergency practice. A retrospective study evaluated the accuracy of helical CT of the chest for predicting blunt traumatic aortic ruptures when periaortic hematoma is used as a positive criterion.

Methods.—The 123 patients had sustained blunt injuries to the chest. Initial chest radiographs showed abnormal findings. All patients underwent CT performed with a HiSpeed Advantage scanner and after a bolus IV injection of contrast material. Aortography was performed if chest CT revealed hemomediastinum (hematoma found in any site of the mediastinum). The retrospective study included 21 patients who had positive

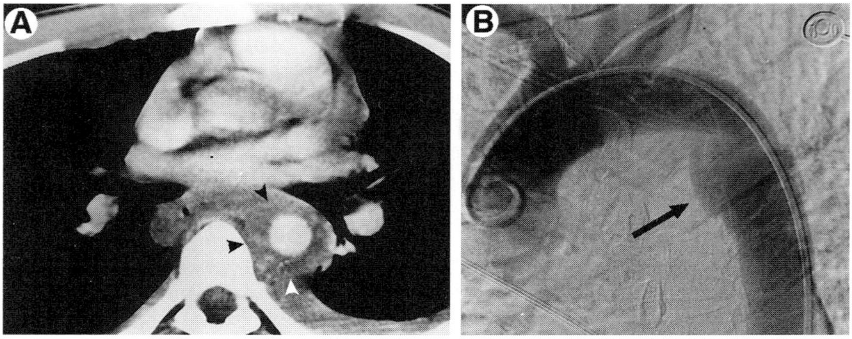

FIGURE 2.—25-year-old man with blunt aortic injury after motor vehicle accident. **A**, enhanced CT scan of chest 10 mm caudal to carina shows thick periaortic hematoma (*arrowheads*) surrounding proximal descending aorta. Periaortic fat is obliterated. **B**, aortogram in left anterior oblique projections shows traumatic aortic rupture at aortic isthmus (*arrow*). (Courtesy of Wong Y-C, Wang L-J, Lim K-E, et al: Periaortic hematoma on helical CT of the chest: A criterion for predicting blunt traumatic aortic rupture. *AJR* 170: 1523-1525, 1998.)

findings for hemomediastinum at CT and who subsequently underwent aortography. The CT scans were independently reviewed by 2 radiologists unaware of the results of aortography and surgical records. Results of CT were compared with those of aortography and surgery (8 patients).

Results.—Eleven of the 21 CT scans that were re-evaluated revealed periaortic hematomas. Eight of the 11 had aortic rupture detected on aortography and confirmed at surgery (Fig 2). The remaining 3 patients with negative aortograms showed no clinical evidence of delayed aortic rupture at a mean follow-up of 4.3 months. None of the 10 patients with CT scans negative for periaortic hematoma and no evidence of aortic rupture on aortography had clinically detected aortic rupture during a mean follow-up of 2 months.

Discussion.—Based on the criterion of periaortic hematoma, the sensitivity, specificity, and negative and positive predictive values of helical CT of the chest for predicting traumatic aortic rupture were 100%, 77%, 100%, and 73%, respectively. Periaortic hematoma is recommended as a positive criterion for predicting traumatic aortic rupture in patients with blunt chest injuries.

► Traumatic aortic rupture is a dramatic, devastating injury that must be diagnosed and treated promptly if the patient is to survive. Clinical clues are rarely (if ever) sufficient to establish the diagnosis of aortic rupture and imaging studies are routinely used both to suggest and to confirm its presence. Chest radiographs have traditionally been used as the primary screening test for evaluating patients suspected of having aortic injury. They have very good sensitivity but relatively poor specificity and other means of screening trauma vicitms have been sought. CT, particularly helical CT, has been increasingly used as an intermediate screening tool interposed between an abnormal chest radiograph and aortography. CT used in this fashion has decreased the number of negative aortograms performed in trauma victims, without, as far as we know, increasing the mortality from undiagnosed and untreated aortic laceration. It has also given us an extraordinary amount of additional information about thoracic and upper abdominal injuries. The problem, according to some, is that as good as CT is, it isn't perfect; CT hasn't completely eliminated negative aortograms. Mirvis et al[1] and Patel et al[2] and others have tried to find ways to increase the specificity of CT in diagnosing traumatic aortic rupture without compromising its sensitivity. These investigators have suggested that not all mediastinal hemorrhage arises from aortic injury. They found that isolated anterior and posterior mediastinal hemorrhage (particularly if centered on a sternal or spine fracture) is usually not associated with aortic injury and should not routinely precipitate an aortogram. Periaortic hemorrhage and blood in the middle and superior mediastinum, however, should be viewed with more caution and further workup to exclude aortic injury is usually indicated. Wong et al. essentially confirm these findings.

Based on the tone of their article, I expected that Wong et al. would unequivocally state that only periaortic hematomas are significant for aortic laceration and need further evaluation; but, in their final paragraph, they write, "In conclusion, we recommend the use of periaortic hematoma as a positive criterion for predicting traumatic aortic rupture." At the present time, periaortic hematoma should be considered a criterion for suspecting aortic injury, but it is by no means the only criterion. Direct CT evidence of aortic laceration is obviously of greatest significance, and periaortic hematoma is also an alarming finding, but even nonperiaortic mediastinal blood may be significant, particularly if it is seen in the superior or middle mediastinum. Will CT ever achieve perfect sensitivity and specificity? I doubt it, but perfection is something to strive for; it is rarely, if ever, attained.

S. Groskin, M.D.

References

1. Mirvis SE, Shanmuganathan K, Miller BH, et al: Traumatic aortic injury: Diagnosis with contrast-enhanced thoracic CT: Five-year experience at a major trauma center. *Radiology* 200:413-422, 1996.
2. Patel NH, Stephens KE, Mirvis SE, et al: Imaging of acute thoracic aortic injury due to blunt trauma: A review. *Radiology* 209:335-348, 1998.

Nontraumatic Rupture of the Thoracic Aorta: Chest Radiographic Features of an Often Unrecognized Condition

Fultz PJ, Melville D, Ekanej A, et al (Univ of Rochester, NY)
AJR 171:351-357, 1998 1–9

Introduction.—Numerous articles have described the radiologic features of traumatic aortic rupture, but few have addressed the radiologic features of nontraumatic thoracic aorta rupture. Radiographs of traumatic and nontraumatic ruptures of the thoracic aorta were compared to identify

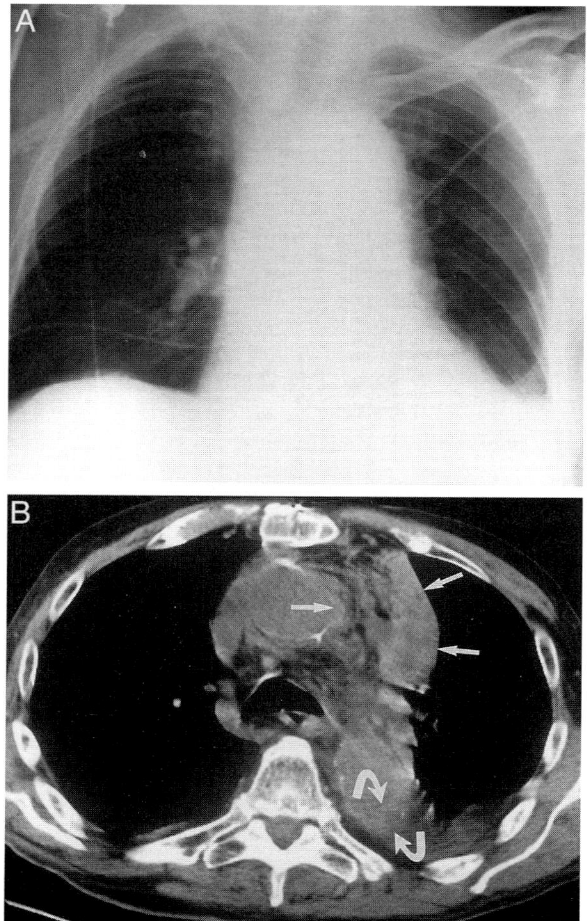

FIGURE 2.—Ruptured DeBakey type III aortic dissection in an 85-year-old man. **A**, chest radiograph shows abnormal aorticopulmonary window region, wide superior mediastinum, enlarged and irregular aortic knob, and descending aortic contour. Note small amount of left pleural fluid. **B**, unenhanced CT scan obtained 2 hours 30 minutes after **A** at level of aorticopulmonary window shows mediastinal hematoma (*straight arrows*) and left chest hematoma. Note acute intramural thrombus (*curved arrows*) in descending thoracic aorta. (Courtesy of Fultz PJ, Melville D, Ekanej A: Nontraumatic rupture of the thoracic aorta: Chest radiographic features of an often unrecognized condition. *AJR* 171:351-357, 1998.)

radiographic features that could help in the rapid detection of nontraumatic mediastinal hemorrhage.

Methods.—Twenty-seven consecutive radiographs taken at admission of patients with hemorrhage from ruptured thoracic aortic aneurysms, aortic dissections, or penetrating aortic ulcers were randomized with radiographs of 23 patients with nonruptured thoracic aneurysms, 20 patients with nonruptured dissections, and 20 controls. Diagnoses were determined by interpreting CT scans, MR images, and findings at surgery, autopsy, or

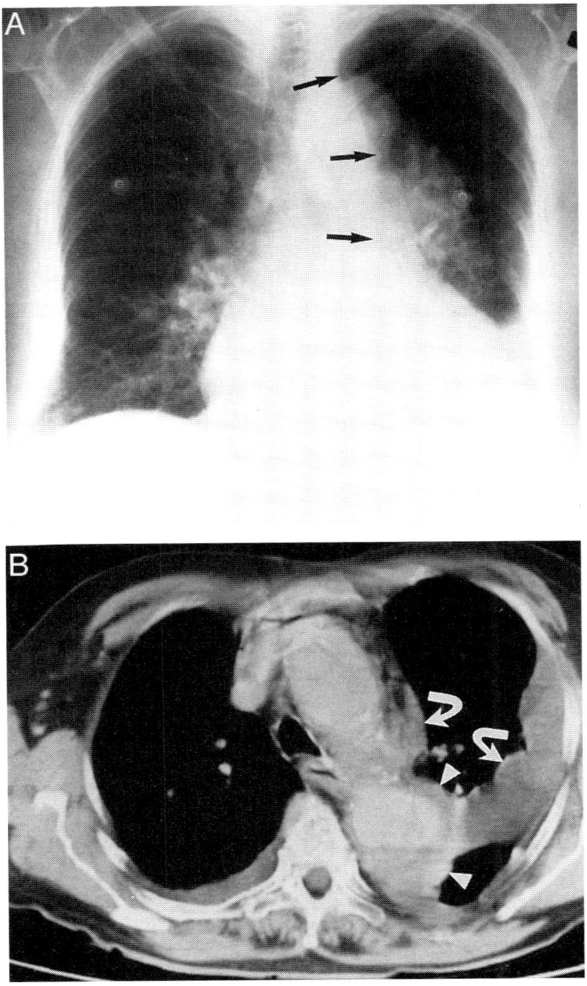

FIGURE 3.—Ruptured thoracic aortic aneurysm in a 55-year-old woman. **A**, chest radiograph shows irregular contour of left paraspinal interface that extends above level of aortic arch (*arrows*). Note wide superior mediastinum and descending aortic contour with left pleural fluid. **B**, CT scan 5 days later shows ruptured proximal descending thoracic aortic aneurysm (*arrowheads*). Hematoma extends into mediastinum and left chest (*curved arrows*). (Courtesy of Fultz PJ, Melville D, Ekanej A: Nontraumatic rupture of the thoracic aorta: Chest radiographic features of an often unrecognized condition. *AJR* 171:351-357, 1998.)

both. Three independent radiologists, unaware of patients' diagnoses, retrospectively reviewed radiographs. Twenty parameters were assessed for each of the 90 radiographs, and observers summarized their findings with final diagnoses. The best predictors of hemorrhage were calculated by means of logistic regression and rank correlation.

Results.—Logistic regression analysis revealed a combination of obscuration or convexity of the aorticopulmonary window (Fig 2) and a displaced left paraspinal interface (Fig 3) as the most helpful predictor of hemorrhage. Rank correlation analysis suggested obscuration or convexity of the aorticopulmonary window, a displaced left paraspinal interface, enlarged aortic knob width, increased thoracic aorta size, an enlarged, obscured, or irregular aortic margin, and left pleural or extrapleural space fluid as potential individual predictors of hemorrhage. Range of observer sensitivities for recognizing hemorrhage were 30% to 59%, and specificities ranged from 83% to 91%. The sensitivities for determining an abnormal from a normal mediastinum in 70 and 20 patients, respectively, were 70% to 90%; sensitivities were 65% to 90%.

Conclusion.—Obscuration or convexity of the aorticopulmonary window and a displaced left paraspinal interface on radiographs may suggest mediastinal hemorrhage. A definitive diagnosis may be established with further imaging.

Scene One

► The squeal of tires, the fingernails-across-the-blackboard sound of metal twisting and shredding, the anguished cries, the smell of gasoline and burning rubber. Next, the shriek of sirens, the flashing lights, and the crackle of tightly controlled voices on the radio. The ER doors explode open, and the attendants race their mangled passenger to Trauma Room One. The patient is inspected, injected, and x-rayed in less than 5 minutes. You quickly but carefully scan the trauma chest film, searching for pneumothorax, hemothorax, thoracic spine fracture, and evidence of aortic injury. The mediastinum looks slightly wide, and a CT scan is immediately done. The study is normal. The patient is stitched, patched, casted, and ultimately discharged.

Scene Two

► An 82-year-old patient in a nursing home complains of chest pain for the 57th time in the last month. Because he is persistent in his complaints (and in his incontinence), the staff send him to the local emergency room for evaluation. He is admitted to the hospital for "failure to thrive." You look at his admitting chest film, talk to a colleague, get another cup of coffee, and dictate, "tortuous aorta. No acute disease." The patient dies the next day; the postmortem diagnosis is aortic dissection with rupture.

Fultz et al remind us that, although not all causes of aortic rupture are dramatic, they are all potentially deadly. An accurate clinical history and a low threshold for proceeding to cross-sectional imaging whenever there is reasonable doubt about the integrity of the aorta are mandatory if we are to have any chance to promptly diagnose and treat these disorders.

S.A. Groskin, M.D.

Possible Causes of Inconclusive Results on CT-guided Thoracic and Abdominal Core Biopsies

Sheiman RG, Fey C, McNicholas M, et al (Harvard Med School, Boston)
AJR 170:1603-1607, 1998 1–10

Introduction.—Although appropriate needle localization within a lesion undergoing biopsy can be ensured by imaging techniques, such as CT and US, inconclusive biopsy results can still occur. Little is known about the possible technical causes of inconclusive percutaneous core biopsy results of a thoracic or abdominal lesion. The frequency of true malignancy of a thoracic or abdominal lesion that was clinically or radiographically suspected of being malignant and that had undergone CT-guided core biopsy with inconclusive results was determined. Possible correctable technical causes for CT-guided core biopsy with inconclusive results were identified.

Methods.—A 20-gauge automatic biopsy system was used in 116 consecutive CT-guided thoracic and abdominal core biopsies, which were retrospectively reviewed. If pathology confirmed malignancy, biopsy results were conclusive (94 patients), and if pathology results were negative for malignancy or were nondiagnostic, results were inconclusive (22 patients) (Table 1). The conclusive and inconclusive biopsy results were compared for lesion volume, location, number of cores, and biopsy technique (paraxial or coaxial). A second biopsy, radiographic follow-up, or surgery were performed to determine malignancy within the group with inconclusive biopsy results.

Results.—Only the biopsy method was identified by regression analysis as a significant factor affecting biopsy outcome. The coaxial method was less likely to yield a conclusive result than was the paraxial method. Lesions obtained by the 2 biopsy methods had similar volumes, locations, and numbers of cores. The 2 methods were equivalent for single-core biopsies. When 2 or more cores were taken, the paraxial method achieved a conclusive result 90% of the time, whereas the coaxial method achieved

TABLE 1.—Summary of Inconclusive Biopsy Results

Location	Inconclusive Biopsy Result			
	Paraxial Method	Coaxial Method	Total (%)	False-Negative Results* (%)
Lung	2/19	5/13	7/32 (22)	4/32 (13)
Pleura and mediastinum	0/5	2/5	2/10 (20)	1/10 (10)
Liver	1/13	2/5	3/18 (17)	2/18 (11)
Kidney	1/9	1/5	2/14 (14)	1/14 (7)
Adrenal gland	0/2	1/4	1/6 (17)	1/6 (17)
Pancreas	1/5	1/4	2/9 (22)	1/9 (11)
Retroperitoneal adenopathy	1/11	2/8	3/19 (16)	2/19 (11)
Miscellaneous†	1/7	1/1	2/8 (25)	2/8 (25)
Total	7/71	15/45	22/116 (19)	14/116 (12)

*Inconclusive biopsy results of tissue shown to be malignant on follow-up.
†Includes lesions of omentum, mesentery, and bowel.
(Courtesy of Sheiman RG, Fey C, McNicholas M, et al: Possible causes of inconclusive results of CT-guided thoracic and abdominal core biopsies. *AJR* 170:1603-1607, 1998.)

a conclusive result 65% of the time. Malignancy was found in 14 of 22 inconclusive biopsy results (65%) at follow-up, indicating an overall false negative rate of 12%.

Conclusion.—Conclusive results will be yielded significantly more often with CT-guided core biopsy performed with 20-gauge automatic biopsy systems and the paraxial method, compared with the coaxial method. Malignancy will exist often enough to warrant follow-up in the event of inconclusive results.

► Percutaneous needle biopsy techniques allow nonsurgical sampling of lesions deep within the thorax and abdomen and represent a quantum leap forward in the management of patients with suspected or documented neoplasm. I have recently started performing percutaneous lung biopsies, and, because the techniques and tools have changed considerably since I was originally taught how to do this, I have been reading everything on this topic that I can get my hands on. I was particularly interested in this article because it addresses 1 of the biggest problems associated with percutaneous needle biopsies: the inconclusive biopsy. For someone just starting out (like me), a nondiagnostic biopsy is a personal affront; it is a strident commentary on my lack of experience and a blaring testimonial to my faulty technique. It makes me feel both angry and guilty.

Sheiman et al. found that the only factor significantly related to an inconclusive biopsy result was the use of a coaxial instead of a paraxial biopsy system. Frankly, this was not what I wanted to hear. I like the coaxial approach to lung biopsies; you position your needle only 1 time and can do multiple biopsies and, because the visceral pleura is only punctured 1 time, the risk of pneumothorax is—at least theoretically—reduced. According to Sheiman and his colleagues, however, not only does using a coaxial approach increase the risk of a nondiagnostic biopsy (probably because of the limited volume of tissue sampled), it also does not reduce the risk of pneumothorax. Intuitively, I find the latter statement difficult to believe, but the numbers in this article support it.

What to do when reality is in conflict with intuition and habit? Go with intuition and habit! I am going to stick with the coaxial biopsy system for a while longer. Someone suggested that I make a slight curve in the tip of the inner coaxial biopsy needle to allow the needle to be directed into different portions of the lesion for sampling. I am going to give this a try. I am also going to be very aggressive in pursuing re-biopsy in patients whose initial biopsies are inconclusive, my injured feelings be damned, as Sheiman et al. found that 64% of lesions whose biopsies were initally inconclusive were malignant when biopsied a second time.

S.A. Groskin, M.D.

Something New

Real-Time CT Fluoroscopy: Usefulness in Thoracic Drainage
Meyer CA, White CS, Wu J, et al (Univ of Maryland, Baltimore)
AJR 171:1097-1101, 1998 1–11

Introduction.—For the interventional radiologist, options for use in imaging-assisted thoracic drainage include fluoroscopy, sonography, and CT. Although CT has advantages in terms of soft-tissue contrast and localization of pleural and mediastinal collections, it is limited by its relatively slow image display time. CT fluoroscopy has been used to guide such procedures as percutaneous lung biopsy. An experience with real-time CT fluoroscopy for guidance of localized pleural and mediastinal air and fluid collections is presented.

Methods.—Over a period of 1 year, the authors used real-time CT fluoroscopy for guidance in 24 thoracic drainage procedures in 20 patients: 14 men and 6 women, age range 25 to 77. The experience included 10 loculated pleural effusions, 2 mediastinal fluid collections, and 12 focal pneumothoraces. All procedures were performed with the use of a CT continuous imaging system in the CT suite. The patient remained in the gantry while the radiologist operated a control panel that was covered with a sterile drape (Fig 1). Drainage was achieved by a modified Seldinger technique or a single-stick trocar technique. CT fluoroscopy was used to confirm optimal catheter placement. After drainage had been carried out,

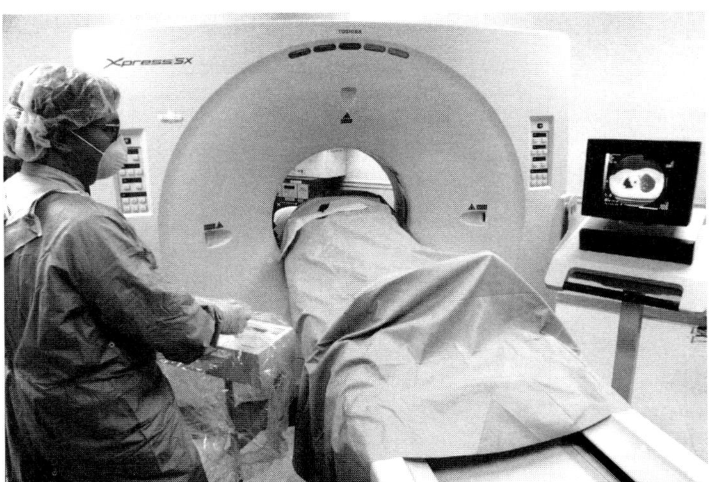

FIGURE 1.—Photograph of CT fluoroscopy system shows gantry, monitor and control panel. Control panel is covered with sterile drape during drainage procedures to allow radiologist to manipulate catheter and adjust controls without compromising sterile technique. (Courtesy of Meyer CA, White CS, Wu J, et al: Real-time CT fluoroscopy: Usefulness in thoracic drainage. *AJR* 171:1097-1101, 1998.)

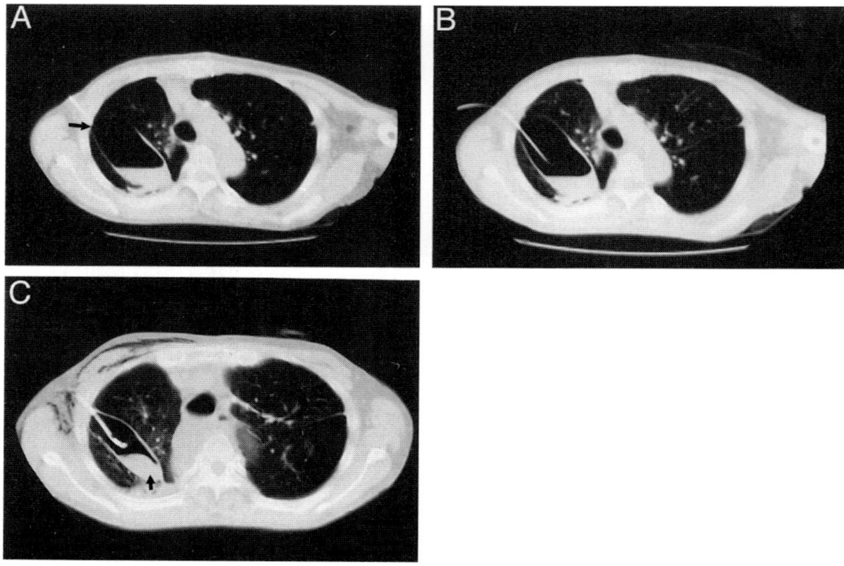

FIGURE 2.—Symptomatic loculated pneumothorax in major fissure in 59-year-old man. The patient had undergone lung volume reduction surgery. Collection was reached by modified Seldinger technique. **A**, CT fluoroscopic image shows 19-gauge Seldinger needle coursing through narrow window adjacent to rib while avoiding lung adjacent to parietal pleura (*arrow*). **B**, CT fluoroscopic image shows placement of 8F catheter that provided symptomatic relief but incompletely drained pneumothorax. C, CT fluoroscopic image obtained after 8F catheter was exchanged for 12F catheter and catheter ports were positioned with CT guidance. Collection is now decompressed. Thrombus (*arrow*) was noted on CT scans before procedure. (Courtesy of Meyer CA, White CS, Wu J, et al: Real-time CT fluoroscopy: Usefulness in thoracic drainage. *AJR* 171:1097-1101, 1998.)

another scan was performed to recheck catheter position and to ensure that no complications had occurred.

Results.—With the use of real-time or interrupted real-time CT fluoroscopic guidance, all 24 collections were successfully reached and drained without complications. Both pneumothoraces and focal fluid collections were successfully evacuated without problem (Fig 2). Real-time CT fluoroscopy was especially useful for rapid tube placement in patients who could not cooperate with breathing instructions or in patients with a narrow access window. The procedures took an average room time of 65 minutes, with an average procedure time of 32 minutes and an average CT fluoroscopy time of 143 seconds.

Conclusions.—Intrathoracic air or fluid collections can be quickly and safely drained under real-time CT fluoroscopic guidance. This technique provides real-time imaging like sonography, but with a wide field of view, improved soft-tissue contrast, and improved depiction of pleural and mediastinal collections. It is especially useful in patients who cannot comply with breath-holding instructions or those in whom access is limited.

► I'm not certain whether this article should be placed in the category of "back in my day, we didn't have it so good" ("We didn't have CT fluoroscopy, we didn't have CT, we didn't even have fluoroscopy—we just moved our patients back and forth in front of a really bright candle . . . "), or whether it should appear under the heading of "I need one right now!" I suspect that both categories are appropriate.

I don't have anything particularly insightful to say about this article or about the CT fluoroscopic equipment described herein, except that it's about time. CT is a terrific imaging technique and a great way to guide percutaneous biopsies and drainage procedures. The exquisitely detailed anatomic information that it provides allows us to pick the best route from the skin surface to the lesion, increasing the safety of procedures while its ability to show us precisely where the tip of our needle or catheter is improves the diagnostic yield and therapeutic efficacy of our procedures. A major drawback to using CT to guide biopsies and drainages was, and to a large extent still is, the lack of direct, real-time feedback about the location of the tip of the needle. The time spent running in and out of the CT suite while images are obtained and reconstructed each time the needle is moved adds significantly to the time required to do the procedure. This, in turn, increases the chance that something will go wrong. CT fluoroscopy is not a panacea, but my friends who have the equipment tell me that it comes pretty close. It is one of the few new technological triumphs that I can honestly say I want and will use, and this article by Meyer et al. supports my position. Now, if I can only convince my chairman.

S.A. Groskin, M.D.

Computer-aided Diagnosis for Detection of Interstitial Opacities on Chest Radiographs

Monnier-Cholley L, MacMahon H, Katsuragawa S, et al (Univ of Chicago)
AJR 171:1651-1656, 1998 1–12

Objective.—The diagnosis of interstitial lung disease on the basis of chest radiographs poses a difficult radiologic challenge associated with large intraobserver and interobserver variation. There is a need for some quantitative method of assessing abnormalities of lung texture. The authors have previously reported the development of a computer-aided technique for diagnosis of pulmonary interstitial infiltrates. They performed an observer test to determine the impact of the computerized scheme on radiologists' interpretations of chest radiographs with interstitial opacities.

Methods.—The study included 20 normal chest radiographs and 20 radiographs showing interstitial opacities. After each film was divided into 4 quadrants and 31 equivocal quadrants were excluded, 80 normal and 49 abnormal quadrants were left for analysis. The films were interpreted by 16 observers, including 6 attending radiologists and 10 residents. The observers interpreted each case as either normal or abnormal, with and without use of the computerized scheme (Fig 7). Observer performance was evaluated by receiver operating characteristic (ROC) analysis.

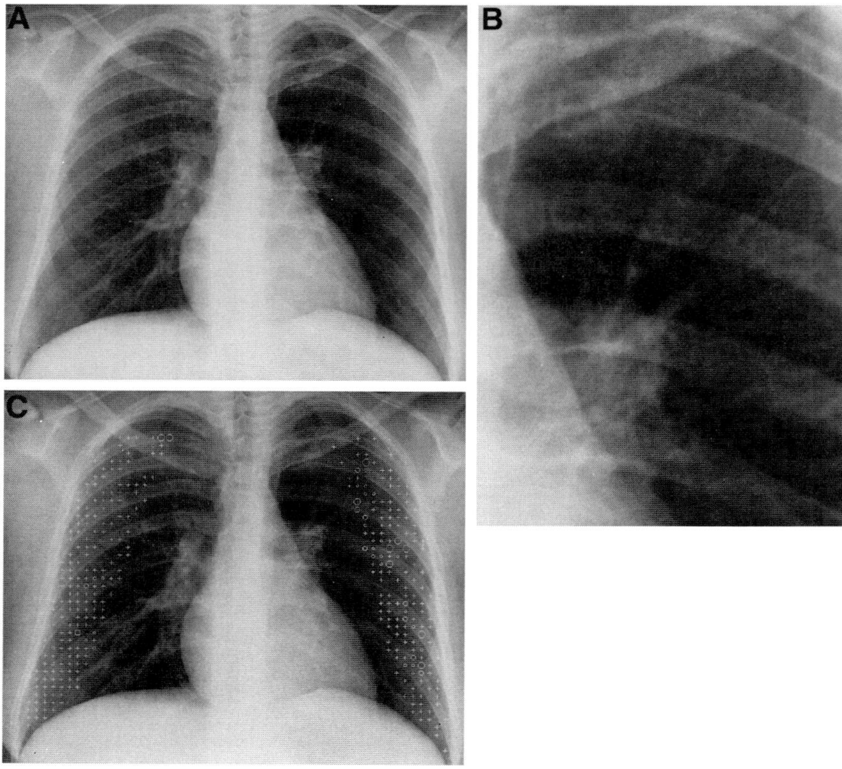

FIGURE 7.—Chest films of a 25-year-old woman with sarcoidosis. **A**, posteroanterior chest radiograph shows fine nodular pattern located mainly in upper lobes. Lung bases are normal. **B**, enlargement of left upper zone of chest radiograph. **C**, computer output superimposed on **A** shows markers that indicate normal (*crosses*), nodular (*circles*), reticular (*squares*), and reticulonodular (*hexagons*) patterns. Several circular icons, particularly in left upper lobe, indicate abnormal nodular pattern. (Courtesy of Monnier-Cholley L, MacMahon H, Katsuragawa S, et al: Computer-aided diagnosis for detection of interstitial opacities on chest radiographs. *AJR* 171:1651-1656, 1998.)

Results.—The computerized scheme significantly improved the observers' diagnostic accuracy. Area under the ROC curve for all observers was 0.970 with computer assistance, compared to 0.948 without. Corresponding values for attending radiologists were 0.972 and 0.960, and for residents they were 0.972 and 0.960. On its own, the computerized scheme had an area under the ROC curve of 0.943. The computerized scheme appeared most useful in confirming normal radiographs, as opposed to supporting the interpretation of an abnormal radiograph.

Conclusions.—A computer-aided diagnostic program can aid in the detection of interstitial opacities on chest radiographs. The computerized scheme appears especially useful in the detection of cases with subtly diffuse abnormalities. The gain in diagnostic accuracy appears greater for less-experienced radiologists.

► In the 1998 Year Book,[1] I commented on an article describing a computer-based technique that will allow radiologists to literally subtract one chest radiograph (the old one) from a second chest radiograph (the new one). The visual information that is left represents the content difference between the 2 radiographs and is the ultimate way to compare old and new chest radiographs. I thought that this was a pretty nifty idea, but it pales in comparison with the computer-based HUD (Heads Up Display) for radiologists described by Monnier-Cholley et al.

Detecting subtle interstitial lung disease on plain chest radiographs is one of the most difficult and frustrating things that we are routinely called on to do; from time to time, we all need a little friendly reassurance and validation. Monnier-Cholley et al developed a computer program that analyzes the radiographic texture of the lungs. The computer-determined textural properties of designated regions of lung are represented by symbols (normal lung=plus sign; reticular opacities=square; nodular opacities=circle; mixed pattern=hexagon), which can be projected onto the chest radiograph. The size of the symbol indicates the extent of the abnormality in that particular area. The computer consultant was particularly helpful for relatively inexperienced viewers but also improved the diagnostic accuracy of experienced staff radiologists. Interestingly, the computer-annotated images were more helpful in confirming that a chest radiograph was normal than in affirming the presence of an abnormality.

Although hard copies of both plain and computer-annotated chest films were used for this study, the authors point out that their program could be incorporated into digital radiographic imaging systems, enabling the viewer to toggle back and forth between the plain and annotated images on a monitor. I wonder how difficult it would be to link the system to a programmable computer voice. Imagine that you've had a really bad day, harassed by clinicians, and beleaguered by medical students (who are all smarter and thinner than you). You put up 1 last chest radiograph, read the requisition ("worked as sandblaster in an asbestos-lined vat in a plant that manufactured fluorescent light bulbs and aircraft parts—r/o interstitial lung disease"), and emit a groan of ultimate anguish. Are those little tiny nodules or dust on your glasses? Are there coarse irregular densities or scratches on the cassette? Help! You push a button, and suddenly all is well. You hear your Mother's voice drifting out of the computer speakers:

"Of course it's normal. You always were such a smart boy, and so good looking too. Here, have a piece of strudel. . . ."

S.A. Groskin, M.D.

Reference

1. 1998 Year Book of Diagnostic Radiology, pp 8-10.

Something Borrowed

Do Radiographic Features of Acute Infection Influence Management of Lower Respiratory Tract Infections in the Community?

Simpson JCG, Hulse P, Taylor PM, et al (Wythenshawe Hosp, Manchester, England; Manchester Royal Infirmary, England)

Eur Respir J 12:1384-1387, 1998 1–13

Introduction.—The term "lower respiratory tract infection" includes such diseases as acute bronchitis and pneumonia. Chest radiographs are ordered to confirm infection, assess response to treatment, identify a complication of infection, and determine underlying pathology, such as a neoplasm. Little is known about the impact of a chest radiograph revealing radiographic features of pneumonia on the subsequent management by the general practitioner. The proportion of chest radiographs performed by general practitioners at 1 institution was identified. The timing and reason for performing the chest radiograph were also identified, as well as the general practitioner's opinion as to whether the result influenced management.

Methods.—A total of 2,538 radiographs performed in patients older than 15 years were requested by general practitioners in a 12-month period. A questionnaire with 9 questions was sent to the general practitioners. It was found that 11 of the chest radiographs (4.4%) showed evidence of a lower respiratory tract infection, and (87%) of these 97 were included in the study.

Results.—It was found that 56 of the patients, or 62%, had the radiograph requested at the second or third visit. Confirmation of infection was the most popular reason that radiographs were performed (45 radiographs or 58%). The general practitioners indicated that the radiograph had affected treatment in 47 patients (48%). It was patients not receiving antibiotics before the radiograph was taken whose treatment was most significantly altered as a result of the radiograph. A radiograph with normal results would have affected management, according to 29 of the general practitioners (32%), most often with respect to antibiotic prescriptions.

Conclusion.—Confirming an infection is the most common reason for ordering a radiograph for patients with suspected lower respiratory tract infection. The results of the radiograph do affect patient treatment, according to general practitioners. Patient management is associated with the wording of the radiologist's report.

► In my darker moments, I often find myself asking the following 2 questions: "Why did they (the clinicians) order that study?" and "Does anyone really read my reports and care about what I say?" (In my darkest moments, these 2 questions are phrased differently: "Are they crazy? My dog knows more about medicine than they do!" and "Either they don't know how to read or they simply don't understand words that contain more than 2 syllables.")

This study by Simpson et al. indicates that sometimes clinicians do have valid reasons for ordering chest radiographs for patients they suspect of having a lower respiratory tract infection (to confirm the presence of pneumonia, assess response to treatment, exclude underlying neoplasm). Furthermore, Simpson and colleagues found that some clinicians do read our reports and that they care enough about what we have to say that they may alter therapy based on our recommendations. In this study, every time the radiologist's report recommended that a patient be referred to the hospital for evaluation, the patient was referred. Also, follow-up radiographs were obtained more commonly when they were recommended in the radiologist's report than when follow-up was not mentioned. As Simpson et al. state, "Radiologists should be conscious of the power of their report in influencing the management of patients." Implied in this statement is our obligation to communicate our findings and recommendations clearly and concisely, without hiding behind jargon, incomprehensible abbreviations, and verbal foliage (hedging).

S.A. Groskin, M.D.

The Utility of Chest Radiography in the Follow-up of Pneumonia

Heaton P, Arthur K (Taranaki Base Hosp, New Plymouth, New Zealand)

N Z Med J 111:315-317, 1998 1–14

Background.—Children hospitalized because of pneumonia often undergo routine postdischarge chest radiographs. However, in the authors' experience, these films rarely reveal any significant abnormalities. There are few data on the need for follow-up radiographs. This retrospective study assessed the clinical value of follow-up chest radiographs in children with pneumonia.

Methods.—The study included all 78 pediatric patients admitted to the authors' hospital for community-acquired pneumonia over a 1-year period. Of these, 13 were excluded because of co-morbidity or age. This left 65 children—38 boys and 27 girls, mean age 3½ years—for analysis. All children underwent posteroanterior and lateral chest x-ray examinations at admission. Follow-up chest radiographs were obtained after discharge in 41 patients. The clinical value of these follow-up chest films was analyzed.

Results.—Admission findings included cough in 79% of the patients, fever in 82%, tachypnea in 82%, and abnormal chest signs in 77%. Sixty-six percent of the patients had elevated C-reactive protein levels, and 65% had leukocytosis. The baseline chest films revealed unilobular or lobar abnormalities in 53% of the patients, bilobar abnormalities in 29%, and diffuse abnormalities in 11%. Follow-up chest radiography was usually performed 4 to 6 weeks after discharge. Of 41 children who had follow-up chest films, 37 had no abnormal signs or symptoms. In 35 of these patients, follow-up findings were normal. The other 2 patients, in whom follow-up films were obtained less than 4 weeks after discharge, showed improvement with residual shadowing. In the 4 patients with continued signs or symptoms, the follow-up radiographs showed either slight resolution or no change from baseline.

Conclusions.—The findings question the routine use of follow-up chest films for children hospitalized because of pneumonia. Only rarely would a continued abnormality in the chest radiograph be the only manifestation of unresolved disease. The authors recommend that follow-up chest films be deferred for at least 4 weeks after discharge in children with community-acquired pneumonia. Follow-up chest films are not necessary in children who have no signs or symptoms at clinical follow-up.

▶ The authors of this modest article set out to determine whether or not kids with pneumonia should have repeat chest radiographs made during or after the completion of treatment. Pediatric patients with pneumonia usually have no other "follow-up" laboratory tests (ie, complete blood cell counts) after completion of antibiotic treatment, so why do we continue to routinely irradiate so many of them? Although I don't know for sure, I suspect that this practice is an illogical extension of the reasonable practice of obtaining follow-up chest radiographs in adult patients with pneumonia. Adults can and do develop bronchogenic carcinoma, and it has long been recognized that a radiographically persistent pneumonia in an adult may actually be an early sign of an underlying tumor (postobstructive pneumonia) or that it (the "pneumonia") may actually be a neoplasm. Radiographic follow-up of pneumonia in adults makes sense because it may lead to the diagnosis of a much more serious underlying disease.

Children, unlike adults, rarely have bronchogenic carcinoma or, for that matter, any other tumor of the lungs or airways that might mimic or predispose them to pneumonia. Although aspirated foreign material, bronchopulmonary sequestration, and other uncommon congenital anomalies may mimic or produce recurrent or persistent pneumonia, these disorders have virtually no malignant potential and do not metastasize. Keeping this major difference between kids and adults in mind, it really doesn't make sense to routinely obtain follow-up chest radiographs in pediatric patients with pneumonia. The authors of this article confirm this impression and recommend that repeat chest radiographs be considered only if the child has persistent symptoms or significant underlying pulmonary disease.

For me, the truly important message of this article is the reminder that kids are unique organisms and not simply little adults. They develop different diseases than do adults, and they often respond both clinically and radiographically to the same diseases in very different ways. It is critical that we remember this. Although I didn't intend to use this commentary as a pitch for pediatrics, I do strongly believe that if our kids are to receive the best possible care, they should be treated by skilled specialists (pediatricians, pediatric nurses, pediatric radiologists, pediatric surgeons) who have been trained to recognize and meet their patients' unique needs. I also believe that when sophisticated management of pediatric disease is necessary, a dedicated pediatric hospital is the best environment for such care.

S.A. Groskin, M.D.

Mass Screening for Lung Cancer With Mobile Spiral Computed Tomography Scanner

Sone S, Takashima S, Li F, et al (Shinshu Univ, Matsumoto, Japan; Matsumoto Research Centre, Asahi, Japan)

Lancet 351:1242-1245, 1998 1–15

Introduction.—Techniques that can diagnose lung cancer at an early stage are needed to reduce mortality. Low-dose spiral CT was evaluated for use in lung cancer screening.

Methods.—Low-dose spiral CT of the chest was performed in 5,483 participants selected from the Japanese general population. The participants were aged 40 to 74 years. The scans were performed using a mobile CT unit in a truck. Scan parameters were: 120 kV peak, 50 mA, 10 mm collimation, and 10 mm/sec table speed. In addition, miniature chest fluorophotography was performed in 3,967 patients. Participants with a smoking history of at least 30 pack-years underwent cytologic assessment of pooled sputum samples. The spiral CT findings were classified as unsatisfactory, normal or showing lung abnormality of little importance, noncancerous lung lesion, noncancerous but suspicious lung lesion, suspicion of lung cancer, indeterminate small nodule (smaller than 3 mm), or extrathoracic abnormality.

Results.—Fifty-nine patients were classified as having noncancerous but suspicious lung lesions, and 84 as having abnormalities suggestive of lung cancer. Fourteen patients (17%) with suspicion of lung cancer proved to have the disease. Two patients with indeterminate small nodules had lung cancer. Eighteen of the 19 cases of cancer were surgically confirmed; the remaining patient refused surgery. Thoracotomy was also performed in 3 patients with inflammatory lesions. The mean tumor size on CT scan was 17 mm. Sixteen of the 19 patients with cancer were in American Joint Committee stage I; the other 3 were in stage IV. Spiral CT had a lung cancer detection rate of 0.48%. All but 4 of the 19 patients with cancer had negative results on miniature chest fluorophotography. There was 1 false negative CT scan. One case of cancer was detected only on sputum cytologic examination.

Conclusions.—Spiral CT performed with a mobile unit is a promising approach to early detection of lung cancers. The cancer detection rate is nearly 10 times higher than that achieved with standard mass screening. The authors plan a 1-year follow-up study of their patients, to include lung cancer mortality compared with that of controls.

► Spiral CT is so devastatingly fast that it can actually allow us to travel back in time. Just look at the picture on page 1244 of the original article. Replace the words "spiral CT scanner" on the side of the van with the words "mass radiography unit" and you have returned to the 1930s, when mobile photofluorography units were used to screen large segments of the population for tuberculosis. At that time, tuberculosis was one of the major life-threatening pulmonary diseases, and bronchogenic carcinoma was still considered a medical curiosity. I am dismayed at our lack of progress in developing effective therapies for bronchogenic carcinoma, and I agree with Sone et al. that early diagnosis and complete surgical resection of the tumor remain a patient's best hope for cure. However, I'm not sure that mass screening with spiral CT is the way to go. The cost per diagnosis (Sone et al. do not mention cost) would almost certainly be quite high, since it would include not only the cost of the screening CT scans (most of which will be normal), but also the cost of the further studies ordered to evaluate abnormalities seen on the "positive" scans. Most of these nodules, densities, and ditzels will ultimately be proven to be benign (in this study, only 1.3% of patients with abnormalities on their CT scans were found to have neoplasms), but because the expedient of obtaining old films for comparison would be of little use (many of the abnormalities seen on the screening CT scans would not be visible on plain chest radiographs), additional CT scans, nuclear scans, biopsies, etc. will be unavoidable. As histoplasmosis is very common in the area in which I practice, I cringe when I think about the number of tiny granulomas we would discover and then be compelled to follow or to biopsy. And what about radiation dose, another issue that Sone et al. don't discuss? What is it per scan and can it be justified in terms of early diagnosis, effective treatment, and lives lengthened or saved?

As I think about it, the solution to the problem of lung cancer is not mass CT screening, sophisticated surgery, powerful new chemotherapeutic agents, or innovative radiation treatment protocols. The solution to the problem of lung cancer is, in most cases, simple: prevent it by preventing smoking. Outlaw smoking or tax it so heavily that the only people who can afford to continue to smoke can also afford to subsidize their own research into the cure for this self-inflicted malady. Wouldn't it be wiser and more humane to spend our dwindling healthcare dollars making sure that pregnant women get adequate prenatal care, and that infants and children receive nutritious meals and are appropriately immunized?

S.A. Groskin, M.D.

Variability in the Detection of Enlarged Mediastinal Lymph Nodes in Staging Lung Cancer: A Comparison of Contrast-enhanced and Unenhanced CT

Cascade PN, Gross BH, Kazerooni EA, et al (Univ of Michigan, Ann Arbor)
AJR 170:927-931, 1998 1–16

Introduction.—CT protocols for staging lung cancer vary. The literature does not contain conclusive evidence regarding whether contrast material should be used for the detection of enlarged mediastinal lymph nodes in

TABLE 1.—Frequency of Observing Zero to 4 or More Enlarged Mediastinal Lymph Nodes With Unenhanced and Contrast-Enhanced CT Summed for 3 Observers

ATS Station	No. of Enlarged Lymph Nodes Observed: Unenhanced CT					Contrast-Enhanced CT				
	0	1	2	3	≥4	0	1	2	3	≥4
1R	149	1	0	0	0	146	3	1	0	0
1L	149	1	0	0	0	147	2	0	1	0
2R	128	10	8	1	3	116	14	10	7	3
2L	145	4	1	0	0	141	6	1	2	0
4R	105	28	8	6	3	104	28	14	3	1
4L	139	6	5	0	0	133	10	6	1	0
5	120	15	13	2	0	117	24	5	4	0
6	127	11	5	5	2	132	9	4	2	3
7	112	32	6	0	0	108	38	4	0	0
8R	133	14	2	1	0	132	14	3	1	0
8L	142	8	0	0	0	144	4	2	0	0
10R	116	21	10	3	0	112	30	6	1	1
10L	146	4	0	0	0	142	4	2	0	0
14R	147	2	1	0	0	146	2	2	0	0
14L	147	1	1	0	1	147	0	2	0	1

Abbreviations: ATS, American Thoracic Society

(Courtesy of Cascade PN, Gross BH, Kazerooni EA, et al: Variability in the detection of enlarged mediastinal lymph nodes in staging lung cancer: A comparison of contrast-enhanced and unenhanced CT. *AJR* 170:927-931, 1998.)

the staging of lung cancer. Intraobserver and interobserver agreement in the detection of enlarged mediastinal lymph nodes was assessed by comparing IV contrast-enhanced and unenhanced CT.

Methods.—Fifty patients with known or suspected bronchogenic carcinoma underwent unenhanced thoracic CT and then contrast-enhanced CT. Thirty-four patients underwent examinations in the nonhelical mode with contiguous 1-cm thick axial tomographic images through the thorax; then contrast material was administered intravenously. Contiguous 1-cm-thick axial tomographic images were taken with the administration of 100 mL of contrast material (diatrizoate meglumine 60% or iohexol 300 mg of iodine per milliliter) for patients undergoing CT of the chest only. After unenhanced imaging of the thorax, patients who underwent helical chest CT received 75 mL of contrast material at a rate of 1.5 mL/per second and were scanned in a superior to inferior direction. Contrast material was administered at a rate of 2.5 mL/per second (150 mL) in patients who underwent helical chest and abdominal CT. Scanning was also done in the superior to inferior direction for this procedure. Patients who underwent helical scanning were asked to hyperventilate and were scanned with a 30-second breath-hold and an 8-second breathe time. All scans were taken with the patient's arm raised for optimal mediastinal assessment free of artifact from the shoulders. Oral contrast material was administered to all patients. American Thoracic Society nodal station designations were assigned by 3 observers.

Results.—Four hundred eighteen enlarged lymph nodes were detected with enhanced CT, compared with 377 detected with unenhanced CT, a significant difference. The numbers of enlarged lymph nodes varied for 5 stations. The numbers were small, with the exception of the right upper paratracheal station (2R) (contrast-enhanced, 68 enlarged lymph nodes; unenhanced, 44; a significant difference). With regard to all stations together, intraobserver agreement between contrast-enhanced and unenhanced procedures was nearly perfect (Table 1). There was no difference for any observer in the proportion of patients with at least 1 enlarged lymph node. Interobserver agreement was nearly perfect for the number of enlarged lymph nodes. One observer detected significantly more patients with at least 1 enlarged lymph node with contrast enhancement at station 2R. There was significantly greater agreement between 2 observers at station 2R with contrast enhancement vs. no enhancement.

Conclusion.—Agreement was high for intraobserver and interobserver interpretations for contrast-enhanced and unenhanced CT. Significantly more enlarged lymph nodes were detected with contrast-enhanced versus unenhanced CT, particularly at station 2R.

► This lovely study is significant for more than trying to determine whether or not the administration of intravenous contrast material facilitates the detection of enlarged mediastinal lymph nodes on CT scans or affects interobserver and intraobserver variability in scan interpretation. It is also significant because it demonstrates how a study should be performed and reported.

I have read a large number of articles describing various techniques for using CT to evaluate patients with bronchogenic carcinoma. Invariably, when I try to apply the authors' protocol, I find that something is missing, which makes it impossible for me to duplicate and use their technique in my practice. The authors may have failed to mention whether intravenous contrast material was used. If contrast material was used, the type of contrast material, the injection rate, the prescan delay time, the direction of scanning, and the total volume of contrast material injected are often not specified. Mention of collimation and pitch may also be notably absent. Is it just my paranoia, or are they trying to keep us from duplicating their work?

Cascade et al. spell it out for us, and I applaud them for their candor and completeness. They tell us exactly what they did, how they did it, why they did it, and what they found. They then tell us how what they found is going to affect their pattern of practice. Short, simple, and to the point. At my institution, we do not routinely use intravenous contrast material when scanning patients with suspected or proven bronchogenic carcinoma. We monitor all studies and obtain supplementary contrast-enhanced images when we believe that the unenhanced images do not adequately demonstrate or exclude the presence of enlarged mediastinal nodes. The findings by Cascade et al. suggest that this is not an unreasonable approach. However, perhaps it is time for us to formally evaluate our own experience. Since we are used to interpreting unenhanced CT images, we could then compare our results with those of Cascade et al. It should be relatively straightforward, since Cascade and colleagues have given us a very workable template to use. Thanks.

S.A. Groskin, M.D.

Thoracic CT in the Intensive Care Unit: Assessment of Clinical Usefulness

Miller WT Jr, Tino G, Friedburg JS (Univ of Pennsylvania, Philadelphia)
Radiology 209:491-498, 1998 1–17

Background.—Despite its imperfections, chest radiography remains the standard for daily imaging studies in the ICU. Chest CT offers greater sensitivity in the recognition of subtle lung parenchymal abnormalities, among its other advantages. However, few studies have examined the value of chest CT in the ICU setting. This retrospective study examined the clinical usefulness of chest CT for ICU patients.

Methods.—The analysis included a total of 108 chest CT scans performed in 85 patients in a surgical, medical, and cardiac ICU of 1 institution. Associated chest radiographs and clinical records were reviewed along with the CT scans. Analysis of the clinical value of CT scans focused on their impact on clinical management or on their ability to answer the clinical question for which they had been performed.

Results.—The analysis included a total of 482 findings: 232 chest radiographic findings and 250 findings demonstrated on CT only. Thus,

TABLE 3.—Comparison of Chest Radiographic and CT Findings

Outcome	No. of Findings
Chest radiographic and CT findings agree	199
Chest radiographic and CT findings disagree	33*
Chest radiographic finding of mild CHF, CT finding of no CHF	19 (58)*
Disagreement about cause of pulmonary opacity	
Chest radiographic finding of atelectasis, CT finding of pneumonia	3 (9)*
Chest radiographic finding of atelectasis, CT finding of pulmonary edema	1 (3)*
Chest radiographic finding of atelectasis, CT finding of carcinoma	1 (3)*
Chest radiographic finding of pneumonia, CT finding of atelectasis	1 (3)*
Chest radiographic finding of contusion, CT finding of pneumonia	1 (3)*
Chest radiographic finding of adult respiratory distress syndrome, CT finding of aspiration pneumonia	1 (3)*
False-positive chest radiographic finding	
Chest radiographic finding of small pneumothorax, CT finding of no pneumothorax	1 (3)*
Chest radiographic finding of lung cavity, CT finding of no cavity	1 (3)*
Chest radiographic finding of pneumopericardium, CT finding of no pneumopericardium	1 (3)*
Chest radiographic finding of mediastinal mass, CT finding of no mediastinal mass	1 (3)*
Chest radiographic finding of chronic obstructive pulmonary disease, CT finding of no chronic obstructive pulmonary disease	1 (3)*
False-negative CT finding of no rib fracture, chest radiographic finding of rib fracture	1 (3)*
CT shows additional findings	250
Small pleural effusion	94 (38)†
Small pneumothorax	14 (6)†
Dependent atelectasis	20 (8)†
Abdominal finding	31 (12)†
Other	91 (36)†

*Number in parentheses is the percentage of disagreement relative to all disagreements.
†Number in parentheses is the percentage of findings relative to all additional CT findings.
Abbreviation: CHF, congestive heart failure.
(Courtesy of Miller WT Jr, Tino G, Friedburg JS: Thoracic CT in the intensive care unit: Assessment of clinical usefulness. *Radiology* 209:491-498, 1998. Radiological Society of North America.)

TABLE 4.—Usefulness of Thoracic CT in the ICU

Finding	No. of Examinations	No. of Examinations With Clinically Important Findings	No. of Examinations That Prompted a Change in Management
New	91 (84)	32 (30)	22 (20)
Affirmation	19 (18)	12 (11)	3 (3)
Excluded	55 (51)	44 (41)	0 (0)
All*	102 (94)	78 (72)	24 (22)†

*Sums of individual columns may not equal the total number because some examinations may have had a combination of new findings, affirmation of previously suspected findings, or exclusion of previously suspected findings.

†Three of these examinations were performed concurrently with abdominal CT examinations that showed the findings. If the examinations with concurrent abdominal CT are excluded, then the total becomes 22 (20%).

Number in parentheses is the percentage of the 108 examinations.

(Courtesy of Miller WT Jr, Tino G, Friedburg JS: Thoracic CT in the intensive care unit: Assessment of clinical usefulness. *Radiology* 209:491-498, 1998. Radiological Society of North America.)

52% of the total number of findings were demonstrated on CT only. Chest CT confirmed 86% of associated chest radiographic findings (Table 3). This figure increased to 93% after exclusion of disagreement regarding mild congestive heart failure. At least one new, clinically relevant finding was made on 30% of the CT scans (Table 4). Important CT findings included mediastinal, chest wall, or retroperitoneal abscesses or postoperative fluid collections; information leading to the detection, staging, or evaluation of malignant lesions; previously unsuspected pneumonia; or pleural effusions (Table 6). In 22% of the cases, thoracic CT led to a change in clinical management.

Conclusions.—Thoracic CT is an important adjunct to bedside chest radiography in ICU patients. Most of these CT scans reveal additional information about the patient's condition, and a significant minority affect clinical management. The findings permit no conclusions about the value of chest CT for the overall ICU population. However, it appears useful for specific indications, especially for evaluation of fever or sepsis of unknown source, evaluation of postoperative complications, characterization of postoperative complications, and detection and staging of malignant thoracic lesions.

► This study confirms what most of us already know: CT is better than AP, portable, semirecumbent, or supine chest radiographs in assessing the chest wall, pleural space, lungs, airways, and mediastinum. The authors correctly point out that 1 imaging test shouldn't be considered superior to another imaging test simply because it demonstrates more abnormalities; it is the significance of the abnormalities detected (their quality) rather than their sheer number (their quantity) that is the truer measure of the value of an imaging examination. In this respect, CT is the clear-cut winner. Thirty percent of the CT scans of the chest obtained in the ICU patients in this study demonstrated abnormalities that were deemed clinically significant; therapy was changed because of these significant findings after 22% of the examinations. I was pleased to note that the authors stressed that their

TABLE 6.—Thirty-eight Clinically Important Findings in 32 Thoracic CT Examinations That Were Unsuspected on Prior Chest Radiographs

Finding	No. of Findings
Mediastinal	13
Postoperative mediastinal fluid collections*	6
Detection, staging, or evaluation of mediastinal malignancy†	4
Cardiac tamponade	2
Sternal wound infection	1
Pulmonary	6
Unsuspected pneumonia or lung abscess	5
Persistent narrowing of airway after stent placement	1
Pleural	4
Large pleural effusion	2
Large pneumothorax	1
Pulmonary entrapment by pleural fibrosis	1
Chest wall	5
Chest wall or paraspinal abscess	3
Vertebral fracture	1
Bone metastasis	1
Other	3
Pulmonary embolism	1
Inadequate position of chest tube	2
Abdominal	7
Hepatic metastasis	4
Retroperitoneal fluid collections	2
Renal mass	1

*Collections around implantable cardiac ventricular assist device, 3 cases (infection proved in 1); collections adjacent to intrathoracic stomach after esophagectomy, 2 cases (esophageal leak proved in 1); and mediastinal collection after cardiac surgery, 1 case.

†Recurrent esophageal carcinoma that invaded the trachea (n = 1), adenoid cystic carcinoma of the trachea (n = 1), lymphoma that compressed the trachea (n =1), and metastatic adenopathy (n = 1).

(Courtesy of Miller WT Jr, Tino G, Friedburg JS: Thoracic CT in the intensive care unit: Assessment of clinical usefulness. *Radiology* 209:491-498, 1998. Radiological Society of North America.)

study population was highly selected and that the results of their study couldn't and shouldn't be generalized to all ICU patients.

One of the findings in this study that caught my attention was the fact that the mortality rate for ICU patients who had CT scans of the thorax was 36%, whereas the mortality rate for all ICU patients was only 9%. Although I believe that the most likely explanation for this is that the patients who had chest CT scans were sicker than those whose clinicians thought they could be managed without CT scans, I can't help but wonder if there might not be another contributing factor. Transporting a critically ill patient and all of the necessary monitoring and life-support equipment from the ICU to the radiology department is no mean feat. Moving that patient from the bed onto and then back off the CT table is also pretty rigorous for both the staff and the patient. Lines and tubes can be compromised, and the patient is certainly subjected to some degree of psychological and physical stress. Does the not-so-simple act of moving the patient for the CT examination contribute to the increased mortality rate described in this article? It may be something to think about the next time you're sitting around with nothing to do while waiting for the next patient to be brought down from the ICU for scanning.

S.A. Groskin, M.D.

Postoperative Portable Chest Radiographs: Optimum Use in Thoracic Surgery

Graham RJ, Meziane MA, Rice TW, et al (Cleveland Clinic Found, Ohio)
J Thorac Cardiovasc Surg 115:45-52, 1998 1–18

Introduction.—An integral part of the postoperative care in thoracic surgery is portable chest radiographs. The role of their routine use has not been documented in terms of efficacy. Little is known about the value of portable chest x-ray studies in patients who had a thoracotomy. The clinical usefulness of portable chest radiographs during the postoperative hospitalization of patients who had thoracotomy was evaluated.

Methods.—Ninety-nine patients had 82 pulmonary resections and 18 other major procedures in a 6-month period. They had 769 portable chest x-ray scans taken, a median of 5 per patient (range 2 to 49). A 3-part survey was conducted with each x-ray scan. In the first part, the survey determined whether the x-ray scan was routine and what the anticipated management would have been if the x-ray scan was not available. In the second part, the radiologist scored the x-ray results as negative, expected findings; minor findings necessitating no intervention; minor findings necessitating intervention; or major findings necessitating intervention (Table 1). In the third part, the x-ray film and interpretation were returned to the surgeon.

Results.—Of the 769 post-operative x-ray scans taken, 731 (95%) were routine and 38 (5%) were nonroutine. There were 106 negative findings (13.8%); 558 minor findings needing no intervention (72.5%); 59 minor findings needing intervention (7.7%); and 46 major findings needing intervention (6.0%). The x-ray findings altered management in 43 of 769

TABLE 1.—Rating of X-ray Findings

Rating	Significance
Negative	No or expected radiographic abnormality
A	Minor radiographic abnormality necessitating no treatment
B	Minor radiographic abnormality necessitating treatment or position adjustment
C	Major radiographic abnormality necessitating treatment or intervention

(Courtesy of Graham RJ, Meziane MA, Rice TW, et al: Postoperative portable chest radiographs: optimum use in thoracic surgery. *J Thorac Cardiovasc Surg* 115:45-52, 1998.)

TABLE 2.—Treatment Plan and Actual Treatment: Routine Portable Chest X-ray Films (n = 731)

	No Change	Add Antibiotics	Adjust Chest Tube
Preop./postop. chest x-ray films			
No change	698	3	1
New chest tube	6		
Add antibiotics	4		1
Add diuretics	4		
Adjust CVP tube	4		
Adjust ET tube	4		
Thoracentesis	2		
Reoperation	2		
Adjust chest tube	1		
Other	4		

Abbreviations: CVP, central venous pressure; *ET*, endotracheal.
(Courtesy of Graham RJ, Meziane MA, Rice TW, et al: Postoperative portable chest radiographs: optimum use in thoracic surgery. *J Thorac Cardiovasc Surg* 115:45-52, 1998.)

studies (5.6%), in 33 of the routine films (4.5%), and in 10 of the nonroutine films (26.3%) (Tables 2 and 3). X-ray findings altered management in 13 minor findings needing no intervention (2.3%), in 22 minor findings needing intervention (37.3%), and in 8 major findings needing intervention (17.4%).

Conclusion.—In terms of management, routine daily portable chest x-ray studies have a minimal impact. Nonroutine x-ray scans more often alter management of patients. If only 1 routine x-ray scan (at a cost of $114) was the limit after the operation, only 133 such studies would have been needed. The cost of care would have been reduced by $725 per patient ($286,000 annually) by eliminating 636 (82.7%) of the x-ray studies. Routine postoperative portable chest x-ray studies can be safely,

TABLE 3.—Treatment Plan and Actual Treatment: Nonroutine Portable Chest X-ray Films (n = 38)

	No Change	Add Antibiotics	Add Antibiotics
Preop./postop. chest x-ray films			
No change	28	4	1
Add antibiotics	1		
Adjust ET tube	1		
Adjust CVP tube	1		
New chest tube	1		
Add diuretics		1	

Abbreviations: ET, endotracheal; *CVP*, central venous pressure.
(Courtesy of Graham RJ, Meziane MA, Rice TW, et al: Postoperative portable chest radiographs: optimum use in thoracic surgery. *J Thorc Cardiovasc Surg* 115:45-52, 1998.)

efficaciously, and cost-effectively eliminated. Nonroutine studies should be ordered only when clinically indicated.

▶ This neatly planned and nicely performed prospective study of patients in a surgical ICU who had undergone elective thoracotomy indicates that routine chest radiographs in this setting cost a great deal, are not particularly useful, and could be done away with without compromising patient care. The authors, radiologists and surgeons, reviewed much of the literature available on the utility of routine chest radiographs, and stressed that their recommendations pertain only to the highly selected population described in this study.

I thought that this study addressed practical issues in a practical fashion and that its conclusions, while perhaps not surprising, made sense. I enjoyed the discussion that followed this article at least as much as I enjoyed the article itself. I was particularly taken by the remarks of Dr. Robert L. Thurer (Boston), who asked Dr. Thomas Rice (Cleveland, Ohio), a surgeon and one of the authors of the paper, " . . . do you think that the interpretation by the radiologist had anything to offer[?] We were all trained to read our own chest x-ray films, and I wonder whether a comparison between the surgeon's reading and the radiologist's reading would show any difference" (see p. 51 of the original article). When I was a pulmonologist, in my ignorance and arrogance, I often asked the same question. I have since found that, for the clinician who is wise enough to read the radiologist's reports and to consult the radiologist in person whenever possible, the radiologist has a great deal to offer. I was heartened to see that Dr. Rice feels the same way: "The radiologist has an important role and we rely on our radiologists quite heavily" (see p. 51 of the original article). Perhaps this attitude of professional respect led to the writing of this multidisciplinary article, or perhaps, the respect was a by-product of the writing of the article. Regardless, as radiologists, surgeons, internists, pediatricians, psychiatrists, we all have too much to do; in order to take the best possible care of our patients we must be willing and able to rely on the expertise of our colleagues.

S.A. Groskin, M.D.

Something Blew

Thin-Section Spiral Volumetric CT for the Assessment of Lobar and Segmental Bronchial Stenoses

Curtin JJ, Innes NJ, Harrison BDW (Norwich Hosp, England)
Clin Radiol 53:110-115, 1998 1–19

Introduction.—Spiral CT has been successful in diagnosing and characterizing stenoses of the trachea and main bronchi. Compared with bronchoscopy, CT is noninvasive and easily repeatable, and it provides information about stenoses that are impassable with a bronchoscope. Thin-section volumetric CT was used to assess lobar and segmental bronchi of 5 patients with known or suspected stenoses of these airways.

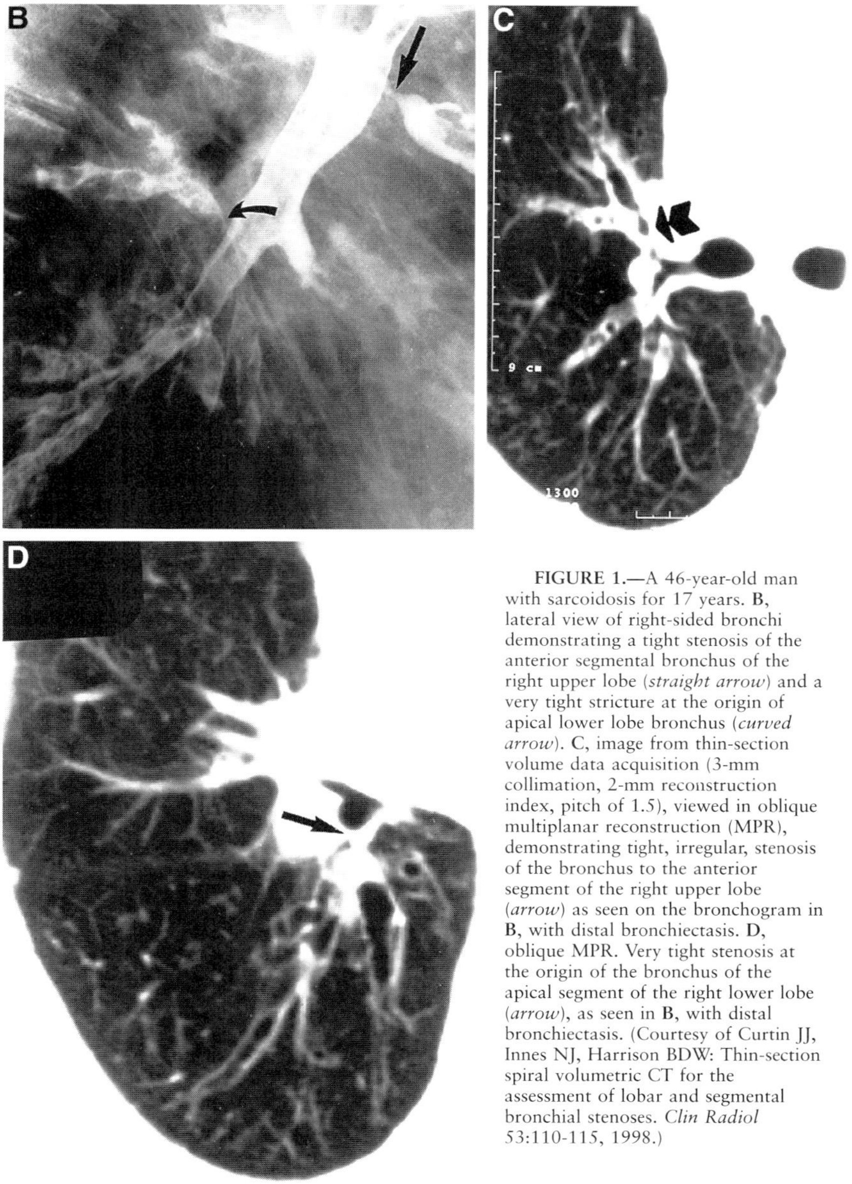

FIGURE 1.—A 46-year-old man with sarcoidosis for 17 years. **B**, lateral view of right-sided bronchi demonstrating a tight stenosis of the anterior segmental bronchus of the right upper lobe (*straight arrow*) and a very tight stricture at the origin of apical lower lobe bronchus (*curved arrow*). **C**, image from thin-section volume data acquisition (3-mm collimation, 2-mm reconstruction index, pitch of 1.5), viewed in oblique multiplanar reconstruction (MPR), demonstrating tight, irregular, stenosis of the bronchus to the anterior segment of the right upper lobe (*arrow*) as seen on the bronchogram in **B**, with distal bronchiectasis. **D**, oblique MPR. Very tight stenosis at the origin of the bronchus of the apical segment of the right lower lobe (*arrow*), as seen in **B**, with distal bronchiectasis. (Courtesy of Curtin JJ, Innes NJ, Harrison BDW: Thin-section spiral volumetric CT for the assessment of lobar and segmental bronchial stenoses. *Clin Radiol* 53:110-115, 1998.)

Methods.—The patients' ages ranged from 46 to 49. Four of the 5 patients had sarcoidosis. All patients underwent high-resolution examination that involved 1.5-mm slices at 10-mm intervals. A volume of tissue was assessed in spiral mode with a slice thickness of 3 mm in 4 patients and

2 mm in 1 patient; a reconstruction index of 2 mm in 4 patients and 1 mm in 1 patient; and a pitch of 1.25 in 2 patients and 1.5 in 3 patients. Tissue volumes varied between 5.8 and 7.2 cm in craniocaudal extent. CT data were compared with previous bronchograms and bronchoscopies.

Results.—Four of 23 lobar bronchi and 42 of 72 segmental bronchi were determined by CT to be stenotic. There was good correlation between bronchograms and CT findings (Fig 1) in 2 patients with sarcoidosis who underwent both examinations. The other 2 patients with sarcoidosis had bronchoscopy 5 years before volumetric CT. The patient with amyloid underwent bronchoscopy 1 year before CT. Comparison between old bronchoscopy or bronchogram investigations and CT showed a high degree of concordance.

Conclusion.—Findings in this small series of patients indicates that thin-section volumetric CT is a promising noninvasive imaging approach that is likely to be useful in the evaluation of lobar and segmental bronchial stenoses.

Volume Rendering of the Tracheobronchial Tree: Clinical Evaluation of Bronchographic Images

Remy-Jardin M, Remy J, Artaud D, et al (Hôpital Calmette, Lille, France)
Radiology 208:761-770, 1998 1–20

Introduction.—The emergence of spiral CT has renewed interest in three-dimensional (3D) medical imaging. These images contain no more data than corresponding series of transverse scans; yet it is thought that the viewer can better appreciate spatial relationships in a 3D display. Volume rendering is a method of producing two-dimensional images that can convey 3D spatial information inherent in a 3D volume data set. The application of the volume-rendering technique to airway disease in 71 consecutive patients with suspected or known airway lesions is described.

Methods.—Seventy-one patients underwent 74 spiral CT examinations (1- to 5-mm section thickness, pitch 1.7 to 2.0) of the tracheobronchial tree. Examinations had to be repeated in 2 patients (transplant recipients) to assess any changes in the anastomoses over time. The procedure was repeated in 1 patient with worsening symptoms. Suspected or known airway lesions consisted of 47 cases of benign tracheobronchial stenosis (group 1), 15 complex airway lesions (group 2), and 12 cases of bronchiectasis (group 3). Overlapping transverse CT scan and volume-rendered bronchographic images were independently compared by 2 radiologists for detection of airway abnormalities and identification of lesion morphology and extent. These data were correlated with bronchoscopic findings.

Results.—Observers graded bronchographic image quality as excellent or good in 73% and 24%, respectively. Three percent of the images were graded as poor in the presence of motion-related artifacts. The trapezoid parameters included window width of -700 to -350 HU, triangular trapezoid shape, parenchymal opacification of 70%, and unshaded algorithm.

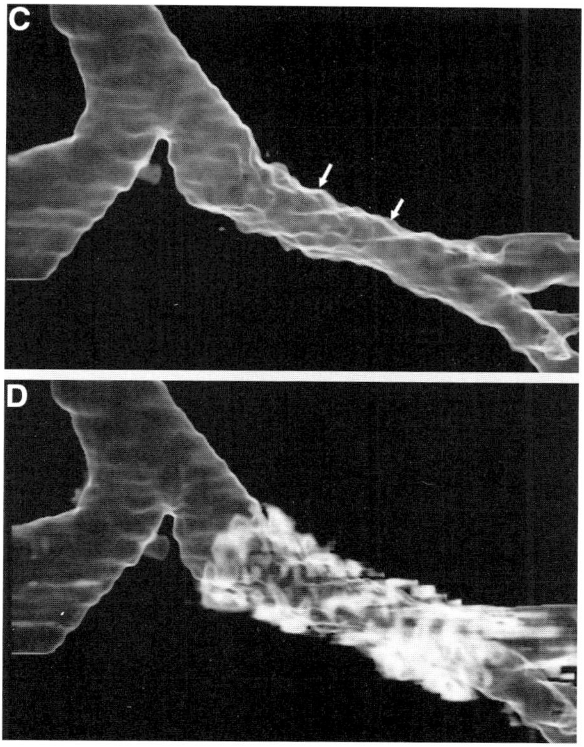

FIGURE 2.—Spiral CT follow-up (2-mm section thickness, pitch 2, 22-second acquisition) of an ischemic stenosis in the left main bronchus treated with an endoprosthesis after left-side single-lung transplantation in a 51-year-old woman. C, anteroposterior view of the bronchographic volume-rendered image demonstrates a mild reduction in the airway diameter at the level of the anastomotic site (*arrows*) (trapezoid position, -600 to -350 HU). **D**, selection of a second trapezoid (trapezoid position, 100 to 400 HU) enables concurrent depiction of the airways and the metallic bronchial stent on the volume-rendered image. (Courtesy of Remy-Jardin M, Remy J, Artaud D: Volume rendering of the tracheobronchial tree: Clinical evaluation of bronchographic images. *Radiology* 208:761-770, 1998. Radiological Society of North America.)

When compared with transverse CT scans, the volume-rendered images (a) gave supplemental diagnostic or morphologic information (Fig 2 and Fig 4) for 23 patients (31%) (16 and 7 patients in group 1 and group 3, respectively), (b) improved confidence in the interpretation of congenital airway abnormalities in 6 patients (8%) from group 2, and (c) corrected interpretive errors in 4 patients (5%) (2 patients each in group 1 and group 2).

Conclusion.—Recognition of mild changes in airway caliber and the understanding of complex tracheobronchial anomalies were enhanced with volume-rendered images.

► The airways have been traditionally considered both clinical and radiologic "blind spots." Fiberoptic bronchoscopy and bronchography revealed new

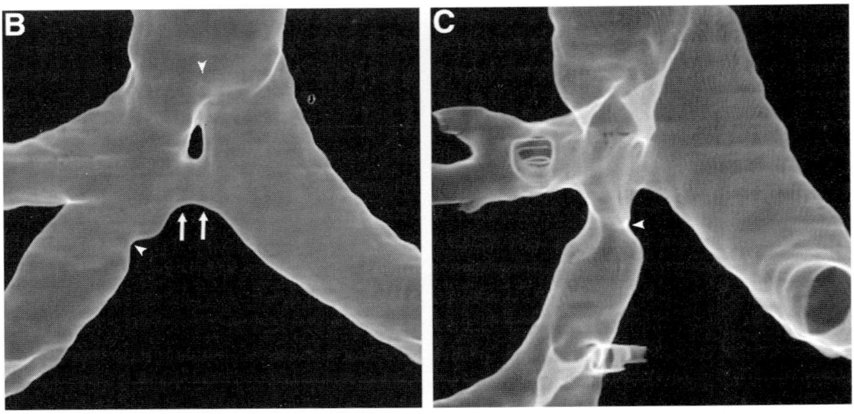

FIGURE 4.—Spiral CT evaluation (2-mm section thickness, pitch 1.5, 18-second acquisition) of a tuberculous fistulous tract in a 75-year-old man. **B**, anteroposterior view of the bronchographic volume-rendered image, which enables correction of the interpretive error with **A**, demonstrates a large fistulous tract (*arrows*) between the right and left main bronchi, 10 mm below the carina (*large arrowheads*) (trapezoid position -600 to -150 HU). Note the presence of a mild mural irregularity (*small arrowheads*) at the level of the initial portion of the right bronchus intermedius, 5 mm below the level of the fistulous tract. C, left posterior oblique view of the bronchographic volume-rendered image provides a synthetic analysis of the asymmetric stenosis (*arrowhead*) of the proximal right bronchus intermedius. (Courtesy of Remy-Jardin M, Remy J, Artaud D: Volume rendering of the tracheobronchial tree: Clinical evaluation of bronchographic images. *Radiology* 208:761-770, 1998. Radiological Society of North America.)

vistas for pulmonologists and radiologists, but both techniques have drawbacks. Both are invasive, both produce a decrease in pO2, both may induce bronchospasm, and both have difficulty assessing airways distal to areas of significant stenosis or obstruction. Also, the favored contrast medium for bronchography, oily Dionosil (which was no treat to work with) is no longer even produced.

CT has shown considerable potential in evaluating both airway form and function. The 2 articles I have included here describe 2 different ways in which volumetric CT can be used to evaluate airway abnormalities. The article by Curtin et al. describes the use of thin-section images displayed in axial and multiplanar 2D formats to depict airway pathology, whereas the article by Remy-Jardin et al. describes an elegant 3D volume-rendering technique that can also be used to display airway abnormalities. Both techniques provide striking images of the airways, and I am not convinced that either technique is truly superior to the other as a diagnostic tool. Pragmatically, the technique described by Curtin et al. seems to be the most applicable to practice settings. The 3-D technique described by Remy-Jardin et al. requires that a technician manually trace the airways of interest on each CT image, erase all other information on each image, and then transfer the final data to a work station for manipulation. This sounds time-consuming and cumbersome, although future software improvements may obviate the need for such "manual" labor.

S.A. Groskin, M.D.

Pulmonary Sarcoidosis: Morphologic Associations of Airflow Obstruction at Thin-section CT

Hansell DM, Milne DG, Wilsher ML, et al (Royal Brompton Hosp, London; Green Lane Hosp, Auckland, New Zealand)

Radiology 209:697-704, 1998 1–21

Introduction.—There is debate on the importance of the prevalence, anatomic site, and prognosis of airflow limitation in patients with pulmonary sarcoidosis. It is not known whether the mechanisms are involvement of the large bronchi or small airways obstruction caused by granuloma or extrinsic peribronchiolar fibrosis. The functional importance of individual CT patterns was determined, and insights into the possible mechanisms responsible for airflow obstruction in sarcoidosis were gained.

Methods.—Forty-five patients had CT examinations in a 2-year period. The patients ranged in age from 22 to 67 years and had epithelioid noncaseating granulomas at lung biopsy, mediastinal node biopsy, extrathoracic site biopsy, or a positive Kveim test result. The scans were scored semiquantitatively for the extent of 5 computed tomography patterns. The functional importance of each pattern was evaluated.

Results.—Decreased attenuation was the most prevalent CT pattern seen in 40 patients, followed by a reticular pattern seen in 37 patients, and a nodular pattern found in 36 patients. The main determinant of functional impairment, particularly airflow obstruction, was a reticular pattern (Fig 4). Airflow obstruction was independently associated with the extent of a reticular pattern, as shown by the inverse relationships with the forced expiratory volume in 1 second, forced expiratory volume in 1 second-forced vital capacity ratio, maximum expiratory flow at 25% above residual volume, and maximum expiratory flow at 50% above residual volume, and the positive relationship with the residual volume-total lung capacity ratio.

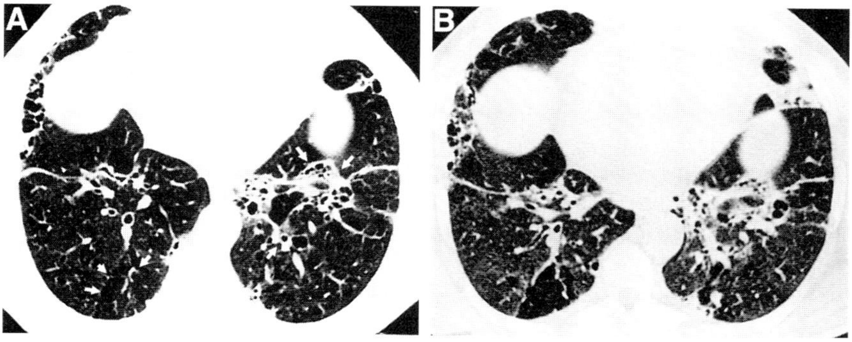

FIGURE 4.—A, Inspiratory CT scan shows a reticular pattern of small cystic air spaces (*arrows*) in the lower lobes. Note the area of decreased attenuation in the posterobasal segment of the right lower lobe (*arrowheads*). B, On the expiratory CT scan, the area of decreased attenuation is more conspicuous. (Courtesy of Hansell DM, Milne DG,Wilsher ML, et al: Pulmonary sarcoidosis: Morphologic associations of airflow obstruction at thin-section CT. *Radiology* 209: 697-704, 1998. Radiological Society of North America.)

Conclusion.—The major morphological association of airflow obstruction is a reticular pattern at CT. Although CT features compatible with small airways disease are common in sarcoidosis, they contribute little to airflow obstruction, particularly in more advanced disease.

► Sarcoidosis is the Lon Chaney, Sr of pulmonary medicine and radiology. It has at least 1,000 different "faces," and despite the fact that it is relatively commonly seen, and even occasionally recognized, it has never been understood. Among the many confusing things that sarcoidosis does, it produces interstitial lung disease that can be associated with either a restrictive or an obstructive functional abnormality. It isn't difficult to explain the restrictive form of pulmonary disease associated with sarcoidosis. Sarcoidosis can produce interstitial fibrosis that leads to decreased pulmonary compliance, reduced lung volumes, and a restrictive abnormality on pulmonary function testing.

Constructing an explanation for the obstructive physiologic abnormality that is sometimes associated with sarcoidosis requires a lot more imagination. Hansell et al, apparently have the required amount of imagination. They also have elegantly demonstrated how effectively data from CT images and physiologic testing can be correlated to shed light on a confusing clinical problem.

Initially, the major focus of radiologic research was radiologic-anatomic and radiologic-pathologic correlation. Today, there is a growing trend to use imaging studies, particularly CT, to perform radiologic-anatomic-pathologic-physiologic correlation. Although I was initially skeptical, I have become progressively more enthusiastic about the ability of CT, particularly high-resolution and inspiratory/expiratory CT, to provide reliable, valuable information about the functional status of the lungs and airways. I doubt that CT scans will replace pulmonary function testing, but, as Hansell et al demonstrated, the ability to correlate anatomic information with functional data can provide some interesting insights into the origins of physiologic abnormalities. I had been taught that the obstructive airways disease associated with sarcoidosis could be attributed to the increased incidence of asthma in these patients (it turns out that patients with sarcoidosis don't develop asthma more frequently than the rest of us) or to endobronchial granulomas. Hansell et al have demonstrated that expiratory airflow obstruction in patients with sarcoidosis is likely related to peribronchial fibrosis, which may actually produce fixed airway narrowing. This observation would explain the failure of patients with sarcoidosis to respond to bronchodilators. I really love it when a new piece of information alters my perspective and suddenly allows me to make sense of what was previously a discordant collection of data and theories.

S.A. Groskin, M.D.

Something Completely Different

Castleman Disease of the Thorax: Radiologic Features With Clinical and Histopathologic Correlation
McAdams HP, Rosado-de-Christenson M, Fishback NF, et al (Duke Univ, Durham, NC; Armed Forces Inst of Pathology, Washington, DC; Uniformed Services Univ of the Health Sciences, Bethesda, Md; et al)
Radiology 209:221-228, 1998 1–22

Background.—Castleman disease, also known as angiofollicular hyperplasia or giant lymph node hyperplasia, is apparently not a distinct entity but a diverse group of rare lymphoproliferative disorders of different histopathologic properties and biologic behavior. Currently, Castleman disease is classified into 2 major subgroups: localized and disseminated. The 2 major histologic variants are hyaline-vascular and plasma cell Castleman disease. The radiologic manifestations of thoracic Castleman disease were correlated with its clinical and histopathologic features.

Methods and Findings.—Thirty patients with pathologically proved Castleman disease were studied. Twenty-four had localized disease, and 6 had disseminated disease. Those with localized disease typically had the hyaline-vascular type, were asymptomatic, and had solitary, well-circumscribed mediastinal masses (Fig 4). At contrast material-enhanced CT, all the lesions enhanced. On MRI, all lesions were found to be heterogeneous, with increased signal intensity on T1- and T2-weighted images. Three patterns on CT or MR scans in 20 patients were evident: a solitary,

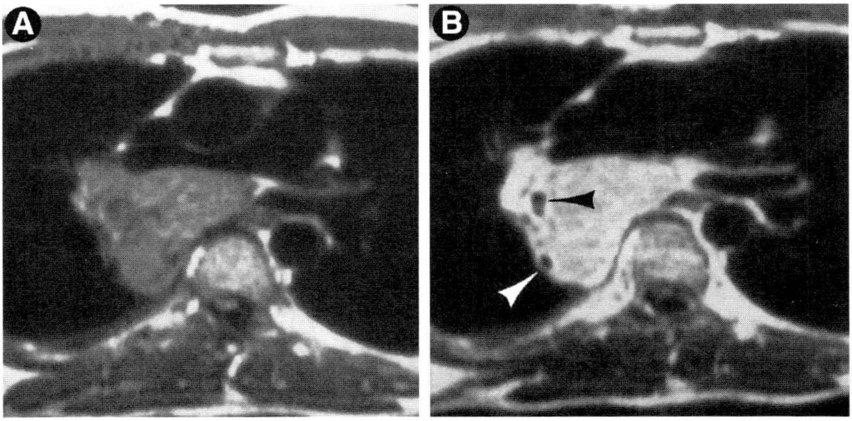

FIGURE 4.—Localized hyaline-vascular Castleman disease in a 25-year-old woman with symptoms of recurrent pneumonia. **A**, Axial MR image (800/72) shows a heterogeneous subcarinal mass. The mass extends into the right hilum and obliterates the bronchus intermedius. **B**, Axial MR image (800/72) obtained after the intravenous administration of gadolinium-based contrast material shows enhancement within the mass. Note the residual lumen of the bronchus intermedius (*black arrowhead*) and the flow void in the peripheral feeding vessel (*white arrowhead*). (Courtesy of McAdams HP, Rosado-de-Chistenson M, Fishback NF, et al: Castleman disease of the thorax: Radiologic features with clinical and histopathologic correlation. *Radiology* 209: 221-228, 1998, Radiological Society of North America.)

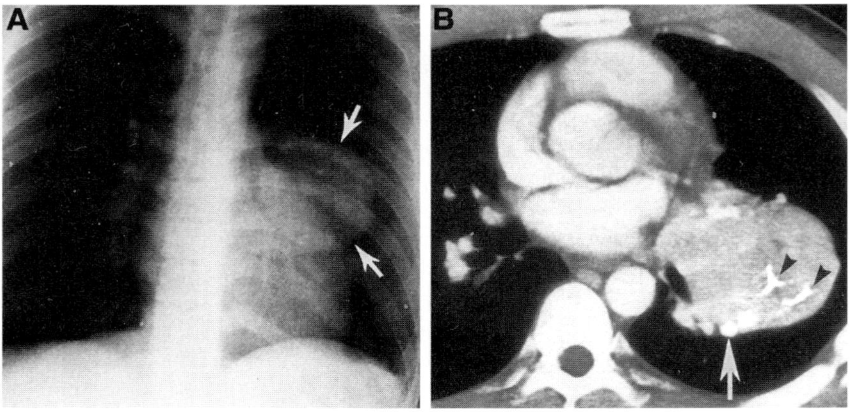

FIGURE 2.—Localized hyaline-vascular Castleman disease in a 28-year-old asymptomatic man. **A**, Posteroanterior chest radiograph shows a lobulated, well-defined mass (*arrows*) in the left hilum. Note the mass effect in the left lower lobe bronchus medial to the mass. The mediastinum is normal, and there is a small left pleural effusion. **B**, Chest CT image (*mediastinal window*) obtained at a later date, after the administration of iodinated contrast material, shows enhancement within the left hilar mass. Note the central calcifications (*arrowheads*) and enhancing vessels (*arrow*) at the periphery of the mass. (Courtesy of McAdams HP, Rosado-de-Christenson M, Fishback NF, et al: Castleman disease of the thorax: Radiologic features with clinical and histopathologic correlation. *Radiology* 209:221-228, 1998, Radiological Society of North America.)

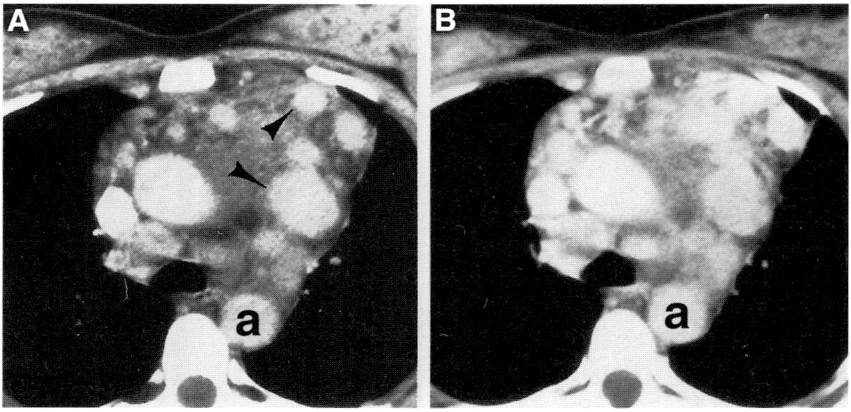

FIGURE 7.—Disseminated hyaline-vascular Castleman disease in a 51-year-old woman with flulike symptoms. **A**, Chest CT image (*mediastinal window*) obtained after the IV administration of iodinated contrast material shows multiple, enlarged lymph nodes (*arrowheads*) within the anterior mediastinum. Right paratracheal nodes are also seen. The lymph node margins are poorly defined. The nodes are homogeneous and have an attenuation similar to that of the descending aorta (*a*). **B**, Chest CT image (*mediastinal window*) obtained at the same level 20 seconds later shows intense enhancement within the lymph nodes, similar to that of the descending aorta (*a*). (Courtesy of McAdams HP, Rosado-de-Christenson M, Fishback NF, et al: Castleman disease of the thorax: Radiologic features with clinical and histopathologic correlation. *Radiology* 209:221-228, 1998, Radiological Society of North America.)

noninvasive mass; a dominant infiltrative mass with related lymphadenopathy; and matted lymphadenopathy without a dominant mass. Of the 6 patients with disseminated Castleman disease, 4 had the plasma cell type, 5 were asymptomatic initially, and 4 had bilateral mediastinal masses on chest radiography. Lesions seen on CT manifested with diffuse mediastinal lymphadenopathy, and all enhanced on contrast-enhanced CT (Figs 2 and 7).

Conclusions.—Localized Castleman disease appears as a solitary, well-circumscribed mediastinal mass or infiltrative mass, with associated lymphadenopathy, on CT or MR images. Disseminated Castleman disease typically occurs with diffuse mediastinal lymphadenopathy.

Intrathoracic Multicentric Castleman Disease: CT Findings in 12 Patients

Johkoh T, Müller NL, Ichikado K, et al (Osaka Univ, Japan; Univ of British Columbia, Vancouver, Canada; Kumamoto Univ, Japan; et al)

Radiology 209:477-481, 1998 1–23

Purpose.—The benign lymphoproliferative disorder, Castleman disease, is associated with lymphoid follicle hyperplasia and occurs in hyaline vascular and plasma cell types. Castleman disease is usually a localized condition, but it also occurs in a multicentric form. The CT findings of 12 patients with intrathoracic multicentric Castleman disease are reported.

Methods.—The patients were 7 women and 5 men, mean age 43 years. All had systemic symptoms, including fatigue. Relevant laboratory findings included anemia, elevated erythrocyte sedimentation rate, and polyclonal hypergammaglobulinemia. All patients underwent diagnostic lymph node biopsy, and open or transbronchial lung biopsy led to a diagnosis of lymphocytic interstitial pneumonitis in 7 of them. Initial thin-section CT scans were reviewed by 2 observers, who reached a consensus regarding the presence and distribution of various CT findings.

Findings.—Bilateral hilar and mediastinal lymph node enlargements were present in all cases. On IV contrast administration, the affected nodes showed mild to moderate enhancement. Parenchymal abnormalities and poorly defined centrilobular nodules were noted on CT scans in all patients. Ten patients had thin-walled cysts, 10 had thickening of the bronchovascular bundles, and 9 had interlobular septal thickening. Subpleural nodules were noted in 6 patients, ground-glass attenuation in 4, air-space consolidation in 1, and bronchiectasis in 1. On pathologic correlation, the CT finding of centrilobular nodules reflected lymphocyte and plasma cell infiltration around the bronchioles, whereas interlobular septal thickening corresponded to infiltration around the interlobular and alveolar septa.

Conclusions.—The CT findings of intrathoracic multicentric Castleman disease include bilateral hilar and mediastinal lymphadenopathy with centrilobular nodular opacities. Lymphocytic interstitial pneumonitis appears to be the pathologic change underlying the parenchymal CT abnormalities. These patients have systemic symptoms and polyclonal hypergamma-globulinemia.

► Castleman disease is 1 of those disorders that everyone knows about but no one ever sees (except, of course, the authors of these 2 articles). I selected these 2 articles for the current YEAR BOOK because they elegantly describe and illustrate the clinical and radiologic findings associated with both the localized and the disseminated forms of Castleman disease. The report by Johkoh et al. is particularly interesting because it describes in detail the patterns of pulmonary parenchymal involvement that may be seen in patients with the disseminated form of the disease. Parenchymal abnormalities were thought to be uncommon in patients with disseminated Castleman disease, but Johkoh et al. found high-resolution CT evidence of lung involvement in all of their patients.

I don't know whether I will ever see another case of Castleman disease (I saw my 1 and only case about 8 years ago); if I do, I hope that I will have the wit to recognize it and to remember these 2 articles.

S.A. Groskin, M.D.

Distinction of Consolidative Bronchioloalveolar Carcinoma From Pneumonia: Do CT Criteria Work?

Aquino SL, Chiles C, Halford P (Wake Forest Univ, Winston-Salem, NC)

AJR 171:359-363, 1998 1–24

Introduction.—About 30% of bronchioalveolar carcinomas (BACs) are of the consolidative type. Certain chest CT findings are reportedly helpful in identifying pulmonary consolidation as BAC. However, there are no data on the use of these characteristics to differentiate between BAC and pneumonia. The CT features of consolidative BAC were compared with those of consolidative infectious pneumonia.

Methods.—The study included 20 patients with consolidative BAC and 20 with infectious consolidative pneumonia for whom chest CT scans were available. Each scan was reviewed by consensus of 2 chest radiologists. In addition to consolidation, the review focused on features such as nodules and ground-glass opacities; the presence of air bronchogram, mucous bronchogram, contrast enhancement, cysts, or cavities within the consolidation; and evidence of pulmonary fibrosis or parenchymal scarring. Data analysis sought to identify any CT patterns that were more specific for 1 disease than the other.

Results.—In the BAC group, all patients had consolidation, most often with a peripheral distribution. Eighteen had multifocality, 16 had associated ground-glass opacities, 14 had air bronchogram, and 11 had coexisting nodules (Fig 1). Findings that were present significantly more often in patients with consolidative BAC were coexisting nodules and a peripheral pattern of consolidation (Table 1). Follow-up CT scans of 7 of 8 patients with BAC showed disease progression.

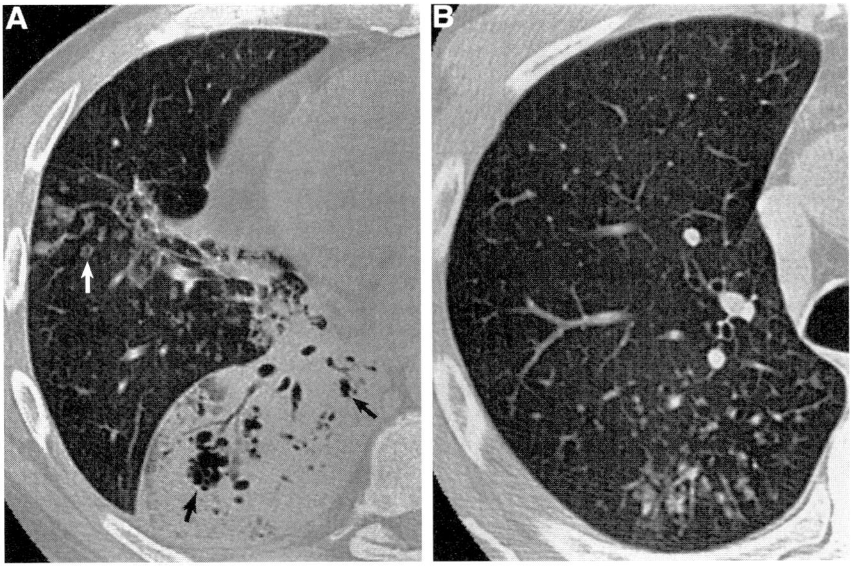

FIGURE 1.—BAC in a 47-year-old man with 6-month history of chronic cough. **A**, CT scan of right lung shows dense consolidation of right lower lobe that contains air bronchogram and numerous cysts (*black arrows*). Note nodules, some of which are cavitary, in middle lobe (*white arrow*). **B**, CT scan of right upper lobe shows more nodules. (Courtesy of Aquino SL, Chiles C, Halford P: Distinction of consolidative bronchioalveolar carcinoma from pneumonia: Do CT criteria work? *AJR* 171:359-363, 1998.)

TABLE 1.—CT Patterns of Consolidative BAC and Infectious Pneumonia

CT Pattern	Number of Patients (%) with BAC	Number of Patients (%) with Pneumonia	*p* value
Nodules	11 (55)	1 (5)	.001
Peripheral distribution	14 (70)	3 (15)	.001
Atelectasis	1 (5)	10 (50)	.003
CT angiogram sign	4/12 (33)	13/16 (81)	.019
Pleural effusion	5 (25)	12 (60)	.054
Mucous bronchogram	0	4 (20)	.106
Adenopathy	3 (15)	8 (40)	.155
Leafless tree	9 (45)	4 (20)	.176
Multifocal	18 (90)	14 (70)	.235
Bulging fissure	5 (25)	2 (10)	.407
Heterogeneous consolidation	5/12 (42)	5/16 (31)	.698
Cysts or cavities	8 (40)	8 (40)	1.000
Consolidation	20 (100)	20 (100)	1.000
Ground-glass opacities	16 (80)	15 (75)	1.000
Air bronchogram	14 (70)	15 (75)	1.000
Low-attenuation consolidation	2 (10)	1/16 (6)	1.000

Abbreviation: BAC, bronchioalveolar carcinoma.
(Courtesy of Aquino SL, Chiles C, Halford P: Distinction of consolidative bronchioalveolar carcinoma from pneumonia: Do CT criteria work? *AJR* 171:359-363, 1998.)

Conclusions.—Certain chest CT findings may be helpful in making the diagnosis of consolidative BAC versus consolidative chest pneumonia. Consolidative BAC should be suspected in adult patients with normal immunity who had a nonresolving peripheral consolidative pneumonia, particularly when associated nodules are present. This diagnosis is almost always made in middle-aged to elderly patients in whom chronic pneumonia has been diagnosed.

► I read this article on a Sunday evening with a growing sense of excitement. Aquino et al. described patients who were identical to a patient whose films I had reviewed and agonized over the previous Friday. I didn't know what my patient had (pneumonia, lymphoma, bronchiolitis obliterans-organizing pneumonia, drug-induced lung disease . . .), but Aquino and her colleagues knew exactly what their patients had. They had the answer, I had their article, tomorrow I would astonish my clinical colleagues with my acumen and perspicacity. I went to bed at one with the universe, in synch with the music of the spheres, balanced and at peace.

Well, despite the peripheral distribution of the consolidation and the presence of pulmonary nodules, my patient didn't have BAC; he had pneumonia and lymphoma, but I still highly recommend this extremely timely and useful article.

The incidence of BAC is increasing, but, because of its protean radiographic manifestations and nonspecific clinical findings, I'm fairly certain that we are not diagnosing it with equally increasing proficiency. (Aquino et al found that the diagnosis of BAC was typically delayed 5 months in their patients.) This head-on comparison of pneumonia and BAC provides us with several practical clues for distinguishing these 2 commonly confused entities (I have found that the presence of nodules is particularly helpful.) I would like to know how patients with pneumonia compared clinically with patients with BAC. Are there any particularly valuable clinical clues to the diagnosis (ie, lack of fever or leukocytosis favoring BAC)? I would also like to know exactly how the diagnosis of pneumonia was established in the patients in the "non-BAC" group. This last question is a matter of great curiosity to me, because I am frequently puzzled by how we and our clinical colleagues go about making a diagnosis of pneumonia.

S.A. Groskin, M.D.

Bullous Sarcoidosis: A Report of Three Cases

Judson MA, Strange C (Med Univ of South Carolina, Charleston)

Chest 114:1474-1478, 1998 1–25

Introduction.—Pulmonary sarcoidosis is highly variable. Most patients have mild or no pulmonary symptoms, minimal pulmonary dysfunction, and no evidence of fibrosis or fibrocystic disease on the chest radiograph. Three patients were seen with bullous emphysema with severe airflow obstruction, but the diagnosis of pulmonary sarcoidosis was not suspected for at least 2 years.

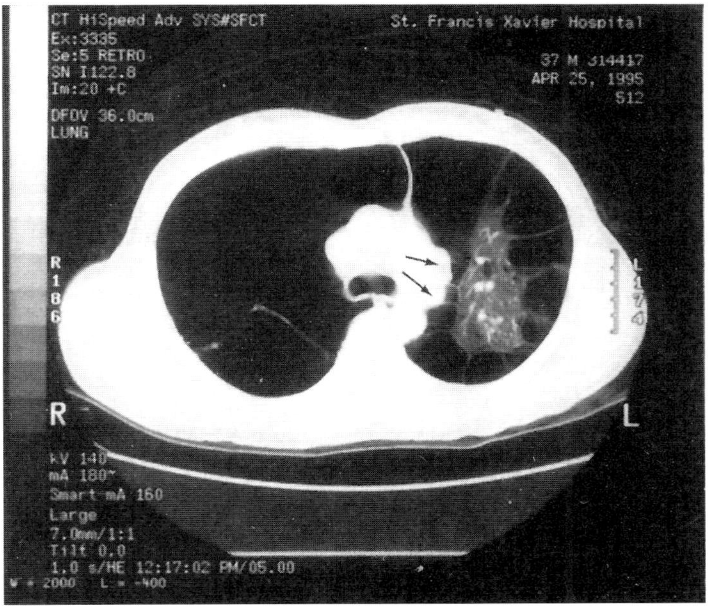

FIGURE 1.—Chest CT scan from patient 1 shows granulomatous lung contraction leaving large peripheral bullae. Note the rounded ispilateral mediastinal adenopathy (*arrows*). (Courtesy of Judson MA, Strange C: Bullous sarcoidosis: A report of three cases. *Chest* 114: 1474-1478, 1998.)

Case 1.—Man, 37, a former smoker of one-half pack of cigarettes daily for 20 years, was referred for bullectomy or lung transplantation. He had a hyperresonant chest, diminished breath sounds, and a prolonged expiratory phase. Extensive bilateral bullous disease with adjacent lung contraction was seen, with a rounded ispilateral mediastinal adenopathy (Fig 1). The CT scan suggested the diagnosis of pulmonary sarcoidosis, and 9 months after referral, the patient received a right single-lung transplant.

Case 2.—Man, 40, was given a diagnosis of emphysema after having progressive dyspnea for 2 years He smoked 1 pack of cigarettes daily from age 14 to age 24 years. He was treated for pneumonia 5 times during the 10 years before his presentation. A calcified mediastinal adenopathy were seen on chest CT scan.

Case 3.—Woman, 48, was a lifelong nonsmoker who had dyspnea on 50 to 100 feet of ambulation. Bullous lung disease and bilateral mediastinal adenopathy were seen on chest CT scan. Her dyspnea was atrributed to asthma and emphysema until the diagnosis of sarcoidosis was considered 16 years later.

Conclusion.—When young patients who have smoked relatively few pack-years are given a diagnosis of emphysema or severe airflow obstruction, the physician should suspect sarcoidosis as the cause of bullous emphysema. The presence of mediastinal adenopathy on a chest radiograph or a CT scan and a history consistent with extrapulmonary sarcoidosis are additional clues. When airspace enlargement is present without surrounding lung fibrosis, bullous emphysema results. The cause of bullous lesions in sarcoidosis is still unknown.

► I selected this article as a companion piece to the article describing the radiologic correlates of obstructive airways disease in patients with sarcoidosis (Abstract 1–21). Judson and Strange describe yet another of the many radiographic manifestations of sarcoidosis-dramatic bullous lung disease that can be, and often is, confused with bullous emphysema. Their speculation about the possible etiologies for ullae in patients with sarcoidosis are interesting and serve as a reminder that sarcoidosis is more than just a disease of the thoracic lymph nodes; it affects the airways, vessels, and the pulmonary interstitium, too.

Sarcoidosis can also involve the central and peripheral nervous system, eyes, heart, kidneys, liver, spleen, esophagus, bowel, skin, bones, joints, salivary glands. I'm not sure what other body parts there are, but I am confident that sarcoidosis also can affect them. So remember, sarcoidosis: It is more than just a lymph node disease, it is a systemic disease.

S.A. Groskin, M.D.

Presentation and Surgical Management of Bronchogenic and Esophageal Duplication Cysts in Adults

Cioffi U, Bonavina L, De Simone M, et al (Univ of Milan, Italy)

Chest 113:1492-1496, 1998 1–26

Introduction.—Bronchogenic and esophageal duplication cysts, which are congenital anomalies of the bronchial tree and foregut, are often asymptomatic in adults. The bronchogenic-type cyst is usually found in the mediastinum around the tracheobronchial tree; it is unilocular and is characterized by a lining of ciliated columnar epithelium and the presence of cartilage. The esophageal duplication type of cyst is close to the esophageal wall, is covered by 2 muscle layers, and has a lining that is squamous, columnar, cuboid, pseudostratified, or ciliated epithelium. Both types of cyst can be complicated by intracystic hemorrhage, perforation, infection, or squamous metaplasia. A retrospective review of surgically treated bronchogenic and esophageal duplication cysts was conducted.

Methods.—There were 27 patients with bronchogenic or esophageal duplication cysts. At initial presentation 10 (37%) were asymptomatic. The most common complaint in symptomatic patients with bronchogenic cysts was chest pain and in patients with a duplication cyst, it was dyspnea. All patients underwent chest x-ray study, barrium swallow, and esophagoscopy. Sixteen patients had a CT scan (Fig 1) and 9 underwent endoscopic US (Fig 4). One patient had MRI (Fig 2).

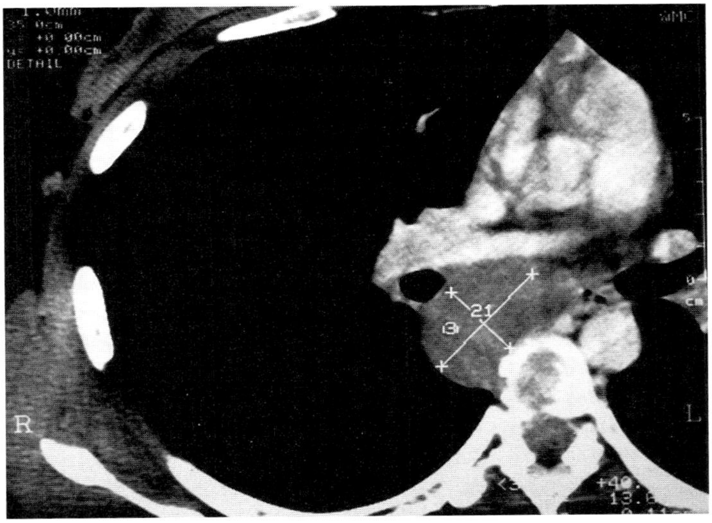

FIGURE 1.—CT scan showing a retrocardiac hypodense mass in a patient affected by bronchogenic cyst close to the right bronchus. (Courtesy of Cioffi U, Bonavina L, De Simone M, et al: Presentation and surgical management of bronchogenic and esophageal duplication cysts in adults. *Chest* 113:1492-1496, 1998.)

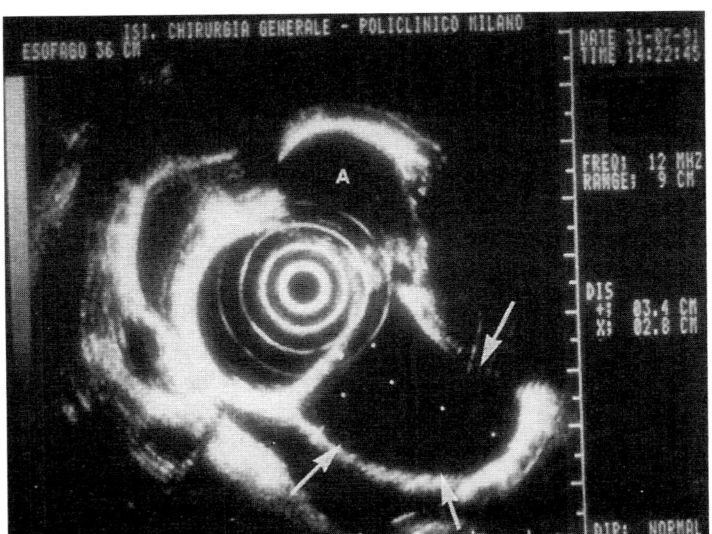

FIGURE 4.—Endoscopic US showing a large hypoechoic mass (*arrows*) of the wall of the esophagus in a patient with esophageal duplication cyst. *Abbreviation*: *A*, aorta. (Courtesy of Cioffi U, Bonavina L, De Simone M, et al: Presentation and surgical management of bronchogenic and esophageal duplication cysts in adults. *Chest* 113:1492-1496, 1998.)

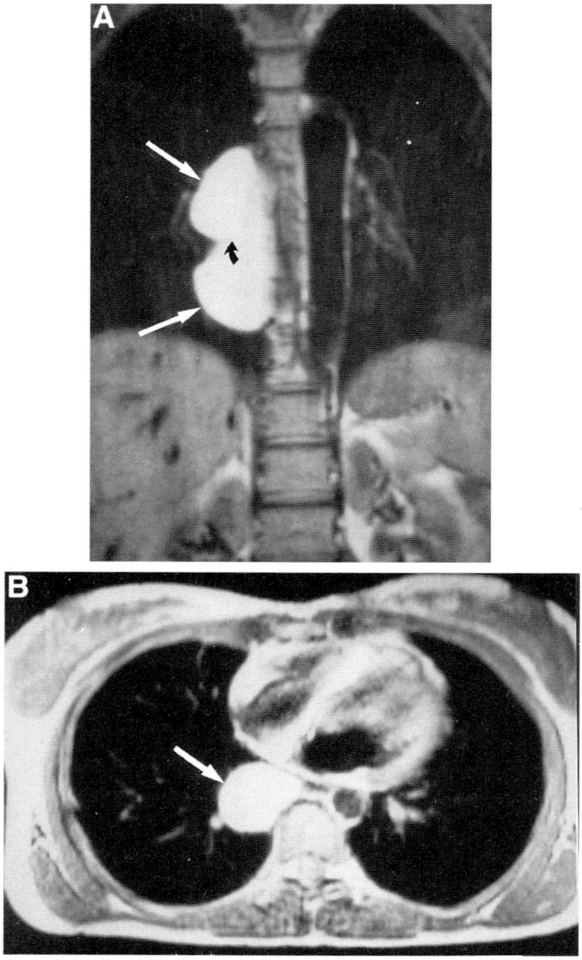

FIGURE 2.—MRI. **A,** Coronal T1-weighted image showing a right mediastinal bilobated bronchogenic cyst (10 × 5 cm) (*white arrows*) with high signal intensity consistent with high protein content. The *black arrow* shows the sept of the cyst. **B,** Axial T2-weighted image of the same bronchogenic cyst (*arrow*) showing decreased signal intensity. (Courtesy of Cioffi U, Bonavina L, De Simone M, et al: Presentation and surgical management of bronchogenic and esophageal duplication cysts in adults. *Chest* 113:1492-1496, 1998.)

Results.—In 26 patients, a complete excision of the cyst was performed, and 1 patient with intrapulmonary cyst had a right upper pulmonary lobectomy. In 23 patients, a posterolateral thoracotomy was performed. In 4 patients, a video-assisted thoracoscopy using a 3-port technique was performed. There was no postoperative morbidity. At a median follow-up of 4 years, all patients except 1, were asymptomatic.

Conclusion.—For bronchogenic and esophageal duplication cysts, surgery is the treatment of choice. The first-line approach in these patients should be video-assisted thoracoscopy.

► Cioffi et al. provide a very concise review of the clinical and radiologic evaluation and treatment of adult patients with bronchogenic and esophageal duplication cysts. Although nothing new or revolutionary is presented, it is helpful to be periodically reminded that (1) even though many patients found to have duplication cysts are initially asymptomatic, over 70% will eventually have symptoms, (2) it is easier to remove an innocuous, uninfected cyst than an angry, infected one, (3) endoscopic US is a great tool for assessing esophageal and periesophageal masses, and (4) the CT density of a bronchogenic cyst can be misleading; Hounsfield numbers as high as 80 may give the false impression that the cyst is a solid mass. The results of surgical resection, either by thoracotomy or via thoracoscopy, are excellent, although cysts may recur if excision is not complete.

S.A. Groskin, M.D.

Case Report: Intradiaphragmatic Bronchogenic Cyst

Rozenblit A, Iqbal A, Kaleya R, et al (Albert Einstein College of Medicine, Bronx, NY; New York Med College)

Clin Radiol 53:918-920, 1998 1–27

Introduction.—Bronchogenic cysts are usually located in the mediastinum or lung parenchyma. It is exceedingly rare to find an intradiaphragmatic location. The case of a patient with a rare bronchogenic cyst located in the left diaphragmatic crus was reported. The diagnostic features of diaphragmatic cysts and the difficulties in localizing the lesion with cross-sectional images were reviewed.

> *Case Report.*—Woman, 64, had had intermittent epigastric pain throughout an 8-year period. The patient had mild epigastric tenderness. She had normal results of upper endoscopy. An extrinsic retrogastric mass was seen in upper gastrointestinal barium studies. A noncontrast abdominal CT showed a 6 × 4–cm, well-defined, soft-tissue density mass in the left suprarenal region, superior and medial to a single limb of the left adrenal gland (Fig 1). Because of a limited acoustic window and unfavorable beam angulation, visualization of the lesion was technically difficult. The MR image showed an intermediate signal on T1-weighted scan and a very bright signal on T2-weighted sequence; however, the MRI could not be completed because of the patient's claustrophobia.

Results.—The site of origin could not be determined before surgery. Because the cyst was located above and medial to the kidney, an adrenal origin was favored. The lesion was believed to arise in the abnormal

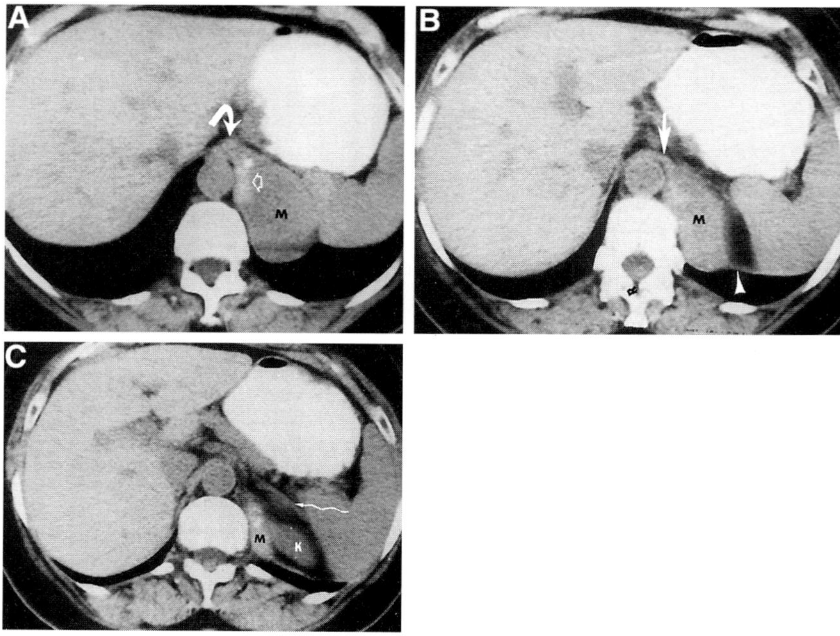

FIGURE 1.—Non-contrast abdominal CT of a 64-year-old woman; 10-mm contiguous sections. **A,** smooth, well-defined soft-tissue mass (*M*) inseparable from the distal esophagus (*curved arrow*). Note peripheral calcification in the mass medially (*open arrow*). **B,** 1 cm below 1A, the diaphragm is seen anteriorly (*arrow*) and posteriorly (*arrowhead*) to the mass (*M*). **C,** 2 cm below 1A, 1 cm caudal to 1B, the inferior portion of the lesion (*M*) is medial to the upper pole of the kidney (*K*). The adrenal gland (*wavy arrow*) is pushed laterally; only a single limb was identified. (Courtesy of Rozenblit A, Iqbal A. Kaleya R, et al: Case report: Intradiaphragmatic bronchogenic cyst. *Clin Radiol* 53:918-920, 1998.)

adrenal limb. The medial adrenal limb was compressed by the diaphragmatic cyst at the time of surgery, and CT could not identify it with the 10 mm–thickness slice used. Because the diaphragm is a thin and curved structure, an intradiaphragmatic lesion is difficult to ascertain with any imaging modality. Nonvisualization of the normal diaphragmatic crus at the level of the lesion that followed dipahragmatic contour suggested the correct diagnosis.

Conclusion.—On CT, a left intradiaphragmatic cyst may resemble an adrenal cyst, and thin sections may be needed for the complete demonstration of the adjacent normal adrenal gland. In the differential diagnosis of cystic peridiaphragmatic mass, a bronchogenic diaphragmatic cyst, although rare, should be included. To confirm the diagnosis, surgical treatment is indicated. US confirmed the cystic nature of the lesion, although this was technically difficult. The lesion was considered cystic, based on the combined imaging characeristics.

► This has to be the strangest location for a bronchogenic cyst that I have heard of (with the possible exception of the base of the tongue and the subcutaneous tissues). The diaphragm is rarely the site of significant pathology and this is a good thing, as we frequently have a difficult time obtaining and interpreting adequate images of the diaphragm when it is. The CT images that accompany this article are quite good, and , as the authors point out, they really do tell the tale.

S.A. Groskin, M.D.

Mediastinal Lipomatosis

Nguyên K, Hoeffel C, Lê LH, et al (Med Diagnostic Ctr, Ho Chi Minh City, Vietnam; Jeanne de'Arc Hosp, Toul Cedex, France)
South Med J 91:1169-1172, 1998 1–28

Introduction.—Mediastinal lipomatosis is a benign condition that features a large amount of mature adipose tissue within the mediastinum. This fat accumulation widens the mediastinum and can lead to diagnostic errors by simulating mass lesions. One patient with a huge mediastinal lipomatosis is described, along with a review of 36 cases previously reported in the literature.

Case Report.—Man, 34, was hospitalized with a 3-month history of dyspnea on exertion; the dyspnea was particularly severe when he walked for a long time or worked hard. His history was negative for steroid intake and thoracic trauma. On physical examination, the patient was in no acute distress, was not obese, and had no apparent abnormalities. A radiograph of the chest revealed a huge enlargement of the mediastinal silhouette that gradually increased from the superior to the inferior mediastinum and had a triangular shape. The borders were well defined and regular. Mediastinal lines were still visualized. There was no narrowing or deviation of the trachea. The cardiac silhouette could not be seen through the mass. Both lungs were well aerated. The relationship of the mass to the heart could not be clarified on the lateral view. A CT scan showed a hypotense and septated large mass of fatty attenuation (-100 to -120 Hounsfield units) that involved the mediastinal space from the level of T3 to the hemidiaphragm. Mediastinal structures were not displaced. The cause of the diffuse mediastinal lipomatosis was not known. Five kilograms of fat was surgically removed to relieve the dyspnea. Pathologic evaluation showed mature fat tissue without nuclear atypia.

Discussion/Conclusion.—Average age of this patient combined with the 36 patients reported in the literature was 28 (range, 3 months to 78 years). The male-to-female ratio was 3:2. Most patients had no symptoms; some experienced thoracic pain, dyspnea, cough, dysphonia, or supraventricular tachycardia. All patients had some evidence of clinical Cushing's syndrome, either primary or iatrogenic. Mediastinal widening is bilateral and may be symmetrical in patients with mediastinal lipomatosis. Differential diagnosis of this finding is limited. CT allowed measurement of the attenuation value of the mass in the patient presented and confirmed its fatty nature.

► Last week I saw a chest radiograph of a young man with AIDS. When I compared his current film with a film made 2 years earlier, I was struck by the marked interval increase in the width of his supra-aortic mediastinum. I immediately called his primary care physician and told her that I believed that her patient had mediastinal lymphadenopathy and, because he had AIDS, that he probably had either tuberculosis or lymphoma. I recommended that a CT scan be obtained. Two days later, the patient's CT scan demonstrated a large amount of fat in the supra-aortic mediastinum, accounting for the abnormality I saw on his plain radiograph.

Several times a year, we encounter patients, brought to the emergency room after falls or motor vehicle accidents, who have widened mediastinal silhouettes caused not by hematoma but by an excessive amount of mediastinal fat or, if you prefer the more elegant term, by mediastinal lipomatosis.

I feel extremely fortunate to have ready access to CT, since it makes the diagnosis of mediastinal lipomatosis (and a number of other mediastinal abnormalities) ridiculously easy. My hat is off to those older, braver radiologists who practiced BC (before CT). They had to grapple with the problem of the widened mediastinum with the aid of only plain films, conventional tomograms, the barium swallow, and their clinical judgment. I recommend that you read Dr. E. Robert Heitzman's book, *The Mediastinum*[1] if you want to see just how far a truly splendid radiologist can go with just those tools.

S.A. Groskin, M.D.

Reference

1. Heitzman ER: *The Mediastinum Radiologic Correlations With Anatomy and Pathology*, ed. 2. Berlin/Heidelberg, Springer-Verlag 1988.

Lentil Aspiration Pneumonia: Radiographic and CT Findings

Marom EM, McAdams HP, Sporn TA, et al (Duke Univ, Durham, NC)

J Comput Assist Tomogr 22:598-600, 1998 1–29

Introduction.—Aspiration of leguminous vegetables may cause a granulomatous pneumonitis, or lentil aspiration pneumonia, that can be detected on radiographs with small, poorly defined nodular opacities. Reported are 2 patients with lentil aspiration pneumonia with nodules as large as 1 cm in diameter on radiographs and CT findings that simulated metastases.

Case 1.—Man, 54, with history of radiation therapy for nasopharyngeal squamous cell carcinoma was seen with a 3-month history of nonproductive cough, a 7-kg weight loss, and general

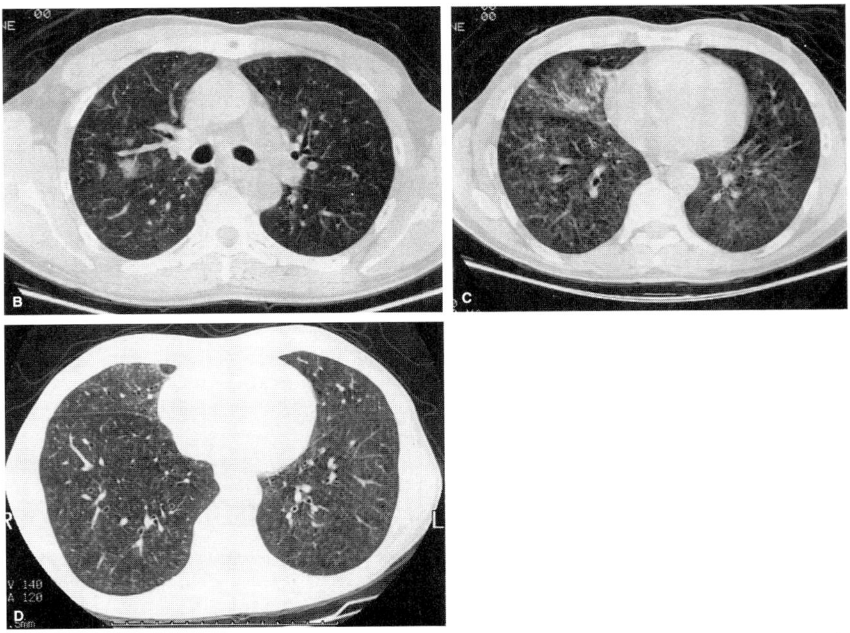

FIGURE 1.—Lentil aspiration pneumonia in a 54-year-old man with esophageal stricture. B, High-resolution CT (1.5-mm collimation, lung window) through the upper lungs shows scattered poorly defined pulmonary nodules up to 10 mm in diameter. C, High-resolution CT (1.5-mm collimation, lung window) through the lower lungs shows diffuse 1- to 3-cm centrilobular nodules and branching opacities (tree-in-bud pattern). Image is degraded by motion. D, High-resolution CT (1.5-mm collimation, lung window) 2 years later shows persistent though improved centrilobular opacities. (Courtesy of Marom EM, McAdams HP, Sporn TA: Lentil aspiration pneumonia: Radiographic and CT findings. *J Comput Assist Tomogr* 22:598-600, 1998.)

malaise. Other than soft-tissue fibrosis in the neck that limited the aperture of his mouth, the remaining physical and laboratory examination findings were within normal limits. A chest radiograph revealed bilateral, poorly defined, nodular opacities in a basilar distribution that were new since a radiograph taken 1 year earlier. Biapical pleural thickening caused by radiation was stable. Chest CT (10-mm slice collimation, 10-mm table increment) revealed multiple bilateral nodules varying from 3 to 10 mm in diameter. High-resolution CT (1.5-mm collimation) obtained at 34 levels revealed scattered, poorly defined 1-cm nodules and smaller centrilobular nodules in the dependent lung. No hilar or mediastinal lymphadenopathy was seen. Fiberoptic bronchoscopy with transbronchial biopsy of the right middle and lower lobe was done to rule out metastases. Pathologic examination showed chronic inflammation and foreign body giant cells engulfing birefringent foreign material that was consistent with lentil particles. All cultures, including those for acid-fast bacilli, were negative at 6 weeks. A barium esophagram revealed aspiration and marked glottic narrowing, which proved on histologic examination to be postradiation fibrosis. After placement of a gastrostomy tube, the patient's symptoms improved. The radiographic opacities gradually resolved, and a chest radiograph was normal at 1-year follow-up. A repeat CT scan 2 years later revealed decreased, yet persistent centrilobular opacities (Fig 1).

Case 2.—Woman, 84, was a smoker with a history of bullous pemphigoid that was treated with corticosteroids. She also had dementia. She was seen with a 2-week history of cough and low-grade fever. She was cachectic, had a temperature of 37.5°C, and had mild inspiratory crackles. A chest radiograph revealed scattered, poorly defined pulmonary nodules up to 1 cm in diameter. Fiberoptic bronchoscopy with transbronchial biopsies and washings was performed to exclude tuberculosis. Nonnecrotizing epithelioid granulomatous inflammation with numerous giant cells and central lentil particles were observed on pathologic examination. At 6 weeks, the specimen was negative for acid-fast bacilli. All cultures were negative.

Conclusion.—Lentil aspiration pneumonia is caused by aspiration of leguminous material and usually occurs in conditions in which aspiration is common. Radiologic findings of lentil aspiration can be challenging to interpret because they can be confused with those of other entities. Biopsy and cultures are required to exclude other diagnoses.

► You may be asking yourself why I decided to include this article in the YEAR BOOK OF DIAGNOSTIC RADIOLOGY. I had 3 very good reasons:

1. Aspiration of liquid or solid material is a substantial cause of morbidity and mortality in both children and adults, and we should be on the lookout for its various radiographic manifestations.
2. One of the radiographic manifestations of lentil aspiration is pulmonary nodules that may mimic metastases. This is a particular problem because patients with certain neoplasms that can metastsize to the lungs (ie, head and neck carcinoma) also have an increased tendency to aspirate.
3. I had never heard specifically of lentil aspiration. I didn't realize that it was a particular problem and that it had its own literature, and I was impressed beyond words that a pathologist could look at a lung biopsy specimen, see typical birefringent particles, and say, "Egad, it's another classic case of lentil aspiration!"

S.A. Groskin, M.D.

Postpneumonectomy Syndrome: Recognition and Management
Valji AM, Maziak DE, Shamji FM, et al (Ottawa Civic Hosp, Ont, Canada)
Chest 114:1766-1769, 1998 1–30

Introduction.—Postpneumonectomy syndrome (PPS) is caused by extreme shift and rotation of the mediastinum after pneumonectomy. It can produce symptomatic proximal airway obstruction and airway trapping.

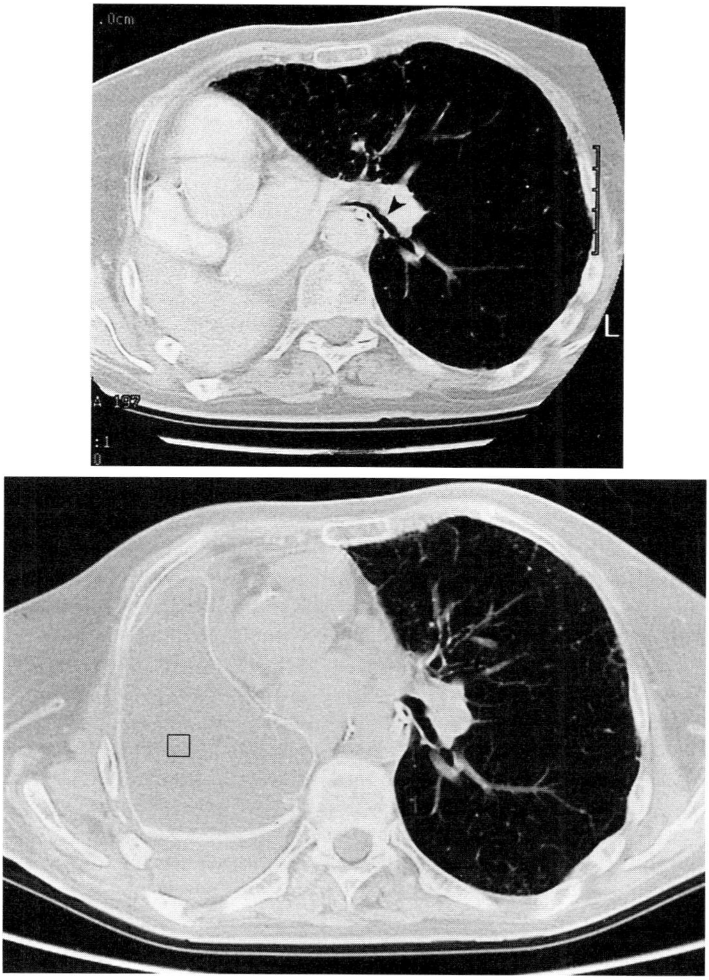

FIGURE 1.—CT scan images of right postpneumonectomy syndrome. **Top,** Contrast-enhanced CT scan demonstrating extrinsic compression of the lower lobe bronchus between the pulmonary artery and the aorta (*arrowhead*). **Bottom,** Mediastinum repositioned with saline solution–filled prosthesis (see box) in the pneumonectomy space. (Courtesy of Valji AM, Maziak DE, Shamji FM: Postpneumonectomy syndrome: Recognition and management. *Chest* 114:1766-1769, 1998.)

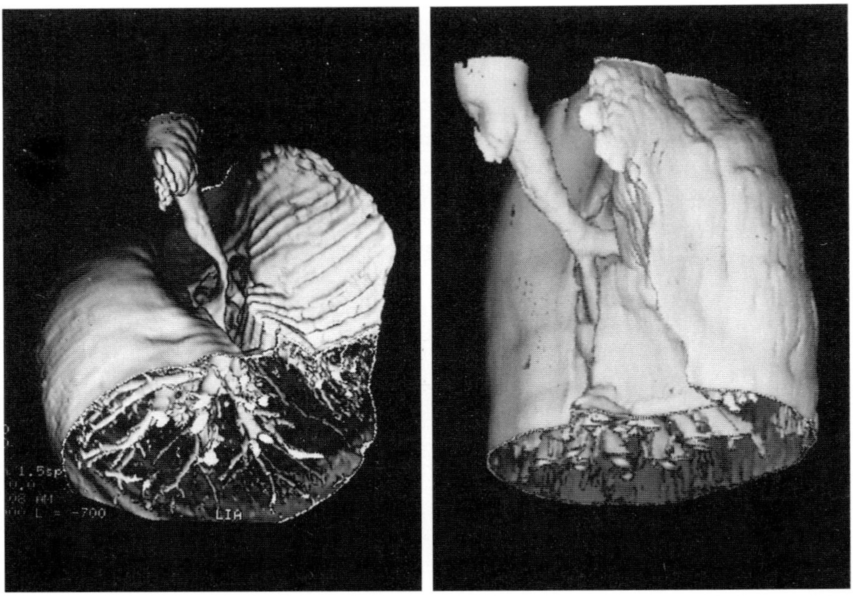

FIGURE 2.—Three-dimensional reconstruction of CT scan images in right PPS before (**left**) and after (**right**) surgical correction. *Abbreviations*: *PPS*, postpneumonectomy syndrome. (Courtesy of Valji AM, Maziak DE, Shamji FM: Postpneumonectomy syndrome: Recognition and management. *Chest* 114:1766-1769, 1998.)

Experience with 5 patients with PPS seen between 1990 and 1997 is reviewed.

Methods.—Of the 5 patients, 4 had previous right pneumonectomy and 1 had left pneumonectomy. All patients were seen because of complaints of dyspnea. There was a median time interval of 21 months (range, 6 months to 9 years) from onset of symptoms to surgical correction after pneumonectomy. Clinical diagnosis of PPS was made with the aid of chest radiographs, 2-dimensional echocardiography, pulmonary function tests, CT scans, and awake fiberoptic bronchoscopy. The earlier incision was reopened. There was a suction noise immediately on entering the pneumonectomy, and the mediastinum fell away from the posterolateral chest wall in 2 patients. No adhesions were seen. In the other 3 patients, the mediastinum was adherent to the chest wall and required lysis of adhesions. After complete mobilization of the mediastinum, anterior pericardiorrhaphy was done before the pericardium was anchored in the parasternal chest wall with nonabsorbable suture. A Silastic prosthesis filled with saline solution was placed to correct overshifting of the mediastinum.

Results.—Mean patient age at pneumonectomy was 46.4, and at a correction of PPS it was 53.8. Morbidity and mortality rates were both 0%. All patients experienced relief of dyspnea. Corrective repositioning of the mediastinum was confirmed with the aid of chest radiographs, CT scans (Figs 1 and 2), and awake fiberoptic bronchoscopy. There was a mean 166.7% (range, 100% to 300%) increase in the cross-sectional diameter of the obstructed bronchus in 4 patients, as determined by CT scan. The measured diameter remained unchanged in 1 patient. The peak expiratory flow rate rose by a mean of 44.2% (range, 40% to 49%) in all 5 patients.

Conclusion.—The diagnosis of PPS should be considered in all patients with progressive dyspnea after pneumonectomy. Repositioning of the mediastinum by means of a prosthesis filled with saline solution and anterior pericardiorrhaphy is a simple procedure and offers immediate and lasting symptomatic relief.

► The other day, 1 of my colleagues called me over to look at the chest radiograph of a patient with "no cardia"—the heart was simply not visible on the radiograph ("no cardia"—sorry, but I couldn't resist). The patient had undergone right pneumonectomy a number of years ago and now complained of increasing dyspnea. The right hemithorax was diminutive and dense, whereas the left lung was markedly hyperinflated, crossing the midline. A CT scan showed the heart huddled in the tiny right postpneumonectomy space. The left lung was hyperinflated, and the left mainstem bronchus was markedly narrowed as it crossed the thoracic spine and aorta.

Valji et al. describe 5 such cases and include a discussion of the pathophysiology, differential diagnosis, and treatment of this syndrome. The radiographs they include are striking and not only demonstrate the significant shift of mediastinal contents and airway narrowing that characterize this process but also, in 1 patient, reveal prominent hyperinflation of the left lower lobe related to attenuation of the left lower lobe bronchus as it passes between the left pulmonary artery and the aorta. The 3-dimensional airway and lung renderings that accompany this article are so wonderful that they almost convinced me that such images might actually be clinically useful. (However, I still favor axial images.)

S.A. Groskin, M.D.

2 Breast Imaging

Introduction

I would like to thank Dr. Anne Osborn for inviting me to join the group of reviewers on the YEAR BOOK OF DIAGNOSTIC RADIOLOGY. For 7 years, Dr. Murray Rebner dedicated time and expertise to this publication and it is with great respect for his legacy that I begin my task. The specialty of breast imaging has expanded over the last 20 years to its present state where many modalities are used in daily practice and are undergoing investigation with the goal of breast cancer detection. Clearly, mammography remains the primary imaging modality, but stereotactic, digital and nuclear imaging, MRI sonographic interventional procedures, and even surgical procedures are changing the way breast cancer is detected, diagnosed, and treated. The articles reviewed in the breast imaging section of this YEAR BOOK present a wide variety of information and will increase our knowledge base as practicing physicians, as well as introducing new concepts and innovations that may shape the way we practice in the future.

The 20 articles chosen for this issue cover areas of interest that include x-ray mammography, sonography, MRI for breast cancer, nuclear imaging, computer-assisted detection (CAD), and interventional procedures including stereotactic and MRI-guided breast biopsy. The first article, however, is not specific to these groups and is focused on what I believe may be one of the most interesting topics in breast cancer at this time, namely that of sentinel lymph node identification. The interest here has much to do with the interactions and education necessary to involve physicians from various branches of medicine in an evolving area of breast cancer diagnosis. As the surgical approach toward this disease has become more conservative, emphasis on the limitation of axillary dissection has motivated some surgeons to learn the procedure of identification and removal of the sentinel lymph node. Krag et al. (Abstract 2–1) address the potential pitfalls and challenges in learning this procedure.

Within the area of general mammography, I chose 2 articles specific to the mammographic appearance of breasts in women taking hormone replacement therapy. Greendale et al. (Abstract 2–2) demonstrate a difference in breast density with the use of estrogen/progestin combination therapy, and Roubidoux et al. (Abstract 2–3) focus on the difficulties in detection of breast cancer in women who are taking hormone replacement therapy. Awareness of the effect of hormone therapy is important to the practice of breast imaging. The third article related to general mammography comes from Kerlikowske et al (Abstract 2–4). This article is educational concerning the issue of intra and inters observer variations in the interpretation of screening mammographic examinations despite the effort of the Breast Imaging Reporting and Data System to standardize these interpretations.

Pisano et al (Abstract 2–5) and Lindfors et al (Abstract 2–6) address the challenging issues of women's response to both "false positive" screening examinations and the choice within the algorithm of breast management between imaging surveillance or percutaneous core biopsy. Both surveys were reassuring in that an overall positive impact may be achieved despite "false positive" interpretations.

The women reported on by Helvie and his group (Abstract 2–7) from Michigan had undergone transverse nectus abdominis musculotaneous flap reconstruction following mastectomies, but all differed from a more random sample in that these 6 women had ductal carcinoma in situ as their initial disease diagnosis. Clearly, this article suggests the need for guidelines for surveillance imaging of the reconstructed breast, at least for women whose disease is not invasive at the time of mastectomy. The Whitman group (Abstract 2–8) present a very simple core biopsy technical innovation which may not be applicable to many patients but, if used properly with 14- or 11-gauge biopsy needles, might benefit the breast imager in daily practice and is included for the purpose of increasing options for percutaneous biopsy.

We are all very aware of the ongoing problem of a dwindling number of available dedicated breast imaging technologists and we strive to find methods to improve our practice. Issues concerning the intrinsic and extrinsic rewards important to the technologists surveyed by Collins and her group (Abstract 2–9) may provide some answers to ways we can attract and keep good technologists working within our practices.

Additional methods of breast cancer detection are addressed in 2 articles, the first by te Brake et al (Abstract 2–10) from the Netherlands. This article outlines nicely some of the process of computer-aided detection (CAD). Clearly, CAD is not a way to diagnosis breast cancer, but it shows promise in serving perhaps as a "second reader" or as a method to alert the radiologist that certain regions of the breast may deserve a second (or even a third!) look. The Fenlon group in Ireland report on their use of scintimammography and demonstrate a positive predictive value of 90% and a negative predictive value of 95% in women with palpable breast masses. The use of nuclear breast imaging varies from practice to practice and many radiologists may not be aware of the diagnostic findings reported using the modality.

The articles on US chosen for this edition are 3, beginning with the *Opinion* by Ferris Hall (Abstract 2–12). The issues and questions raised by this thoughtful work concerning the increasing use of breast US and concerns over who is performing these studies deserve our attention. An additional question raised by Dr. Dianne Georgian-Smith (personal communication) is that of the need for a study that actually demonstrates the benefits of breast US (similar to the Breast Cancer Detection Demonstration Project). How often does US of a palpable mass which is "negative" miss a cancer? How often are women reassured that "there is nothing there" by non image-trained physicians who may have suboptimal machines in their offices? The article on microbubble intravenous contrast injection used to differentiate benign from malignant breast lesions (Abstract 2–13) is of interest, but, to echo Dr. Rebner's statement from last year's YEAR BOOK, "it appears that we are not quite at the point where ultrasound can accurately differentiate benign from malignant lesions". The third article raises the very controversial question of screening for breast cancer with sonography. The work of Kolb et al (Abstract 2–14) is impressive because of the large sample group scanned and the assumed expertise required for the individual examinations. Resurrecting the idea of whole breast screening for breast cancer with sonography raises many questions including issues of accreditation for both physicians and technologists, requirements for machinery used, and the significant question of the time involved for these examinations. It will be very interesting to follow the results of other investigators in this specialized field.

The articles on diagnostic imaging of the breast with MRI include work focused on the use of dynamic contrast imaging (Abstract 2–15), identifying ductal carcinoma in situ (Abstract 2–16) and adapting to the 0.5 T open architecture MR imaging system (Abstract 2–17). There exists today a vast array of opinions from many experts in this field including types of magnets used, the design of breast coils, the sequences utilized, whether 1 breast or 2 is examined simultaneously, the subtraction technique, and the benefits of dynamic contrast imaging to enhance image evaluation. This is an evolving area of investigation and exciting material is coming from all directions.

The final articles are those addressing interventional procedures and begins appropriately with the excellent work from Dr. Liberman and her group in New York (Abstract 2–18), reporting on the retrieval of calcium using an 11-gauge directional vacuum-assisted breast biopsy device. Many ask, "is bigger better?", and with improvement in diagnosis, without a significant increase in complication rates, this may prove to be the case. Next year, I plan to include work on the use of the very large core biopsy devices (the Advanced Breast Biopsy System and the Site Select). Intervention within the high-field strength magnet environment brings many challenges including type of magnet used (open or closed bore) and the availability of instruments. Not only do biopsy instruments have to be non ferro-magnetic, but even those that are compatible within the magnet need to create as little image artifact as possible. These challenges are significant and Daniel et al. (Abstract 2–19) and Schorn et al. (Abstract 2–20) elaborate on a few of these problems. Clearly, I consider this to be a major realm of investigation encompassing detection, diagnosis, and possibly, even treatment of breast cancer and look forward to reporting on the emerging methodologies and advancements in this technologically rich branch of breast imaging.

I certainly hope this year's selection of articles is of interest to you. The field of breast imaging is growing all the time and the challenge to stay current with all its many aspects is somewhat daunting.

Robyn L. Birdwell, M.D.

The Sentinel Node in Breast Cancer: A Multicenter Validation Study

Krag D, Weaver D, Ashikaga T, et al (Univ of Vermont, Burlington; Sylvester Cancer Ctr, Miami, Fla; Arkansas Cancer Research Ctr, Little Rock, et al)

N Engl J Med 339:941-946, 1998 2–1

Objective.—Sentinel node resection offers a possible alternative to axillary lymph node dissection in selected patients with breast cancer and the complications and psychologic distress associated with it. In preliminary studies, probe-guided resection of the sentinel node using radioactive tracers has been found to identify regional metastases. A multicenter trial of sentinel node evaluation in patients with breast cancer is reported.

Methods.—The study included 443 women with invasive breast cancer who had negative results on examination of the ipsilateral axilla and a treatment plan that included axillary lymph node dissection. Before surgery, technetium-99m sulfur colloid, 37 MBq, was injected into the breast around the tumor or biopsy cavity. A gamma probe was then used to identify hot spots corresponding to the sentinel node. After radioactive sentinel nodes were removed, the patients underwent complete axillary lymphadenectomy. The investigators compared the pathologic findings of the sentinel nodes with those of the remaining axillary nodes.

TABLE 1.—Rate of Technical Success in Identifying a Hot Spot, According to Surgeon, Before Incision

Surgeon No.	No. of Patients	Success Rate (%)*	Exact 95% Binomial Confidence Interval
1	51	98.0	89.6-100.0
2	51	98.0	89.6-100.0
3	51	98.0	89.6-100.0
4	50	98.0	89.4-100.0
5	49	95.9	86.0-99.5
6	47	95.7	85.5-99.5
7	43	79.1	64.0-90.0
8	33	93.9	79.8-99.3
9	30	83.3	65.3-94.4
10	22	81.8	59.7-94.8
11	16	87.5	61.7-98.5
Total	443	93.2†	90.5-95.4

*P = .001 by Fisher's exact test for the comparison of technical-success rates among surgeons.
†Hot spots were identified in 413 of the 443 patients.

(Reprinted by permission of *The New England Journal of Medicine* from Krag D, Weaver D, Ashikaga T, et al: The sentinel node in breast cancer: A multicenter validation study. *N Engl J Med* 339: 941-946.)

Results.—Hot spots were successfully identified in 93% of the patients (Table 1). Sentinel node evaluation was 97% accurate in predicting the positivity or negativity of the axillary nodes. The procedure had a specificity of 100%, a positive predictive value of 100%, a negative predictive value of 96%, and a sensitivity of 89%. Eight percent of sentinel nodes were located outside the axilla, and 11% outside level 1 nodes. Of all positive sentinel nodes, 3% were found in nonaxillary locations. The various participating surgeons had comparable false negative rates. The number of positive sentinel nodes was significantly correlated with the number of positive nonsentinel nodes.

Conclusions.—This study validates the use of sentinel node biopsy to predict the presence or absence of axillary lymph node metastases in patients with breast cancer. However, the procedure is technically complex, and the success rates may vary between surgeons and with patient characteristics. False negative results are most likely to occur in lesions located in the lateral half of the breast.

▶ The most significant prognostic indicator for invasive breast cancer is the presence or absence of metastatic tumor in regional lymph nodes. Axillary lymph node dissection with complete nodal removal at levels I and II is a standard part of the surgical treatment of invasive breast cancer at this time. However, this procedure is not without morbidity, including complications of lymphedema, numbness, seroma formation, and restriction of shoulder mobility. For women with breast cancers assessed as T1 lesions, only 20% to 30% will have axillary metastases. Therefore, the concept of sentinel lymph node (SLN) biopsy, originally reported by Cabanas in 1977 and widely used for melanoma staging, is now under intense scrutiny for breast cancer.[1,2] The SLN is the first lymph node (or up to 4 nodes) along the afferent lymphatic tumor drainage pathway. The importance of the SLN is its status (tumor present or not) may reflect that of the nodes upstream. Therefore, if the SLN is negative for tumor, no further axillary dissection may be necessary. Early studies report a technical success rate of 66% to 100% correlating results of SNL biopsy with axillary dissection with reported sensitivity of 85% to 100%, specificity of 100%, and accuracy at 95% to 100%.[4,5]

This excellent work by Krag et al is a multicenter study of the method as used by 11 surgeons in a variety of practice settings and demonstrates that the procedure, indeed, can be technically challenging and that one can expect success rate variation. The literature reports a variety of methods for the mapping of SLNs, including radionuclide injection (with and without lymphoscintigraphy) and intraoperative vital blue dye injection with direct visual observation of the lymphatic uptake of the dye. As this procedure is being learned, it is imperative to add the SLN biopsy to that of the standard axillary dissection to correlate the accuracy of the SLN findings with that of the standard axillary dissection finding. No doubt next year's YEAR BOOK will reflect the important advances and, hopefully, the gradual consensus as to the method of this procedure. Equally important during this time of changing standards is the vital roll of education, which needs to be directed toward all arms of medicine related to this procedure, including radiologists, nuclear medicine physicians, and surgeons with clearly defined protocols including intraoperative communication.

R.L. Birdwell, M.D.

References

1. Cabanas RM: An approach for the treatment of penile carcinoma. *Cancer* 39:456-466, 1977.
2. Krag DN, Meijer SJ, Weaver DL, et al: Minimal-access surgery for staging of malignant melanoma. *Arch Surg* 130:654-660, 1995.
3. Morton DL, Wen DR, Wong JH, et al: Technical details of intraoperative lymphatic mapping for early stage melanoma. *Arch Surg* 127:392-399, 1992.
4. Giuliano AE, Jones RC, Brennan M, et al: Sentinel lymphadenectomy in breast cancer. *J Clin Oncol* 15:2345-2350, 1997.
5. Veronesi U, Paganelli G, Galimberti V, et al: Sentinel node biopsy to avoid axillary dissection in breast cancer with clinically negative lymph nodes. *Lancet* 349:1864-1867, 1997.

Effects of Estrogen and Estrogen-Progestin on Mammographic Parenchymal Density

Greendale GA, for the Postmenopausal Estrogen/Progestin Interventions (PEPI) Investigators (Univ of California, Los Angeles; Wake Forest School of Medicine, Winston-Salem, NC; Johns Hopkins Univ, Baltimore, Md; et al)

Ann Intern Med 130:262-269, 1999 2–2

Introduction.—Mammographic density appears to be a strong, independent risk factor for the development of breast cancer. Earlier reports analyzing the relationship between postmenopausal use of hormones and mammographic density have been limited to observational trials, convenience samples, or uncontrolled clinical trials. The effects of placebo, conjugated equine estrogen (CEE), and CEE combined with 1 of 3 progestin regimens on mammographic density in 307 of 875 women from the Postmenopausal Estrogen/Progestin Interventions Trial are described.

Methods.—Seven ambulatory centers participated in this 3-year, multicenter, double-blind, randomized, placebo-controlled trial. Each woman underwent a baseline mammogram and at least 1 follow-up mammogram. Participants had not taken estrogen for at least 5 years before baseline and did not have breast implants. Patients were randomized to treatment with either (1) placebo, (2) CEE, 0.625 mg/day, (3) CEE plus cyclic medroxyprogesterone acetate (MPA), 10 mg/day for 12 days per month, (4) CEE plus daily MPA, 2.5 mg/day, or (5) CEE plus micronized progesterone (MP), 200 mg/day for 12 days per month. Women were observed for changes in mammographic density, according to American College of Radiology Breast Imaging Reporting and Data System grades.

Results.—Nearly all increases in mammographic density occurred in the first year. At 12-month follow-up, the percentage of women with density grade increases was 0%, 3.5%, 23.5%, 19.4%, and 16.4%, respectively, in the placebo, CEE, CEE plus cyclic MPA, CEE plus daily MPA, and CEE plus cyclic MP groups. At the 12-month time point, the odds of increased mammographic density were 13.1, 9, and 7.2, respectively, for CEE plus cyclic MPA, CEE plus daily MPA, and CEE plus cyclic MP, compared with CEE alone.

Conclusion.—Increasing mammographic density may be an important marker for increased risk of breast cancer in women taking estrogens and estrogen-progestins.

► This randomized double-blind placebo-controlled trial of the effect of estrogen alone and of estrogen plus progestin on breast density as judged mammographically adds weight to the anecdotal and reported effect of hormone replacement therapy on mammographically assessed breast tissue density.[1] The authors found that, over the 3 years of follow-up, approximately 8% of the patients using estrogen only and 19% to 24% of those using the estrogen and progestin mixture had a demonstrated increase in mammographic density based on the BI-RADS categorization, moving from 1 category of density to the next higher category. When compared with women treated with estrogen only, the estrogen/progestin users had a 7- to 13-fold increased risk of development of denser breasts. There is consistent evidence that greater mammographic density increases the risk of breast cancer both by potentially masking a lesion and by mechanisms not yet clearly understood.[2,3] This information is important for breast imagers, particularly because hormone replacement therapy is used more and more in the United States for its protective effect on heart disease and osteoporosis.

R.L. Birdwell, M.D.

References

1. Kaufman Z, Garstin WI, Hayes R, et al: The mammographic parenchymal patterns of women on hormonal replacement therapy. *Clin Radiol* 43:389-392, 1991.
2. Laya MB, Gallagher JC, Schreiman JS, et al: Effect of postmenopausal hormonal replacement therapy on mammographic density and parenchymal pattern. *Radiology* 196;433-437, 1995.
3. Saftlas AF, Hoover, RN, Brinton LA, et al: Mammographic densities and risk of breast cancer. *Cancer* 67:2833-2838, 1991.

Breast Cancer in Women Who Undergo Screening Mammography: Relationship of Hormone Replacement Therapy to Stage and Detection Method

Roubidoux MA, Wilson TE, Orange RJ, et al (Univ of Michigan Hosps, Ann Arbor; Towsley Ctr, Ann Arbor, Mich; Univ of Utah, Salt Lake City; et al)
Radiology 208:725-728, 1998 2–3

Introduction.—Hormone replacement therapy has been reported to decrease the sensitivity of screening mammography and to increase the risk of breast cancer. Higher breast cancer stage and increased rates of palpable cancer, as well as false negative mammograms, may result if the accuracy

TABLE 1.—Cancer Stages in Women Who Received Hormone Replacement Therapy Versus Those in Women Who Did Not Receive Hormone Replacement Therapy

Cancer Stage*	HRT Group (n = 58)	Non-HRT Group (n = 57)
0	15 (26)	19 (33)
I	28 (48)	24 (42)
T1a	4 (7)	2 (4)
T1b	7 (12)	8 (14)
T1c	17 (29)	14 (25)
II	13 (22)	11 (19)
III	2 (3)	2 (4)
IV	0 (0)	1 (2)
Nodal metastases	11 (19)	13 (23)

Note: Numbers in parentheses are percentages.

*P = .75 for differences between the hormone replacement therapy group and the non–hormone replacement therapy group in the number of women with stage I, II, III, or IV cancer. P = .65 for differences between the hormone replacement therapy group and the non–hormone replacement therapy group in the number of women with nodal metastasis.

Abbreviation: HRT, hormone replacement therapy.

(Courtesy of Roubidoux MA, Wilson TE, Orange RJ, et al: Breast cancer in women who undergo screening mammography: Relationship of hormone replacement therapy to stage and detection method. *Radiology* 208:725-728, 1998. Radiological Society of North America.)

of the mammograms is affected by hormone replacement therapy. Cancers found in women who had screening mammography were evaluated. Women who use hormone replacement therapy were compared with those who do not.

Methods.—One hundred fifteen women with breast cancer, ranging in age from 55 to 65, who had at least 1 screening mammogram within the last 24 months before diagnosis were studied. Their history of hormone replacement therapy was retrospectively reviewed, and a statistical analysis was performed.

Results.—Of the 58 women who received hormone replacement therapy, 15 (26%) had stage 0 cancer, 28 (48%) had stage I, 13 (22%) had stage II, and 2 (3%) had stage III (Table 1). Among the 57 women who did not receive hormone replacement therapy, 19 (33%) had Stage 0 cancer, 24 (42%) had stage I, 11 (19%) had stage II, 2 (4%) had stage III, and 1 (2%) had stage IV. Mammography alone detected cancers in 38 of the women who did not receive hormone replacement therapy (67%) and in 38 of those who did receive hormone replacement therapy (66%). Five women in the non–hormone replacement therapy group (9%) and 4 in the hormone replacement therapy group (7%) had false-negative mammograms.

Conclusion.—There were no significant differences in cancer stages or in the number of mammographically detected cancers or false-negative mammograms between the group who received hormone replacement therapy and the group that did not among the screened women in whom breast cancer developed.

▶ This retrospective review of 115 cases of breast cancer in women in whom at least 1 screening mammogram was obtained 24 months before diagnosis of breast cancer included those who received hormone replacement therapy (n = 58) and those who did not (n = 57). The breakdown of breast cancer stages was similar in the 2 groups, and there was a similar rate of false negative mammograms in the 2 groups. The subgroup of women taking hormone replacement therapy included those using estrogen alone and those using estrogen in combination with progesterone, without separation of the 2 hormone replacement therapy types. As discussed in the article by Greendale et al. (see article elsewhere in the YEAR BOOK) the type of therapy may affect breast density differently. Although not all cancers were detected on screening mammograms, all of these women had undergone screening examinations at least 24 months before the detection of their cancer, and there were very similar numbers in both subgroups with respect to ultimate cancer detection by mammography alone, by palpation alone, or by mammography and palpation. Although this is not truly an evaluation of cancers detected by screening mammography, it is helpful as a part of the evolving body of data concerning the limitations based on examinations, both physical and radiologic, in the detection of breast cancer in women undergoing hormone replacement therapy. There were no significant differences between groups as to the stages of cancer or positive findings of axillary lymph nodal involvement. Focus on the choice of whether hormone replacement therapy is used continues to lie primarily with each woman and her physician. However, the more aware we are of the limitations in diagnosis and the possibilities of the relationship between estrogen alone and estrogen and progestin combinations, the more patients may benefit.

R.L. Birdwell, M.D.

Variability and Accuracy in Mammographic Interpretation Using the American College of Radiology Breast Imaging Reporting and Data System

Kerlikowske K, Grady D, Barclay J, et al (Univ of California, San Francisco)
J Natl Cancer Inst 90:1801-1809, 1998 2–4

Introduction.—Several trials have reported considerable variability among radiologists in interpretations of mammograms. Several trials were limited by the small numbers of screening examinations reviewed, the small numbers of cancers detected, and the selection of difficult mammograms for review. Described in the largest investigation to date is intraobserver and interobserver agreement in interpretation of screening mammography and accuracy of mammography using the American College of Radiology Breast Imaging Reporting and Data System (BI-RADS).

Methods.—Mammographic examinations were randomly selected on the basis of original mammographic interpretation and cancer outcome from 71,713 screening examinations between April 1985 and February

TABLE 3.—Agreement Between Two Radiologists Interpreting Screening Mammography Films Using the Breast Imaging Reporting and Data System

	All Readings (n = 2,578) Agreement			Cancer (n = 302) Agreement			No Cancer (n = 2,276) Agreement			
Parameter	Observed, %	Expected, %*	κ (95% Confidence Interval)	Observed, %	Expected, %*	κ	Observed, %	Expected, %*	κ	P†
Finding/no finding	84	54	0.66 (0.63-0.69)	86	69	0.54	84	58	0.62	.21
Primary finding‡	66	23	0.56 (0.52-0.60)	71	30	0.58	64	22	0.54	.36
Breast density§	75	39	0.59 (0.55-0.62)	77	41	0.62	74	39	0.58	.39
Assessment category‖	78	48	0.58 (0.55-0.61)	65	34	0.46	80	54	0.56	.02
Recommendation¶	83	58	0.59 (0.56-0.63)	71	46	0.47	84	66	0.55	.13

*Expected agreement by chance alone.

†Comparison of κ statistic in cancer and no cancer group. All P values are two-sided.

‡The following 9 findings were possible: mass, calcification, density, focal asymmetric density, multiple bilateral masses, multiple bilateral calcifications, multiple bilateral calcifications and masses, architectural distortion, and other findings (n = 222 cancer group; n = 500 no cancer group).

§The following 4 categories were possible: entirely fatty, scattered fibroglandular tissue, heterogeneously dense, and extremely dense (n = 302 cancer group; n = 145 no cancer group).

‖The following 5 categories were possible: normal, normal with benign finding; incomplete, additional evaluation needed; suspicious abnormality; and highly suggestive of malignancy.

¶The following 5 categories were possible: normal interval screening, additional view, US, fine-needle aspiration, and biopsy.

(Courtesy of Kerlikowske K, Grady D, Barclay J: Variability and accuracy in mammographic interpretation using the American College of Radiology Breast Imaging Reporting and Data System. *J Natl Cancer Inst* 90:1801-1809, 1998, by permission of Oxford University Press.)

1995. The final sample consisted of 1,563 normal examinations, 786 abnormal examinations with no detected cancer, and 267 abnormal examinations with detected cancer. Films were read independently by 2 radiologists using BI-RADS. Cancer status was ascertained by contacting the women's physicians and by linkage to the regional Surveillance, Epidemiology, and End Results Program.

Results.—Agreement between radiologists in reporting findings was moderate when cancer was present and substantial when cancer was not present. Agreement was moderate in assigning an assessment category; it was significantly lower in the presence of cancer than when cancer was not present (Table 3). There was a 2-fold greater chance of agreement in reporting the presence of a finding and mammographic assessment in examinations with less dense breasts. Agreement was higher on repeat readings by the same radiologist than on interpretations between radiologists. Sensitivity of mammography was lower when BI-RADS was used than when the original system of mammographic interpretation was used. The positive predictive value of mammography was higher with BI-RADS.

Conclusion.—There was considerable variability in the interpretation of mammographic examinations. Variability and accuracy of mammograms were neither improved nor reduced with the use of BI-RADS.

► With the Mammography Quality Standards Act issuing the final regulations in April 1999, all breast imagers are now required to conform to categories determined by the BI-RADS for mammographic assessment, including standardization of terms and recommendations for follow-up screening or diagnostic tests. This large study of randomly selected mammographic examinations chosen on the basis of original mammographic interpretation and cancer outcome from 71,713 screening examinations performed in the mobile screening program at the University of California in San Francisco from April 1985 to February 1995 included 786 abnormal screening examinations with no cancer detected, 267 abnormal examinations with cancer detected, and 1,563 normal examinations. The authors used the BI-RADS classification to determine intraobserver and interobserver agreement in interpreting screening mammographic examinations. They also compared the accuracy of mammographic interpretation based on the BI-RADS system with the accuracy of their original system for mammographic interpretation. They found that agreement was higher on repeat readings by the same radiologist than between radiologists and that the sensitivity of mammography was lower with BI-RADS than with their original system of mammographic interpretation. However, they found that the positive predictive value of mammography was higher with the BI-RADS system.

Overall, despite the efforts at standardization of categorization of findings, which was at least in part the motivation for the Mammography Quality Standards Act issued by Congress in 1992, this large study found considerable variability in the interpretation of mammographic examinations. Unfortunately, variability and accuracy of the practice of reading mammograms have neither improved nor significantly diminished with the use of BI-RADS.

It appears that the human element and intraobserver variability in perception and interpretation continue, as has been reported in many areas of radiology (and is not specific to breast imaging!).[1-3]

R.L. Birdwell, M.D.

References

1. Elmore JG, Wells CK, Lee CH, et al: Variability in radiologist's interpretations of mammograms. *N Engl J Med* 331:1493-1499, 1994.
2. Garland LH: Studies of the accuracy of diagnostic procedures. *AJR* 82:25, 1959.
3. Felson B, Morgan WKC, Bristol LJ, et al: Observations on the results of multiple readings of chest films on coal miner pneumoconiosis. *Radiology* 109:19, 1973.

Screening Behavior of Women After a False-Positive Mammogram

Pisano ED, Earp J, Schell M, et al (Univ of North Carolina, Chapel Hill)

Radiology 208:245-249, 1998 2–5

Background.—As the number of women undergoing mammography increases, so does the number of false-positive results. There is little information on the effects of a false-positive mammogram on the patient's compliance with recommendations for annual screening mammography. The impact of a false-positive mammogram leading to an open biopsy on the patient's subsequent screening behavior was examined retrospectively.

Methods.—Forty-three women, aged 50 or older, who had an abnormal mammogram followed within 6 months by a benign result on an open surgical biopsy were included in the study. A random sample of 136 women—including women with normal mammograms who did not have biopsies and women with abnormal mammograms for whom a 6-month follow-up mammogram was recommended—served as the control group. Information on subsequent screening behavior and other variables was gathered by means of a structured telephone interview.

Results.—The study and control groups were similar in terms of age, race, marital status, education, and income. The women with false-positive mammograms were more likely to believe that they had a high susceptibility to breast cancer and were more likely to say that they intended to undergo annual screening mammography in future years.

Conclusions.—Having a false-positive mammogram followed by an open surgical biopsy does not make women less likely to return for subsequent screening mammographic examinations. The experience of a false-positive mammogram may even increase patients' intentions to have regular screening. Recommendations for a breast biopsy should be considered in the context of their impact on the individual patient.

▶ There was a great deal of consternation, certainly among the breast imagers with whom I work, after the article entitled "Ten Year Risk of False Positive Screening Mammograms and Clinical Breast Examinations" appeared in the April 16, 1998, issue of *The New England Journal of Medicine*.[1]

Would women stop having mammograms? Lumping mammography and clinical examinations together, these authors estimated that, among women who do not have breast cancer, 18.6% will undergo a biopsy after 10 mammograms (approximately 10 years) and 6.2% after 10 clinical breast examinations. It was stated that physicians should educate women about the risk of a false positive result of a screening test for breast cancer. This may be an appropriate conclusion, but the present paper by Pisano et al. elucidates some reassuring findings. Their telephone interview study of a retrospective cohort revealed two significant differences between those women who had an abnormal mammogram leading to a surgical biopsy and those women who had not had a surgical biopsy. Study patients were more likely than control patients to plan to undergo screening mammography annually in the future, and they believed that they had an increased susceptibility to breast cancer. It is conceivable that this perception of an increased susceptibility to breast cancer might be the motivating force for women to plan for annual mammography in the future. In any case, those women who might have appeared most likely to shy away from this screening tool did not, in fact, change their personal practice of planning for regular mammography.

R.L. Birdwell, M.D.

Reference

1. Elmore JG, Barton MB, Moceri VM, et al: Ten-year risk of false positive screening mammograms and clinical breast examinations. *N Engl J Med* 338:1089-1096, 1998.

Short-Interval Follow-up Mammography Versus Immediate Core Biopsy of Benign Breast Lesions: Assessment of Patient Stress

Lindfors KK, O'Connor J, Acredolo CR, et al (Univ of California, Sacramento; Univ of California, Davis; Woodland Clinic, Calif)

AJR 171:55-58, 1998 2–6

Introduction.—Periodic mammographic surveillance is effective in the management of clinically occult and probably benign lesions. It has been suggested that needle biopsy be used instead of periodic mammography to allay patient anxiety. The stress experienced by women undergoing surveillance mammography for benign lesions was compared with stress levels of women undergoing core biopsy of benign lesions.

Methods.—A retrospective postal survey was mailed to 174 women with probably benign breast abnormalities that were stable at short-interval follow-up mammography and 116 women in whom a core biopsy of the breast was performed with benign findings. The survey questioned participants about the stress related to the diagnostic experience as well as about who advised them of the results of their breast imaging studies and the information these professionals provided.

TABLE 1.—Self-Reported Overall Stress of Experience by Two Groups of Women

Group	None	A Little	Moderate	Very	Extreme	Total
Core biopsy	5 (9)	16 (28)	27 (47)	9 (16)	1 (2)	58 (100)
Surveillance	21 (26)	34 (43)	21 (26)	2 (3)	2 (3)	80 (100)

*Values are numbers of patients. Numbers in parentheses are percentages rounded to whole numbers.
(Courtesy of Lindfors KK, O'Connor J, Acredolo CR, et al: Short-interval follow-up mammography versus immediate core biopsy of benign breast lesions: Assessment of patient stress. *AJR* 171:55-58, 1998.)

Results.—Eighty surveys were returned by women who underwent short-interval follow-up mammography, and 58 were returned by women who underwent core breast biopsy. Self-reported overall stress experienced by women who underwent biopsy was significantly higher than that reported by women in the follow-up mammography group (Table 1). The level of anxiety was not influenced by the patient's perception of the probability that the lesion represented carcinoma. There was no significant difference among women who discussed their mammogram results with a radiologist and those who were notified by their primary care provider.

Conclusion.—Short-interval follow-up mammography is acceptable in the evaluation of lesions that are probably benign and does not increase the patient's anxiety about outcome. Stress associated with the notification of mammography results was not related to the physician's specialty.

► The question addressed here is one that has been speculated upon by many of us in the field, namely, that of patients' insistence on more percutaneous breast biopsies rather than the waiting and following method of short-interval imaging surveillance. This survey-based retrospective study included women who either had been followed up with surveillance mammography at a short interval or had undergone a benign core biopsy. Stress-related questions in the survey related to the diagnostic experience and which medical specialist advised the women of the results. Women who had core biopsy reported more "moderate to extreme" stress than those undergoing surveillance ("no stress" was indicated by 26% of those undergoing surveillance compared with 9% with the core biopsy). The biopsy group differed from the surveillance group in income (higher) and age (younger). More women in the biopsy group indicated a change in attitude/practice, with 19% of this group saying that they would improve adherence to a regular mammography schedule compared with only 7% of the surveillance group who indicated the same change in practice. Brenner and Sickles[1] have shown an 8:1 ratio of the cost of core biopsy to the cost of mammographic surveillance. The clearly established guidelines set by Sickles[2] in 1991 for BI-RADS category 3 "probably benign lesions" should encourage breast imagers to continue to rely on surveillance for appropriately chosen lesions. This study gives some reassurance that patient anxiety will not be increased by this approach. I was interested to note that stress levels of the 2 groups of women were not affected by which medical group or person conveyed the pertinent medical information. The supposition has been that a dedicated breast imager would be more knowledgeable concerning the likelihood of a lesion being "probably benign" and could reduce a patient's stress. This proved not to be the case in this study. Perhaps the established rapport with the primary care provider may be as helpful as consultation with the breast imaging expert in alleviating stress, both when abnormal results are presented and when alternative recommendations are discussed.

R.L. Birdwell, M.D.

References

1. Brenner RJ, Sickles EA: Surveillance mammography and stereotactic core breast biopsy for probably benign lesions: A cost comparison analysis. *Acad Radiol* 4:419-425, 1997.
2. Sickles EA: Periodic mammographic follow-up of probably benign lesions: Results in 3,184 consecutive cases. *Radiology* 179:463-468, 1991.

Mammographic Appearance of Recurrent Breast Carcinoma in Six Patients With TRAM Flap Breast Reconstructions

Helvie MA, Wilson TE, Roubidoux MA, et al (Univ of Michigan, Ann Arbor)

Radiology 209:711-715, 1998 2–7

Background.—Transverse rectus abdominis musculocutaneous (TRAM) flap reconstruction of the breast after mastectomy is becoming popular for patients with breast cancer. The mammographic appearance of locally recurrent carcinoma in mastectomy patients with TRAM flap reconstructions is described.

Methods.—The patients were 6 women who had been treated for breast carcinoma with mastectomy and TRAM flap reconstruction. The median time from diagnosis of breast cancer to recurrence was 42 months; the mean age at recurrence was 48. The 8 carcinomas were palpable in 5 of the patients, and carcinoma was identified by screening mammography in the sixth patient. Patients' records and mammograms were reviewed to characterize the recurrences.

Findings.—Mammography identified all 8 recurrences, which consisted of 4 masses, 2 pleomorphic microcalcifications, and 2 masses with calcifications (Fig 2). Half the recurrences were in the upper central portion of the breast. Before TRAM flap reconstruction, all 6 patients had a diagnosis of multifocal ductal carcinoma in situ (DCIS). All 8 of the recurrences were invasive ductal carcinoma, and 2 patients had positive axillary lymph nodes.

Conclusions.—The mammographic appearance of the recurrences in these patients was similar to that of primary breast cancer. Given that all the patients originally had multifocal DCIS, these patients may be at greater risk of local recurrence after TRAM flap reconstruction.

► The TRAM flap reconstruction technique after mastectomy was originally described by Hartrampf et al.[1] in 1982 and its acceptance in the United

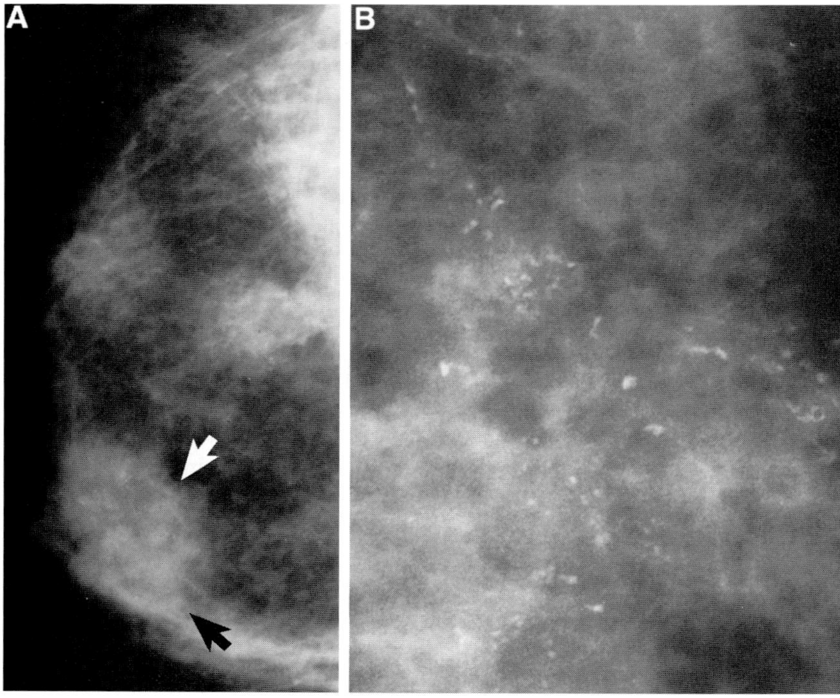

FIGURE 2.—A, Mediolateral oblique mammogram of a 50-year-old woman demonstrates a 4 × 3-cm area of pleomorphic calcifications with associated soft-tissue density (*arrows*) in the lower central portion of TRAM flap reconstructed breast. B, Magnification mammogram shows the ductlike distribution of calcifications. Histologic examination revealed invasive adenocarcinoma with mucinous features and ductal carcinoma in situ. (Courtesy of Helvie MA, Wilson TE, Roubidoux MA, et al. Mammographic appearance of recurrent breast carcinoma in six patients with TRAM flap breast reconstructions. *Radiology* 209:711-715, 1998. Radiological Society of North America.)

States is increasing, in part because of the issue of the safety of silicone breast implants for reconstruction. There are no imaging guidelines for the surveillance of the TRAM flap–reconstructed breasts. Local breast cancer recurrence has been reported to be uncommon and may be adequately assessed by means of physical examination. This retrospective review was of women treated with mastectomy and TRAM flap reconstruction in whom local recurrences developed from 1995 to 1997. All 8 cancers identified (in 6 patients) were in women whose initial diagnosis was extensive or multifocal DCIS (noninvasive tumors). All 8 local recurrences were invasive, and 2 of them were associated with positive axillary nodes. In only 1 of these patients was the diagnosis made on a screening mammogram performed at an institution other than the one reporting these findings. In cases in which mastectomy and reconstruction are performed for invasive cancers, any recurrent lesions are treated as a manifestation of systemic disease.[2,3] Therefore, the standard of examination for recurrences focused on clinical rather than image-based detection appears appropriate. However, for this subpopulation of women whose initial disease was DCIS, treatment of the invasive recurrence may positively affect survival and may be improved only with more aggressive imaging surveillance. Perhaps a standard recommendation outlining guidelines for the reconstructed breast should be issued. Note is made by the authors that technical imaging of the TRAM flap was not difficult, despite the mean breast thickness of 6 to 7 cm (normally 4 to 5 cm) because of the fatty nature of the autologous tissue itself.

R.L. Birdwell, M.D.

References

1. Hartrampf CR, Scheflan M, Black PW: Breast reconstruction with the transverse abdominal island flap. *Plast Reconstr Surg* 69:216-224, 1982.
2. Gilliland MD, Barton RM, Copeland EM III: The implications of local recurrence of breast cancer as the first site of therapeutic failure. *Ann Surg* 197:284-287, 1983.
3. Harris JR, Lippman ME, Veronesi U, et al: Breast cancer. *N Engl J Med* 327:390-398, 1992.

Coaxial Core Needle Biopsy Under Mammographic Guidance: Indications and Applications

Whitman GJ, Kopans DB, McCarthy KA, et al (Univ of Texas, Houston; Harvard Med School, Boston; Albany Med School, NY)

AJR 171:67-70, 1998 2–8

Background.—A method of mammographically guided coaxial core needle biopsy that allows removal of multiple biopsy specimens from large areas of calcification is described.

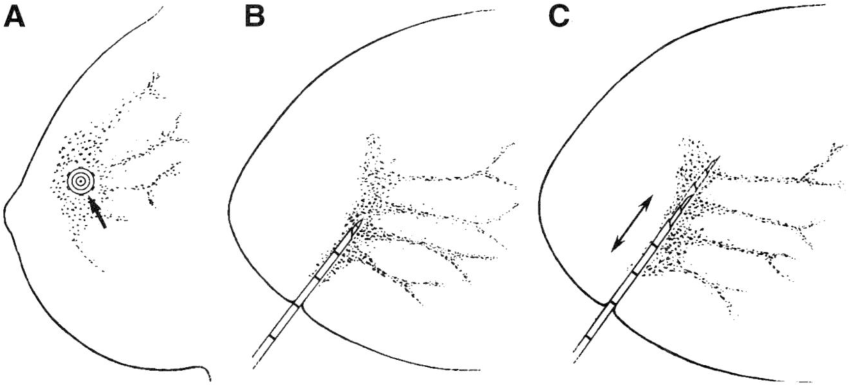

FIGURE 1.—Line drawings illustrate mammographically guided coaxial core needle biopsy technique. **A**, With mediolateral approach, introducing needle (*arrow*) is inserted to pass through targeted lesion. **B**, While breast is compressed in craniocaudal projection, needle tip is placed in targeted tissue. **C**, With tip of introducing cannula in targeted lesion, biopsy needle can be introduced repeatedly (*arrow*), allowing multiple samples to be obtained. (Courtesy of Whitman GJ, Kopans DB, McCarthy KA, et al. Coaxial core needle biopsy under mammographic guidance: Indications and applications. *AJR* 171:67-70, 1998.)

Methods.—Twelve procedures were performed in 11 women (mean age, 55). The targeted area was positioned in a fenestrated alphanumeric compression device to allow a mediolateral or lateromedial position. A 15-gauge introducing cannula was inserted through the targeted lesion (Fig 1). The breast was then repositioned and recompressed in a craniocaudal projection, and the 16-gauge biopsy needle was placed in the targeted tissue. With the needle, it was possible to retrieve multiple samples (mean, 13.7 per patient) without repositioning of the patient or the cannula.

Findings.—The indications for biopsy were large microcalcifications in 11 cases and a 4-cm poorly defined mass in 1 case. In 3 procedures needle biopsy found ductal carcinoma in situ (DCIS), but surgical biopsy revealed invasive ductal carcinoma in addition to DCIS.

Conclusions.—The technique described is effective for sampling diffuse or segmental calcifications that would be difficult to target under stereotactic guidance. Furthermore, patients need not be prone, which allows the evaluation of lesions that could not be identified stereotactically (ie, periareolar calcifications).

► This technical innovation demonstrates the use of a coaxial approach involving a 15-gauge outer cannula and a 16-gauge core biopsy instrument to sample mammographically detected lesions by means of the alphanumeric compression device and a standard mammographic machine. The authors suggest this method for cases in which there are very large regions of calcifications where the placement of this coaxial system may be easily altered and cover a larger region or for those lesions for which the prone table does not appear appropriate. I agree with the authors that the use of a 16-gauge core biopsy instrument is not appropriate for accuracy of lesion diagnosis and that if this alternative procedure is used, the coaxial core needle biopsies should be performed with 14- or 11-gauge biopsy needles.[1]

R.L. Birdwell, M.D.

Reference

1. Nath ME, Robinson TM, Tobon H, et al: Automated large-core needle biopsy of surgically removed breast lesions: Comparison of samples obtained with 14-, 16-, and 18-gauge needles. *Radiology* 197:739-742, 1995.

Mammographic Technologist Job Satisfaction: What Radiologists Need to Know—Results of a Large National Survey

Collins J, Prue LK, Leahy-Gross KM, et al (Univ of Wisconsin, Madison)

Radiology 207:473-480, 1998 2–9

Background.—How satisfied are mammographic technologists with their jobs? And what factors correlate with job satisfaction? A national survey was performed to measure job satisfaction.

Methods.—The authors created a 29-item survey that addressed the work environment, benefits (including salary), experience, education, and overall job satisfaction. The survey was mailed to 5,000 mammographic technologists, 1,503 of whom (30%) responded. The authors compared these results with a similar 1987 survey of general radiologic technologists.

Findings.—In total, 1,249 respondents (83.1%) indicated that they were at least partly satisfied with their jobs (mean rating 3.4 on a 5-point scale, with 5 signifying very satisfied). This percentage is similar to the 1987 survey of general radiologic technologists, 86% of whom reported being satisfied with their jobs. Overall job satisfaction was significantly correlated with gaining enjoyment from working with other technologists (93%) and radiologists (85.3%). Other factors significantly related to increased job satisfaction included a higher rate of pay, more vacation days, and reimbursement for the costs of continuing medical education.

Conclusions.—Overall, mammographic technologists are satisfied with their jobs. Being aware of and working to improve the intrinsic (ie, working relationships) and extrinsic (ie, benefits) rewards identified can improve job satisfaction, which can affect job performance and perhaps improve patient care.

► According to Locke,[1] job satisfaction is defined as "the pleasurable emotional state resulting from the appraisal of one's job as achieving or facilitating the achievement of one's job values; job dissatisfaction is the unpleasurable emotional state resulting from the appraisal of one's job as frustrating or blocking the attainment of one's job values or as entailing disvalues." Specifically in the area of breast imaging, additional requirements for the technologist have escalated and may, in fact, be burdensome to those technologists practicing in groups where there is no reimbursement for the required continuing medical education costs. A total of 1,500 technologists across the United States responded to 29 questions. Some of the findings reported from this survey that are of particular potential benefit to the radiologist or administrators who employ technologists are those alerting awareness to intrinsic and extrinsic rewards. Of the intrinsic rewards, the single most statistically significant positive statement linked to job satisfaction involved a good working relationship with the radiologist. Equally important were the extrinsic rewards important to job satisfaction, which included rate of pay, vacation days, and reimbursement for the required continuing education costs. Dissatisfaction included the time required for quality assurance and paperwork. From a recent companion survey sent by our institution to the Society of Breast Imagers, we found that in 1996 17% of the tracking of abnormal mammograms was done by technologists alone, whereas in 1999 only 8% of practices reported tracking handled by technologists alone.[2] Some of this shift in responsibility has gone to other members of the breast-imaging department, and some practices report the use of full-time quality assurance personnel. This is costly to the institutions but may improve the job satisfaction of the technologist, who continues to be our single most important ambassador between the patient and the radiologist.

R.L. Birdwell, M.D.

References

1. Locke EA: What is job satisfaction? *Organizational Behav Hum Performance* 4:309-336, 1969.
2. Birdwell RL, Ikeda, DM, Brenner RJ: Methods of compliance with Mammography Quality Standards Act regulation for tracking positive mammograms: Results of a survey of the Society of Breast Imaging Fellows. *AJR* 172:691-696, 1999.

Automated Detection of Breast Carcinomas Not Detected in a Screening Program

te Brake GM, Karssemeijer N, Hendriks JHCL (Radboud Univ Hosp, Nijmegen, The Netherlands)
Radiology 207:465-471, 1998 2–10

Background.—Computer-aided diagnostic systems have the potential to increase the ability of mammographers to detect breast cancers. Several groups are attempting to design pattern-recognition techniques for the detection of mammographic abnormalities. One automated system was evaluated for its ability to detect early signs of cancer that were missed in a breast cancer screening program.

Methods.—The automated system was based on a neural network programmed to recognize the presence of spicules or masses in mammograms. The system was applied to a set of 75 mammograms from 65 women with subtle circumscribed masses, stellate lesions, and architectural distortions. All these mammographic abnormalities were missed by 2 radiologists in a breast cancer screening program. The analysis also included contralateral mammograms from the same patients, which yielded a total of 142 normal mammograms.

Results.—The automated system detected an early sign of cancer in 34% of the cases and had a specificity of 1 false-positive finding per image. When the system was set to a specificity of 3 false-positive findings per image, it detected 60% of the cancers. One half of the cases classified as screening errors were detected at a specificity of less than 0.5 false-positive findings per image. A detection scheme based on both mass and spicule detection showed similar performance in interval and screening-detected carcinomas. This detection scheme was superior to schemes based on detection of spicules only or of masses only for the combined group of interval and screening-detected carcinomas and for the group consisting only of screening-detected carcinomas. Tumors classified as screening errors were detected with a greater specificity than those classified as minimal signs.

Conclusions.—An automated detection system can detect many breast cancers that were missed in a screening mammography program and has specificity levels of less than 1 false-positive finding per image. The specificity level required for effective computer-aided detection is unclear. However, the capability of an automated detection system to signal early malignant signs to the radiologist could lead to the detection of many missed cancers. Further studies of this hypothesis are needed.

► Computer-aided detection (CAD) is not a tool for interpretation but shows promise for alerting the breast imager to look again at areas on the mammogram that may be "hiding" abnormalities. The system designs are based on pattern-recognition algorithms that are "taught" to the computer and encompass normal and abnormal findings, including characteristics for masses and calcifications.[1] The system marks the patterns recognized as abnormal on the mammogram image that is projected on a screen on a specialized mammography viewbox. The sensitivity threshold of the CAD system can be altered because, although the system must be sensitive for cancer detection, we must continue to limit the number of false positives generated by screening mammography. Counting the number of areas of a test set of mammograms assessed as stable (or "normal") over more than a 12-month period by a dedicated mammographer that result in a positive "hit" from the CAD system has determined specificity of the systems in test situations.

This study evaluated mammograms with later proven cancers that were not detected in a screening program by 2 radiologists and reported that 34% of 65 cases resulted in a positive "hit" by the CAD system with a specificity of 1 false positive "hit" per image. When the threshold was decreased to 3 false positive "hits" per image, 60% of the missed cancers were detected. This exciting technology of CAD is being actively investigated, and 1 commercial company now has FDA approval. No company is claiming that these products should take the place of the radiologist (thank goodness!), but they may be beneficial, particularly in the dense breast, by alerting the radiologist to an area that she or he may want to review. It will be exciting to see this technology mature and to determine, if possible, what types of detection errors versus possible errors of interpretation are found in these retrospectively "missed" cancers.[2] Of particular interest to me are those cases in which, even in retrospect, expert imagers cannot detect a lesion that would have resulted in a recommendation for biopsy. Can we learn new cancer mammographic patterns that would allow us to detect cancer even earlier than we can now from the very computers we "taught"?!

R.L. Birdwell, M.D.

References

1. Patrick N, Chan HP, Shiner B, et al: Computer-aided breast mass detection: False positive reduction using breast tissue composition, in Do K, Giggler ML, Nishikawa RM, Schmidt RA (eds): *Digital Mammography 1996* (International Congress Series 1119). Amsterdam, Elsevier Science, 1996, pp 373-378.
2. Bird RE, Wallace TW, Yankaskas BC: Analysis of cancers missed at screening mammography. *Radiology* 184:613-617, 1992.

Tc-99m Tetrofosmin Scintigraphy as an Adjunct to Plain-Film Mammography in Palpable Breast Lesions

Fenlon HM, Phelan N, Tierney S, et al (Univ College Dublin)
Clin Radiol 53:17-24, 1998 2–11

Background.—According to recent reports, scintimammography can differentiate benign from malignant breast lesions with a sensitivity and specificity similar to that of contrast-enhanced MRI. Tc-99m tetrofosmin was used as the imaging agent in women with palpable breast masses and compared the results with those of plain-film mammographic and pathologic examination.

Methods.—The subjects were 44 women (mean age 51) each of whom had a palpable breast mass that required fine needle aspiration biopsy (FNAB). All patients underwent Tc-99m tetrofosmin scintimammography, and the 38 patients who were more than 35 years old also underwent 2-view mammography on the same day. Then, within 7 days, patients underwent FNAB, and appropriate candidates were referred for surgery.

Findings.—FNAB identified malignant disease in 21 patients (47.7%). At surgery, these patients were found to have invasive ductal carcinoma (n = 20) or mucinous carcinoma (n = 1). In all but 1 of the patients with carcinoma (95.2%), Tc-99m tetrofosmin scintimammography also had positive results. The 1 false negative result occurred in a patient who could not be optimally positioned because of severe rheumatoid arthritis. In comparison, 21 of the 38 patients who underwent 2-view mammography had FNAB-proved carcinoma, but images revealed carcinoma in only 17 (81%) of these 21 patients. The 4 false negative plain-film mammographic findings occurred in 2 women with dense breasts (Fig 3) and 2 women with prior breast surgery. FNAB results were benign in 23 patients (52.3%). All but 2 of the patients with benign lesions (91.3%) also had negative results on Tc-99m tetrofosmin scintimammography. The 2 false positive results occurred in a patient with proliferative dysplasia and in a patient with hypervascular fibroadenoma. In comparison, 17 of the 38 patients who underwent 2-view mammography had FNAB-proved benign disease, but images appeared benign in only 14 (82.4%) of these 17 patients. The 3 false positive plain-film mammographic findings occurred in 2 patients with a postoperative fibrofatty change and in 1 patient with a radial scar in a dense breast. In addition, in 7 cases dense breast parenchyma or previous surgery or radiotherapy obscured the results of mammography. In all 7 cases, however, the lesions were correctly identified by Tc-99m tetrofosmin scintimammography. The sensitivity, specificity, positive predictive value, and negative predictive value of scintimammography were 95.2%, 91.3%, 90.9%, and 95.5%, respectively. Comparable values for plain-film mammography were 81%, 82.4%, 85%, and 77.8%.

Conclusions.—Tc-99m tetrofosmin scintimammography was more accurate than plain-film mammography in differentiating benign from malignant tumors in patients with palpable breast lesions. It is particularly useful for patients with dense breasts, for patients who have previously

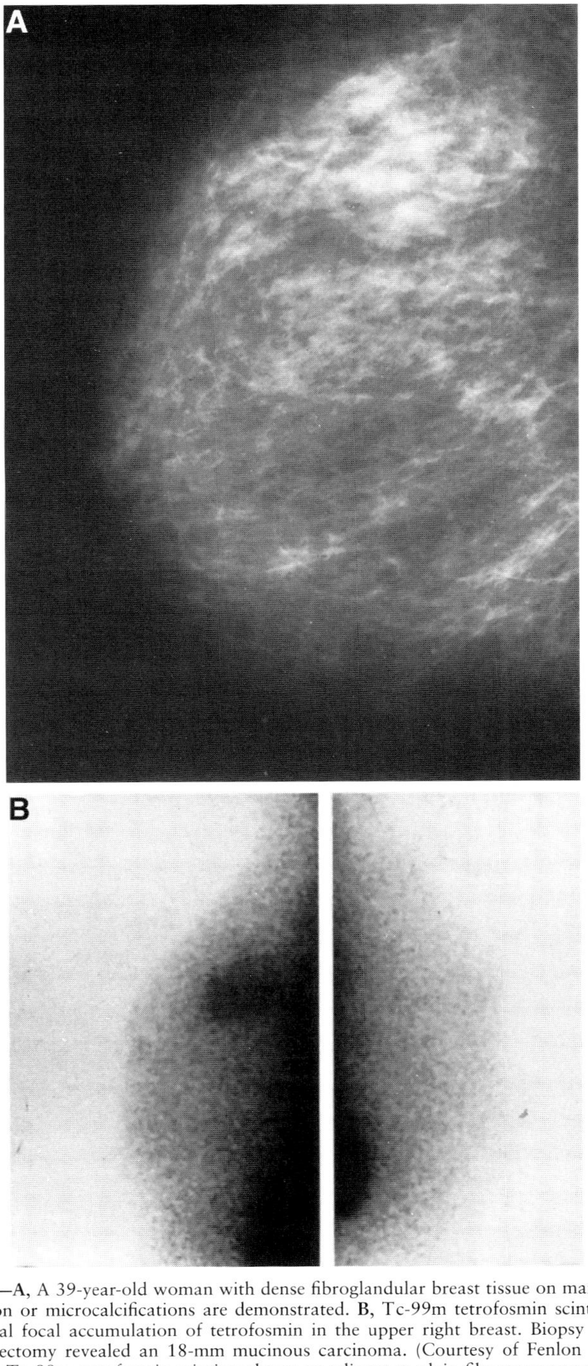

FIGURE 3.—**A**, A 39-year-old woman with dense fibroglandular breast tissue on mammography. No focal mass lesion or microcalcifications are demonstrated. **B**, Tc-99m tetrofosmin scintimammography reveals abnormal focal accumulation of tetrofosmin in the upper right breast. Biopsy and subsequent segmental mastectomy revealed an 18-mm mucinous carcinoma. (Courtesy of Fenlon HM, Phelan N, Tierney S, et al: Tc-99m tetrofosmin scintigraphy as an adjunct to plain-film mammography in palpable breast lesions. *Clin Radiol* 53: 17-24, 1998.)

undergone surgery or radiotherapy, and for patients in whom plain film mammographic results are indeterminate.

► Although mammography is clearly the imaging modality for screening of the breast in age-appropriate women, experts continue to investigate possible roles of alternative imaging, either for different types of breast lesion or for specific subpopulations of women. In particular, young women, women with very large breasts and difficult physical examination, and women with very dense breasts are thought by some investigators to qualify for consideration of scintimammography. Scintimammography may be "an accurate, noninvasive alternative for differentiating benign from malignant breast lesions with quoted sensitivity and specificity similar to contrast enhanced MR mammography," but these authors from Ireland compare their results between plain film mammography and scintimammography.[1-3] They looked at 21 patients with palpable masses that were later proved malignant and 17 patients with benign palpable masses. On mammography, the malignant lesions were seen in only 81%, whereas 95 % of those 21 patients had positive scintimammograms. In the 17 patients with benign lesions, 82% had benign appearances on plain-film mammography, but the other 18% had suspicious mammographic findings. Negative scintigraphy was found in 91% of these 17 patients. The authors reported a positive predictive value of 90% and a negative predictive value of 95%, encouraging numbers for those who use scintimammography. This article, however, does not present a comparison with contrast-enhanced MR; nor was the less expensive modality of ultrasonography. Clearly, if one is using x-ray mammography as the "gold standard," we are well aware that at least 11% of the time a palpable malignant lesion may be present in the face of a negative mammogram. Supplementary techniques are necessary for further evaluation of patients with palpable masses, and US has been used routinely in many practices in the United States. For those who choose or have easy access to scintimammography, it appears that it too may play a role as a supplementary technique.

R.L. Birdwell, M.D.

References

1. Lee VW, Sax EJ, McAneny DB, et al: A complementary role for thallium-201 scintigraphy with mammography in the diagnosis of breast cancer. *J Nucl Med* 34:2095-2100, 1993.
2. Campeau RJ, Kronemer KA, Southerland CM: Concordant uptake of Tc-99m Sestamibi and Tl-201 in unsuspected breast tumour. *Clin Nucl Med* 17: 936-937, 1992.
3. Khalkali I, Mena I, Jouanne E, et al: Prone scintimammography in patients with suspicion of carcinoma of the breast. *J Am Coll Surg* 178:491-497, 1994.

Sonography of the Breast: Controversies and Opinions
Hall FM (Harvard Med School, Boston)
AJR 169:1635-1636, 1997 2–12

Background.—The use of breast US has increased dramatically in the past few years. Some of the issues that exist with respect to breast sonography are discussed.

Indications for Breast Sonography.—Initially, breast US was used to determine whether a palpable mass was cystic or solid. Current indications call for its use also in evaluating nonpalpable masses identified by mammography. Core biopsies are easy to perform under US guidance; however, this ease has resulted in too many biopsies of non-palpable breast nodules in BI-RADS category 3, which previously would have been followed "at short intervals with" mammography for 6 months. A great controversy exists as to whether breast US should be used to differentiate benign and malignant solid breast masses. This author leans toward including US when mammography reveals solid breast masses that are probably benign and basing therapy (follow-up or biopsy) on the US indications. Breast sonography is particularly useful in confirming that no mass exists when results of physical examination are equivocal. Also, sonography should be confined to the area of palpatory or mammographic concern; to image the entire breast is to perform screening, which is a low-yield examination.

Utilization Patterns.—Initially, breast US was ordered mainly by breast surgeons. Currently, primary care physicians or even patients themselves are the ones requesting the service. This leads to the situation in which the breast imager may be the first physician to examine patients and discuss the procedure. In addition, many technologists accredited in general sonography lack training and education in mammography, and the current certification requirements in mammography do not include breast sonography.

► I included this *Opinion* primarily because of the excellent points raised by Dr. Hall. Issues including the rapid increase in use of breast US, the appropriate indications for sonography, and the fact that more and more of the examinations may be being performed by individuals not specifically educated in the area of breast US need our attention. In addition to those excellent points made by Dr. Hall, I am particularly concerned about the role played by those technologists who are accredited in the field of mammography but working in breast imaging departments with breast US. How are these women educated? What agency accredits them? If a technologist is trained as a general sonographer, there is some training in breast US. However, many breast US machines are within the breast-imaging department where the mammographically accredited technologists are not required to have any training in breast US. The American College of Radiology is looking into these questions, and we should have some direction in the very near future.

Personal communication with Dr. Dianne Georgian-Smith at the University of Washington led to an additional point that should be of interest to breast imagers. It is important that we recognize the need for a project demonstrating the benefits and capabilities of breast sonography. This study could be similar to the establishment of the Breast Cancer Detection Demonstration Project (BCDDP) by the American Cancer Society, cosponsored by the National Cancer Institute, in the 1970s.[1] Should such a project be started for breast sonography? Would such a project possibly result in increased governmental control of breast US as we have seen in mammography?

R.L. Birdwell, M.D.

Reference

1. Beahrs OH, Shapiro S, Smart C, et al: Report of the working group to review the National Cancer Institute–American Cancer Society Breast Cancer Detection Demonstration Project. *J Natl Cancer Inst* 62:639-698, 1979.

Effects of a Microbubble Contrast Agent on Breast Tumors: Computer-assisted Quantitative Assessment With Color Doppler US—Early Experience

Huber S, Helbich T, Kettenbach H, et al (Lainz Hosp, Vienna; Univ Hosp, Vienna; German Cancer Research Ctr, Heidelberg, Germany)

Radiology 208:485-489, 1998 2–13

Introduction.—The characteristic features of neovascularity in malignant lesions can be demonstrated by color Doppler US. The detection of low-volume blood flow can be improved by intravascular contrast agents by increasing the signal-to-noise ratio. A new agent is a galactose-based US contrast agent, which contains microbubbles that are maintained during passage through the pulmonary vascular system. Image-based, computer-assisted analysis was used to quantify contrast agent enhancement. This method allowed quantification of color pixel density in a selected region of interest and recalculation of theoretic local flow velocities. The study sought to determine whether contrast agent-enhanced images are diagnostically more valuable than unenhanced images and whether the enhancement kinetics carry additional information.

Methods.—Before and after intravenous injection of a microbubble contrast agent, 47 patients, aged 23 to 61, underwent color Doppler US. To objectively evaluate the increase in the number of color Doppler US signals, the potential additional differential diagnostic information, and the transit time of the microbubble bolus, a 3-minute computer-assisted assessment of the color pixel density was used.

Results.—For carcinomas, the peak color pixel density at contrast agent–enhanced color Doppler US was 14.3% ± 8.1. For benign lesions, the peak color pixel density was 9.3 ± 4.9. Carcinomas had a shorter time to peak enhancement (39 seconds ± 20) when compared with benign tumors, which had a time of 71 seconds ± 48. The final color pixel density was equal or close to the baseline values. The accuracy of color Doppler US was 62%, the specificity was 79%, and the sensitivity was 55%, when the median for peak color pixel density as a threshold was 13%. The sensitivity rose to 84%, the specificity dropped to 57%, and the accuracy rose to 76% when the median time to peak was 50 seconds.

Conclusion.—Carcinomas and benign lesions behave differently in degree, onset, and duration of Doppler US enhancement after injection of a microbubble contrast agent. The value of these criteria is still limited for prospective diagnosis by high interindividual variability and temporal variations in the Doppler US signal.

► These authors are investigating frequency shift Doppler US before and after intravenous injection of a positive contrast agent. The microbubbles in this intravenously injected contrast agent may improve the detection of low-volume blood flow, which may be found in malignant tumors by increasing the signal-to-noise ratio. These authors used image-based computer-assisted analysis and, with that method, looked at the "color pixel density" (CPD) in a selected region of interest in both benign and malignant breast lesions. They report a difference in the peak CPD from baseline level to maximum between carcinomas and benign lesions. They also found that this peak was achieved more rapidly in carcinomas than in benign lesions. These findings may be physiologically similar to the dynamic scanning used to evaluate the wash in and ultimate wash out of gadolinium in enhanced MRI scanning for breast cancer and may relate to the neovascularity that is more common in malignant than in benign lesions.[1,2]

Efforts to improve the ability to differentiate benign and malignant breast lesions with US suffer in both techniques and interpretations.[3-6] Although this study is no exception, it is encouraging and provides anticipation of further work differentiating between malignant and benign lesions with the use of a microbubble contrast agent.

R.L. Birdwell, M.D.

References

1. Daniel BL, Yen Y-F, Glover GH, et al: Breast disease: Dynamic spiral MR imaging. *Radiology* 209:499-509, 1998.
2. Liu P-F, Debatin JF, Caduff RF, et al: Improved diagnostic accuracy in dynamic contrast enhanced MRI of the breast by combined quantitative and qualitative analysis. *Br J Radiol* 71:501-509, 1998.
3. Carson PL, Adler DD, Fowlkes JB, et al: Enhanced color flow imaging of breast cancer vasculature: Continuous wave Doppler and three-dimensional display. *J Ultrasound Med* 11:377-385, 1992.
4. Cosgrove DO, Kedar RP, Bamber JC, et al: Breast disease: Color Doppler US in differential diagnosis. *Radiology* 189:99-104, 1993.
5. Lee S-K, Lee T, Lee K-R, et al: Evaluation of breast tumors with color Doppler imaging: A comparison with image-directed Doppler ultrasound. *J Clin Ultrasound* 23:367-373, 1995.
6. Birdwell RL, Ikeda DM, Jeffrey SS, et al: Preliminary experience with power Doppler imaging of solid breast masses. *AJR* 169:703-707, 1997.

Occult Cancer in Women With Dense Breasts: Detection With Screening US—Diagnostic Yield and Tumor Characteristics

Kolb TM, Lichy J, Newhouse JH (New York; Columbia Univ, New York)
Radiology 207:191-199, 1998 2–14

Background.—The sensitivity of mammography is reduced in women with predominantly fibroglandular breasts or areas of dense breast tissue. Previous studies have not shown US to be an effective method of breast cancer screening; it is generally accepted that the main role of US in breast cancer is the evaluation of palpable or mammographically identified breast masses. Current US technology, however, provides increased spatial and contrast resolution. The use of bilateral screening US was evaluated for the detection of occult breast masses and cancer in women with dense breasts in whom mammographic and physical examination findings were normal.

Methods.—The prospective study included 11,220 consecutive women (mean age, 59 years) undergoing mammography and physical examinations. From this group, 3,626 women with dense breasts and normal mammographic and physical examination findings were identified. These patients underwent screening US performed by a physician who used a broad-band transducer centered at 7.5 MHz. The results were analyzed to

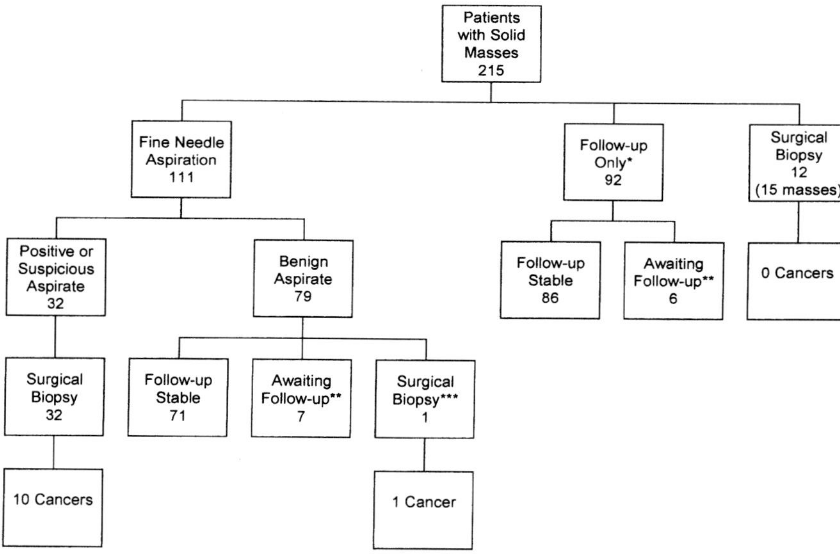

FIGURE 2.—Diagnostic pathway for solid masses detected with US alone. Biopsy or follow-up may have been performed in multiple masses in a single patient. *Follow-up consisted of at least 1 additional US examination performed 4 to 6 months after the initial examination. †For the purposes of this study, all patients who were awaiting follow-up were considered to have benign masses. ‡One patient with a normal fine-needle aspiration result was recommended for surgical biopsy because of a discordant appearance on US scans. She was found to have an invasive lobular cancer. (Courtesy of Kolb TM, Lichy J, Newhouse JH: Occult cancer in women with dense breasts: Detection with screening US—Diagnostic yield and tumor characteristics. *Radiology* 207:191-199, 1998. Radiological Society of North America.)

determine the frequency of breast cancer and other masses detected by US only and to compare the characteristics of those cancers with cancers detected by mammography or physical examination.

Results.—Thirty-nine percent of the women had a level of breast density that could obscure a breast cancer; this figure was even higher in premenopausal women and in those receiving hormone replacement therapy. Eleven cancers in 11 women were identified by US alone, which yielded a prevalence of 0.3% (Fig 2). As breast density increased, so did the number of cancers detected by US only, but this trend was not statistically significant. The US-detected cancers were similar in mean surgical size and stage to nonpalpable cancers detected by mammography. They were smaller and lower in stage than the palpable cancers detected in the remainder of the population. For women with dense breast tissue, the use of US increased the overall cancer detection rate by 17% and increased the number of tumors detected with imaging studies alone by 37%.

Conclusions.—Screening US can identify otherwise occult cancers in women with dense breasts. The US-detected cancers are similar in size and stage to mammographically detected, nonpalpable cancers. Further evaluation of screening US is needed in larger groups of women. However, the additional costs and false positive rate of this study must be evaluated before screening US comes into widespread use.

► In the late 1970s and early 1980s, there was a ripple of excitement through the world of breast imaging that whole-breast water bath US machines could replace mammography for the screening of symptom-free women. Apparently many practices invested in these machines, and certainly one would imagine that women were quite pleased to have the opportunity to lie prone in a comfortable position without compression and without the fear of irradiation and to have a resulting report that attested that all was well in the breast! The work of Kopans and Sickles[1,2] in the early 1980s showed that this tool was not technologically capable of finding small cancers and, in particular, that microcalcifications were not consistently detected. The concept of US screening for breast cancer, therefore, was laid to rest with a lot of disappointment. Now we are beginning to see a resurrection of the concept of screening sonography in the symptom-free patient as presented in this article by Kolb and his group in New York. The key factors here are a physician-driven examination with a hand-held transducer, marked improvement in sonographic technology, and time. The study was well organized with a differentiation of breast density as determined mammographically with the Breast Imaging Reporting and Data System scale resulting in the assignment of women into 3 groups, groups 1 and 2 being the most specific for comparison. Women in group 1 had breasts that were described as either heterogeneously dense or dense with negative physical examination findings whereas group 2 had the same description of breast density but a palpable or mammographically identified mass. The truly "screened" group (group 1) numbered 3,626 and constituted 32% of all women examined in this study. Specific attention is given to the solid masses, with 279 solid masses reported in 215 women in group 1. The mean image size was 9.1 mm (range, 3-30 mm). One hundred thirty-seven of these solid masses were subjected to either biopsy with fine-needle aspiration, surgical biopsy, or both in the patients screened.

Among the 3,626 women screened, there were 11 surgically proven cancers in 11 women. Note is made that these cancers were smaller and of a lower stage than the 64 palpable cancers that were diagnosed in the other groups. What about the time these examinations took? The authors reported on 100 consecutive bilateral screening US examinations from the application of gel to the end of the examination and described the mean time for completion as about 4 minutes! This article raises concerns about the availability of US in the breast imaging department, the expertise of those performing the examination, and the equipment used. Many in this country continue to practice without immediate availability of US to complete the diagnostic work-up. Do we need to require US machines in breast imaging departments if, indeed, those practices are indicated as diagnostic "full-service" departments? What about technologists? Within general sonography there are accreditation programs, and in breast imaging mammography technologists are accredited, but there is no specific breast US accreditation (or educational programs) for mammography-qualified technologists. Who should be in charge of accreditation, and, how much additional time can be expected from the physician's schedule for direct focused hand-held physician-guided US? These are difficult questions, provoking many different responses that we can look forward to reading in the future.

R.L. Birdwell, M.D.

References

1. Kopans DB, Myer GE, Lindfors KK: Whole breast ultra sound imaging: four years follow-up. *Radiology* 157:505-507, 1985.
2. Sickles EA, Philly RA, Callen PW: Breast cancer detection with sonography and mammography: comparison using state of the art equipment. *AJR* 140:843-845, 1983.

Improved Diagnostic Accuracy in Dynamic Contrast Enhanced MRI of the Breast by Combined Quantitative and Qualitative Analysis

Liu P-F, Debatin JF, Caduff RF, et al (Zurich Univ, Switzerland)
Br J Radiol 71:501-509, 1998 2–15

Introduction.—The diagnostic performance of conventional mammography is still limited, particularly in the assessment of dense parenchyma, breast implants, or postoperative scarring. The detection of breast malignancy is improved with dynamic 3-dimensional gradient echo MRI. However, the diagnostic criteria remain poorly defined. The diagnostic performances of various quantitative and qualitative MRI criteria used to characterize breast lesions were ascertained by retrospectively reviewing 120 histopathologically verified breast lesions. An optimized, integrated

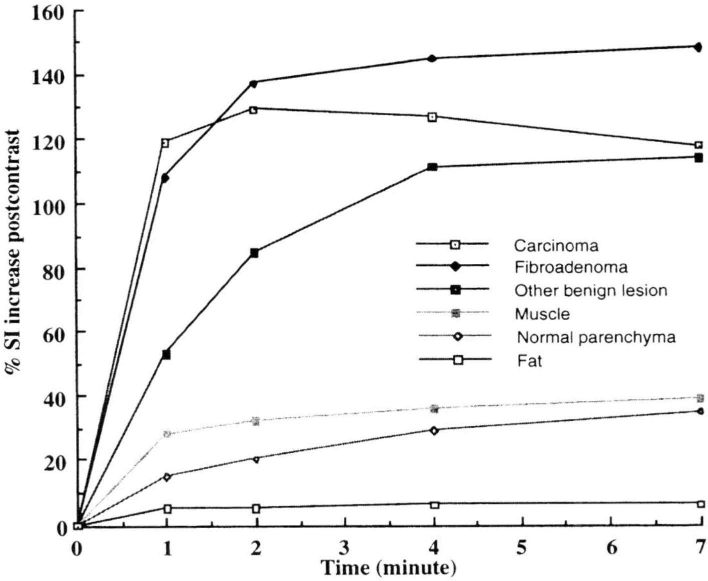

FIGURE 1.—Enhancement profiles for various lesions and normal tissues. (Courtesy of Liu P-F, Debatin JF, Caduff RF, et al: Improved diagnostic accuracy in dynamic contrast enhanced MRI of the breast by combined quantitative and qualitative analysis. *Br J Radiol* 71: 501-509, 1998.)

diagnostic MR-interpretation strategy was developed for detecting breast cancer.

Methods.—The features of 120 histopathologically verified lesions were retrospectively reviewed on contrast enhanced, dynamically acquired, "3-dimensional" gradient echo images. The review was conducted before and 1, 2, 4, and 7 minutes after injection of 0.2 mmol kg gadoterate-meglumine (Gd-DOTA). There were 70 malignant lesions and 50 benign lesions, and their quantitative criteria, based on relative signal intensity measurements and qualitative morphological features—including margins, lesion shape, and enhancement patterns—were analyzed.

Results.—Quantitative assessment of enhancement profiles was most accurate when analysis was based on early 1-minute measurements (Fig 1). The sensitivity in detecting breast cancer was 83% and the specificity was 66% when there was a 90% threshold. Sensitivity was 83% and specificity was 54% when assessment was based on qualitative morphological analysis alone. There was a sensitivity of 93%, a specificity of 74%, and an accuracy of 85% when the quantitative and qualitative assessments were combined. Lesions with early enhancement and 1 or more morphological signs of malignancy were considered malignant. Benign lesions were those without early enhancement and with no morphological signs of malignancy.

Conclusion.—Basing the interpretation on both quantitative and qualitative criteria can improve results from dynamic contrast enhanced breast MRI.

► These authors report on optimization of the dynamic contrast enhanced breast MRI based on a combination of both quantitative and qualitative criteria. There is tremendous ongoing evolution in the field of breast cancer detection involving MRI following the injection of gadolinium. Clearly, while sensitivity has been reported as very high, specificity remains a problem. Differences in opinion concerning, in particular, the use of dynamic contrast imaging to evaluate the rapidity of contrast uptake by lesions in the breast and to differentiate benign and malignant disease result in many different methodologies, reported in the literature.[1,2] Qualitative morphological evaluation is critical for any imaging modality, but many believe that the addition of dynamic imaging may further improve specificity. In 1998, the United States Public Health Services Office on Women's Health sponsored the International Working Group for Breast MRI held in March and September in Tyson's Corner, Virginia. This international gathering was divided into 5 groups focused on the following issues: lesion diagnosis, local breast cancer staging, high-risk screening, dedicated systems, and biopsy and interventional procedures. The goal of this gathering was to brainstorm and potentially avoid constant reinvention of the wheel from institution to institution. This was a well-organized effort on the part of all involved and well-coordinated by Dr. Steve Harms, the scientific director of the program. The simplest summary agreed upon by most of the participants is that MRI of the breast with gadolinium enhancement for the detection of breast cancer is truly in its infancy. A tremendous amount of work is necessary on many fronts. Work should focus on recognizing the patterns of abnormalities detected with this modality, identifying populations at highest risk for the disease who may benefit from this modality, communicating directly with vendors to coordinate the needs for specific machines and tools, and evaluating how best to adapt interventional procedures to the environment of the high field-strength magnets. In the next few years, we will see this area of breast imaging literally explode with projects furthering the refinement of the techniques, providing a lexicon for the improvement in communication of imaging findings, and—perhaps the singlemost important goal—improving specificity.

R.L. Birdwell, M.D.

References

1. Harms SE, Flamig DP, Evans WP, et al: MR imaging of the breast: Current status and future potential. *AJR* 163:1039-1047, 1994.
2. Daniel BL, Yen Y-F, Glover GH, et al: Breast disease: Dynamic spiral MR imaging. *Radiology* 209:499-509, 1998.

MR Imaging of Mammographically Detected Clustered Microcalcifications: Is There Any Value?

Westerhof JP, Fischer U, Moritz JD, et al (Georg-August-Universität, Göttingen, Germany)

Radiology 207:675-681, 1998 2–16

Introduction.—Benign calcifications cannot always be distinguished from malignant calcifications in mammography. Previous studies have shown a higher sensitivity for invasive cancers with contrast material-enhanced MR imaging of the breast. However, for ductal carcinomas in situ, the sensitivity and specificity have been lower. Sixty-three patients with isolated clustered microcalcifications detected at mammography were retrospectively reviewed.

Methods.—Dynamic MR imaging of the breast was performed on 63 women, aged 31 to 84 years, who had mammographically suspicious clustered microcalcification before surgical biopsy. A 1.5 T unit and a 2-dimensional fast low-angle shot sequence with a flip angle of 80 degrees were used to perform MR imaging. Before and 5 times after administration of gadopentetate dimeglumine, 32 axial sections, 4 mm thick and without interval gaps, were acquired. The standard of reference was the histologic findings.

Results.—Biopsy findings verified 33 patients with ductal carcinomas in situ, 13 patients with proliferative fibrocystic disease, 8 patients with nonproliferative fibrocystic disease, 5 patients with T1 invasive carcinomas, and 4 patients with sclerosing adenosis. A sensitivity of 45% and a specificity of 72% were found with contrast material-enhanced dynamic MR imaging. The overall accuracy was 56% in differentiating benign and malignant microcalcifications.

Conclusion.—In mammographically suspicious clustered microcalcifications, MR imaging of the breast is not reliable in differentiating benign and malignant breast disease, and the imaging has no effect on treatment.

► One issue related to contrast-enhanced MR imaging of the breast is the detection of ductal carcinoma in situ (DCIS), which often presents itself as microcalcifications on mammography.[1] These authors used a 1.5 T unit with 2-dimensional enhanced imaging to evaluate 63 patients with mammographically suspicious clusters of microcalcifications. The authors examined both breasts simultaneously and subtracted precontrast images from the corresponding postcontrast images. Some investigators believe that the subtraction technique is limited in lesion morphology evaluation, due to loss of fine detail on the subtracted images. The authors' overall accuracy, 56%, in differentiating benign from malignant microcalcifications isn't much better than is commonly achieved with mammographic assessment. These authors identified DCIS in 22 of their 33 patients (67%), compared to Orel et al., who identified approximately 72% of DCIS.[2] Contrast enhanced MRI for breast cancer clearly is evolving (as seen in other articles included in this volume of the YEAR BOOK but the difficulties in diagnosing DCIS may be one of our greatest challenges.

R.L. Birdwell, M.D.

References

1. Bassett LW: Mammographic analysis of calcifications. *Radiol Clin North Am* 30:93-105, 1992.
2. Orel SG, Mendonca MH, Reynolds C, et al: MR imaging of ductal carcinoma in situ. *Radiology* 202:413-420, 1997.

Breast Cancer: Gadolinium-enhanced MR Imaging With a 0.5-T Open Imager and Three-Point Dixon Technique

Daniel BL, Butts K, Glover GH, et al (Stanford Univ, Calif)

Radiology 207:183-190, 1998 2–17

Introduction.—Contrast material-enhanced MR imaging can detect breast cancer with exceptional sensitivity. However, the widespread application of diagnostic MR imaging of the breast has been slowed by the lack of easy, accurate MR-guided biopsy techniques. The role of MR imaging in the diagnosis and treatment of breast cancer might be greatly expanded by open-architecture MR imaging systems that allow improved access to the breast. An alternative method of obtaining water-specific T1-weighted images of the breast is the Dixon technique, which is based on the relative phase difference between fat and water. Whether 3-point Dixon imaging could provide fat-nulled images of contrast-enhanced breast cancer in a 0.5 T open MR system was determined.

Methods.—Ten women with 12 breasts that had lesions and 1 healthy volunteer participated in this imaging study. Real and imaginary source images were obtained with an interleaved gradient-echo sequence with a repetition time of 550 msec and echo times of 12.8, 19.8, and 26.8 msec. The sagittal plane with a 90-degree flip angle, 256 × 192 matrix, 3-4.5 mm section thickness, and acquisition time of 10 minutes 54 seconds were used to obtain 24 to 28 sections. To generate water-specific, fat-specific, and combined images from the raw image data, a 3-point Dixon reconstruction algorithm was used.

Results.—Nine of the 12 lesions had histopathologic proof available. When compared to extended 2-point Dixon and fat-suppressed images, 3-point Dixon images were superior. They were also superior to images generated by means of subtraction of 3-dimensional fast spoiled gradient-echo images obtained before contrast material injection. No phase-unwrapping errors occurred that caused incorrect decomposition of breast fat or glandular tissue. However, there were subtle phase-unwrapping errors that caused mismapping of small peripheral sections of the chest wall or skin. Because of a chemical shift of silicone resulting in an indeterminate accumulation of phase with the 71-Hz echo spacing required for

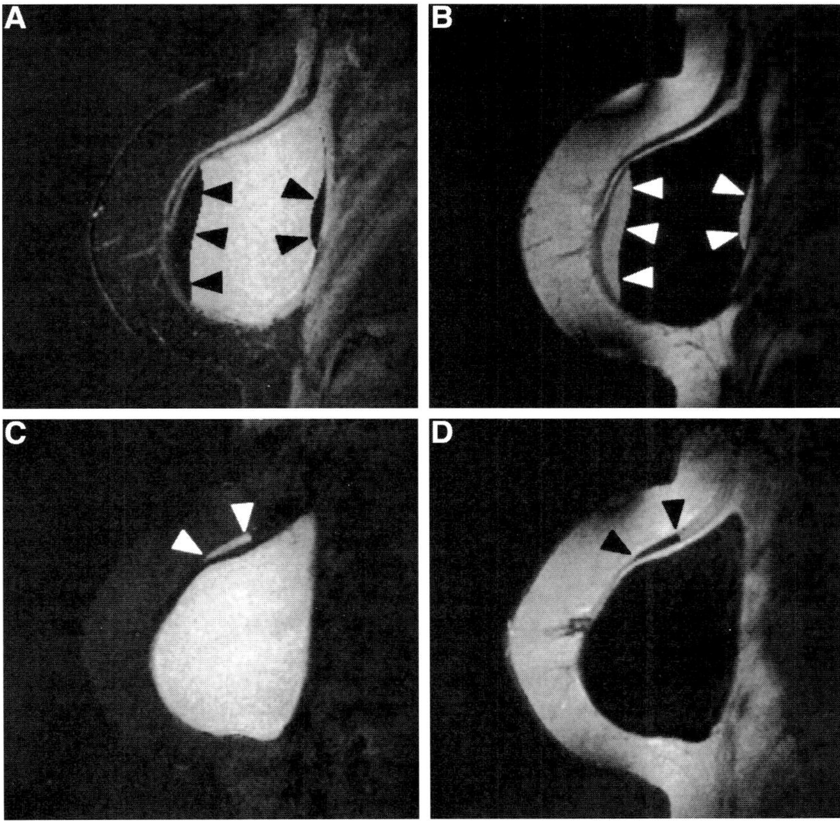

FIGURE 3.—Effect of echo spacing on 3-point Dixon images in a 47-year-old patient with a subpectoral silicone implant. **A**, Water-specific and **B**, Fat-specific 3-point Dixon images obtained with an echo spacing of 7.0 msec (2π = 71 Hz) show clear separation of fat and glandular (water) tissue. However, decomposition errors occurred in the silicone implant (*arrowheads*). **C**, Nonsilicone- and **D**, Silicone-specific 3-point Dixon images obtained with an echo spacing of 15.2 msec (**D**only) (2π = 33 Hz) clearly show silicone separate from nonsilicone tissues, except for a small decomposition error in the pectoral muscle (*arrowheads*). Imaging parameters. 0.5 T, repetition time msec = 550 or 800 (**D**only), 90 degrees flip angle, 256 × 192 matrix, 4-mm section thickness, 0.5-mm gaps between sections, and 20-cm field of view. (Courtesy of Daniel BL, Butts K, Glover GH, et al: Breast cancer: Gadolinium-enhanced MR imaging with a 0.5-T open imager and three-point Dixon technique. *Radiology* 207:183-190, 1998. Radiological Society of North America.)

the separation of fat and water, there were 11 mismapping errors in 1 woman who had a silicone implant (Fig 3).

Conclusion.—Three-point Dixon imaging provides a robust technique for creating fat-nulled images of enhancing breast lesions in the 0.5-T open MR environment. In regions of B_0 heterogeneity, water-specific 3-point Dixon images are successful and superior to fat-suppressed images. Water-specific 3-point Dixon images are also less susceptible to motion artifact than subtraction images are.

► The Interventional Group of the International Working Group on Breast MRI, which met in Virginia in 1998, focused on breast biopsy and intervention, with specific attention to lesion visualization, localization, and instrumentation. Specific to lesion visualization and localization is the magnet design. Dr. Daniel and his group at Stanford, working in the areas of both diagnostic and interventional MRI of the breast, have recognized major benefits in the open-architecture MR imaging system designed by GE. This is a "double doughnut" imager with a vertically open gap that allows access to the patient from both sides. One of the primary issues in moving to this magnet from the 1.5 T is that of a decrease in field strength. The 0.5 T open-architecture MR imaging system increases patient access, but provides a challenge in adaptation of the imaging sequences. Specific to the success of the use of the open imager, then, is the creation of new sequences and recognition of both breast findings and the artifacts from biopsy instruments on those sequences.[1,2] This group has found that the 3-point Dixon imaging sequence provides excellent fat-nulled images of enhancing breast lesions in the 0.5 T open MR environment.[3,4] Progress in the field of interventional MRI has been significantly hindered by the problem of adequate biopsy tools (see Dr. Daniel's second article in this section of the YEAR BOOK [Abstract 2–19]). Dr. Stuart Gould in London (personal communication) has performed lumpectomies and mastectomies in the open access magnet and reports that a number of instruments commonly used in the operating room are safe to use in the magnet. However, many new instruments must be created and one of the greatest disappointments in breast intervention MRI work has been the limited performance of the core biopsy needles presently available.[5] Clearly, with only 13 of these open access imagers up and running throughout the world, this environment can provide only some of the answers to the many questions of biopsy and interventional procedures for the breast using MRI.[6]

R.L. Birdwell, M.D.

References

1. Kuhl CK, Kreft BP, Hauswirth A, et al: MR mammography at 0.5 Tesla. I. Comparison of image quality and sensitivity of MR mammography at 0.5 and 1.5 T. *Rofo* 162:381-389, 1995.
2. Kuhl CK, Kreft BP, Hauswirth A, et al: MR mammography at 0.5 Tesla. II. The capacity to differentiate malignant and benign lesions in MR mammography at 0.5 and 1.5 T. *Rofo* 162:482-491, 1995.
3. Dixon TW: Simple proton spectroscopic imaging. *Radiology* 153:189-194, 1984.
4. Glover GH, Schnieder E: Three-point Dixon technique for true water/fat decomposition with B subzero inhomogenity correction. *Magn Reson Med* 18:371-383, 1991.
5. Harms SE, Flamig DP, Hessley KL, et al: MR imaging of the breast with rotating delivery of excitation off resonance: Clinical experience with pathologic correlation. *Radiology* 187:493-501, 1993.
6. Personal communication, 1999.

Calcification Retrieval at Stereotactic, 11-Gauge, Directional, Vacuum-assisted Breast Biopsy

Liberman L, Smolkin JH, Dershaw DD, et al (Mem Sloan-Kettering Cancer Ctr, New York)

Radiology 208:251-260, 1998 2–18

Introduction.—Stereotactic, 14-gauge, automated, large-core breast biopsy is an accurate and cost-effective alternative to surgical biopsy for the diagnosis of nonpalpable breast lesions. However, it is limited in assessing calcifications. Stereotactic, directional, vacuum-assisted breast biopsy is being increasingly used for the diagnosis of indeterminate or suspicious lesions identified at mammography and may provide better retrieval and characterization of calcification, most likely as a result of the larger size of each specimen and the ability of the vacuum-assisted device to acquire tissue outside of the line of fire. An 11-gauge probe would allow for more accurate placement of a localizing marker but is more expensive than the 14-gauge probe. However, the 11-gauge probe may decrease the frequency of histologic underestimates in lesions containing atypical ductal hyperplasia and ductal carcinoma in situ, and it obtains larger tissue specimens. The usefulness of 11-gauge, directional, vacuum-assisted biopsy for calcific lesions was evaluated.

Methods.—There were 112 calcific lesions in 80 women, aged 31 to 85 years, who had stereotactic, 11-gauge directional, vacuum-assisted biopsy. Each lesion had a mean of 14 specimens. Identification of calcifications on radiographs of specimens defined calcification retrieval. Lesions that yielded atypical ductal hyperplasia at stereotactic biopsy and carcinoma at surgery were considered to be atypical ductal hyperplasia underestimates. Lesions that yielded ductal carcinoma in situ at stereotactic biopsy and

TABLE 5.—Calcification Retrieval at Stereotactic Breast Biopsy

Study	No. of Lesions With Calcifications Retrieved at 14-Gauge, Automated, Large-Core Breast Biopsy	No. of Lesions With Calcifications Retrieved at Directional, Vacuum-Assisted Breast Biopsy	
		14-Gauge	11-Gauge
Liberman et al (5)	65/72 (90)	...	...
Lee et al (12)	133/151 (88)	...	...
Liberman et al (29)	...	50/55 (91)*	...
Meyer et al (32)	118/130 (91)	106/106 (100)†	...
Jackman et al (37)	1,122/1,196 (94)	1,195/1,209 (99)	720/723 (>99)‡

Note: The numbers in parentheses are percentages.

*The frequency of calcification retrieval was 19/24 (79%) in the first half of the 8-month study and 31/31 (100%) in the second half.

†$P<.001$

‡The frequency of retrieving calcifications was significantly higher for 14-gauge, directional, vacuum-assisted biopsy than it was for 14-gauge, automated, large-core biopsy ($P<.001$ and it was significantly higher for 11-gauge, directional, vacuum-assisted biopsy than it was for 14-gauge, automated, large-core biopsy ($P<.001$) but was not significantly different for 11- versus 14-gauge, directional, vacuum-assisted biopsy ($P=.15$).

(Courtesy of Liberman L, Smolkin JH, Dershaw DD, et al: Calcification retrieval at stereotactic, 11-gauge, directional, vacuum-assisted breast biopsy. *Radiology* 208:251-260, 1998. Radiological Society of North America.)

TABLE 6.—ADH and DCIS Underestimates at Stereotactic Breast Biopsy

Study	No. of Underestimated Cases With 14-Gauge, Automated, Large-Core Breast Biopsy	No. of Underestimated Cases With Directional, Vacuum-Assisted Breast Biopsy	
		14-Gauge	11-Gauge
ADH underestimates			
Jackman et al (6)	9/16 (56)*	...	...
Liberman et al (17)	11/21 (51)†	...	...
Burbank (28)	8/18 (44)	0/8 (0)‡	...
Jackman et al (31, 38)	26/54 (48)§	13/74 (18)§	4/31 (13)§
This study	...	...	1/10 (10)‖
DCIS underestimates			
Jackman et al (6)	8/43 (19)*	...	...
Liberman et al (16)	3/15 (20)†	...	...
Burbank (28)	9/55 (16)#	0/32 (0)#	...
This study	...	...	1/21 (5)**

*Note:*The numbers in parentheses are percentages.
*Mean of 8 specimens per lesion.
†Mean of 5 specimens per lesion.
‡P=.03. Mean of 17 specimens per lesion for 14-gauge, automated, large-core breast biopsy and mean of 27 specimens per lesion for 14-gauge, directional, vacuum-assisted breast biopsy.
§The frequency of ADH underestimates was significantly lower for 14-gauge, directional, vacuum-assisted breast biopsy than it was for 14-gauge, automated, large-core breast biopsy (P<.001). It also was significantly lower for 11-gauge, directional, vacuum-assisted breast biopsy than it was for 14-gauge, automated, large-core breast biopsy (P=.002). A lower frequency of ADH underestimates was observed for 11-gauge versus 14-gauge, directional, vacuum-assisted breast biopsy; however, this difference was not statistically significant (P=.76). The mean numbers of specimens obtained per lesion were 10 for 14-gauge, automated, large-core breast biopsy; 16 for 14-gauge, directional, vacuum-assisted breast biopsy; and 14 for 11-gauge, directional, vacuum-assisted breast biopsy.
‖Mean of 14 specimens per lesion. None of the 5 cases in which all calcification were removed was underestimated.
#P=.02. Mean of 19 specimens per lesion for 14-gauge, automated, large core breast biopsy and a mean of 27 specimens per lesion for 14-gauge, directional, vacuum-assisted breast biopsy.
**Mean of 14 specimens per lesion. None of the 12 cases in which all calcifications were removed was underestimated.
(Courtesy of Liberman L, Smolkin JH, Dershaw DD, et al: Calcification retrieval at stereotactic, 11-gauge, directional, vacuum-assisted breast biopsy. *Radiology* 208:251-260, 1998. Radiological Society of North America.)

infiltrating carcinoma at surgery were considered to be ductal carcinoma in situ underestimates.

Results.—In 51 lesions, all calcifications were removed with stereotactic, 11-gauge, directional, vacuum-assisted biopsy (46%). Some calcifications were removed in 55 lesions (49%). No calcifications were removed in 6 lesions (5%). In lesions 5 mm or smaller, in calcifications with amorphous morphology, and if the probe was fired outside the breast, there was significantly more likelihood of a failure to retrieve calcifications. In 1 of 10 lesions that yielded atypical ductal hyperplasia, surgery revealed ductal carcinoma in situ (10%) at stereotactic biopsy. In 1 of 21 lesions that yielded ductal carcinoma in situ at stereotactic biopsy, surgery revealed infiltrating carcinoma. When all calcifications were removed, no underestimation occurred.

Conclusion.—There was successful calcification retrieval in 106 of 112 lesions (95%) with stereotactic, 11-gauge, directional, vacuum-assisted biopsy. Histologic underestimation was infrequent. Directional, vacuum-assisted breast biopsy obtained larger tissue specimens, had a higher rate of calcification (Table 5), and had a lower likelihood of atypical ductal hyperplasia and ductal carcinoma in situ underestimation (Table 6) than automated, large-core biopsy.

► The benefits of the directional vacuum-assisted breast biopsy device are many, including the now available 11-gauge needle that allows larger tissue samples. The single entry of the probe, as well as the vacuum-assistance that allows the device to acquire tissue outside the direct line of fire and to suction blood from the biopsy cavity, are also major advances in percutaneous biopsy methodology. This article is one of many from Dr. Liberman and her group in the field of stereotactic percutaneous breast biopsy and outlines the use of the 11-gauge needle to increase the positive retrieval of calcifications. Obtaining calcifications increases the chance that the target lesion has been sampled, and it is hypothesized that the 11-gauge needle will decrease the number of samples that "underestimate" the pathology.[1-4] In this study, only 1 of the 10 lesions in which the 11-gauge biopsy yielded ADH proved to be ductal carcinoma at surgery, and 1 of the 21 lesions of ductal carcinoma in situ proved to be infiltrating carcinoma at open surgical biopsy. The authors make some important technical observations, 1 relating to the potential differences between the 2 prone tables on the market. With the needle in the "postfire" position, the Mammotest made by Fischer apparently controls the depth of the needle placement by depressing a lever and manually advancing the probe driver, whereas the LoRad StereoGuide controls the depth by turning a dial. Dr. Liberman's group found that if you place the needle in a postfire position using the LoRad table, this may limit the force that can be applied to pierce the lesion. In contrast, Drs. Parker and Klaus have not reported any problems in lesion piercing when placing the probe in the postfire position using the Fischer table.[5] A second technical point is that the "air gap" technique helps to allow tissue acquisition in breasts that compress to a very thin volume.[6,7] In brief, a reversed compression paddle is placed between the far side of the breast and the breast support plate and the apertures of both compression paddles are aligned. When the probe is placed in the postfire position, it will displace breast tissue through the aperture on the far side of the breast, rather than striking the paddle or the plate.

The literature thus far does not indicate significant complications associated with vacuum-assisted biopsy; Burbank reported 1% complication rates for both 11-and 14-gauge stereotactic vacuum-assisted biopsies.[8] Those active in the field suggest that perhaps more aggressive measures to achieve hemostasis, including the use of lidocaine with epinephrine for deep anesthesia, as well as wrapping the chest with a 6-inch rubber elastic bandage for 24 hours after 11 vacuum-assisted biopsy, may be the better part of valor. Is bigger better? As long as there is an increase in accurate diagnoses and no significant increase in complication rate, maybe the answer is yes. However, at what point is bigger too big? We will include in next year's YEAR BOOK further reports of the truly large-core biopsy now available, in which 2 cm (and even 3 cm!) cylinders are advanced into the breast for lesion removal.

R.L. Birdwell, M.D.

References

1. Liberman L, LaTrenta L, Van Zee KJ, et al: Stereotactic core biopsy of calcifications highly suggestive of malignancy. *Radiology* 203:673-677, 1997.
2. Parker SH, Burbank F, Jackman RJ, et al: Percutaneous large-core breast biopsy: A multi-institutional study. *Radiology* 193:359-364, 1994.
3. Liberman L, Cohen MA, Dershaw DD, et al: Atypical ductal hyperplasia diagnosed at stereotactic core biopsy of breast lesions: An indication for surgical biopsy. *AJR* 164:1111-1113, 1995.
4. Jackman RJ, Burbank FH, Parker SH, et al: Atypical ductal hyperplasia diagnosed by 11-gauge, directional-assisted breast biopsy: How often is carcinoma found at surgery? *Radiology* 205:325A, 1997.
5. Parker SH, Klaus AJ: Performing a breast biopsy with a directional, vacuum-assisted biopsy instrument. *Radiographics* 17:1233-1252, 1997.
6. Parker SH, Burbank F: A practical approach to minimally invasive breast biopsy. *Radiology* 200:11-20, 1996.
7. Burbank F: Stereotactic breast biopsy: Its history, its present, and its future. *Am Surg* 62:128-150, 1996.
8. Burbank F: Stereotactic breast biopsy: Comparison of 14-gauge and 11-gauge Mammotome probe performance and complications rates. *Am Surg* 63:988-995, 1997.

Breast Lesion Localization: A Freehand, Interactive MR Imaging–guided Technique

Daniel BL, Birdwell RL, Ikeda DM, et al (Stanford Univ, Calif; Presbyterian Hosp and Imaging Ctr, Charlotte, NC)
Radiology 207:455-463, 1998 2–19

Background.—Breast cancer detection can be performed with high sensitivity using contrast-enhanced MRI. The authors describe an experience in which rapid, interactive MRI guidance of needle placement in the freely suspended breast was performed beneath the platform of a commercially available open breast coil with the patient in a prone position.

Methods.—Before MRI-guided needle localization, diagnostic contrast-enhanced MRI was performed. A 1.5-T imager was used with an open-frame platform configuration phased-array breast coil. On the localization day, the patient was positioned prone on the open breast coil. In the first 4 cases, the breast was stabilized with moldable thermoplastic mesh (Fig 1). On the basis of preliminary images, the table was repositioned so that the target lesion was in the image plane. A rapid set of 5 guidance images was obtained, and further adjustments were made if necessary. An MRI-compatible needle was inserted and advanced incrementally. After each manipulation, another set of guidance images was obtained. After the needle reached its target, methylene blue dye was injected and a hookwire was deployed (Fig 4). Diagnostic whole-breast MRI was performed to document the final trajectory of the hookwire. The distance from the hookwire to the lesion was measured on mammograms or US images.

Results.—This MRI-guided localization technique was used to localize 19 breast lesions in 17 women, aged 38 to 70. All hookwires were placed

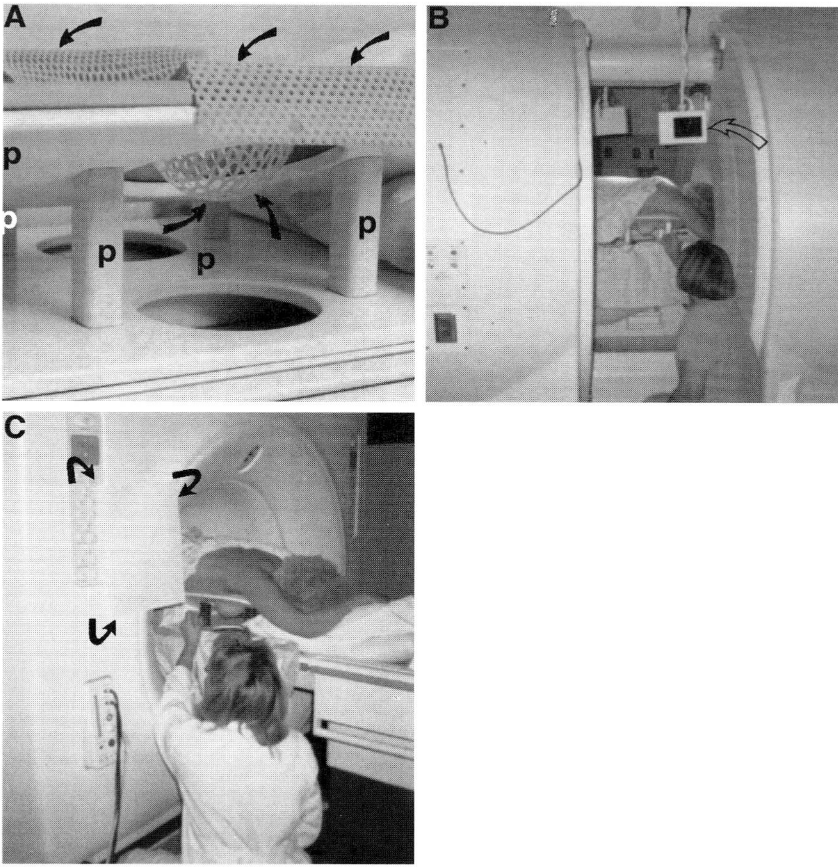

FIGURE 1.—Open-platform breast coil (*p*). **A,** Photograph shows thermoplastic mesh that is molded around the breasts as the patient (removed for photograph) is in the prone position on the coil. Once hardened, the mesh (*arrows*) creates a rigid exoskeleton that fixes the breast in place. Fenestrations in the mesh allow good visualization of the breast and many sites for needle access from many angles. **B,** Photograph demonstrates that in the open 0.5-T MR imager, the physician has direct access to the breast for needle placement without removing the patient from the imager. The progress of the needle is monitored on MR images displayed on the small viewing screen (*arrow*) located on the magnet shroud over the patient within the magnet bore. **C,** Photograph demonstrates that localization with a conventional, closed-bore 1.5-T system is performed with the patient partially removed from the bore for needle access. The progress of the needle is checked by briefly returning the patient to the center of the bore for MR imaging. A video projector that displays the MR images on a small screen (*arrows*) on the magnet shroud facilitates the procedure by allowing the physician to remain with the patient at all times. (Courtesy of Daniel BL, Birdwell RL, Ikeda DM, et al: Breast lesion localization: A freehand, interactive MR imaging-guided technique. *Radiology* 207:455-463, 1998. Radiological Society of North America.)

within 9 mm of the target lesions. Lateral, circumareolar, and tangential approaches were used to reach these lesions. The procedure time was less than 1 hour in all cases and averaged 17 minutes. All procedures were well tolerated.

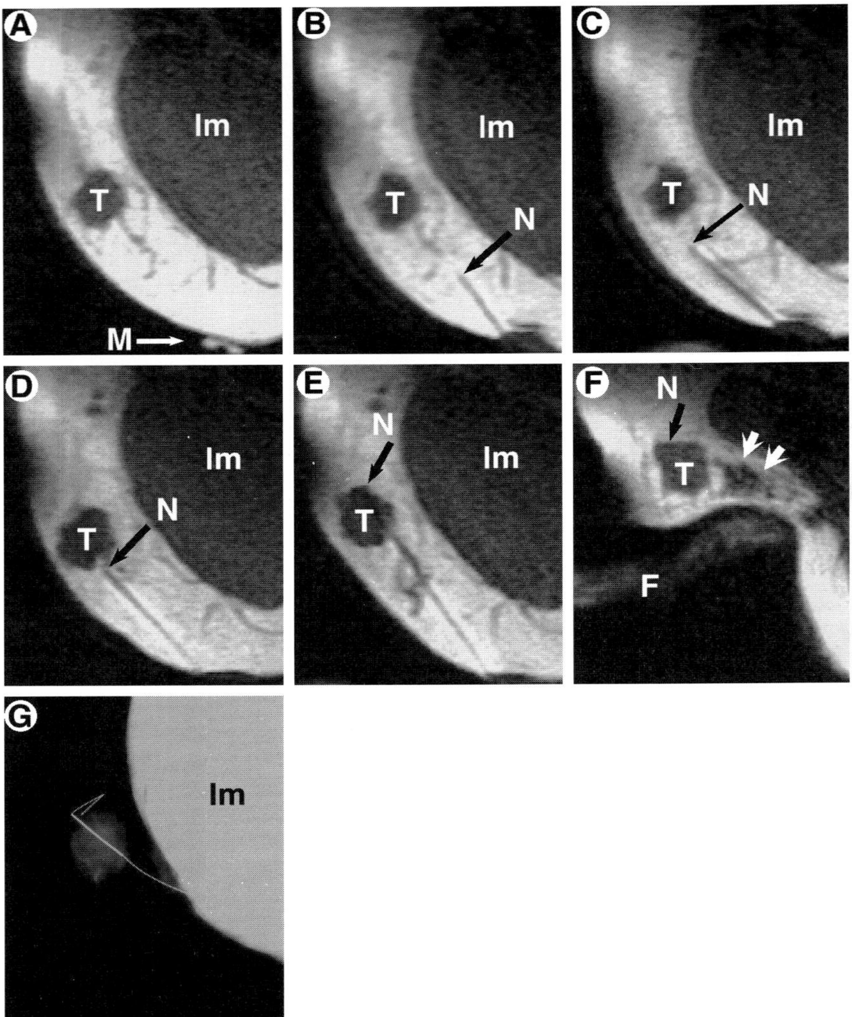

FIGURE 4.—MR imaging-guided preoperative hookwire localization in a 57-year-old woman; 0.5-T, vertically open imager. **A,** Preliminary T1-weighted axial fast spin-echo image (300/14 [effective]) shows a target mass (*T*) that is lateral to a single-lumen silicone implant (*Im*). A small marker (*arrow, M*) filled with dilute copper sulfate was taped to the areolar margin, the planned skin entry site for a circumareolar approach. **B-E,** Axial fast spin-echo images (300/14 [effective]) repeatedly obtained with identical imaging parameters between successive manipulations of the needle (*arrow, N*) toward the target. The needle remained tangential to the implant (*Im*) surface to prevent puncture; this trajectory is impossible with lateral grid-compression plate devices. Despite substantial motion of the target lesion (*T*), the needle was easily directed into the mass within a few minutes by using these images for interactive guidance. **F,** Axial fast spin-echo image (300/14 [effective]) obtained while compressing the breast after deploying the hookwire. The tip of the stiffener of the wire (*N, black arrow*) remained centered in the target lesion (*T*). A small hematoma (*white arrows*) that was noted along the wire after removal of the localizing needle from the mass was easily controlled with firm manual pressure. Note the radiologist's fingers (*F*) compressing the anterior part of the breast without removing the patient from the breast coil. **G,** Radiograph of the mastectomy specimen shows the hookwire traversing the target lesion lateral to the implant (*Im*). Histopathologic analysis revealed a 2.5-cm infiltrating ductal carcinoma. (Courtesy of Daniel BL, Birdwell RL, Ikeda DM, et al: Breast lesion localization: A freehand, interactive MR imaging-guided technique. *Radiology* 207:455-463, 1998. Radiological Society of North America.)

Conclusions.—This method of MRI-guided breast lesion localization, using a commercially available open-platform breast coil, accurately positioned needles in 19 breast lesions. The advantages of the method include better access and visualization, use of commercially available coils, no need for stereotactic positioning devices, motion compensation, similar configuration for both diagnosis and biopsy, and patient comfort. The accuracy of this technique was similar to that of freehand, US-guided preoperative needle localizations.

► This is an extension of the work reported previously from the Stanford group under the direction of Dr. Daniel in which breast lesions are localized in a freehand fashion with interactive MRI. These 19 MRI-guided breast lesion needle localizations were performed before surgical biopsy procedures in either a 1.5-T closed bore magnet or, later in the study, in a 0.5-T open imager. Ten of the lesions were visible on either mammograms or ultrasonograms, and the ultimate position of the wire placed with MR guidance was corroborated with the imaging modality that was used initially to image the lesion. The freehand approach increased the access to the breast and allowed different needle trajectories. The procedures were simple and accurate, and no special stereotactic equipment was required. The open imager was more efficient in that the patient did not have to be moved in and out of the magnet bore. Breast compression has been encouraged and the Schorn article (Abstract 2–20) is an example of one of the prototype compression devices undergoing investigation. Schnall et al.[1] believed that compression was necessary to prevent motion of the target lesions, but Dr. Daniel and his group found this not to be a specific problem because of the interactive rapid imaging approach used to incrementally advance the needle to the target lesion. One of the other arguments in favor of the freehand approach without compression is that the configuration of the breast during the diagnostic MRI is the same as that during the imaging-guided lesion localization. This makes target identification, particularly of small lesions or lesion with somewhat subtle characteristics, more easily accomplished if they can be identified with the T1-weighted fast spin-echo sequences without the initial injection of gadolinium at the time of the needle localization procedure. Daniel and his group no longer use the stabilizing mesh described in the article. This method proved more problematic than helpful. All breast interventional procedures are now performed by the free-hand technique.

Two other investigators have reported the use of nongrid techniques similar to that used by Dr. Daniel's group, but in both of these methods the patient was required to move out of the imaging coil because the breast could not be accessed within the closed type of breast coil used.[2,3] This is a major benefit of the dedicated open breast coil that Dr. Daniel and his group use.

R.L. Birdwell, M.D.

References

1. Schnall MD, Orel SG, Connick TJ: MR-guided biopsy of the breast. *Magn Reson Imaging Clin N Am* 2:585-589, 1994.
2. Davis PL, Julian TB, Staiger M, et al: Magnetic resonance imaging detection on wire localization of an "occult" breast cancer. *Breast Cancer Res Treat* 32: 327-330, 1994.
3. Brenner RJ, Shellock FG, Rothman BJ, et al: Technical note: Magnetic resonance imaging–guided preoperative breast localization using "freehand technique." *Br J Radiol* 68:1095-1098, 1995.

Compression Device to Reduce Motion Artifacts at Contrast-enhanced MR Imaging in the Breast

Schorn C, Fischer U, Döler W, et al (Klinikum der Georg-August-Universität Göttingen, Germany)

Radiology 206:279-282, 1998 2–20

Background.—The contrast enhancement pattern is an important diagnostic indicator for assessing breast lesions on MRI. The subtraction technique for obtaining increased conspicuity of lesion enhancement is popular but is vulnerable to motion artifacts. A simple compression device was developed, using commercially available breast surface coils, to reduce motion artifacts on routine diagnostic breast MR images.

Methods.—The prototype compression device for a bilateral breast surface coil was tested on 157 patients. Resultant images were compared with those obtained with simple ventral stuffing of the bottom of the coil in 181 patients.

Findings.—Compression decreased the proportion of MR examinations with severe motion artifacts from 11% to 2%. The compression device made the subtraction technique more effective in ensuring more lesion conspicuity.

Conclusions.—This compression device significantly reduced motion artifacts. Severe artifacts were almost completely prevented. Because the degree of compression was not too great, it was not uncomfortable for the patients. Contrast material uptake was not affected. The routine use of this compression device can improve image quality.

► This article reports a prototype compression device for a bilateral breast surface coil tested on 157 patients. This group of authors used the subtraction technique, felt by some investigators to limit image interpretation. However, using this new breast compression prototype, the reduction of breast motion was likely very beneficial for better evaluation of the imaging findings, even with the subtraction technique. In my experience, women don't like having their breasts compressed. If further investigation of MRI in breast imaging demonstrates success in the evaluation of the breast in the prone position using dedicated breast coils without the need for compression, this might be a good thing. However, we have much to learn and should remain open to all viable alternatives.

R.L. Birdwell, M.D.

3 Musculoskeletal System

Introduction

This year I decided to divide the articles according to subject matter by anatomic location, and I have included separate sections on tumors and miscellaneous conditions.

A number of articles discuss the use of MR in the diagnosis of patients with suspected fractures or the detection of unsuspected fractures utilizing MR imaging. The cost effectiveness of MR imaging in patients with suspected hip fractures is particularly important in these days of cost containment, and Dr. Rubin and colleagues (Abstract 3–4) have addressed this issue.

Imaging of anterior cruciate ligament injuries by MRI is well established, but two articles here discuss different aspects of anterior cruciate ligament injuries, namely, intercondylar notch width and the relationship of cruciate ligament tears and combined ligament injuries.

I hope all radiologists are familiar with the Ottawa Ankle Rules. The use of these well-established criteria will decrease the number of unnecessary ankle radiographs in the emergency room. It is important that we utilize these rules so that films ordered by generalists and nurse practitioners can be used in a cost effective manner.

The spine is an area of great controversy and the largest number of articles chosen involve the spine; these include interventional as well as diagnostic articles. The subject of discography has been included with the very controversial article by Milette and colleagues.

Miscellaneous subjects include an article on bone mineral density measurements and another on the use of PET scanning in the management of soft tissue sarcomas round out the chosen articles.

Murray K. Dalinka, M.D.

Shoulder

Neuropathic Arthropathy of the Shoulder

Hatzis N, Kaar TK, Wirth MA, et al (Univ of Texas, San Antonio)
J Bone Joint Surg Am 80-A:1314-1319, 1998 3–1

Purpose.—Neuropathic arthropathy of the shoulder is a rare condition with a variable presentation. In many cases, the shoulder symptoms eclipse the neurologic deficits. A 28-year experience with neuropathic arthropathy of the shoulder is reviewed, with emphasis on the patterns of clinical presentation.

Patients.—The experience included 6 men, average age 47. The shoulder of the dominant extremity was involved in 3 patients, and 1 patient had bilateral involvement. Five patients reported an acute onset of shoulder symptoms, usually after minor trauma to the previously normal shoulder. In each case, the pain was relatively mild. Neurologic symptoms were present in all patients, including motor weakness in 5. All had sensory changes, including decreased sensation to light touch in 5 patients and dissociative sensory loss in 1.

Findings.—Resorption of the humeral head was apparent on radiographs of all 7 involved shoulders. In 3 patients with serial radiographs, the average time from onset of symptoms to radiographic evidence of humeral head resorption was 13 days (Fig 1). Four patients showed resorption of the glenoid or osseous debris about the soft tissues. MRI demonstrated a central cord syrinx in 5 patients; the remaining patient had chronic alcoholism. The diagnosis of syringomyelia was made an average of 67 months after onset of symptoms, with a range of 10 to 180 months. Four of the patients underwent 1 or more shoulder operations before the diagnosis of neuropathic arthropathy was made.

Discussion.—Neuropathic arthropathy of the shoulder is a rare condition that is most often associated with syringomyelia. However, the diagnosis is often delayed for months to years. The presentation usually consists of shoulder swelling and pain, stiffness, or loss of motion. Radiographs show extensive and rapid destruction of the proximal aspect of the humerus and glenoid. Treatment should be nonoperative, with a focus on preservation of function; shoulder arthrodesis is contraindicated.

► This article describes 6 patients with neuropathic arthropathy of the shoulder and reviews the clinical, radiologic and therapeutic aspects of this entity. It is important to note that this is a frequently missed diagnosis and that rapid destruction of the shoulder is common.

M.K. Dalinka, M.D.

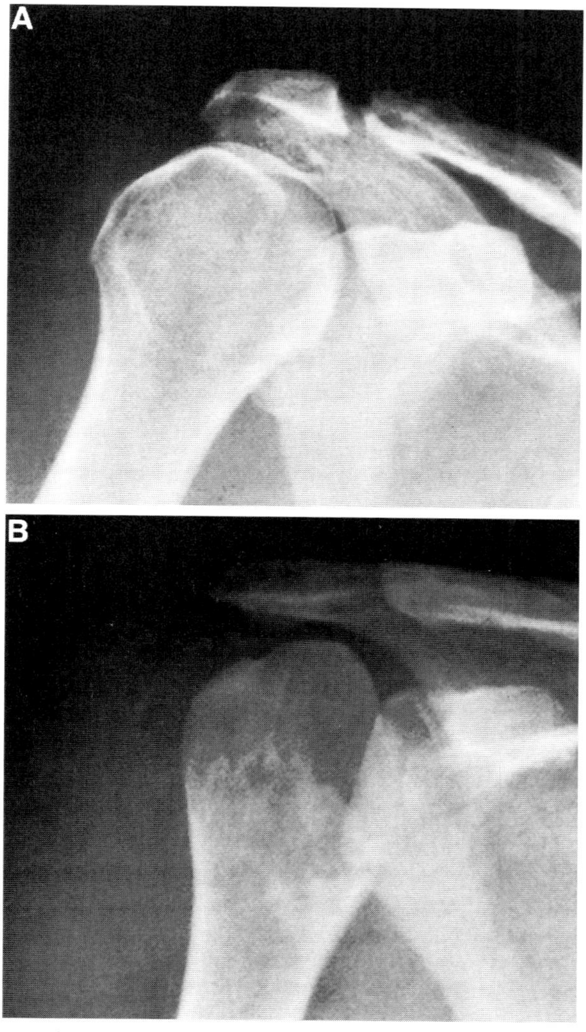

FIGURE 1.—**A**, Radiograph, made when the patient was first seen, showing mild degenerative changes involving the acromioclavicular joint. **B**, Radiograph, made 3 weeks after the initial presentation, showing resorption of nearly 50% of the humeral head. (Courtesy of Hatzis N, Kaar TK, Wirth MA, et al: Neuropathic arthropathy of the shoulder. *J Bone Joint Surg Am* 80-A:1314-1319, 1998.)

Occult Fractures of the Greater Tuberosity of the Humerus: Radiographic and MR Imaging Findings

Mason BJ, Kier R, Bindleglass DF (Univ of Oklahoma, Oklahoma City; Bridgeport Hosp, Conn)

AJR 172:469-473, 1999 3–2

Purpose.—There are many possible causes of fracture of the greater tuberosity of the humerus, including seizures, glenohumeral dislocations, and forced abduction with impaction of the tuberosity on the acromion. Minimally displaced greater tuberosity fractures may not be visible on conventional shoulder radiographs. The radiographic and MRI findings of 12 cases of clinically occult greater tuberosity fractures are presented, including the findings in the rotator cuff.

Methods and Findings.—The 12 patients all had weakness in abduction and external humeral rotation. All were undergoing shoulder MRI for suspected rotator cuff problems. Radiographically, the greater tuberosity was best seen on anteroposterior radiographs with the joint in external rotation. The MRI scans identified abnormal signal in the distal supraspinatus tendon in every case (Fig 2). The results were consistent with a partial tear in 7 patients and tendinosis in 5. Accompanying tears of the infraspinatus tendon were present in 3 patients. However, none had a full-thickness rotator cuff tear. A review of the initial radiographs in 11 patients showed subtle, previously unrecognized greater tuberosity fractures in 9 cases. Suboptimal radiographic technique was used in 2 of these patients. In most of the remaining cases, good radiographic technique had been used, but subtle cortical irregularities and radiolucencies were not appreciated prospectively.

Discussion.—This series underscores the importance of recognizing 1-part fractures of the greater tuberosity of the humerus. Appreciation of subtle findings on radiography will eliminate unnecessary MRI examination as symptoms may simulate those of a rotator cuff tear.

▶ The authors report a series of cases with subtle greater tuberosity fractures that were detected on MR and missed on plain films. This is sometimes a very subtle plain film diagnosis and many times the patients are referred in without the original plain films. The clinical findings in these patients simulate a rotator cuff tear and often the rotator cuff is abnormal but not torn. The increasing use of MR has shown that subtle fractures in unusual locations are often picked up on MRI in patients presenting with chronic pain.

M.K. Dalinka, M.D.

Suggested Reading

Robbins ML, Wilson MG, Sella EJ: MR imaging of anterosuperior calcaneal process fractures. *AJR* 172:475-479, 1999.

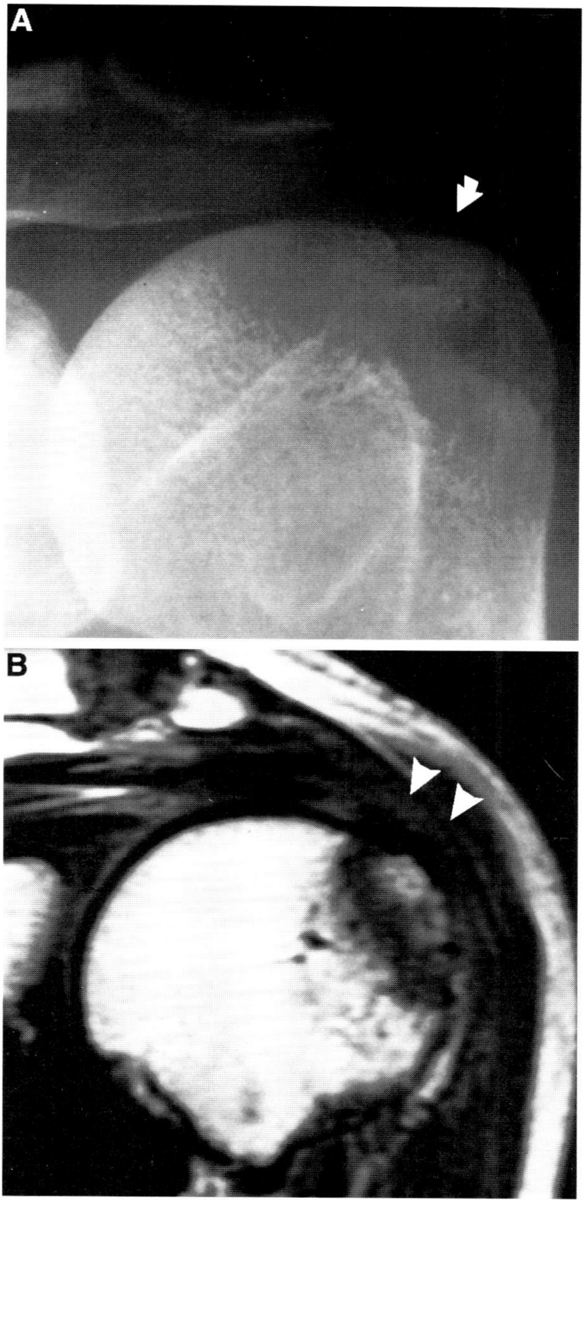

(Continued)

FIGURE 2 (cont.)

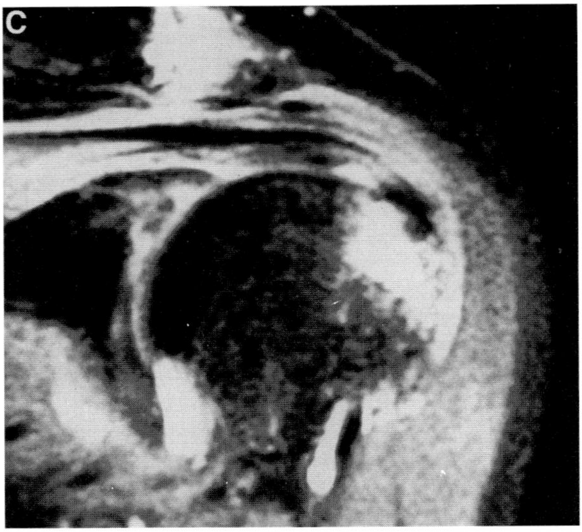

FIGURE 2.—54-year-old man with acute shoulder pain after hyperabduction injury to shoulder 4 days before MR imaging. **A**, Conventional radiograph shows cortical radiolucency in region of greater tuberosity (arrow) that was initially not appreciated. **B** and **C**, Oblique coronal T1-weighted spin-echo (B) and fat-suppressed T2-weighted fast spin-echo (C) MR images show ill-defined linear area of abnormal signal in region of greater tuberosity (arrow) consistent with bone marrow edema. No discrete fracture is seen in these images. Supraspinatus tendon has heterogeneous signal distally (arrowheads), consistent with partial-thickness tear. Patient is currently being treated conservatively. (Courtesy of Mason BJ, Bindleglass DF: Occult fractures of the greater tuberosity of the humerus: Radiographic and MR imaging findings. *AJR* 172:469-473, 1999.)

Pelvis and Hip

Contrast Enhanced Magnetic Resonance Imaging for Femoral Neck Fracture

Kamano M, Narita S, Honda Y, et al (Baba Mem Hosp, Osaka, Japan; Osaka City Univ, Japan)
Clin Orthop 350:179-186, 1998 3–3

Background.—A variety of methods for predicting which patients will have avascular necrosis after femoral neck fracture have been described. Preoperative evaluation of the vascular status of the femoral head is needed to determine appropriate treatment. The value of contrast-enhanced fat saturation MRI in the assessment of perfusion of the femoral head in the acute phase after intracapsular fracture was investigated.

Methods.—Twenty-nine patients underwent contrast-enhanced fat saturation MRI after acute femoral neck fracture. To monitor for the development of avascular necrosis, the patients were followed up with T1- and T2-weighted spin echo MRI without fat saturation. Mean time from injury to initial MRI was 24.5 hours. Average patient age at the time of injury was 69 years. Mean follow-up time was 26.9 months.

Findings.—Three distinct patterns of femoral head enhancement emerged in the acute phase after fracture. In 6 patients, the head showed no enhancement (type 1); in 12 patients, the head showed partial enhancement (type 2); and in 11 patients, the whole femoral head was well enhanced (type 3). Avascular necrosis developed in all patients with the type 1 pattern, in about half of those with the type 2 pattern, and in none with the type 3 pattern. Overall, the predictive value of this method was only 59% because of the uncertainty in patients with the type 2 pattern.

Conclusions.—Contrast-enhanced MRI accurately predicts the development of avascular necrosis in patients with type 1 and 3 enhancement. However, its overall predictive value is only 59%. Further study is needed before this method can be recommended for routine clinical use.

► In the past, multiple nuclear medicine articles were written on attempts to predict osteonecrosis in patients following femoral neck fractures. Some of these articles conclude that such studies could predict the development of osteonecrosis while others refuted these results. Similar studies were performed to predict ischaemic necrosis of the scaphoid. These studies seem to have fallen by the wayside. The results of this paper are interesting, but I am skeptical because the overall predictive value in this case was only 59%. In addition, the main interval from fracture to the initial MRI examination was 24 hours, but the authors do not mention the period from time of the injury to the time of surgery. The articles below are recommended for additional reading.[1-3]

M.K. Dalinka, M.D.

References

1. Speer KP, Spritzer CE, Harrelson JM, et al: Magnetic resonance imaging of the femoral head after acute intracapsular fracture of the femoral head. *J Bone Joint Surg* [Am] 72-A:98-103, 1990.
2. Frandsen PA, Andersen E, Madsen F, et al: Garden's classification of femoral neck fractures: An assessment of inter-observer variation. *J Bone Joint Surg [Br]*, 70-B:588-90, 1998.
3. Lang P, Mauz M, Schörner W, Schwetlick G, et al: Acute fracture of the femoral neck: Assessment of the femoral head perfusion with gadopentetate dimeglumine-enhanced MR imaging. *AJR*: 160:335-341, 1993.

Magnetic Resonance Imaging: A Cost-effective Alternative to Bone Scintigraphy in the Evaluation of Patients With Suspected Hip Fractures

Rubin SJ, Marquardt JD, Gottlieb RH, et al (Univ of Rochester, NY)

Skeletal Radiol 27:199-204, 1998 3–4

Background.—The cost associated with hip fractures is significant. Diagnosis can be difficult, because history and physical evaluations often yield unreliable findings, and plain film assessment is often either falsely negative or equivocal. Delayed diagnosis can result in increased morbidity and prolonged hospitalization. Though both radionuclide bone scintigraphy (RBS) and MRI are relatively accurate in diagnosing occult hip fractures early, it is unclear which procedure is more cost-effective.

Methods.—The medical records of all 40 patients seen in an emergency department during 4.5 years who had clinically suspected hip fracture, with either negative or equivocal plain films, and either a subsequent bone scan or MRI were reviewed. Twenty-one patients had bone scans, and 19, MRI. The theoretical cost analysis was based on current charges.

Findings.—Mean time to diagnosis was 2.24 days for patients undergoing bone scanning and 0.37 days for those undergoing MRI. Twenty patients having bone scans were hospitalized, compared with 13 having MRI. Mean time to surgery was at least 1 day longer in patients undergoing bone scanning. Because of the diagnostic delay, RBS was associated with greater patient costs than MRI.

Conclusions.—MRI may have additional value over RBS in obtaining anatomical information about the extent and orientation of the fracture and may be more accurate in diagnosing femoral neck fractures in patients with advaned hip arthritis. Compared with RBS, MRI shortens the time to diagnosis of occult hip fractures, reduces the hospital admission rate, and decreases time to surgery. Thus, MRI is a more cost-effective diagnostic modality at centers that perform RBS after 48 hours or longer.

► This retrospective study concludes that MRI is a cost-effective method of making the diagnosis of hip fractures in patients with equivocal or negative plain films. This conclusion was true despite the fact that the authors did a complete MRI examination. It is possible to do a limited examination at decreased cost to exclude the possibility of fracture. Bogost and colleagues have demonstrated that occult pelvic fractures and bone or soft-tissue abnormalities were found in the majority of patients who did not have hip fractures.[1]

M.K. Dalinka, M.D.

Reference

1. Bogost GA, Lizerbram EK, Crues JV, et al: MR imaging in evaluation of suspected hip fracture: Frequency of unsuspected bone and soft-tissue injury. *Radiology* 197:263-267, 1995.

Knee

Articular Cartilage Changes Seen With Magnetic Resonance Imaging-Detected Bone Bruises Associated With Acute Anterior Cruciate Ligament Rupture

Johnson DL, Urban WP Jr, Caborn DNM, et al (Univ of Kentucky, Lexington)
Am J Sports Med 26:409-414, 1998 3–5

Background.—Anterior cruciate ligament (ACL) rupture has long been associated with subsequent development of degenerative arthritis. Recent research shows that a significant proportion of patients with ACL rupture will subsequently show radiographic evidence and experience clinical symptoms of osteoarthritis, despite ligament reconstruction. There is often no association between knee stability and the development of degenerative arthritis. Occult subchondral bone lesions, present in more than 80% of patients with complete ruptures, can be hidden by overlying articular cartilage on direct arthroscopic assessment. Despite the high prevalence of these lesions, the histologic changes in the adjacent articular cartilage have not been well documented.

Methods.—Ten patients with acute ACL ruptures were studied. All had geographic bone bruises at the sulcus terminalis on the lateral femoral condyle documented preoperatively by MRI. A 3-mm diameter trephine biopsy of the articular cartilage and subchondral bone overlying the bone bruise was performed at the time of ACL reconstruction. Articular cartilage and subchondral bone specimens were stained with hematoxylin and eosin and toluidine blue.

Findings.—Significant arthroscopic and histologic articular cartilage irregularities were seen in all patients in the area overlying the bone bruise. An arthroscopic examination of the articular cartilage showed softening, fissuring, or overt chondral fracture. Histologic assessment showed degeneration of the chondrocytes and loss of toluidine blue staining in the articular cartilage. Necrosis of osteocytes in the subchondral bone and empty lacuna were also documented.

Conclusions.—The exact histologic changes in the articular cartilage overlying a geographic bone bruise caused by acute ACL tear were documented. A geographic bone bruise documented using MRI indicates substantial damage to normal articular cartilage homeostasis.

► In this important study, the authors performed biopsies on articular cartilage in 10 patients with geographic bone contusions and ACL tears. The results show that all of these patients had injuries to the articular cartilage. Prior studies of animals show that alterations in the articular cartilage occur even when the cartilage has a normal gross appearance. It is well known that patients with ACL tears may develop osteoarthritis even if they are stable and have early reconstructions. The authors postulate that the articular cartilage injury at the time of the ACL tear may determine the long-term outcome of the patient. Please note that these results can not be extrapolated to patients with reticular contusions, which frequently disappear without sequelae.

M.K. Dalinka, M.D.

MR Imaging of Knees Having Isolated and Combined Ligament Injuries

Rubin DA, Kettering JM, Towers JD, et al (Univ of Pittsburgh, Pa; Westmoreland Regional Hosp, Greensburg, Pa)
AJR 170:1207-1213, 1998 3–6

Introduction.—Clinical evaluation and MRI are both less accurate in the diagnosis of meniscal tears in patients with isolated anterior cruciate ligament (ACL) tears than in patients with no ligamentous injuries. However, MRI is more sensitive than physical examination in detecting meniscal tears in patients with torn ACLs. Clinical evaluation is complicated in patients with severe trauma, who may have numerous soft-tissue injuries around the knee, with or without dislocation. The accuracy of MRI in the diagnosis of ligament tears was evaluated in patients with varying degrees and numbers of ligamentous injuries.

Methods.—The investigators reviewed 340 knee MRIs from 388 consecutive patients who went on to knee arthroscopy or arthrotomy. The patients were 229 males and 109 females with a median age of 31 years. The scans were interpreted by radiologists, who used standard criteria for the diagnosis of ligamentous injuries and meniscal tears. The interpreters had access to the clinical findings. The radiologic findings were compared with the operative diagnosis for the anterior and posterior cruciate ligaments, the collateral ligaments, and patellar tendon, and the menisci. Three different scoring systems for the cruciate ligaments were evaluated, given the difficulty in diagnosing partial injuries to these structures.

Results.—With all 3 scoring systems, the sensitivity of MRI in the diagnosis of ACL tears was 93%, with a specificity of 93% to 96%. MRI offered a sensitivity of 93% for isolated ACL tears, 83% for ACL tears when both the ACL and posterior cruciate ligament (PCL) were torn, 100% for isolated PCL tears, and 83% for PCL tears when both the ACL

TABLE 4.—Accuracy of Magnetic Resonance Imaging for Revealing Meniscal Tears, Stratified by Anterior Cruciate Ligament Status

		Lateral Meniscus			Medial Meniscus	
ACL Status	Knees (*n*)	Sensitivity	Specificity	Knees (*n*)	Sensitivity	Specificity
Intact	208	90 (78-95)	92 (87-95)	202	98 (93-99)	90 (83-95)
Torn	122	83 (71-91)	91 (82-96)	114	84 (72-92)	79 (68-88)
p		NS	NS		.006	NS

Sensitivity and specificity are percentages. Numbers in parentheses are 95% confidence intervals.
Abbreviations: ACL, anterior cruciate ligament; *NS*, not significant.
(Courtesy of Rubin DA, Kettering JM, Towers JD, et al: MR imaging of knees having isolated and combined ligament injuries. *AJR* 170:1207-1213, 1998.)

and PCL were torn. Surgery revealed tearing of more than 1 supporting structure in 6% of cases.

The incidence of medial meniscus tears was 49% in knees with all ligaments intact, 46% in knees with 1 ligament torn, and 37% in knees with 2 or more structures torn. The sensitivities of MRI for medial meniscal tears in these 3 groups were 98%, 89%, and 57%, respectively. The results were similar on analysis of patients with ACL tears (Table 4). The rate of lateral meniscus tears was 23% in knees with all ligaments intact, 43% in knees with 1 ligament torn, and 47% in knees with 2 or more structures torn. The sensitivity of MRI for lateral meniscal tears was 89% in knees with intact ligaments vs. 78% in knees with 2 or more structures torn, and 90% in knees with an intact ACL vs. 83% in knees with a torn ACL. However, the differences in sensitivities were nonsignificant.

Conclusions.—The diagnostic accuracy of MRI is reduced in knees with multiple ligament injuries. Specificity for ligamentous tears is significantly reduced in such knees, as is the sensitivity for medial meniscus tears. Nonetheless, MRI scanning continues to be a valuable diagnostic procedure, particularly if the physical examination is difficult or incomplete. Partial ACL tears are difficult to diagnose; however, clinically significant ACL injuries can be recognized with high specificity and sensitivity.

► Rubin and colleagues have shown that MR accuracy decreases as the number of injuries in the knee increases. However, MR is still more accurate than clinical examination in these patients and often complements a difficult or incomplete examination.

M.K. Dalinka, M.D.

The Relationship Between Intercondylar Notch Width of the Femur and the Incidence of Anterior Cruciate Ligament Tears: A Prospective Study

Shelbourne KD, Davis TJ, Klootwyk TE (Methodist Sports Medicine Ctr, Indianapolis, Ind)

Am J Sports Med 26:402-408, 1998 3–7

Background.—Recent research has sought to identify factors predisposing athletes to arterior cruciate ligament (ACL) injury. Women have been found to experience ACL tears at a greater rate than men, possibly because of differences in the intercondylar notch width of the femur. The relationship between intercondylar notch width of the femur and the incidence of ACL tears was studied prospectively.

Methods.—Seven hundred fourteen consecutive patients undergoing autogenous patellar tendon graft ACL reconstructions were studied. Intercondylar notch width was measured during surgery. Patients were divided into groups based on notch width: 15 mm or less and 16 mm or greater.

Findings.—The mean notch width in women was 13.9 mm, and in men, 15.9 mm. Notch width in height groups for women and men did not differ significantly. With height and weight as covariates, notches were signifi-

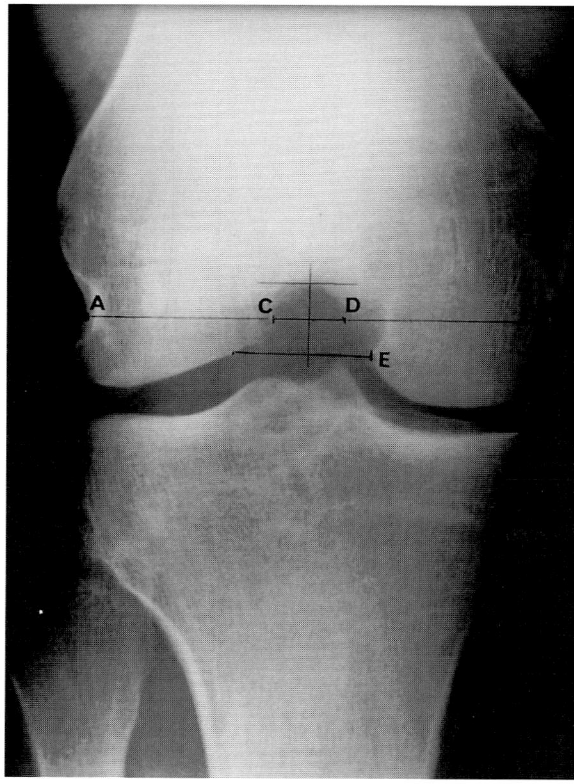

FIGURE 1.—The method used to measure femora condyle width and intercondylar notch width. A line is drawn across point "E," which corresponds to the medial meniscal rim on the medial femoral condyle. Another line is drawn at the level of the apex of the intercondylar notch. The width of the notch (distance from point "C" to point "D") is measured at one half of the notch height. The femoral condyle width is also measured at one half of the notch height (distance from point "A" to point "B"). (Courtesy of Shelbourne KD, Davis TJ, Klootwyk TE: The relationship between intercondylar notch width of the femur and the incidence of anterior cruciate ligament tears: A prospective study. *Am J Sports Med* 26:402-408, 1998.)

cantly narrower in women than in men. Within notch-width groups, there was no significant difference in contralateral tear rates between women and men. After reconstruction with equally sized 10-mm autografts, the graft tear rate did not differ significantly between men and women (Fig 1).

Conclusions.—Notch width affects the ACL tear rate. There is no sex difference that predisposes women with 10-mm ligament grafts to a greater likelihood of ACL tearing. Patients with narrower notches have a greater incidence of tearing the contralateral ACL.

► The authors have examined over 700 patients with ACL reconstructions, measured the width of the intercondylar notch and the notch width index, and determined that the incidence of ACL tears can be related to the notch width. The authors conclude that tears of the opposite ACL are more common in patients with narrow notches, and recommend obtaining routine standing posteroanterior views of the knee to evaluate notch width. The authors did not test the reproducibility of the notch-width measurement nor did they determine or make suggestions about what can be done for patients with narrow notches. The authors believe that a narrow intercondylar notch reflects a smaller ACL and that this may be the reason for increased ACL tears in these patients.

M.K. Dalinka, M.D.

Magnetic Resonance Imaging of Articular Cartilage in the Knee: An Evaluation With Use of Fast-Spin-Echo Imaging

Potter HG, Linklater JM, Allen AA, et al (Hosp for Special Surgery, New York)

J Bone Joint Surg Am 80-A:1276-1284, 1998 3–8

Purpose.—Surgery for acute and chronic chondral lesions has focused on chondral flap debridement, drilling of the subchondral bone, abrasion or microfracture, and perichondral graft insertion. Newer techniques, including autologous cartilage implantation and mosaicplasty, have spurred demand for more accurate techniques of assessing articular cartilage lesions. This technique, preferably noninvasive, would be useful both in diagnosis and treatment monitoring. MRI was compared with arthroscopy for the detection, grading, and localization of chondral lesions in the knee.

Methods.—The study included 88 patients (mean age, 38) who underwent MRI followed by arthroscopy of the knee for suspected meniscal or ligamentous injury. MRI examination of the articular cartilage in the sagittal, axial, and coronal planes was performed using 3 sequences. The sequences included fast-spin-echo images with a repetition time of 3,500 to 5,000 msec; a short effective echo time of 30 to 34 msec; an echo train length of 8 to 10; a bandwidth of 20.8 to 31.3 kHz; 2 excitations; and a slice thickness of 3.5 to 4.0 mm. For sagittal images, a matrix of 512×256, a field of view of 15 to 16 cm, and a scan time of 4.5 minutes were used; for axial images, a matrix of 512×256, a field of view of 14 to 15 cm, and a scan time of 4.0 minutes; and for coronal images, a matrix of 256×256, a field of view of 12 to 13 cm, and scan time of 4.0 minutes. An additional sagittal fast-spin-echo sequence with frequency-selective fat suppression was used as well. Two readers prospectively interpreted the images in blinded, independent fashion, confirming chondral lesions in at least 2 planes. Scans showing a uniform thickness of the intermediate signal intensity band between the subchondral plate and joint fluid were considered to indicate intact articular cartilage. The findings were compared with those of the arthroscopic assessment of articular cartilage.

Results.—A total of 248 articular cartilage lesions were identified on arthroscopy. Interobserver variability was minimal. In the detection of chondral lesions, MRI had a sensitivity of 87%, with a specificity of 94%, accuracy of 92%, a positive predictive value of 85%, and a negative predictive value of 95%. Sensitivity was lowest for lesions on the lateral tibial plateau, with a high rate of false negative results. Lesions of the patellar facets and trochlea were recognized with high sensitivity and specificity.

Conclusions.—Using fast-spin-echo sequences with a high-resolution matrix, MRI was highly accurate in assessing the articular cartilage of the knee. Close attention to technique, including higher resolution, is needed to detect subtle chondral injuries. Readers may tend to overdiagnose chondral softening. The MRI pulse sequence used in this study can be used along with most arthroscopic classification systems, which are also designed to evaluate morphologic changes of the chondral surface. Limitations of this study include possible selection bias and the fact that the MRI data were available to surgeons.

► The authors compare MRI with fast-spin-echo proton density weighted images and a fat-saturated sagittal sequence with findings at arthroscopy. Blinded readers had a Kappa value of 0.93 and values of 0.88 and 0.89 compared to arthroscopic findings, an almost perfect agreement. This is an amazing statistic. The authors do not state whether they used high-speed gradients for their proton density images or whether they used the minimum second echo time for the images. These techniques have been shown to decrease the blurring typically present in fast-spin-echo imaging.

M.K. Dalinka, M.D.

Failure of Clinical Methods in Assessing Graft Integrity After Anterior Cruciate Ligament Reconstruction: An Athroscopic Evaluation

Passler JM, Babinski K, Schippinger G (Univ of Utah, Salt Lake City)

Arthroscopy 15:27-34, 1999 3–9

Introduction.—Endoscopic anterior cruciate ligament reconstruction utilizing the central third of the patellar tendon has yielded excellent results. The KT-1000 arthrometer has been used in the assessment of outcomes after anterior cruciate ligament reconstruction. Patients who had subjectively stable knees after anterior cruciate ligament reconstruction but had insufficient or nonexistent grafts were reviewed to determine whether objective clinical tests such as with the KT-1000 device could detect instability.

Methods.—Twenty-four symptomatic patients underwent knee arthrosocopy after a bone–patellar tendon–bone autograft anterior cruciate ligament reconstruction. The patients had pain, swelling, catching, or locking before surgery. One patient had subjective instability. Arthroscopic findings were compared with the subjective and objective clinical findings, including those from the KT-1000 arthrometer examination.

Results.—An insufficient graft by arthroscopic examination was found in 13 of 24 patients. Physical examination on KT-1000 detected only 5 of these patients. Subjective and objective clinical criteria, as well as the

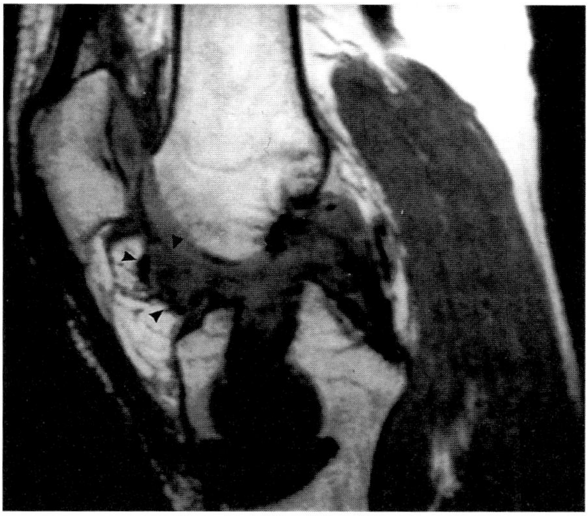

FIGURE 6.—Sagittal T1-weighted gradient-echo sequence: 1 year after anterior cruciate ligament reconstruction. Artifacts in the proximal tibia resulting from metal fixation of the distal bone block. The graft is not visible. Posterior to the fat pad (*arrows*) is an ovoid area 1 cm in diameter with hypointense signal pattern, which is identified as cyclops tumor by arthroscopy. (Courtesy of Passler J, Babinski K, Schippinger G: Failure of clinical methods in assessing graft integrity after anterior cruciate ligament reconstruction: An athroscopic evaluation. *Arthroscopy* 15:27-34, 1999.)

KT-1000 criteria, showed the other 8 patients have stable knees without significant degenerative changes or lack of motion. Excellent or good Orthopädische Arbeitsgruppe Knie score was found in 7 of the 8 patients who maintained a high level of function. Lack of an intact graft was confirmed in 2 patients who had preoperative MRI (Fig 6).

Conclusion.—Despite the lack of a functioning anterior cruciate ligament graft, a subset of patients appear to have stable knees. In detecting graft integrity after anterior cruciate ligament reconstruction, standard clinical and KT-1000 criteria for anterior cruciate ligament–deficient knees have limitations. When graft integrity is in question, arthroscopy or MRI may be necessary.

► In this study, clinical examination and KT-1000 arthrometer testing failed to detect instability in patients with failed anterior cruciate ligament grafts who had symptoms severe enough to necessitate arthroscopic surgery. Most of the patients in this study had full range of motion, a high level of function, and were without degenerative changes, despite the graft failure. The authors could not explain why the knee was stable in the presence of the torn reconstructed ligament. MR images were performed only in 2 patients, and they were both correct. Preoperative MRI would have arrived at the diagnosis before arthroscopy; and may eliminate the need for arthroscopy in many cases.

M.K. Dalinka, M.D.

Spine

Predictive Signs of Discogenic Lumbar Pain on Magnetic Resonance Imaging With Discography Correlation

Ito M, Incorvaia KM, Yu SF, et al (Hokkaido Univ, Sapporo, Japan; State Univ of New York, Syracuse)

Spine 23:1252-1260, 1998 3–10

Background.—The correlations between pathologic findings on MRI and pain reproduction by provoked diskography have not been thoroughly documented. Various pathologic parameters seen on MRI in patients with diskogenic lumbar pain were assessed and correlated with diskography findings.

Methods and Findings.—One hundred one lumbar disks in 39 patients were assessed by MRI and pain provocation diskography. Radial tears were commonly seen on MRI in disks with concordant pain on diskography, although the presence of such tears did not reliably predict a painful disk on diskography. A high-intensity zone on T2-weighted images was a relatively reliable predictor of pain. However, the statistical values were lower than those previously reported. Massive degeneration and severe disk height loss, which were rare in these patients, were good predictors of pain on disk injection.

Conclusions.—Lumbar intervertebral disks with posterior combined anular tears are likely to produce pain. However, these signs are of limited value for predicting diskogenic lumbar pain.

► This is an interesting article addressing the important subjects of diskography and diskogenic low back pain. The authors compared the findings on MRI to the results of the reproduction of concordant symptoms on diskography. The authors found that massive disk degeneration was a reliable predictor of pain reproduction but was rarely present. Radial tears were common in MRI but had a low specificity and low positive predictive value. The presence of a high-intensity zone on MRI was a reliable predictor of pain. In addition, diskography was more accurate than MRI in detecting disruption of the outer anulus. Most importantly, the authors found that it was not possible to characterize the correlation between many morphology features on MRI and the clinical symptoms as meaningful.

M.K. Dalinka, M.D.

Development of Vertebral Fractures in Patients With Multiple Myeloma: Does MRI Enable Recognition of Vertebrae That Will Collapse?

Lecouvet FE, Vande Berg BC, Michaux L, et al (Univ of Louvain, Brussels; Mont-Godinne Univ Hosp, Yvoir, Belgium)

J Comput Assist Tomogr 22:430-436, 1998 3–11

Background.—Vertebral compression fractures occur in 50% to 70% of patients with multiple myeloma (MM), and spinal cord compression occurs in 10% to 15%. Systemic antiresorptive treatment with bisphosphonate-compounds has been advocated to decrease the incidence of fractures. Recent research showed that the pattern of bone marrow involvement on MRI may be relevant in detecting patients with stage 3 MM who are at high risk for fracture. The relationship between the presence and size of focal marrow abnormalities on MRI in vertebral bodies and subsequent vertebral fractures in patients with MM was investigated.

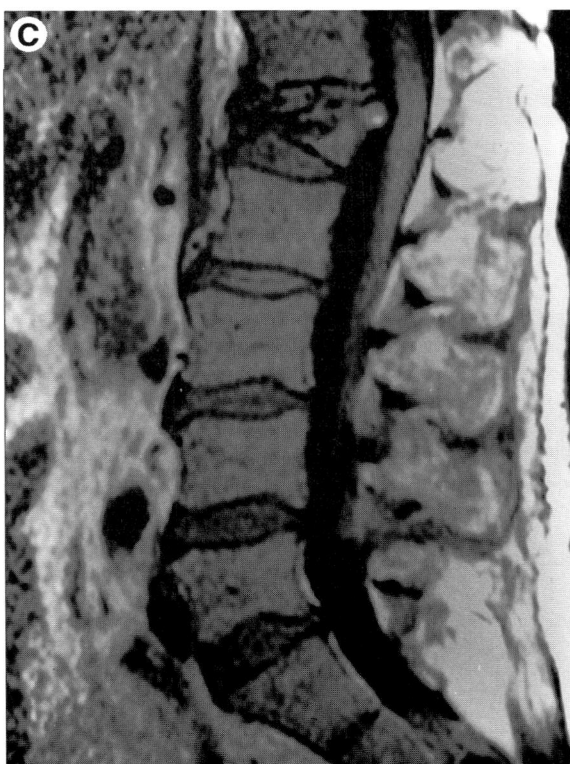

FIGURE 1.—A 52-year-old man with stage 3 multiple myeloma. Absence of vertebral lesion observed at MRI before fracture occurrence. T1-weighted (350/20 TR/TE). C, corresponding T2-weighted GE (500/27; flip angle 30°). (Courtesy of Lecouvet FE, Vande Berg BC, Michaux L, et al: Development of vertebral fractures in patients with multiple myeloma: Does MRI enable recognition of vertebrae that will collapse? *J Comput Assist Tomogr* 22:430-436, 1998.)

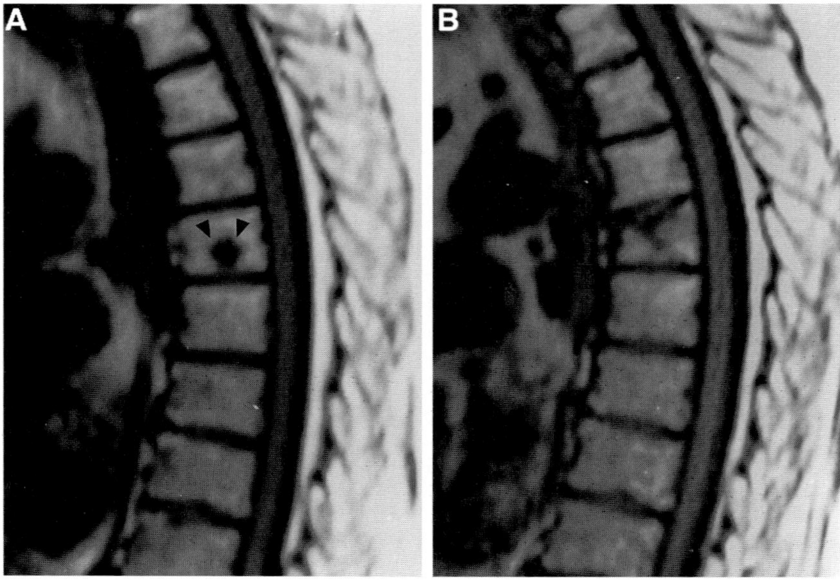

FIGURE 2.—A 49-year-old woman with stage 3 multiple myeloma. Preexisting vertebral lesion observed at MRI before fracture occurrence. **A**, T1-weighted (350/20 TR/TE) sagittal MR image of the thoracic spine shows rounded area of low signal intensity within the T5 vertebra (*arrowheads*) compatible with focal myelomatous involvement. **B**, T1-weighted (350/20 MR) MR image obtained 5 months later shows compression fracture of the T5 vertebral body. (Courtesy of Lecouvet FE, Vande Berg BC, Michaux L, et al: Development of vertebral fractures in patients with multiple myeloma: Does MRI enable recognition of vertebrae that will collapse? *J Comput Assist Tomogr* 22:430-436, 1998.)

Methods and Findings.—One hundred seventy-nine follow-up MR images of the thoracic and lumbar spine, obtained prospectively in 37 patients with stage 3 MM, were analyzed. One hundred thirty-one vertebral bodies fractured during follow-up. Sixty-three percent of these fractures appeared in vertebrae previously free of focal bone marrow abnormality at MRI, and 37% appeared in vertebrae in which focal lesions were present on the previous MR study. The size of the lesions preceding fractures did not differ significantly from the size of contemporary lesions that did not fracture (Figs 1 and 2).

Conclusions.—Pre-existing focal vertebral marrow lesions found on MRI appear to be unrelated to the subsequent development of vertebral fractures. A diffuse myeloma-induced bone resorption, rather than focal osteolysis, may be the main cause of bone weakening and fractures. Increased osteoclastic resorption is associated with the widespread dissemination of myeloma cells, because of the synthesis of various osteoclast-activating factors. The current findings raise doubts about the value of prophylaxis with local stabilization procedures, such as orthopedic fixation or cement vertebroplasty, to prevent further vertebral compression fractures in vertebral bodies with focal lesions in patients with MM.

► These authors have written many papers in this area and the interested reader is referred to their other articles on vertebral compression fractures in multiple myeloma. This article appears to be a follow-up to earlier articles[1,2] and the results are surprising and seemingly contradictory. The key word is "potential," used in the second part of the previous article. There is a lack of correlation between focal marrow lesions and the subsequent development of vertebral fractures.

M.K. Dalinka, M.D.

References

1. Lecouvet FE, Vande Berg BC, Maldague BE, et al: Vertebral compression fractures in multiple myeloma. Distribution and appearance at MR imaging. *Radiology* 204:195-199, 1997.
2. Lecouvet FE, Malghem J, Michaux L, et al: Vertebral compression fractures in multiple myeloma. Assessment of fracture risk with MR imaging of spinal bone marrow. *Radiology* 204:201-205, 1997.

Acute Nontraumatic Spinal Epidural Hematomas: An Important Differential Diagnosis in Spinal Emergencies

Alexiadou-Rudolf C, Ernestus R-I, Nanassis K, et al (Univ of Thessaloniki, Greece)

Spine 23:1810-1813, 1998 3–12

Introduction.—Fewer than 1% of spinal epidural space-occupying lesions are spontaneous spinal epidural hematomas (SSEHs), a rare spinal emergency that can be difficult to recognize. Good outcomes require an accurate diagnosis and prompt surgical decompression. Most cases occur in the lumbar region and dorsal to the spinal cord. The typical history is acute, nontraumatic onset of local pain, with signs of spinal cord compression occurring within hours. The differential diagnosis includes spinal abscess, tumor, ischemia, transverse myelitis, and acute vertebral disk disease, but the time spent on diagnostic tests may reduce the chance of a good outcome. Five patients with SSEH, with their clinical outcomes after spinal decompression, are reported.

Patients and Outcomes.—The patients were 3 men and 2 women, mean age 72. Four of the patients had acute back pain and paresthesia in both legs, with rapidly progressive paraplegia and loss of sensory function in the legs; the remaining patient had incomplete cauda equina syndrome. The diagnosis was made with spinal CT or MRI in 4 patients, and with lumbar myelography in 1. One patient who underwent spinal decompression within 12 hours after onset of symptoms had almost complete normalization of neurologic deficits. Good results were also achieved in the patient with cauda equina syndrome, who went to surgery within 48 hours. Two patients operated on after 12 hours had no neurologic improvement; surgery was not attempted in 1 patient referred 72 hours after onset of symptoms.

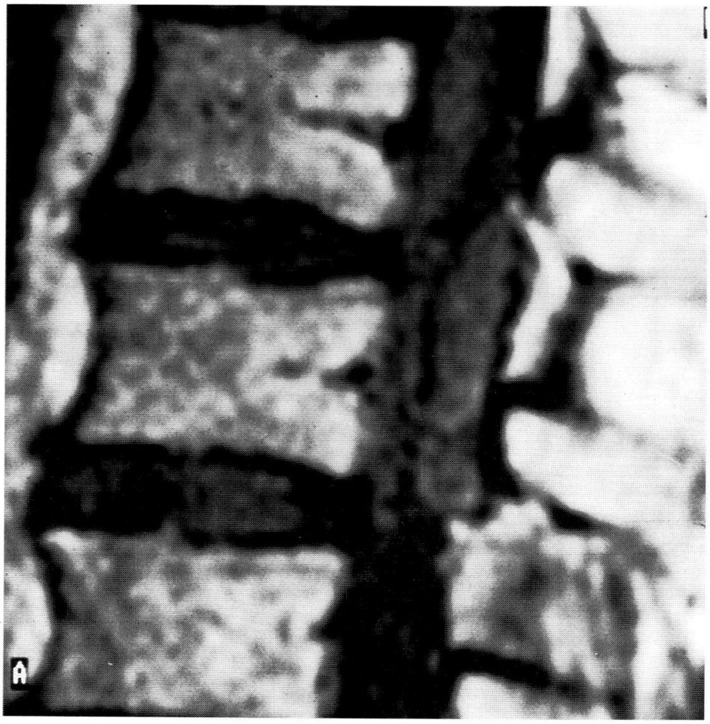

FIGURE 1.—T1-weighted magnetic resonance image of a spontaneous spinal epidural hematoma in patient 3. The hematoma is localized at D12 dorsal to the spinal cord. The epidural location is verified because cerebrospinal fluid (*black*) is present between the hematoma and the spinal cord. (Courtesy of Alexiadou-Rudolf C, Ernestus R-I, Nanassis K, et al: Acute nontraumatic spinal epidural hematomas: An important differential diagnosis in spinal emergencies. *Spine* 23: 1810-1813, 1998.)

Discussion.—Patients with SSEH present with rapidly progressive sensorimotor paralysis or cauda equina syndrome. The prognosis is strongly dependent on the timing of surgical decompression. Good postoperative function can be expected only if the patient is operated on within 12 hours after onset of symptoms. MRI is the diagnostic method of choice and shows signal behavior identical to that of intracerebral hematoma (Fig 1). Spinal MRI should be performed as quickly as possible to avoid diagnostic delays.

► This article points out the importance of recognizing this uncommon syndrome so that rapid intervention can reverse the clinical symptoms. This series is not large, but knowledge of the characteristic symptoms, coupled with the typical MRI manifestations, should enable one to make the diagnosis.

M.K. Dalinka, M.D.

No Association Between Peridural Scar and Outcome After Lumbar Microdiscectomy

Nygaard ØP, Kloster R, Dullerud R, et al (Univ Hosp of Tromsø, Norway; Ullevaal Hosp, Oslo, Norway)

Acta Neurochir (Wien) 139:1095-1100, 1997 3–13

Background.—Peridural scar formation after laminectomy has been linked to nerve root compression and tethering, which may cause radicular pain and disability. However, recent reports have suggested that the association between peridural fibrosis and persistent radicular pain is debatable. This MRI study evaluated the relationship between postoperative scarring and the clinical outcomes of lumbar microdiskectomy for herniated disks.

Methods.—Over a 2-year period, the investigators performed microdiskectomy for unilateral single-level disk herniation in 100 patients. At 1 year's follow-up, contrast-enhanced MRI was performed in 16 patients in whom surgery was classified as unsuccessful and in a random sample of patients in whom surgery was successful. The final analysis included 50 patients, representing 14 failures and 40 successes. The mean time from surgery to MRI was 16 months. Each scan was evaluated for the presence of an enhancing scar at the level of surgery and graded for the presence or absence of scarring within the spinal canal, degree of enhancement as scored by Glickstein and Sussmann, and the amount of scarring. Scar enhancement was graded with respect to the signal intensity of fat. The MRI scans were interpreted in independent, blinded fashion by 2 neuroradiologists.

Results.—Most patients had Glickstein score 2 scarring, with 25% to 50% of the circumference filled with scar tissue. Interobserver agreement was rated good for the amount of scar formation and moderate for intensity of contrast enhancement. The success or failure of surgery was unrelated to the amount or contrast enhancement of peridural scar formation. Peridural scarring was unrelated to any aspect of clinical outcome, including patient satisfaction scores.

Conclusions.—This study does not confirm previous reports linking peridural scar formation to persistent radicular pain after diskectomy. Neither the amount of scarring nor the intensity of scar tissue enhancement on MRI is associated with the 1-year outcomes of surgery. The conclusion is the same with different systems for the classification of scarring.

► This article compares contrast-enhanced MRIs in symptomatic patients and in asymptomatic patients after microdiskectomy. The authors conclude that peridural scar has no relationship with patient outcome after 1 year. This finding is a contradistinction to those of earlier articles on the subject.

M.K. Dalinka, M.D.

Spondylodiskitic Abscesses: CT-guided Percutaneous Catheter Drainage

Staatz G, Adam GB, Keulers P, et al (Univ-Hosp of the RWTH Aachen, Germany)

Radiology 208:363-367, 1998 3–14

Introduction.—Infectious spondylitis may involve bone, disks, the epidural space, or the paraspinal soft tissues, with paraspinal abscesses observed in up to three fourths of the cases. Abscesses must be treated immediately to prevent spinal deformity or neurologic damage. Patients with neurologic complications, epidural abscesses, failure of conservative therapy, and other indications need surgical treatment. Percutaneous drainage under CT guidance has been used for the treatment of abscesses outside the spinal canal. This study examined the use of CT-guided percutaneous catheter drainage of spondylodiskitic abscesses as an alternative to surgery.

Methods.—Over a 7½-year period, the investigators performed percutaneous catheter drainage of 33 spondylodiskitic abscesses in 21 patients. The patients were 16 men and 5 women, mean age 59.5. Drainage was indicated for abscesses larger than 1 to 2 cm that were located intradiskally, paravertebrally, or within the psoas muscle and were causing increased laboratory markers of inflammation. Drainage was not performed in patients in whom solid paravertebral or paraspinal granulation tissue was associated with small, low-attenuating fluid collections or in those in whom epidural or intrathecal abscesses were causing spinal cord compression. Drainage catheters remained in place for as long as secretion was apparent and irrigation revealed purulent or turbid fluid. Follow-up, including routine CT scans, continued for at least 6 months.

Results.—There were 9 intradiskal, 12 paravertebral, and 12 psoas muscle abscesses. All were successfully drained, with no complications. Evacuation of the abscess cavity was followed by clinical improvement over a period of days, with subsidence of pain and inflammatory markers. There were no recurrences, although 9 of the 21 patients required 2 or 3 drainages. A specific organism was identified in 76% of the patients, most frequently *Mycobacterium tuberculosis* and *Staphylococcus aureus.*

Conclusions.—CT-guided percutaneous drainage appears to be a safe and efficient alternative to surgery for the management of spondylodiskitic abscesses. Paravertebral and intradiskal abscesses can be managed by catheter drainage; surgery is required for patients with epidural abscesses causing neurologic compromise, impingement of the spinal cord or cauda equina, or spinal instability. The causative organism must be isolated to ensure correct diagnosis and proper treatment of the spondylodiskitis. This technique could be particularly valuable for critically ill patients or those at high risk of surgical complications.

► The authors show that paraspinal and intradiskal infections can be successfully drained in the absence of surgery. This procedure is an effective alternative to surgical therapy. The authors of course exclude patients with epidural or intrathecal abscess formation and spinal cord compression. CT-guided drainage seems to be ideal for this procedure.

M.K. Dalinka, M.D.

The Association of Radiographically Detected Vertebral Fractures With Back Pain and Function: A Prospective Study

Nevitt MC, Ettinger B, Black DM, et al (Univ of California, San Francisco; Kaiser Permanente Med Care Program, Oakland, Calif; Univ of Minnesota, Minneapolis)

Ann Intern Med 128:793-800, 1998 3–15

Introduction.—About one third of vertebral fractures in elderly women are evaluated medically, which suggests that most vertebral fractures are not symptomatic. Attitudes about back pain in older women and access to health care may determine whether vertebral fractures receive medical attention. The effect of incident vertebral fractures on back pain and back-related functional limitations was assessed prospectively in a large community-based sample of elderly women who underwent serial spinal radiography and annual assessment of back pain and disability.

Methods.—Seven thousand two hundred twenty-three white women aged 65 and older underwent lateral spine radiographs at baseline and at follow-up examinations an average of 3.7 years later. Prevalent and incident radiographic vertebral fractures were evaluated by quantitative morphometry. Participants completed annual questionnaires regarding the frequency and severity of back pain, disability in performing activities involving the back, days of bed rest, and days of activity limited by back pain.

Results.—In women without a vertebral fracture at baseline, those with at least 1 incident vertebral fracture were more likely to experience increased back pain, back disability, at least 1 day of bed rest because of back pain, and 7 days of limited activity because of back pain per year. In women with a fracture at baseline, those with an incident vertebral fracture were at increased risk for back pain, back disability, at least 1 day of bed rest, and 7 days of limited activity yearly. Women with incident fractures had nearly 10 additional limited activity days and 1-2 days of bed rest yearly. New vertebral fractures not receiving medical attention were correlated with increased back pain and functional limitation.

Conclusion.—New vertebral fractures, even those not detected clinically, were correlated with substantial increases in back pain and functional limitation.

Clinical Significance.—New vertebral fractures, even painful ones, are typically unrecognized by older women and their physicians. Older women with back pain and accompanying decreased functional ability should be assessed for vertebral osteoporosis.

▶ This important article discusses the frequency of undetected vertebral fractures in elderly women and the associated morbidity. The authors make a strong case for the performance of bone densitometry in elderly patients with new-onset back pain.

M.K. Dalinka, M.D.

Selective Cervical Spine Radiography in Blunt Trauma: Methodology of the National Emergency X-Radiography Utilization Study (NEXUS)

Hoffman JR, Wolfson AB, Todd K, et al (Univ of California, Los Angeles; Univ of Pittsburgh, Pa; Emory Univ, Atlanta, Ga)

Ann Emerg Med 32:461-469, 1998 3–16

Introduction.—Most victims of multiple blunt trauma undergo radiographic imaging of the spine, prompted by fears of missed cervical spine injury. As a result of this practice, a large number of patients are exposed to x-rays, at high overall cost, to detect cervical spine injuries in a few. Studies have suggested certain clinical characteristics are associated with a minimal risk of cervical spine injuries. A design of a large, nationwide study to test these criteria—the National Emergency X-Radiography Utilization Study (NEXUS)—is reported.

NEXUS Methods.—At study centers, all blunt trauma victims will be assessed for 4 criteria associated with a low risk of cervical spine injury before spinal imaging studies are performed. The criteria are: absence of neurologic abnormalities, with normal alertness and no focal deficits;

BOX.—Instructions to Participating Physicians

1. Altered neurologic function is present if *any* of the following is present: (a) Glasgow Coma Scale score of 14 or less; (b) disorientation to person, place, time, or events; (c) inability to remember 3 objects at 5 minutes; (d) delayed or inappropriate response to external stimuli; or (e) any focal deficit on motor or sensory examination. Patients with none of these individual findings should be classified as having normal neurologic function.
2. Patients should be considered intoxicated if they have either of the following: (a) a recent history of intoxication or intoxicating ingestion; or (b) evidence of intoxication on physical examination. Patients may also be considered to be intoxicated if tests of bodily secretions are positive for drugs that affect level of alertness, including a blood alcohol level greater than .08 mg/dL.
3. Midline posterior bony cervical spine tenderness is present if the patient complains of pain on palpation of the posterior midline neck from the nuchal ridge to the prominence of the first thoracic vertebra, or if the patient evinces pain with direct palpation of any cervical spinous process.
4. Patients should be considered to have a distracting painful injury if they have any of the following: (a) a long bone fracture; (b) a visceral injury requiring surgical consultation; (c) a large laceration, degloving injury, or crush injury; (d) large burns; or (e) any other injury producing acute functional impairment. Physicians may also classify any injury as distracting if it is thought to have the potential to impair the patient's ability to appreciate other injuries.

(Courtesy of Hoffman JR, Wolfson AB, Todd K, et al: Selective cervical spine radiography in blunt trama: Methodology of the national emergency x-radiography utilization study (NEXUS). *Ann Emergency Med* 32:461-467, 1998.)

absence of evidence of intoxication; absence of posterior midline cervical spine tenderness; and absence of other distracting, painful injuries (Box). After this assessment, the decision to perform spine imaging is up to the discretion of emergency department (ED) clinicians. However, no spinal imaging studies may be performed before the presence or absence of the low-risk criteria have been documented. The studies may not be performed without proper forms, which can be generated only after data entry has been completed, although data entry should never interfere with patient care. Patients may be designated "unstable" if such delay is deemed inappropriate.

No rigid definitions of the low-risk criteria will be supplied to ensure their wide applicability. When spinal imaging is performed, it should include at least 3 standard views: cross-table lateral, anteroposterior, and open-mouth odontoid. Oblique views, flexion-extension views, cervical CT, or other studies may be performed as indicated. All images obtained, including inpatient studies, will be used to make the diagnosis. To prove the criteria clinically reliable, they will need to have negative predictive value and sensitivity of 100%. Patients who meet 1 or more of the criteria and are diagnosed as having cervical spine injury will be considered true positives; those who meet none of the criteria but do have cervical injury will be considered false negatives.

Discussion.—A prospective, multicenter trial of this type is essential to determine whether clinical judgment can identify all cervical spine injuries in multiple trauma patients, at the same time reducing the number of radiographic spinal studies performed. To reach the target level of statistical significance, a sample size of nearly 50,000 patients will be required. If the selective criteria prove effective, they may cut the number of blunt trauma patients requiring radiographic studies by one third. This could save nearly $60 million per year, as well as avoid radiation exposure and risk of thyroid malignancy. Sources of bias must be carefully avoided, including workup bias.

► Although one could find a number of criticisms, I believe it is an ambitious and worthwhile project. For those who practice with busy EDs in level 1 trauma centers, it is hard to see how to enforce refusing studies in unstable patients until certain forms are completed. A tremendous commitment by the heads of the emergency and trauma services is necessary to see that the forms are completed in a timely fashion.

M.K. Dalinka, M.D.

Usefulness of MRI in Isolated Upper Cervical Spine Fractures in Adults

Vaccaro AR, Kreidl KO, Pan W, et al (Thomas Jefferson Univ, Philadelphia)
J Spinal Disord 11:289-293, 1998 3–17

Objective.—More than 15% of adult patients hospitalized for spinal injury have isolated fractures of the upper cervical spine. MRI has come into widespread use for evaluation of the spinal cord in trauma patients. This study analyzed the value of routine MRI in patients with isolated upper cervical spine fracture.

Methods.—During a 36-month period, all patients with isolated upper cervical spine fracture at a regional spinal cord injury center underwent MRI to identify potentially unstable ligamentous injuries. Studies were performed regardless of the patients' neurologic examination results. To be included in the study, patients had to have undergone MRI within 48 hours of the traumatic event. Fifty-five of 132 patients with upper cervical spine injury met this criterion. A radiologist and orthopedic surgeon independently reviewed the scans and studied and compared the findings with those of the neurologic examination. The impact of the MRI scans on the patients' clinical management was analyzed.

Results.—Ninety-three percent of patients had no neurologic deficit on physical examination. None of these patients were found to have ligamentous, disk, or spinal cord lesions on MRI. In all 4 patients with neurologic evidence of cervical spine injury, MRI precisely identified the location of the injury. For the neurologically intact patients, MRI did not affect the treatment plan. The MRI finding of ligamentous disruption also did not affect treatment, as these patients were already undergoing external immobilization. In 1 of the 4 patients with neurologic abnormality, the MRI finding of cord compression and edema led to spinal stabilization.

Conclusions.—For patients with isolated cervical spine fracture, routine MRI scanning does not appear to be indicated in the absence of neurologic abnormalities. It is not a cost-effective screening device, and it provides no new information relevant to patient management. It may be used in patients considered for stabilization procedures involving potential risk to the extracranial vessels. MRI scanning is useful in localizing the spinal cord lesion in patients with neurologic deficits.

► This article concludes that patients with isolated upper cervical spine fractures without a neurologic deficit do not require an MRI. In the authors' series of 55 patients with upper cervical spine fractures, only 4 had symptoms. Those without a neurologic deficit had no ligamentous, discal, or cord-disease on cervical MRI imaging. The authors later state that the identification of ligamentous disruption did not influence treatment. This is a difficult statement to make when the authors saw no ligamentous injury in these patients without symptoms. MR influenced treatment in only 1 of the 4 patients with symptoms.

The major problem is the lack of follow-up. How many of these patients later developed symptoms and required further therapy? It is well known that patients with upper cervical spine injuries who present in the ER are frequently without neurologic deficit, because most of the patients with severe neurologic injury of the upper cervical spine do not survive.

M.K. Dalinka, M.D.

Cervical Spine Degenerative Diseases: An Evaluation of Clinical and Imaging Features in Surgical Decisions

Soo MYS, Tran-Dinh HD, Dorsch NWC, et al (Westmead Hosp, NSW, Australia)

Australas Radiol 41:351-356, 1997 3–18

Purpose.—Imaging studies play an important role in treatment decision-making for patients with cervical myelopathy and radiculopathy caused by spinal degenerative disease. CT myelography (CTM) and MRI can demonstrate the degree of spinal cord compression and other abnormalities. It has been suggested that the best indicator of a good surgical result in patients with compressive myelopathy is the transverse cord area at the level of maximal compression. However, the significance of radiologic evidence of cord compression in patients with spondylotic myelopathy and radiculopathy is unknown. This study evaluated the clinical value of these radiologic parameters in surgical decision-making for patients with cervical spine degenerative disease.

Methods.—The retrospective study included 44 patients undergoing cervical CTM, including 20 with clinical spondylotic myelopathy and 24 with radiculopathy. On review of the CTM scans, the level of maximal spinal cord compression was identified (Fig 2). If the scans showed uniform degenerative disease across several levels, then cord compression was measured at C5/C6. Duration of illness was defined as the time from symptom onset to the time of CTM.

Results.—Twenty-seven patients underwent surgery. Spinal cord area differed significantly between patients who did and did not undergo decompressive surgery. Mean cord area in patients with myelopathy undergoing decompressive surgery was 50.8 mm^2. All patients with myelopathy had tight canal stenosis involving 1 particular level. In patients with diffuse spondylosis, the degrees of stenosis in the maximally affected area was the main determinant of the need for surgery. Symptom severity was significantly associated with both the likelihood of surgery and with cord area. Older patients were more likely to undergo surgery; age was negatively correlated with cord area. Two thirds of patients undergoing surgery had soft tissue and bone changes leading to canal stenosis. A few patients had abnormal signals within the affected cord, which did not affect the likelihood of surgery.

Conclusions.—In patients with spondylotic myelopathy, the reduction in transverse cervical cord area at the level of maximal compression—as demonstrated by CTM—is a key factor in surgical decision-making. Clinical variables, including age, duration of illness, and number of levels involved, seem less important. The results suggest that developmental narrowing plays a role in the genesis of spondylotic myelopathy. This study is unique because the decision whether to perform surgery is used as an endpoint.

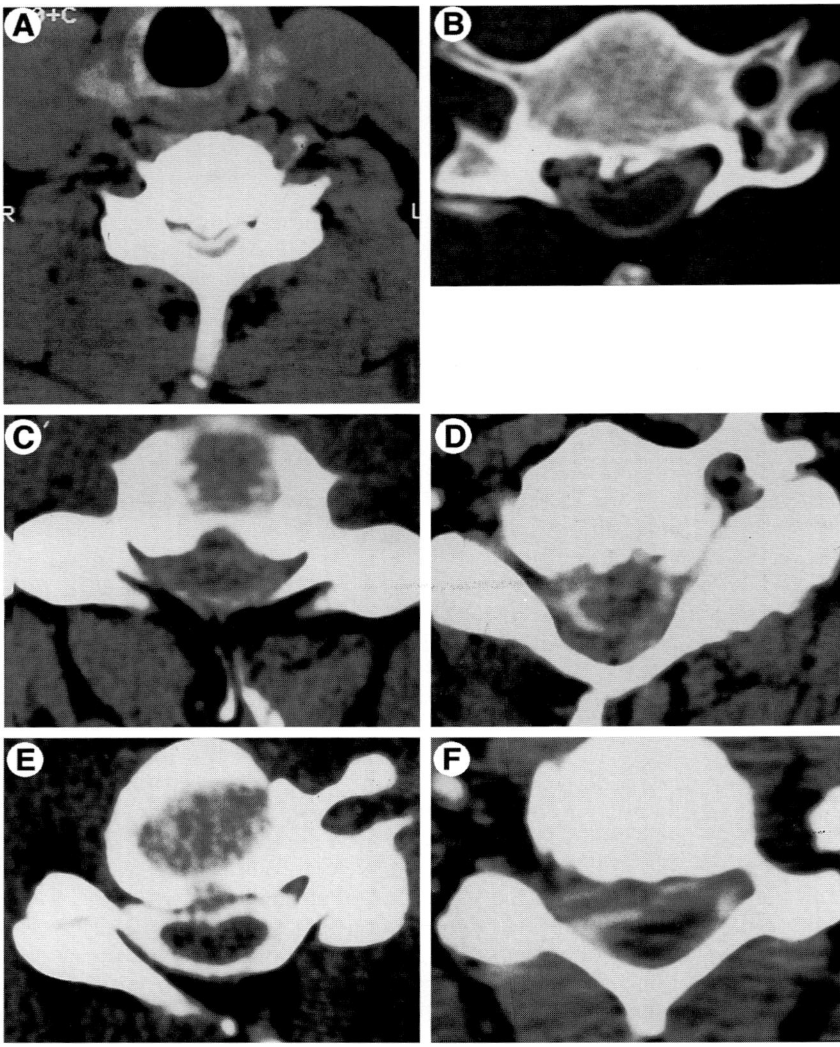

FIGURE 2.—A, Banana-shaped compressed cord. B, Deformed and compressed cord caused by posterior osteophyte. C, Thecal sac and cord deformity caused by bilateral uncovertebral spurs. D, Posterior disk bulge and flaval ligament hypertrophy creating uniform cord compression. E, Virtually normal-shaped cord with some anterior thecal sac narrowing. F, Unilateral thecal sac and cord deformity caused by a posterolateral disk protrusion on the right side. (Courtesy of Soo MYS, Tran-Dinh HD, Dorsch NWC, et al: Cervical spine degenerative diseases: An evaluation of clinical and imaging features in surgical decisions. *Australas Radiol* 41:351-356, 1997).

► This interesting article from Australia evaluates 44 patients retrospectively with surgery as the end point or gold standard. The authors concluded that the decreased area of the spinal cord was the most important criteria for decompressive surgery in patients with spondylotic myelopathy. In their series, there was no association between the duration of symptoms and the decision to operate. Abnormal signal within the affected spinal cord did not alter management strategies.

M.K. Dalinka, M.D.

Differentiating Lumbar Disc Protrusions, Disc Bulges, and Discs With Normal Contour but Abnormal Signal Intensity: Magnetic Resonance Imaging With Discographic Correlations

Milette PC, Fontaine S, Lepanto L, et al (Centre Hospitalier de l'Université de Montréal)

Spine 24:44-53, 1999 3–19

Introduction.—MRI and CT reports use identical terminology in describing lumbar disk abnormalities, which are based on the morphology of the disk contour with the terms *normal, bulge, protrusion*, and *extrusion*. To investigate the fundamental characteristics of common lumbar disk abnormalities, MRIs were correlated with the anatomic and clinical findings of diskography to assess the validity of a particular nomenclature. An attempt was made to define the anatomic and clinical differences between disk protrusions, disk bulges, and disc with normal contour but abnormal signal intensity on T2-weighted MRIs.

Methods.—Forty-five patients, ranging in age from 22 to 64 years, who had low back pain, with or without radiating pain to the lower extremities, for 2 to 34 years, were studied. MRIs were evaluated for central and peripheral signal characteristics, height, contour, and nerve-root compression. Degrees of disk degeneration, disruption, and pain reproduction were used to classify diskograms.

Results.—Disk disruptions extending into or beyond the outer anulus on diskograms and loss of intervertebral height or abnormal signal intensity on MRIs were found. Stage 2 or 3 anular disruptions were associated with all 23 protrusions (100%) and 12 of 15 disk bulges (80%). Most had similar or exact reproduction of pain during disk injection. With respect to degree of disk degeneration, extent of disruptions, or presence of diskogenic pain, there were no significant differences between disk protrusion, disk bulges, and disks with normal contour but abnormal signal.

Conclusion.—Symptomatic tears extending into or beyond the outer anulus are highly predicted by loss of disk height or abnormal signal intensity in patients with chronic low back pain. Disk protrusions or disk bulges do not represent disks with significantly different internal architecture, nor do they represent symptomatic tears.

► This article was written by members of a well-known neuroradiology group and was extremely disturbing. Selected patients with MR findings of disk degeneration, disk protrusions, and disk bulges underwent diskography. The reproduction of pain by disk injection was extremely high in all cases, and the positive predictive value for disk disruption was greater than 80% with any of these findings. Considering the high incidence of asymptomatic disk protrusions, bulges, and degeneration in the population, this finding is astounding and requires independent confirmation in a large number of patients.

M.K. Dalinka, M.D.

Foot and Ankle

A Pooled Analysis of the Ottawa Ankle Rules Used on Adults in the ED

Markert RJ, Walley ME, Guttman TG, et al (Wright State Univ, Dayton, Ohio)
Am J Emerg Med 16:564-567, 1998 3–20

Objective.—The Ottawa ankle rules were developed as an aid to clinical decision-making in emergency evaluation of ankle and foot injuries. The goal is to identify patients in whom radiography can be avoided without compromising patient outcomes. In the original rules, ankle radiography is recommended in patients with pain near the malleoli and with at least 1 of the following: age 55 or older, inability to bear weight, and bone tenderness. Foot radiography is recommended for patients with midfoot pain and bone tenderness. The rules were later modified to eliminate age as a criterion for ankle radiography. The recommendation for foot radiography was changed to pain in the midfoot plus inability to bear weight and bone tenderness at the navicular or base of the fifth metatarsal. An analysis of pooled data from 7 previous studies of the Ottawa ankle rules was performed.

Findings.—With radiography as the gold standard, the Ottawa ankle rules showed excellent performance in ruling out a fractured ankle or foot, with a combined sensitivity of 97% or higher and negative predictive value of greater than 99%. However, with specificity of 31% to 63% and positive predictive value of less than 20%, they performed poorly in ruling in a fracture.

Conclusions.—Available data suggest that the Ottawa ankle rules are a useful clinical practice guideline for the diagnosis of ankle and foot injuries in adult patients in the emergency department (ED). The rules are highly effective in ruling out foot or ankle fracture—when the findings are negative, fracture is highly unlikely. Ankle or foot radiographs are recommended only for patients who satisfy the Ottawa criteria. However, the rules should not be used to rule in fracture. In the busy ED environment, use of the Ottawa ankle rules shifts the emphasis from examination of a radiograph to examination of the patient.

▶ This article pooled the results of 7 large studies on the use of the Ottawa ankle rules and it shows how effective the rules can be in eliminating unnecessary radiographs. The American College of Radiology appropriateness guidelines also recommend the use of these rules before ordering ankle or foot radiographs in the emergency room.

Unfortunately, these rules are often not followed. There are a number of reasons for this: ordering of films by triage nurses, decompression by a busy emergency room, and patient demand. In addition, we often see ankle and foot radiographs ordered when only 1 is necessary. We are hopeful that a decrease in unnecessary examinations will occur in the future as it did for skull and rib films.

M.K. Dalinka, M.D.

The Snowboarder's Foot and Ankle

Kirkpatrick DP, Hunter RE, Janes PC, et al (North Country Orthopaedic Surgery and Sports Medicine, Queensbury, NY; Orthopaedic Associates of Aspen and Glenwood, Colo; Summit-Vail Orthopaedics and Sports Medicine, Frisco; et al)

Am J Sports Med 26:271-277, 1998 3–21

Background.—The popularity of snowboarding is increasing. Definite patterns of injury have been reported in ankle trauma sustained during snowboarding. Fractures of the lateral process of the talus, a fracture pattern previously believed to be rare, have been noted. The current prospective study determined the type and distribution of foot and ankle snowboarding injuries.

Methods and Findings.—Data on 3,213 snowboarding injuries occurring between 1988 and 1995 were analyzed. Four hundred ninety-one (15.3%) were ankle injuries, and 58 (1.8%) were foot injuries. Forty-four percent of the ankle injuries were fractures, and 52% were sprains. Fifty-seven percent of the foot injuries were fractures, and 28% were sprains. The remainder were soft-tissue injuries, contusions, or abrasions. Boot

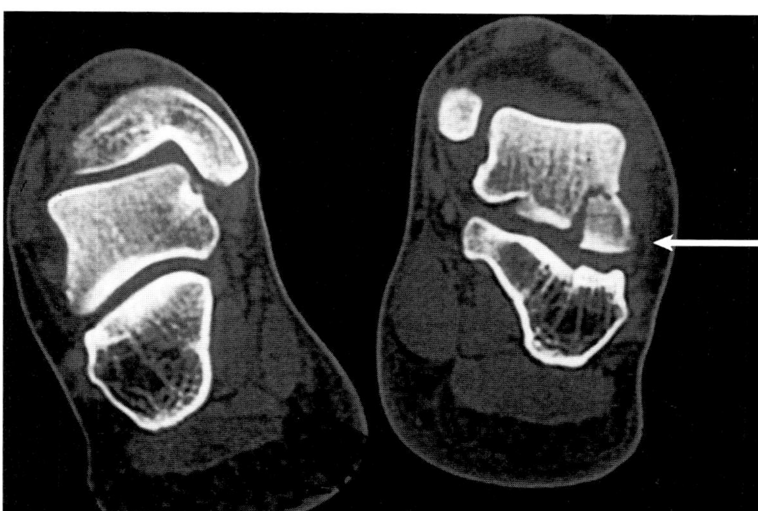

FIGURE 3.—C, a CT scan of the ankle shows a displaced interarticular fracture of the lateral processes (*arrow*); the opposite foot shows normal anatomy. (Courtesy of Kirkpatrick DP, Hunter RE, Janes PC, et al: The snowboarder's foot and ankle. *Am J Sports Med* 26:271-277, 1998.)

type was not correlated with overall foot or ankle injury rate, however. Significantly fewer ankle sprains occurred in patients wearing hybrid boots, and fewer fractures of the talar lateral process occurred in patients wearing soft boots. The number of fractures of the lateral process of talus was surprisingly high, constituting 2.3% of all snowboarding injuries, 15% of all ankle injuries, and 34% of all ankle fractures. Many of these fractures were not apparent on plain radiographs and the diagnosis was made by CT (Fig 3).

Conclusions.—Clinicians must maintain a high index of suspicion for occult fractures in patients with anterolateral ankle pain in snowboarders. Subtle fractures that may need surgical treatment should not be mistaken for anterior talofibular ligament sprains.

▶ This article points out the frequency of foot and ankle injuries in snowboarders. Fractures of the lateral process of the talus are not uncommon in snowboarders and are difficult to see on routine radiography. These fractures are best diagnosed by CT. Awareness of this injury should lead to earlier diagnosis and a decrease in late morbidity.

M.K. Dalinka, M.D.

Tumors

Chondromyxoid Fibroma of Bone: A Clinicopathologic Review of 278 Cases

Wu CT, Inwards CY, O'Laughlin S, et al (Mayo Clinic and Mayo Found, Rochester, Minn)

Hum Pathol 29:438-446, 1998 3–22

Background.—Chondromyxoid fibroma is a rare, benign bone tumor, with a classic histologic picture of stellate or spindle-shaped cells arranged in lobules on a myxoid background. Chondromyxoid fibroma is histologically similar to chondroblastoma, which may cause diagnostic difficulties. A large series of patients with chondromyxoid fibroma was reviewed.

Patients.—The study included 278 patients with chondromyxoid fibroma: 145 males and 132 females. The average age was 31 years, with about half the patients being in the second or third decade of life. Forty-seven percent of tumors were found in the long bones, 30% in the flat bones, 17% in the bones of the hands and feet, and 5% in the skull and facial bones. The small bones of the feet were affected 5 times more often than the bones of the hand, and the lower limbs nearly 6 times more often than the upper limbs.

There were 32 known local recurrences, with 30% of the recurrences showing soft-tissue tumor nodules. Two patients had malignant transformation of chondromyxoid fibroma.

Radiographic Findings.—Review of radiographs in 192 cases showed that tumors affecting the long bones were usually eccentric. The metaphysis was solely involved in 68% of tumors; it was involved in 88% of long bone tumors overall. The matrix was purely radiolucent in 87% of tumors.

Ninety percent showed cortical thinning, whereas 85% showed cortical expansion. Part of the cortex was missing in about half the cases.

Pathologic Findings.—Fifteen percent of tumors were associated with reactive new bone formation, although not enough to suggest a bone-forming tumor. Nine percent of tumors were associated with secondary aneurysmal bone cysts. Soft-tissue extension was noted in 31% of cases, trabecular bone permeation in 9%, and cortical permeation in 0.4%. In most cases, the myxoid matrix appeared solid and pale blue, without the liquefaction associated with myxoid changes in chondrosarcoma. However, 39% of tumors were associated with focal liquefactive change. Eighteen percent included tumor cells with bizarre histologic features; this finding was more common in tumors involving the small bones of the hands and feet.

Discussion.—Chondromyxoid fibroma is a very rare bone tumor most commonly affecting the proximal tibia. Its name indicates chondroid differentiation, and focal hyaline cartilage is found in about one fifth of cases; however, hyaline cartilage of the type seen in chondroma or chondrosarcoma is rarely observed. Chondromyxoid fibroma may be associated with microscopic foci of calcification, which are probably unrecognized on radiographs. More than 10% of cases may show mitotic figures. The distinction between chondroblastoma and chondromyxoid fibroma is difficult to make, but does not appear clinically significant. The authors use the former term for epiphyseal lesions and the latter for metaphyseal lesions.

► This article provides a very nice review of a large number of cases of an unusual neoplasm. The authors' series was almost three fourths of the total number of previously reported cases.

M.K. Dalinka, M.D.

Accuracy of CT-Guided Needle Biopsy of Musculoskeletal Neoplasms

Dupuy DE, Rosenberg AE, Punyaratabandhu T, et al (Massachusetts Gen Hosp, Boston)

AJR 171:759-762, 1998 3–23

Background.—With an accuracy of 98%, open biopsy is considered the gold standard for obtaining diagnostic tissue of connective tumors. However, open biopsy can be risky and difficult. Although needle biopsy and fine-needle aspiration are less painful, less hazardous, and usually do not require general anesthesia or hospitalization, their accuracy rates are only 61% to 96%. The accuracy of CT-guided biopsy of musculoskeletal neoplasms was determined.

Methods.—From 1992 through 1994, 176 core-needle biopsies and 45 fine-needle aspirations were performed, using CT guidance, in patients with musculoskeletal lesions. Biopsy diagnosis was compared with final diagnosis at the time of definitive treatment.

Findings.—Needle biopsy had an accuracy of 93%, and fine-needle aspiration had an accuracy of 80%. Both techniques had a complication rate of less than 1%. The accuracy rate was 87% for primary malignancy, 75% for round-cell lesion, 94% for local recurrence, and 100% for metastatic carcinoma. Mismatch rates in soft-tissue and bone lesions were similar. Accuracy was reduced for round-cell lesions (20%) and lesions in the spine or perivertebral region (20%). Eight percent of the patients had specimens that were nondiagnostic or insufficient.

Conclusions.—Needle biopsy is efficient, safe, and convenient in the approach to musculoskeletal lesions. With reasonable expertise in musculoskeletal radiology and pathology, CT guidance can markedly improve the positive yield rate, allowing access to tumors in locations that are hard to reach.

► This article is from a topnotch group with considerable expertise in musculoskeletal radiology and pathology. The results are extremely encouraging because of the high accuracy and low complication rate of fine-needle aspiration and core biopsy under CT guidance. This is an excellent area of radiologic growth for those whose hospitals offer expertise in musculoskeletal radiology, cytology, and musculoskeletal pathology.

M.K. Dalinka, M.D.

Evaluation of Fluorodeoxyglucose Positron Emission Tomography in the Management of Soft-Tissue Sarcomas

Lucas JD, O'Doherty MJ, Wong JCH, et al (St Thomas' Hosp, London)

J Bone Joint Surg Br 80-B:441-447, 1998 3–24

Background.—Metastases after the treatment of soft-tissue sarcomas are common, with about one third of patients developing local or distant recurrences (particularly to the lung). Local recurrences can be evaluated with magnetic resonance imaging (MRI) and computed tomography (CT), but identifying distant metastases is difficult because of their wide possible distribution. This study compared the utility of ^{18}F-fluorodeoxyglucose (FDG) PET with that of MRI and CT in detecting local and distant metastases in patients with soft-tissue sarcoma.

Methods.—The subjects were 62 patients (34 men and 28 women, mean age at diagnosis, 50 years 11 months) with soft-tissue sarcoma. Liposarcoma (n = 18) and synovial sarcoma (n = 12) were the most common tumors. Patients were evaluated with whole-body FDG (350 MBq) PET, contrast-enhanced T1-weighted MRI of the local site, and contrast-enhanced CT of the chest to identify distant metastases, a mean of 3 years, 2 months after primary tumor treatment. Recurrences were confirmed histologically.

Findings.—For the detection of local recurrence, there were 72 FDG PET scans for comparison with 67 MRI scans. FDG PET indicated 14 true positive findings, 3 false positive findings, and 5 false negative findings, for a sensitivity of 73.7% and a specificity of 94.3%. Magnetic resonance imaging indicated 15 true positive findings, 2 false positive findings, and 2 false negative findings, for a sensitivity of 88.2% and a specificity of 96%. For the detection of distant recurrence, there were 70 FDG PET scans for comparison with 70 CT scans of the chest. Fluorodeoxyglucose PET indicated 13 true positive findings, 0 false positive findings, and 2 false negative findings, for a sensitivity of 86.7% and a specificity of 100%. CT indicated 15 true positive findings, 2 false positive findings, and 0 false negative findings, for a sensitivity of 100% and a specificity of 96.4%. Furthermore, the whole-body FDG PET scan identified 13 additional areas of distant metastases. Lung metastases were also present in 7 cases. Distant areas included the thigh, arm, liver, ribs, left adrenal gland, retroperitoneum, lymph node, spine, and anterior chest wall.

Conclusions.—The specificity and accuracy of whole-body FDG PET in identifying local and distant recurrences were comparable to those of MRI and CT. PET is attractive because it is a 1-step procedure that images the entire body, and indeed PET identified distant metastases that might not be found with CT. Nonetheless, the most prudent approach to staging disease and identifying metastases seems to be a combination of MRI, CT, and FDG PET.

► This retrospective analysis of FDG PET suggests that this technique may be valuable in the detection of metastatic disease. However, PET was inferior to CT in detecting lung metastases and inferior to MRI in detecting local recurrence. The authors believe that PET is of considerable value in detecting extra-pulmonary visceral spread and may enable the evaluation of local and distant recurrences with a single study. These results are preliminary and require more data for confirmation.

I am intrigued by the fact that there were 15 local recurrences and all of them had been treated with marginal excision. This emphasizes the point that soft-tissue malignancies should be handled by an oncologic surgeon, and marginal excision is usually not the treatment of choice for malignant soft-tissue tumors.

M.K. Dalinka, M.D.

T1-weighted Magnetic Resonance Imaging in Breast Cancer Vertebral Metastases: Changes on Treatment and Correlation With Response to Therapy

Brown AL, Middleton G, Macvicar AD, et al (Royal Marsden NHS Trust, Sutton, Surrey, England)

Clin Radiol 53:493-501, 1998 3–25

Objective.—The spine is the most common site of skeletal metastases in patients with metastatic breast cancer. Metastatic breast cancer is considered an incurable disease, although multiple treatment options are available. MRI is sensitive for the detection of skeletal metastases, but its value in assessing treatment response is unknown. A single T1-weighted spinal MRI scan was evaluated for use in assessing treatment response in patients with spinal metastases from breast cancer. Patterns of morphologic change in the MRI appearance of vertebral metastases were assessed as well.

Methods.—The investigators reviewed 552 MRI's of the spine performed in patients with breast cancer over a 6-year period. Of these, a total of 109 scans in 41 patients detected vertebral metastases from biopsy-confirmed breast cancer. The number of scans per patient ranged from 2 to 7; the minimum interval between scans was 1 month. During the interval between scans, the patients underwent systemic or local therapy for vertebral metastases. Sagittal T1-weighted scans were evaluated in blinded fashion by 2 radiologists. Vertebral metastases were recognized by the finding of focally decreased signal intensity within the bone marrow. For each lesion, T1-weighted signal intensity before and after treatment was classified as low homogeneous, low heterogeneous, or high homogeneous. Treatment responses were categorized according to criteria of the International Union Against Cancer as disease regression, no change, and disease progression.

Results.—In a total of 68 intervals between scans, the number of lesions increased in 47% of the cases, remained unchanged in 53%, and decreased in none. Lesion size increased in 43% of the cases, remained unchanged in 54%, and decreased in 3%. In 65% of the intervals, lesion signal intensity remained unchanged. Almost all new metastases developing between MRI scans demonstrated low homogeneous signal intensity.

The overall response—evaluated by clinical, biochemical, radiographic, and scintigraphic findings—was disease progression in 57%, no change in 24%, and disease remission in 19%. In 63% of the intervals, the MRI response to therapy and the overall response to therapy were the same. Changes in T1-weighted signal intensity were unrelated to overall response to therapy, either systemic therapy or local radiotherapy.

Conclusions.—This study describes the morphologic MRI changes of vertebral metastases from breast cancer in response to treatment. The results suggest that T1-weighted spinal MRI predicts overall progression of metastases in 79% of the cases and stable disease in 75%, which compares favorably with other evaluation techniques. T1-weighted spinal MRI offers a quick and efficient technique for assessing response to treatment of metastatic breast cancer and can differentiate between patients with progressive disease and those with stable or regressing disease. As MRI scans were performed when clinically indicated in this study, a prospective trial is needed to tell whether MRI can distinguish between stable disease and disease remission.

► These authors present a retrospective review of cases in which MR was performed only when clinicians thought it was clinically indicated. The MRI accurately predicted progression in 79% of cases and stable disease in 75%. The clinical response to therapy and its concordance with radiographic and scintigraphic findings predicted progression in 81% of cases and stability in

72%. This is not a statistically significant improvement. A randomized prospective evaluation is necessary before accepting the authors' conclusions.

M.K. Dalinka, M.D.

Miscellaneous

Review of 3,530 Referrals for Bone Density Measurements of Spine and Femur: Evidence That Radiographic Osteopenia Predicts Low Bone Mass

Ahmed AIH, Ilic D, Blake GM, et al (Guy's Hosp, London)
Radiology 207:619-624, 1998 3–26

Background.—The goal of bone mineral density (BMD) measurement is to identify osteopenia at an early stage, thus preventing deterioration and the development of osteoporosis. The relationship between BMD measurement and the initial reason for referral to a BMD screening service was investigated.

Methods and Findings.—Of 3,530 women referred for BMD screening, referral letters for 3,479 were classified by screening indication. Mean BMD in each indication group was compared with the age-matched value from the local normal range. The most common reason for referral, present in the letters of 700 women, was to help guide decision making about hormone replacement treatment. The group referred because of radiographic evidence of osteopenia had the highest proportion of women with osteoporosis.

Conclusions.—In this series, radiographic evidence of osteopenia was a good predictor of osteoporosis. Osteopenia screening appears to be justified for such women, and for other women at high risk and those seeking a rationale for preventive therapy.

► The authors found that the best predictor of bone mass was the radiologic diagnosis of osteopenia. This is somewhat surprising because the plain film is unreliable in making this diagnosis in the absence of compression fractures. In this study, the history of previous fracture was less predictive of low bone mass than radiographically evident osteopenia, despite the known high intra- and interobserver error rate in the radiologic diagnosis of osteopenia. It is interesting that bone density measurements were ordered mainly by general practitioners in this study from England; in our institution, almost all studies are requested by specialists.

M.K. Dalinka, M.D.

Multifocal Osteonecrosis

LaPorte DM, Mont MA, Mohan V, et al (Johns Hopkins Univ, Baltimore, Md)
J Rheumatol 25:1968-1974, 1998 3–27

Background.—Osteonecrosis is debilitating when confined to 1 joint (most typically the hips, knees, or shoulders), but when it spreads to multiple sites, its effects can be devastating. These authors evaluated the clinical, demographic, and radiographic characteristics of patients with multifocal osteonecrosis to determine factors that could lead to earlier diagnosis and better treatment.

Methods.—Over 20 years, the authors evaluated 1,056 patients with osteonecrosis. Of these, 32 (3%; 8 men and 24 women, mean age 34) had multifocal osteonecrosis, defined as lesions at 3 or more separate anatomic sites. The demographic and clinical data of these 32 patients were analyzed, including the patients' use of corticosteroids, alcohol, and tobacco and any comorbid diseases. The time course of the disease was examined to identify which joints were affected first and to evaluate symptoms. Plain radiographs and MRI were used to determine where the lesions were and their presenting stage.

Findings.—All but 2 of the patients (94%) had used or were using corticosteroids; these 2 patients had a coagulopathy. Corticosteroids were used in 13 patients with systemic lupus erythematosus, 5 with inflammatory bowel disease, 3 renal transplant recipients, 4 patients with malignancy, 3 with pulmonary disease, 3 with glaucoma, and 1 with spinal stenosis. Also, 10 patients (32%) were smokers, and 4 (8%) had a history of alcohol use. The total number of osteonecrotic lesions was 201, for a mean of 6.3 lesions per patient. Each of the patients had bilateral lesions at the femoral head, and all but 2 patients had bilateral knee lesions (these 2 patients had unilateral knee involvement). Osteonecrosis was also very common at the shoulder (28 patients) and ankle (8 patients). Most patients (22, or 69%) had multiple joint or hip symptoms when first seen, but 8 patients (25%) were first seen with only knee symptoms. The hips were affected first in 41% of patients, second in 34%, and third in 35%. The knees were affected first in 35% of patients, second in 22%, and third in 40%. The shoulders were affected first in 13% of patients, second in 34%, and third in 25%. Symptoms were present in all the knees involved, in 92% of the shoulders involved, but in only 78% of the hips. Radiographs showed that most of the joints (77%) were at a pre-collapse stage.

Conclusions.—Patients with osteonecrosis of the knee, shoulder, or ankle must be evaluated for multifocal disease, because about half these patients will have involvement at other anatomic sites. The hip was not symptomatic in all patients, but all patients had hip involvement, so all patients with osteonecrosis should be evaluated for hip lesions. The high use of corticosteroids in these patients suggests that these drugs are strongly associated with multifocal osteonecrosis.

► The major value of this article is in the large number of patients studied and in the attempt at putting a new twist on an old subject. The demographic data are interesting and important. The authors stress the bilaterality of osteonecrosis and its incidence, which is best gauged by MR (plain films and nuclear medicine studies underestimated this occurrence). The authors' experience is similar to my own in that the vast majority (94%) of patients with multifocal osteonecrosis were on steroids.

The authors suggest that patients with osteonecrosis in areas other than the hip should have MRIs to determine the presence or absence of osteonecrosis elsewhere. In these days of cost containment, it may be difficult to justify this, particularly when there are few data available on the effectiveness of early treatment. In the hip (for which more data are available), considerable controversy remains.

M.K. Dalinka, M.D.

4 Pediatric Radiology

Introduction

I am pleased to welcome two expert super-specialist contributors to the pediatric radiology chapter of the 1999 YEAR BOOK OF DIAGNOSTIC RADIOLOGY. Dr. Alan Oestreich of Cincinnati Children's Hospital, brings a fresh and incisive style to the pediatric musculoskeletal selections and comments. Dr. Tina Young Poussaint of Boston Children's Hospital, adds practical experience and perspective to the neuroradiological selections and comments.

Five categories are again used, although slightly modified from last year: neurological, musculoskeletal, respiratory/vascular, gastrointestinal, and genitourinary. Among the "hot topics" from these categories are: MR findings of perinatal asphyxia and hypoxic encephalopathy that have outcome predictive value; MR lymphangiography for vascular anomalies; voiding US with echo enhancement for vesicoureteric reflux; and gadolinium-enhanced MR imaging for childhood pyelonephritis.

There are many other noteworthy topics in each category. The neurological category includes articles on cytotoxic edema and neonatal stroke; frontoethmoidal encephaloceles; hydrocephalus and craniosynostosis; CNS candidiasis; subdural empyema; cerebral vasculopathy with cervicofacial hemangioma; intracranial ependymomas; MR in idiopathic growth hormone deficiency; and PET imaging of sickle cell cerebral vasculopathy. The musculoskeletal category includes wonkon the metacarpal sign in Rett syndrome; vagaries of human sternal development; heterogeneous Klippel-Feil syndrome; enhanced MRI of dysplastic hip sequelae; US of patellar abnormalities, of Perthes' disease, and in sickle cell crisis; MRI of sacroiliitis; enhanced MRI of juvenile chronic arthritis; imaging vagaries of Langerhans' cell histiocytosis; Little Leaguer's shoulder; MRI measurement of rotation in scoliosis; and coronal classification of scoliosis. The respiratory/vascular category includes articles on MRI of the left circumflex aortic arch; the braided bronchus; cogenital thymic cysts; roentgenography in adenoidal obstruction; probable cytomegalovirs-caused Wilson-Mikity syndrome; ehrlichiosis; congenital pyriform fossa sinus and acute supportive thyroiditis; and "status asthmaticus" presentation and tracheal schwannoma. The gastrointestinal category includes discussions of interstitial cells of Cajal and neonatal intestinal pseudo-obstruction; gastric cystic duplication and recurrent pancreatitis; intestinal malrotation in polysplenia/asplenia syndromes; imaging of complicated Meckel diverticula; CT of retropsoas hernia; MRI of nonperforated acute appendicitis; and dynamic enhanced MRI of infantile hepatic hemangioendothelioma. The genitourinary category includes wonkon VCUG in ureteral sciatic hernia; testicular cystic dysplasia and multicystic renal dysplasia; color Doppler US and scintigraphy of the acute scrotum; imaging of nephroblastomatosis; and genetics and imaging of second malignant neoplasms.

Read! It should stimulate ever more learning. It can change your life.

Lionel W. Young, M.D.

Neurological

Prediction of Neuromotor Outcome in Perinatal Asphyxia: Evaluation of MR Scoring Systems

Barkovich AJ, Hajnal BL, Vigneron D, et al (Univ of California, San Francisco)
AJNR 19:143-149, 1998 4–1

Background.—MRI has been reported to be useful in the early assessment of brain injury in asphyxiated neonates. Although scoring systems have been developed to evaluate imaging findings and compare them with clinical outcome, none of the investigators have devised and compared scoring systems using different imaging sequences to assess asphyxia in the first days after birth. A scoring system for the evaluation of perinatal asphyxia as seen on MR images was presented.

Methods.—The basal ganglia (BG) score, watershed (W) score, combined BG and W (BG/W) score, and the summation score of BG and W scores were derived. Three MR sequences (T1-weighted, first-echo T2-weighted, and second-echo T2-weighted) were obtained for each patient for each scoring system. Neuromotor examinations were done when the infants were 3 and 12 months of age. Cognitive development was tested at 12 months.

Findings.—The most useful score for predicting neuromotor outcome at 3 and 12 months, as well as cognitive outcome at 12 months, was the BG/W score obtained with the first-echo T2-weighted sequence. T1-weighted and first-echo T2-weighted sequences were more strongly associated with outcome in patients undergoing imaging in the first postnatal week; and second-echo T2-weighted sequences were more strongly associated with outcome in patients imaged in the second postnatal week.

Conclusion.—Using the BG/W score, MRI can accurately discriminate between patients with good and poor neuromotor and cognitive outcomes at 3 and 12 months. The first-echo T2-weighted sequence appears to discriminate best between infants with good and poor outcomes at 3 and 12 months.

► The authors propose an MR scoring system for predicting neuromotor outcome in infants with perinatal asphyxia. The scoring system is worthwhile for identifying infants at risk, especially when therapeutic interventions are available. In future studies, diffusion imaging should be correlated with this MR scoring system because diffusion-weighted imaging has great sensitivity for detecting hypoxic ischemic abnormality in a neonatal brain.[1] The reader is referred to 2 other articles in which MR predictive value is emphasized. In 1,[2] the abnormal MR signal in the internal capsule in hypoxic ischemic encephalopathy is reported, and in the other[3] various MR patterns are described. D_2-receptor imaging with ^{123}I-iodobenzamide brain SPECT is another noteworthy functional imaging method.[4]

T. Young Poussaint, M.D.
L.W. Young, M.D.

References

1. Cowan FM, Pennock JM, Hanrahan JD, et al: Early detection of cerebral infarction and hypoxic-ischemic encephalopathy in neonates using diffusion weighted magnetic resonance imaging. *Neuropediatrics* 25:172-175, 1994.
2. Rutherford MA, Pennock JM, Counsell SJ, et al: Abnormal magnetic resonance signal in the internal capsule predicts poor neurodevelopmental outcome in infants with hypoxic-ischemic encephalopathy. *Pediatrics* 102:323-328, 1998.
3. Kuenzle C, Baenzier O, Martin E, et al: Prognostic value of early MR imaging in term infants with severe *perinatal asphyxia. Neuropediatrics* 25:191-200, 1994.
4. Kapucu LO, Koc E, Gucuyener K, et al: D_2 receptor imaging with iodine-123-iodobenzamide brain SPECT in infants with hypoxic-ischemic brain injury. *J Nucl Med* 39:1703-1706, 1998.

MR of Hypoxic Encephalopathy in Children After Near Drowning: Correlation With Quantitative Proton MR Spectroscopy and Clinical Outcome

Dubowitz DJ, Bluml S, Arcinue E, et al (Huntington Med Research Insts, Pasadena, Calif; Schulte Research Inst, Santa Barbara, Calif; Huntington Mem Hosp, Pasadena, Calif; et al)
AJNR 19:1617-1627, 1998 4–2

Objective.—Hypoxic encephalopathy in children commonly occurs as a result of near drowning. Although this condition has been studied by quantitative MR spectroscopy, the accompanying MRI changes remain uncertain. The MRI findings in children with hypoxic encephalopathy caused by near-drowning were studied, including their relationship to the findings of proton MR spectroscopy and to clinical outcome.

Methods.—The study included 22 children (mean age, 3.5 years) admitted to the pediatric ICU after near-drowning. The patients underwent a total of 47 combined cerebral MRI and quantitative proton MR spectroscopic studies using a 1.5 T MRI machine. These studies were reviewed by 2 radiologists who were unaware of the MR spectroscopic findings and final clinical outcome. Variables evaluated on the MRI scans included edema, basal ganglia changes, cortical changes, focal hemorrhage, and infarction. The 2 standard locations for quantitative, short-echo time proton MR spectroscopy were the posterior parieto-occipital lobes in the gray matter and the deep parietal lobe in the white matter.

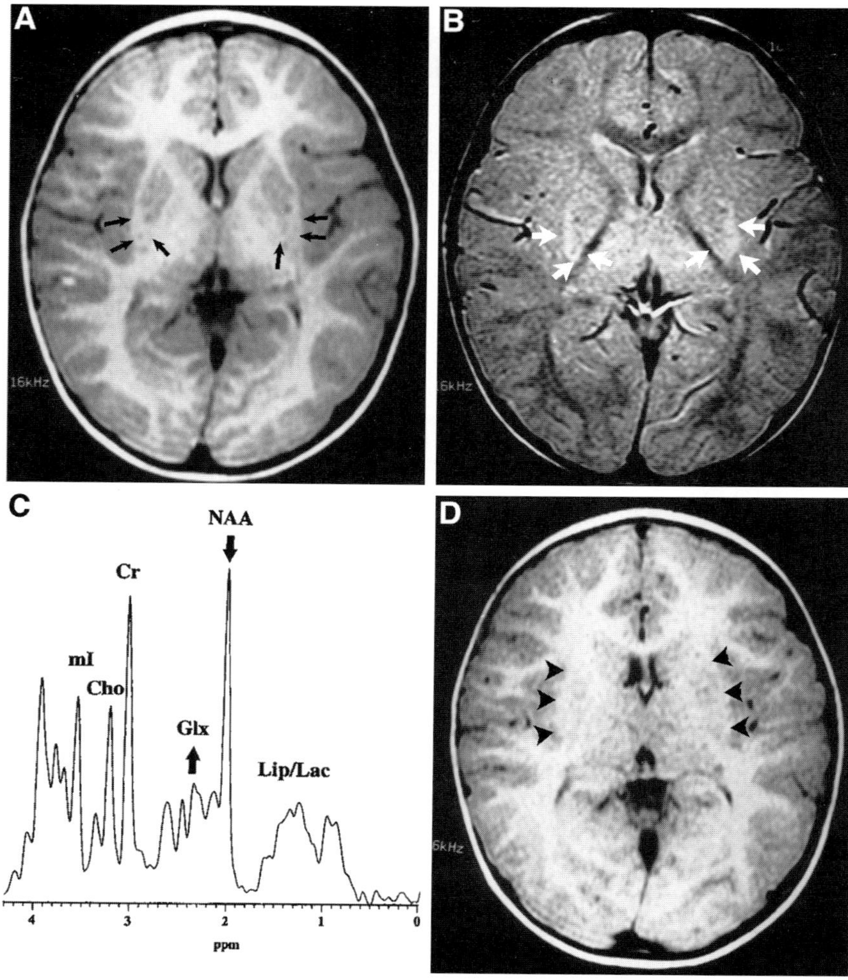

(*Continued*)

Results.—The outcome was rated good in 6 patients; 4 were left in a persistent vegetative state and 12 died. Of the 6 children with good outcomes, 5 were shown to have abnormal and indistinct basal ganglia margins when first studied a mean of 2 days after submersion. Four were shown to have loss of the normal posteromedial margin of the lentiform nuclei. Cortical abnormalities were detected in all patients in a persistent vegetative state. These included subcortical lines on the baseline studies of 3 patients and focal T2 hyperintensity in the fourth. Subsequent studies showed changes including cerebral atrophy and brain stem infarcts. Seventy-eight percent of T1-weighted images showed indistinct basal ganglia margins, an early sign of anoxia-ischemia (Fig 2). This finding was some-

FIGURE 2 (cont.)

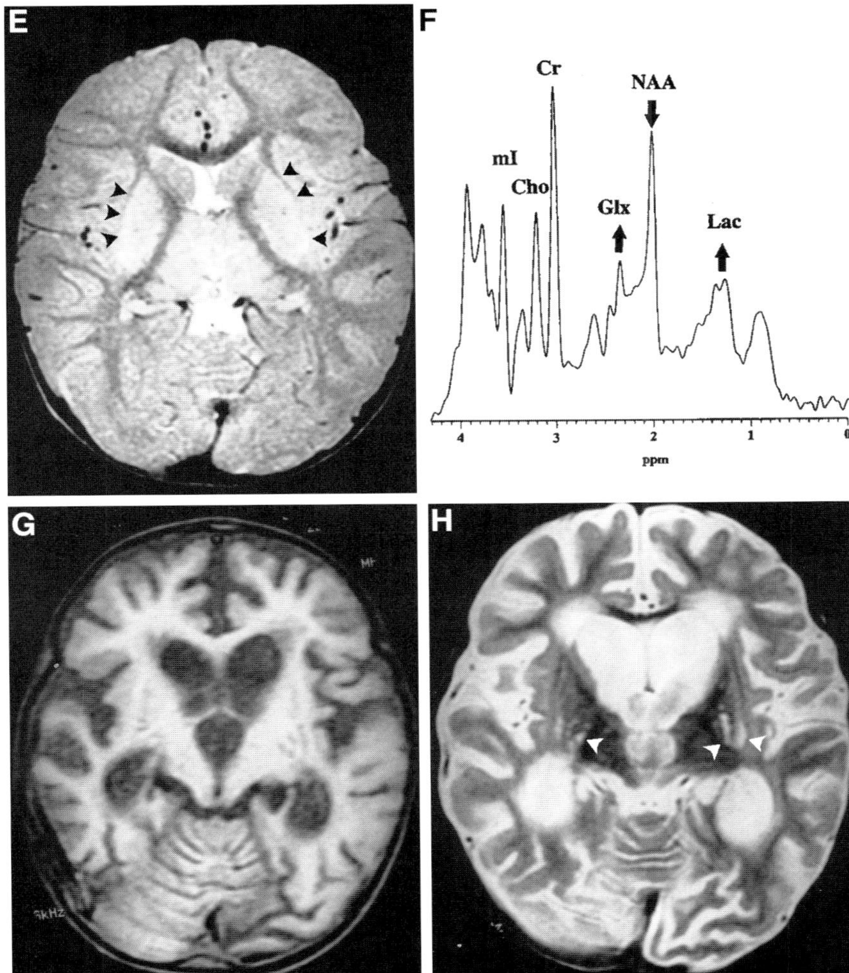

(Continued)

times reversible in cases of mild hypoxia. Patients with basal ganglia T2 hyperintensities, which progressed from a patchy to diffuse distribution, had poor outcomes. Patchy high T2 signal in the cortex, subcortical lines, and brain stem infarcts were all specific but insensitive indicators of poor outcome.

Conclusion.—MRI provides useful information in the evaluation of children with near-drowning, especially if interpreted in combination with MR spectroscopy. Both studies provide better predictive information after day 3. The MRI findings associated with hypoxic encephalopathy include

FIGURE 2 (cont.)

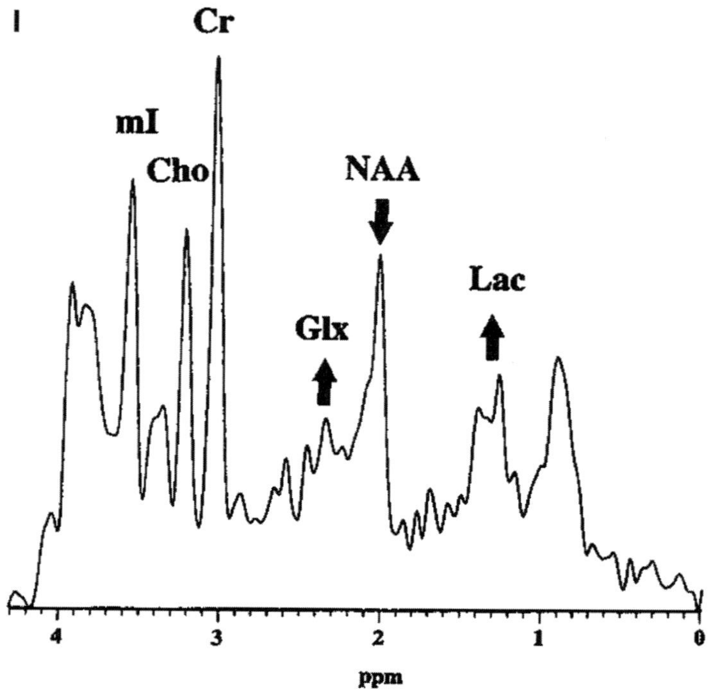

FIGURE 2.—Progression of basal ganglia changes in a 19-month-old boy who remained in a permanent vegetative state. **A** and **B**, Axial spin-echo T1-weighted (600/20) (**A**) and proton density–weighted (3000/30) (**B**) MR images on day 1 show indistinct margins of lentiform nuclei (*arrows*, **A**) and high signal intensity peripherally (*arrows*, **B**). **C**, Gray matter spectrum (1500/30, with a mixing time of 13.7) on day 1 shows reduced *N*-acetylaspartate (*NAA*) and elevated glutamine/glutamate (*Glx*). The peak superimposed on the lipid and macromolecular resonances (*Lip/Lac*) may indicate excess lactate (a difficult diagnosis on this spectrum in isolation, but confirmed on the later examination at day 3). **D** and **E**, Axial spin-echo T1-weighted (600/20) and T2-weighted (3000/90) MR images on day 3. The lentiform nuclei are seen less clearly on the T1-weighted image (*arrowheads*, **D**) and have diffuse signal intensity on the T2-weighted image (*arrowheads*, **E**). **F**, Gray matter spectrum on day 3 shows considerably reduced NAA and elevated Glx and lactate. **G** and **H**, Axial spin-echo T1-weighted (600/20) (**G**) and T2-weighted (2500/90) (**H**) MR images at 3 months show diffuse atrophy and chronic changes in the basal ganglia with focal T2 high signal intensity changes in the posterior aspect of the lentiform nuclei bilateral (*arrowheads*, **H**). **I**, Gray matter spectrum (1500/30, with a mixing time of 13.7) at 3 months shows almost absent NAA and elevated Glx and lactate. *Abbreviations*: *mI*, *myo*-inositol; *cho*, choline; *cr*, creatine. (Courtesy of Dubowitz DJ, Bluml S, Arcinue E, et al: MR of hypoxic encephalopathy in children after near drowning: Correlation with quantitative proton MR spectroscopy and clinical outcome. *AJNR* 19:1617-1627. Copyright 1998 by American Society of Neuroradiology.)

focal and generalized edema, basal ganglia changes, cortical abnormalities, and brain stem infarcts. Where MR spectroscopy is unavailable, these findings will aid in recognizing hypoxic encephalopathy, predicting outcomes, and planning management.

► This excellent article advocates use of MRI and MR spectroscopy in evaluating children afflicted by near drowning. MR spectroscopy findings correlated with MRI findings have been shown to be useful in infants with hypoxic-ischemic encephalopathy.[1-3] The application of MR diffusion-weighted imaging in near-drowning patients and correlation of its findings with MRI and MR spectroscopy findings will be interesting future research in the near-drowning hypoxic-ischemic encephalopathy scenario.

T. Young Poussaint, M.D.

References

1. Penrice J, Kady EB, Lorek A, et al: Proton magnetic resonance spectroscopy of the brain in normal preterm infants and early changes after perinatal hypoxia-ischemia. *Pediatr Res* 40:6-14, 1996.
2. Ross B, Kreis R, Ernst T: Clinical tools for the 90s: Magnetic resonance spectroscopy and metabolite imaging. *Eur J Radiol* 14:128-140, 1992.
3. Kreis R, Arcinue E, Ernst T, et al: Hypoxic encephalopathy after near-drowning studied by quantitative 1H-magnetic resonance spectroscopy. *J Clin Invest* 97:1142-1154, 1996.

Lasting Cytotoxic Edema as an Indicator of Irreversible Brain Damage: A Case of Neonatal Stroke

Rumpel H, Ferrini B, Martin E (Univ Children's Hosp Zurich, Switzerland)
AJNR 19:1636-1638, 1998 4–3

Purpose.—Cellular swelling, or cytotoxic edema, is a common feature of diverse brain disorders of varying mechanisms. The extent of swelling and its impact on cell and tissue survival have an important effect on diagnosis and treatment. A case of neonatal stroke in the territory of the left middle cerebral artery (MCA) was presented, illustrating the predictive value of cytotoxic edema.

Case Report.—Boy, 5 days, was admitted for evaluation of right-sided seizures after a normal pregnancy and delivery. T2-weighted MR images showed a hyperintense ischemic lesion in the left MCA territory. Snapshot fast low-angle shot imaging with a diffusion-weighting preparation period was used to calculate the apparent diffusion coefficient of water. This coefficient was 78% of baseline in the temporal part of the MCA territory lesion, compared with a near normal value in the frontal zone. By age 3 months, the patient had asymmetric muscle tone with spontaneous movements in the legs. Follow-up T2-weighted images showed partial recovery of the frontal part of the lesion, accompanied by atrophy of the cortex, subcortical white matter, and portions of the lenticular nucleus. In contrast, a cystic infarction had developed in the temporal part of the lesion (Fig 1).

Discussion.—The separate zones of cellular swelling noted on these T2-weighted images depict areas with differing degrees of cytotoxic edema

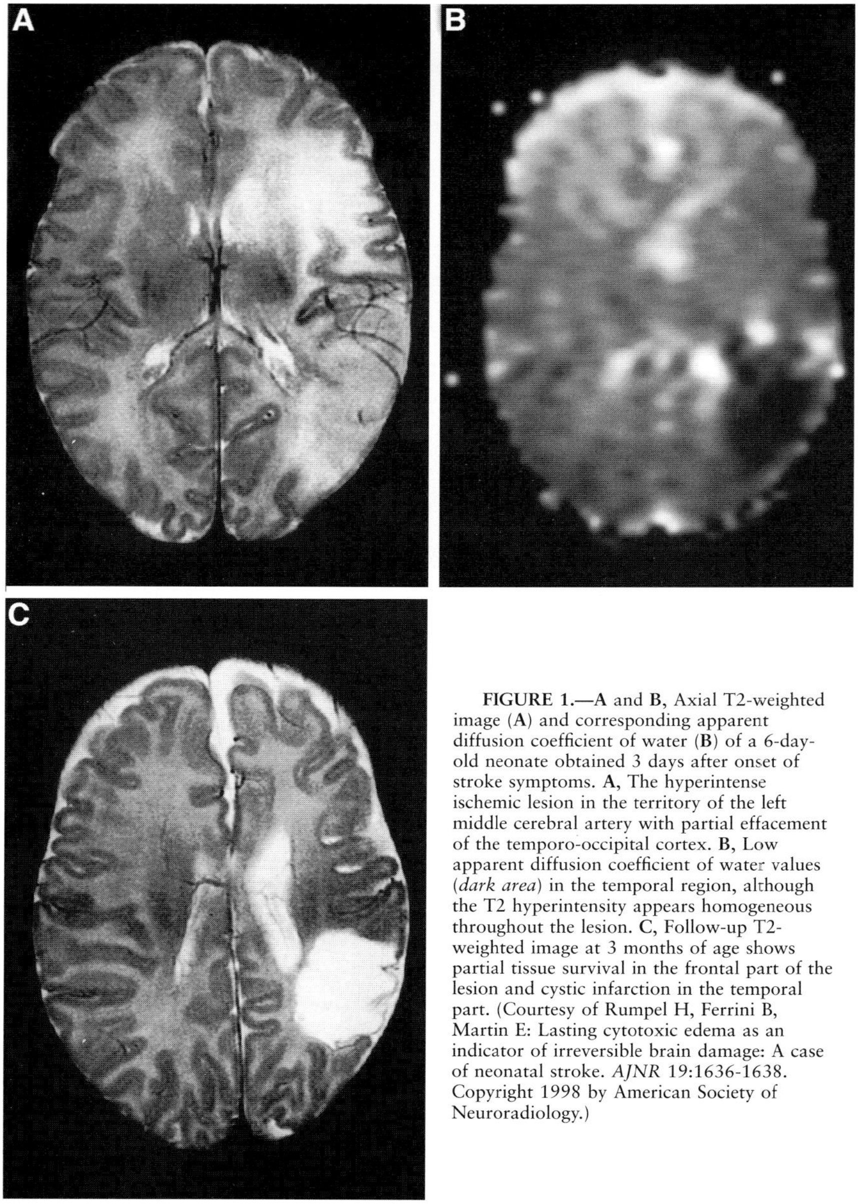

FIGURE 1.—A and B, Axial T2-weighted image (A) and corresponding apparent diffusion coefficient of water (B) of a 6-day-old neonate obtained 3 days after onset of stroke symptoms. A, The hyperintense ischemic lesion in the territory of the left middle cerebral artery with partial effacement of the temporo-occipital cortex. B, Low apparent diffusion coefficient of water values (*dark area*) in the temporal region, although the T2 hyperintensity appears homogeneous throughout the lesion. C, Follow-up T2-weighted image at 3 months of age shows partial tissue survival in the frontal part of the lesion and cystic infarction in the temporal part. (Courtesy of Rumpel H, Ferrini B, Martin E: Lasting cytotoxic edema as an indicator of irreversible brain damage: A case of neonatal stroke. *AJNR* 19:1636-1638. Copyright 1998 by American Society of Neuroradiology.)

and differing prognoses. The near-normal finding in the frontal zone probably reflects the compensating effects of interstitial space; thus the apparent diffusion coefficient of water is normal although the T2 is prolonged. In the temporal part, the persistently reduced apparent diffusion

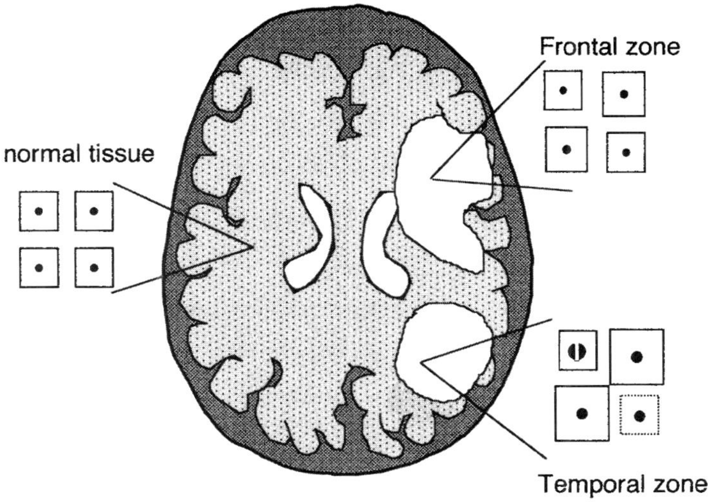

FIGURE 2.—Schematic diagram of the extracellular to intracellular volume fraction based on 4 cells for normal tissue, the frontal zone, and the temporal zone. In the time scale of MR imaging, observation focuses on isotropic diffusion through both compartments. On the basis of image contrast of T2 hyperintensity and the apparently normal apparent diffusion coefficient of water of the frontal part of the lesion, one could judge the slight swelling of the cells and the enlargement of interstitial space in such a way that the volume fraction remains seemingly normal. In the temporal part of the lesion, the low apparent diffusion coefficient of water together with an elevated T2 suggests severe cellular swelling combined with cell lyses (*dotted square*) and/or apoptosis (*divided dot*), leading to a decreased extracellular volume of increased tortuosity, albeit partially compensated by an accumulation of free interstitial fluid. (Courtesy of Rumpel H, Ferrini B, Martin E: Lasting cytotoxic edema as an indicator of irreversible brain damage: A case of neonatal stroke. *AJNR* 19:1636-1638. Copyright 1998 by American Society of Neuroradiology.)

coefficient of water reflects more pronounced cellular swelling, with increased extracellular fluid resulting from previously lysed cells (Fig 2). This theory is supported by the greater preservation of gray-white interfaces in the frontal zone and by the difference in MRI appearance at 3 months' follow-up.

► MR diffusion-weighted imaging is being more widely used in stroke. The zonular edema findings of MR diffusion imaging, as described in this article, should be helpful in determining which lesions may result in irreversible ischemic injury. The simplified explanation given for this complex phenomenon as schematically diagrammed in Figure 2 is attractive. Recent supportive data by the lead author in an animal model is referenced below.[1]

T. Young Poussaint, M.D.

Reference

1. Rumpel H, Nedelcu J, Aguzzi A, et al: Late glia swelling after acute cerebral hypoxia-ischemia in the neonatal rat: A combined magnetic resonance and histochemical study. *Pediatr Res* 42:54-59, 1997.

Morphologic Study of 120 Skull Base Defects in Frontoethmoidal Encephalomeningoceles

Boonvisut S, Ladpli S, Sujatanond M, et al (Mahidol Univ, Bangkok, Thailand; Queen Sirikit Natl Inst of Child Health, Bangkok, Thailand)

Plast Reconstr Surg 101:1784-1795, 1998 4–4

Introduction.—Frontoethmoidal encephalomeningocele is a herniation of the brain and meninges through a congenital bone defect of the skull base located at the junction of the frontal and ethmoidal bones. This endemic deformity is most commonly seen in South and Southeast Asia. It rarely occurs in Western Europe, Japan, Australia, or North America. Between 1992 and 1996, 120 patients with a diagnosis of frontoethmoidal encephalomeningocele were examined to detail fully the morphology of the bony defects at the frontoethmoidal junction and the surrounding area and to propose a more precise classification than what is currently used.

Methods.—Patients underwent a thorough history and detailed physical examination of the affected parts. Findings of a plastic surgeon, neurosurgeons, and an ophthalmologist were documented, together with standard photography of the face and calvarium and radiologic skull studies. Forty patients underwent 3-dimensional CT scans. Radiologists described precise bony defects.

Results.—The multidisciplinary approach revealed more types of defects than previously reported. There were single or multiple external openings

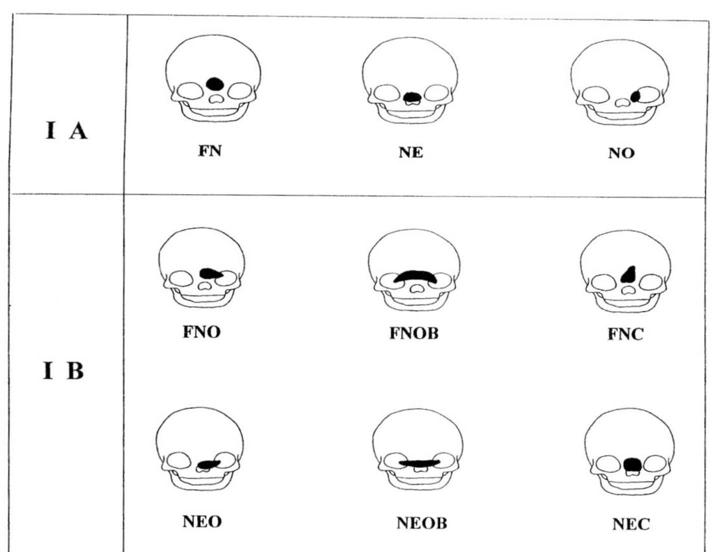

FIGURE 1.—Schematic drawings show skull defects in type IA, IB, and 9 subtypes. *Abbreviations*: *F*, frontal; *N*, nasal; *E*, ethmoidal; *O*, orbital; *B*, bilateral; *C*, cephalad. (Courtesy of Boonvisut S, Ladpli S, Sujatanond M, et al: Morphologic study of 120 skull base defects in frontoethmoidal encephalomeningoceles. *Plast Reconstr Surg* 101:1784-1795, 1998.)

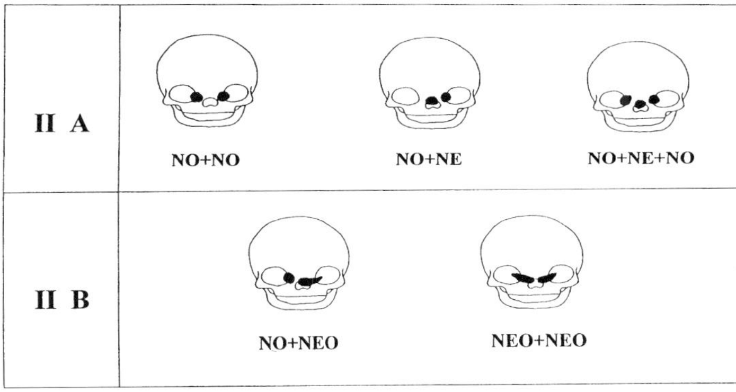

FIGURE 2.—Schematic drawings show skull defects in type IIA, IIB, and 5 subtypes. *Abbreviations*: *N*, nasal; *E*, ethmoidal; *O*, orbital. (Courtesy of Boonvisut S, Ladpli S, Sujatanond M, et al: Morphologic study of 120 skull base defects in frontoethmoidal encephalomeningoceles. *Plast Reconstr Surg* 101:1784-1795, 1998.)

(Figs 1 and 2) in the area between the frontal, nasal, ethmoidal, and orbital bones. Findings were categorized into types: type I, a single external opening between frontal, nasal, ethmoidal, and orbital bones; type IA, opening limited to between 2 bones of the area (Figs 3 and 4); type IB, opening extended transversely or cephalad to involve adjacent structures; type II, multiple external openings in the region; type IIA, all openings

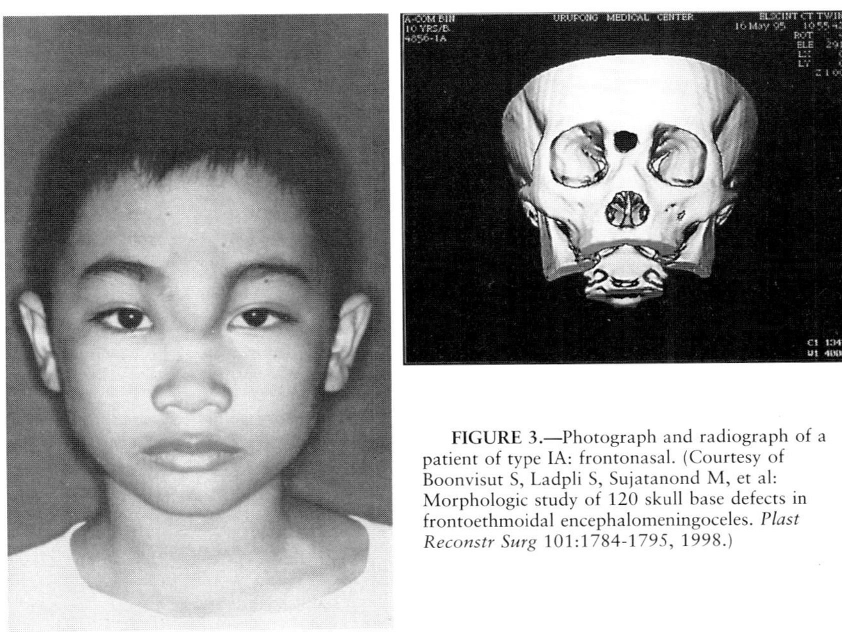

FIGURE 3.—Photograph and radiograph of a patient of type IA: frontonasal. (Courtesy of Boonvisut S, Ladpli S, Sujatanond M, et al: Morphologic study of 120 skull base defects in frontoethmoidal encephalomeningoceles. *Plast Reconstr Surg* 101:1784-1795, 1998.)

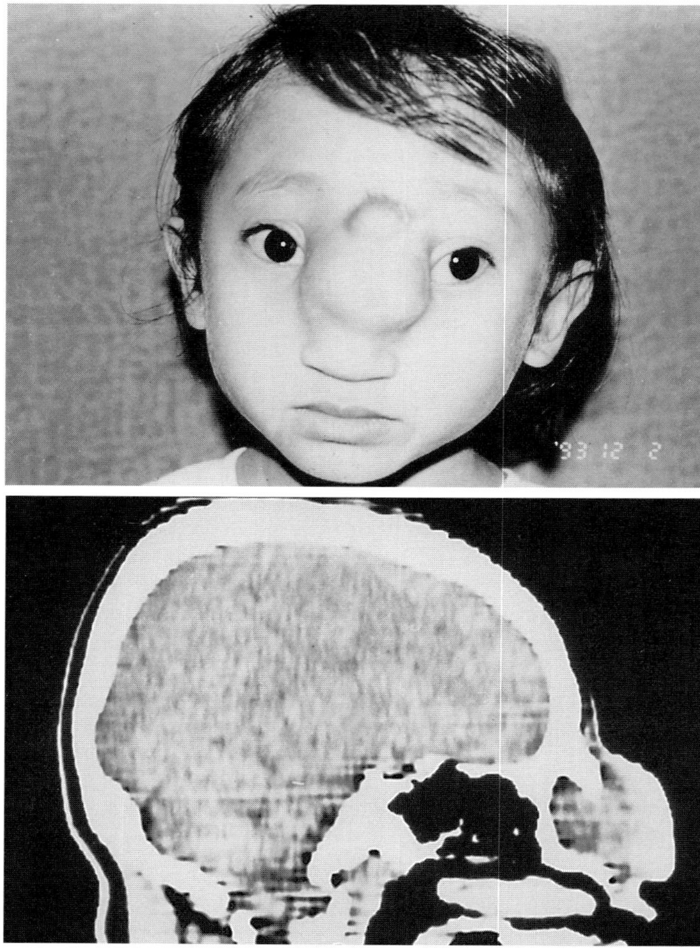

FIGURE 4.—Photograph and radiograph of a patient of type IA: nasoethmoidal. (Courtesy of Boonvisut S, Ladpli S, Sujatanond M, et al: Morphologic study of 120 skull base defects in frontoethmoidal encephalomeningoceles. *Plast Reconstr Surg* 101:1784-1795, 1998.)

limited types; and type IIB, one or more openings extended type(s) that involve adjacent structures. There were 14 subtypes: 3 in type IA, 6 in type IB, 3 in type IIA, and 2 in type IIB.

Conclusion.—A new classification of frontoethmoidal encephalomeningocele was developed from a series of 120 patients seen over a 5-year period by 1 team. Malformations may be a single defect or multiple defects and can be limited to 2 adjacent bones or extend to involve neighboring areas.

► Such a large series of young patients with frontoethmoidal encephaloceles is rare in North America, but common in Southeast Asia.[1] The result of this analysis is a new, more complete classification of frontoethmoidal encephaloceles. In 3-dimensional CT imaging of these patients, knowledge of this classification should be helpful in sorting out anatomical/bony detail. MRI may also be useful.[2]

T. Young Poussaint, M.D.

References

1. Richards CGM: Frontoethmoidal meningoencephalocele: A common and severe congenital abnormality in South East Asia. *Arch Dis Child* 67:717, 1992.
2. Zinreich SJ, Borders JC, Eisele DW, et al: The utility of magnetic resonance imaging in the diagnosis of intranasal meningoencephaloceles. *Arch Otolaryngol* 118:1253, 1992.

Hydrocephalus and Craniosynostosis

Cinalli G, Sainte-Rose C, Kollar EM, et al (Université René Descartes, Paris; Leeds Gen Infirmary, Leeds, England)

J Neurosurg 88:209-214, 1998 4–5

Background.—Intracranial CSF volume may be increased by dilation of the ventricular cavities and dilation of the pericerebral spaces, both of which can be observed before or after craniofacial surgery. Both may be static or evolve to cause symptomatic intracranial hypertension. Each of these variations was correlated with types of craniosynostosis.

Methods.—In this retrospective study, 1,727 patients with craniosynostosis were classified as having either nonsyndromic or syndromic disease. Surgery for cranial deformity was performed in 1,297 patients, 95% of whom had a postoperative follow-up of 5 years.

Findings.—Intracranial CSF hydrodynamics were abnormal in 8.1% of the patients. There were 3 types of CSF hydrodynamic disturbance: progressive hydrocephalus with ventricular dilation, nonprogressive ventriculomegaly, and dilation of the subarachnoid spaces. Hydrocephalus was much more common in patients with syndromic craniosynostosis than in those with isolated craniosynostosis. Hydrocephalus was a constant feature in patients with kleeblattschädel. Patients with Crouzon's syndrome were much more likely to have hydrocephalus than those with other syndromes. Ventricular dilation was very common in Apert's syndrome, although it was almost never progressive. Venous sinus obstruction or chronic tonsillar herniation, or both, occurred in most patients with syndromic craniosynostosis (Fig 1 and Table 1).

Conclusion.—Although hydrocephalus is rare in patients with nonsyndromic craniosynostosis, it is relatively common in patients with syndromic craniostenosis, especially those with Crouzon's or Apert's syndrome. In addition, it is a constant finding in patients with kleeblattschädel deformity.

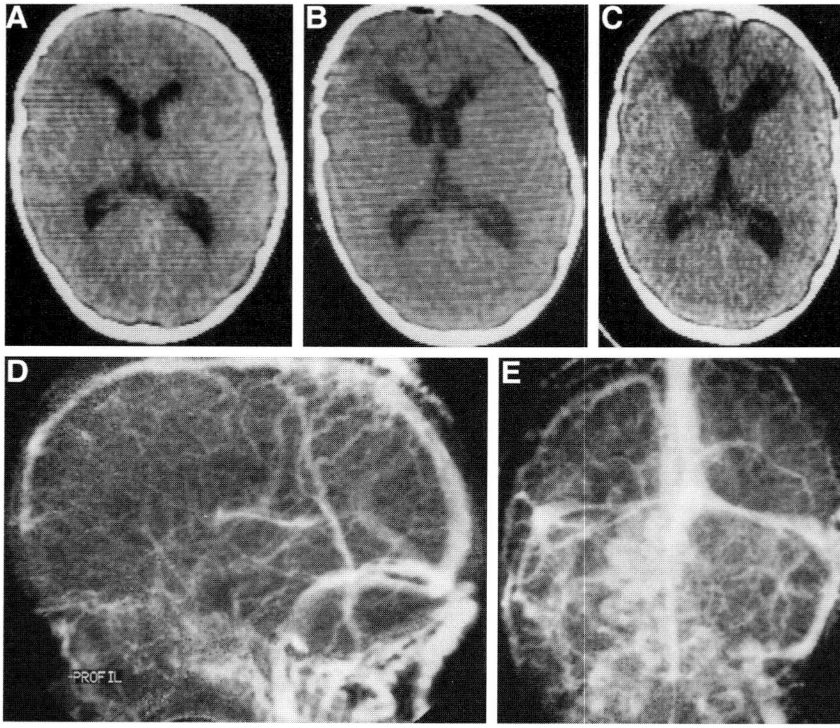

FIGURE 1.—Imaging data obtained in a patient with oxycephaly. **A**, Preoperative CT scan obtained when the patient was 5 years old. **B**, Postoperative CT scan obtained 2 weeks after forehead advancement. Note the increased ventricular size and the signs of transependymal resorption. **C**, CT scan obtained 4 months after forehead advancement. There is a significant additional increase in ventricular size, which is more marked at the level of the frontal horns, with periventricular lucency. **D**, Angiogram, lateral view, showing stenosis of both jugular foramina. Note the significant transdiploic collateral circulation at the level of the sagittal sinus in the parietal region and at the level of the posterior fossa. **E**, Angiogram, posterior view, showing hypoplasia of both lateral sinuses, stenosis of both jugular foramina, and a marked collateral circulation. (Courtesy of Cinalli G, Sainte-Rose C, Kollar EM, et al: Hydrocephalus and craniosynostosis. *J Neurosurg* 88:209-214, 1998.)

► This useful report of a large series of patients with craniosynostosis describes the substantially increased incidence of hydrocephalus in syndromic craniosynostosis as compared with its rarity in nonsyndrome craniosynostosis. The article includes an excellent description of the pathophysiologic mechanisms that may be involved in several forms of syndromic craniosynostosis. The subject of the inability to accurately diagnose increased intracranial pressure by calvarial signs alone has been a subject of recent articles that address possible surgical excesses in patients with nonsyndromic craniosynostosis.[1,2,3] More important imaging in craniosynostosis is the use of CT and angiography for demonstration of hydrocephalus and vascular impingement.

T. Young Poussaint, M.D.
L.W. Young, M.D.

TABLE 1.—Patients Presenting Stable or Progressive Dilation of Cerebral Ventricles or Pericerebral CSF Spaces in a Series of 1,727 Cases of Craniosynostosis

Type of Craniosynostosis	No. of Patients: Ventricular Dilation	Pericerebral Fluid Collection	Average Age (mos) at Shunt Insertion	VP Shunt	Subduroperitoneal Shunt	Total CSF Diversions
Crouzon's syndrome	36	3	12.3	22	3	25
Apert's syndrome	35	37	13	5	4	9
Pfeiffer's syndrome	5	0	13	5	0	5
Opitz syndrome	1	0	2	1	0	1
Antley-Bixler's syndrome	0	1	13	0	1	1
complex	3	1	15	3	1	4
brachycephaly	1	3	10	1	3	4
scaphocephaly	0	3	7.3	0	3	3
trigonocephaly	0	2	6	0	2	2
oxycephaly	1	0	60	1	0	1
total	82	50	NA	38	17	55

Abbreviation: NA, not applicable.
(Courtesy of Cinalli G, Sainte-Rose C, Kollar EM, et al: Hydrocephalus and craniosynostosis. *J Neurosurg* 88:209-214, 1998.)

References

1. Fernbach SK: Craniosynostosis 1998: Concepts and controversies. *Pediatr Radiol* 28:722-728, 1998.
2. Tuite GF, Evanson J, Chong WK, et al: The beaten copper cranium: A correlation between intracranial pressure, cranial radiographs, and computed tomographic scans in children with *craniosynostosis. Neurosurgery* 39:691-699, 1996.
3. McAlister WH: Invited commentary: Posterior deformational plagiocephaly. *Pediatr Radiol* 28:727-728, 1996.

Central Nervous System Candidiasis in Very Low–Birth-Weight Premature Neonates and Infants: US Characteristics and Histopathologic and MR Imaging Correlates in Five Patients

Huang C-C, Chen C-Y, Yang H-B, et al (Natl Cheng Kung Univ, Tainan, Taiwan; Tri-Service Gen Hosp and Natl Defense Med Ctr, Taipei, Taiwan; Chang Gung Children's Hosp, Kaohsiung, Taiwan)
Radiology 209:49-56, 1998 4–6

Background.—Systemic candidal infection carries high morbidity and mortality in very low–birth-weight infants. Early diagnosis of CNS candidiasis is essential but may be difficult. The CT and MRI findings on CNS candidiasis have been reported. This study evaluates the cranial US characteristics of CNS candidiasis, including correlation with histopathologic, MRI, and clinical findings.

Methods.—Of 76 consecutive very low–birth-weight premature newborns and infants with systemic candidiasis, 1 neonate and 4 older infants

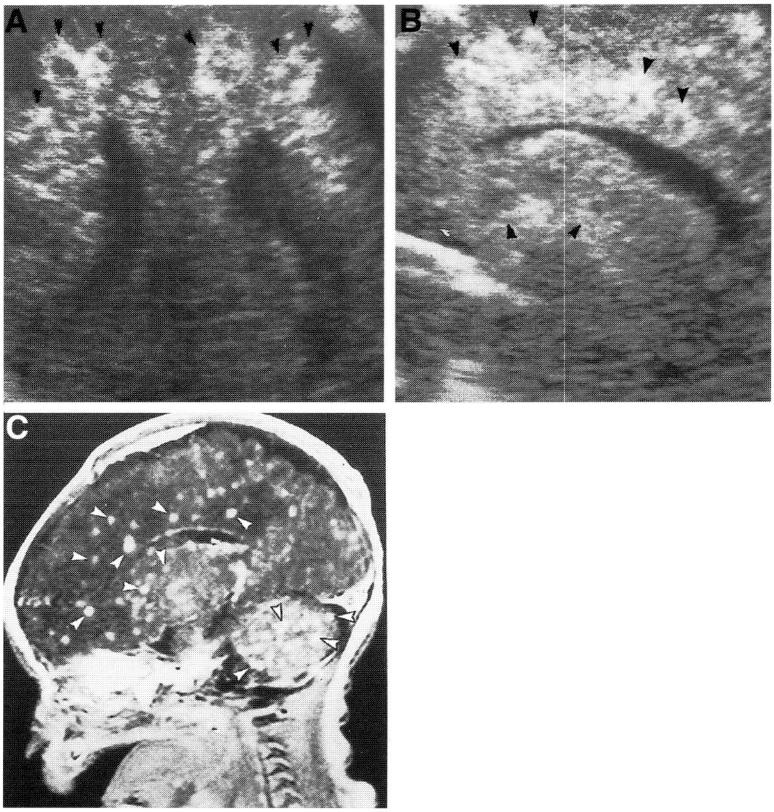

(*Continued*)

were found to have CNS involvement. All underwent cranial US using a real-time US imaging unit with a 5.0- or 7.5-9 MHz transducer. In 2 patients, MRI using a 1.5-T unit was performed within 1 week after US.

Results.—On US, 4 patients had parenchymal abnormalities and 3 had ventricular lesions. Four patients had multiple echogenic, rimlike microabscesses throughout the subcortical, periventricular, and basal ganglia areas (Fig 1). Two had confluent macroabscesses, which appeared in the periventricular regions and/or thalami as echogenic masslike lesions with hypoechoic centers. Two patients had ventricular dilatation, 3 had increased ependymal echogenicity, 2 had intraventricular echogenic septa, and 2 had a lumpy choroid plexus or debris (Fig 4). The US findings were highly correlated with the MRI and autopsy findings, although MRI better depicted the histologic changes in the posterior fossa than did US.

Conclusion.—High-resolution cranial US may be useful in the diagnosis of CNS candidiasis in very low birth weight newborns and infants. The US findings in this series suggest that CNS involvement may take parenchymal and ventricular forms. The US signs of CNS candidiasis are nonspecific

FIGURE 1 (cont.)

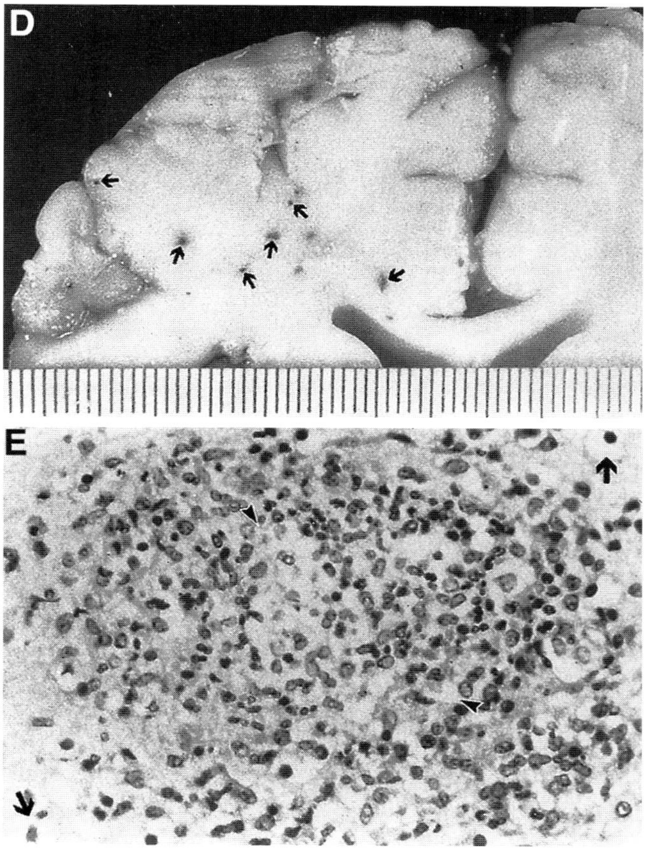

FIGURE 1.—Disseminated candidal microabscesses in a 103-day-old premature infant (gestational age, 29 weeks). A, Posterior, angled, coronal US image obtained through the bodies of the lateral ventricles shows multiple, small, rimlike hypoechoic lesions (*arrowheads*) with irregular echogenic borders in the bilateral periventricular and subcortical regions. B, Oblique parasagittal US image obtained through the body of the lateral ventricle shows multiple, small, rimlike hypoechoic lesions with irregular echogenic borders in the periventricular and subcortical regions (*upper arrowheads*) as well as in the basal ganglia (*lower arrowheads*). C, Corresponding parasagittal contrast-enhanced T1-weighted MR image (600/15, 1 signal acquired) shows disseminated enhancing nodules (*arrowheads*) with perifocal hypointense edema in the subcortical and periventricular areas, basal ganglia, and cerebellum. D, Autopsy specimen of the brain shows that the microabscesses (*arrows*) are well demonstrated as multiple, small, dark greenish lesions in the subcortical and periventricular areas of the brain. Scale is in millimeters. E, Photomicrograph of a microabscess reveals that the center is mildly necrotic with leukocytic infiltration (*arrowheads*) and surrounded by proliferating endothelial cells and reactive gliotic cells. The microabscess is bordered by astrocytes with edematous changes (*arrows*); hematoxylin-eosin; original magnification, ×500. (Courtesy of Huang C-C, Chen C-Y, Yang H-B, et al: Central nervous system candidiasis in very low–birth-weight premature neonates and infants: US characteristics and histopathologic and MR imaging correlates in five patients. *Radiology* 209:49-56, 1998. Radiological Society of North America.)

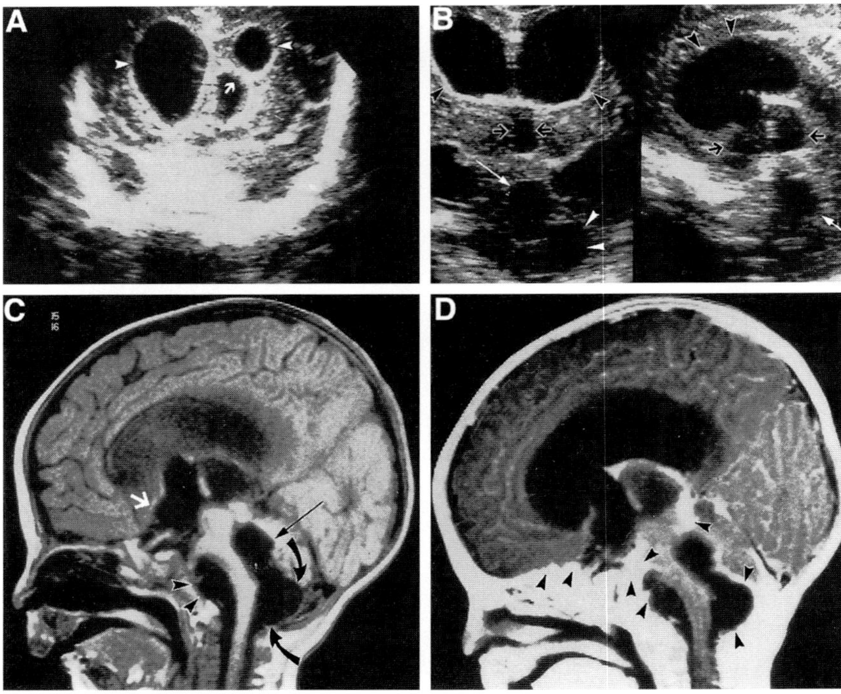

FIGURE 4.—US images obtained in a 161-day-old infant (gestational age, 26 weeks) with ventricular CNS candidiasis demonstrate the limitation of far-field resolution in 5.0-MHz US in the detection of basal exudates and trapped subarachnoid spaces of the posterior fossa. **A**, Anterior, angled coronal US image shows dilatation of the bilateral ventricles (*arrowheads*) and a thick strand (*arrow*) extending across the frontal horn of the right lateral ventricle. **B**, Midsagittal (**right**) and coronal (**left**) US images show marked dilatation of the lateral ventricles (*black arrowheads*), third ventricle (*black arrows*), and fourth ventricle (*white arrow*). The posterior fossa subarachnoid space (*white arrowheads* in **left** image) is also dilated. **C**, Unenhanced midsaggital T1-weighted MR image (600/15, 1 signal acquired) shows dilatation of the prepontine cistern (*arrowheads*) and the cisterna magna (*curved black arrows*), with resultant dilatation in the third (*white arrow*) and fourth (*straight black arrow*) ventricles and brain stem compression. **D**, The corresponding contrast-enhanced T1-weighted image (600/15, 2 signals acquired) shows diffuse enhancement of the basal cisterns (*arrowheads*) both supratentorially and infratentorially. The dilated arachnoid spaces seem to be trapped in the posterior fossa. (Courtesy of Huang C-C, Chen C-Y, Yang H-B, et al: Central nervous system candidiasis in very low–birth-weight premature neonates and infants: US characteristics and histopathologic and MR imaging correlates in five patients. *Radiology* 209:49-56, 1998. Radiological Society of North America.)

and include ventriculomegaly, irregularity and thickening of the ventricular walls, intraventricular strands and debris, and a lumpy choroid plexus. The differential US diagnosis includes intracranial hemorrhage, periventricular leukomalacia, brain abscess, and bacterial ventriculitis.

► The recognition of characteristic, if not specific, sonographic findings of rare CNS candidiasis is a significant contribution, as its diagnosis in very low–birth-weight premature neonates and infants may be difficult. Characteristic high-resolution US imaging findings of candidiasis in affected neonates should enable earlier diagnosis and treatment and better prognosis. Other articles on CNS candidiasis are listed below.[1,2]

T. Young Poussaint, M.D.

References

1. Lai PH, Lin SM, Pan HB, et al: Disseminated miliary cerebral candidiasis. *AJNR* 18:1303-1306, 1997.
2. Johnson SC, Kazzi NJ: Candida brain abscess: A sonographic mimicker of intracranial hemorrhage. *J Ultrasound Med* 4:237-239, 1993.

Subdural Empyema in 10 Infants: US Characteristics and Clinical Correlates

Chen C-Y, Huang C-C, Chang Y-C, et al (Tri-Service Gen Hosp and Gen Defense Med Ctr, Taipei, Taiwan; Natl Cheng Kung Univ, Tainan, Taiwan; Chang Gung Children's Hosp, Kaohsiung, Taiwan; et al)

Radiology 207:609-617, 1998 4–7

Background.—Subdural empyema (SDE) is rare in young infants and is usually a complication of purulent meningitis. However, its sequelae may be more severe than in other age groups. Because the clinical manifestations of SDE in young infants are often indistinguishable from those of other CNS infections, making an early clinical diagnosis of SDE is difficult. The US characteristics of SDE and its differentiation from reactive subdural effusion (RSE) in infants with meningitis were reported.

Methods and Findings.—The images of 10 infants with SDE, with or without RSE complicating meningitis, were correlated with clinical findings and compared with US and MR images from 4 infants with meningitis and RSE. On US, 15 of 16 SDEs in the group of 10 infants were heterogeneous to hyperechoic convexity collections. Twelve SDEs showed hyperechoic strands. Other findings included a thick, echogenic inner membrane, present in 9 SDEs; increased echogenicity of pia-arachnoid and exudates in the subarachnoid space in 16; mass effect in 16; and loculated extra-axial collections in 2. Findings on MR images correlated well with US and surgical results. At CT, SDE was misread as RSE in 1 patient because of the absence of inner membrane contrast material enhancement. Clinical outcomes were associated with the degree of brain damage consequent to meningitis and the chronicity of SDE. In 7 patients, RSEs were anechoic. An inner membrane was noted in 6 and increased pia-arachnoid echogenicity in 4 (Fig 1).

Conclusion.—Because characteristic clinical SDE manifestations are lacking in infants, this diagnosis may be overlooked and appropriate treatment delayed. High-resolution US, with its improved near-field resolution, is useful for the early diagnosis of SDE and for differentiating SDE from benign RSE in infants with bacterial meningitis.

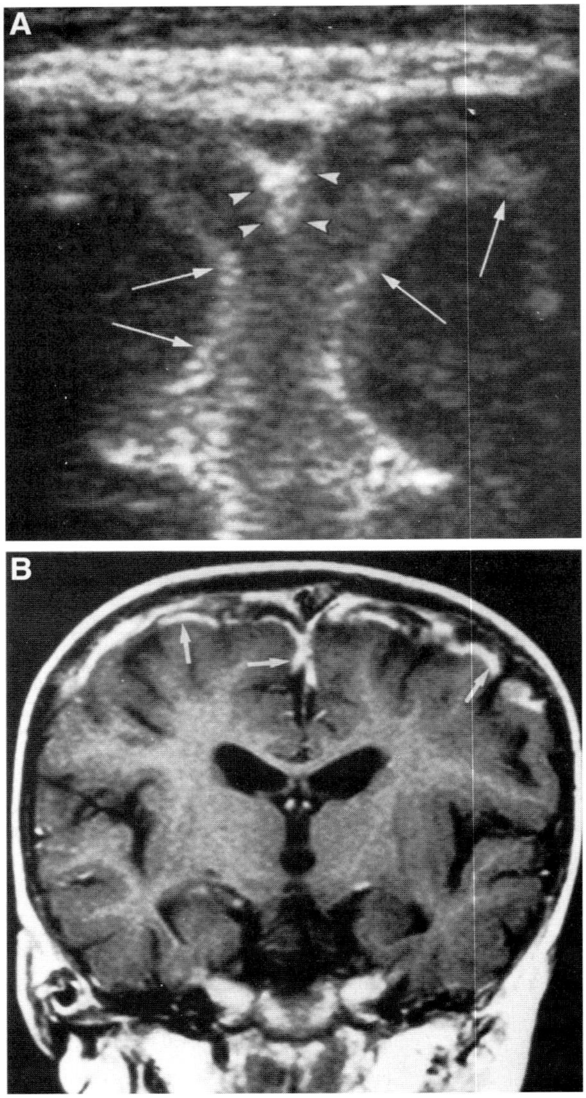

FIGURE 1.—*Neisseria meningitidis* meningitis complicated with bilateral subdural empyema in a 7-month-old girl. **A**, Coronal US scan of the superior frontal region shows hyperechoic extra-axial collections and increased echogenicity of the pia-arachnoid (*arrows*). The falx cerebri (*arrowheads*) was thick. **B**, Corresponding Gd-enhanced coronal T1-weighted (600/15, 2 signals acquired) MR image shows enhanced extra-axial collections and pia-arachnoid (*arrows*) over the superior frontoparietal convexities. (Courtesy of Chen C-Y, Huang C-C, Chang Y-C, et al: Subdural empyema in 10 infants: US characteristics and clinical correlates. *Radiology* 207:609-617, 1998. Radiological Society of North America.)

► This article emphasizes US characteristics helpful in the early diagnosis of SDE and distinguishes it from RSE in infants with meningitis. US is also easily used for follow-up in these patients. The corroboration of MRI may be necessary in some cases, but MRI does not distinguish SDE from nonpurulent RSE. Another recent article reports the compatibility of US and CT in imaging complications of acute bacterial meningitis.[1]

T. Young Poussaint, M.D.
L.W. Young, M.D.

Reference

1. Smyth A, Cairns J: Ultrasound diagnosis of subdural abscess complicating meningitis. *Trop Doct* 27:54-55, 1997.

Cerebral Vasculopathy and Neurologic Sequelae in Infants With Cervicofacial Hemangioma: Report of Eight Patients

Burrows PE, Robertson RL, Mulliken JB, et al (Children's Hosp, Boston; Yale Univ, New Haven, Conn)

Radiology 207:601-607, 1998 4–8

Background.—Infantile hemangiomas are common, but few have been associated with malformative anomalies. The association of cerebral arterial anomalies and progressive cerebral arterial occlusive disease in infants with facial hemangiomas was investigated.

Methods.—The cases of 8 infants given a diagnosis of cervicofacial hemangioma and intracranial arterial anomalies were reviewed. Findings on cranial CT, MRI, MR angiography, and catheter angiography were assessed.

Findings.—Additional congenital anomalies associated with cervicofacial hemangioma were found in 5 children. Seven were treated with corticosteroids or interferon-α2a. In 4 of 7 patients, serial imaging showed progressive cerebrovascular occlusive changes. In 4 other children, all treated with pharmacotherapy, there were MRI findings of cerebral infarction. All 4 had consistent, acquired neurologic symptoms (Fig 1).

Conclusion.—Intracranial anomalies can be associated with cervicofacial hemangioma. Aneurysmal and occlusive changes can be progressive and lead to cerebral infarction. The association between occlusive cerebrovascular disease and pharmacologic treatment may be causal.

► This article describes the important association of cervicofacial hemangiomas with cerebral arterial anomalies, including occlusions, stenoses, hypoplastic arteries and moya-moya phenomena. This association is relevant and must be searched for by imaging examinations. The findings of occlusive disease and aneurysmal change can lead to infarction and may be associated with seizures and developmental delay. Another recent article on this topic is listed.[1]

T. Young Poussaint, M.D.

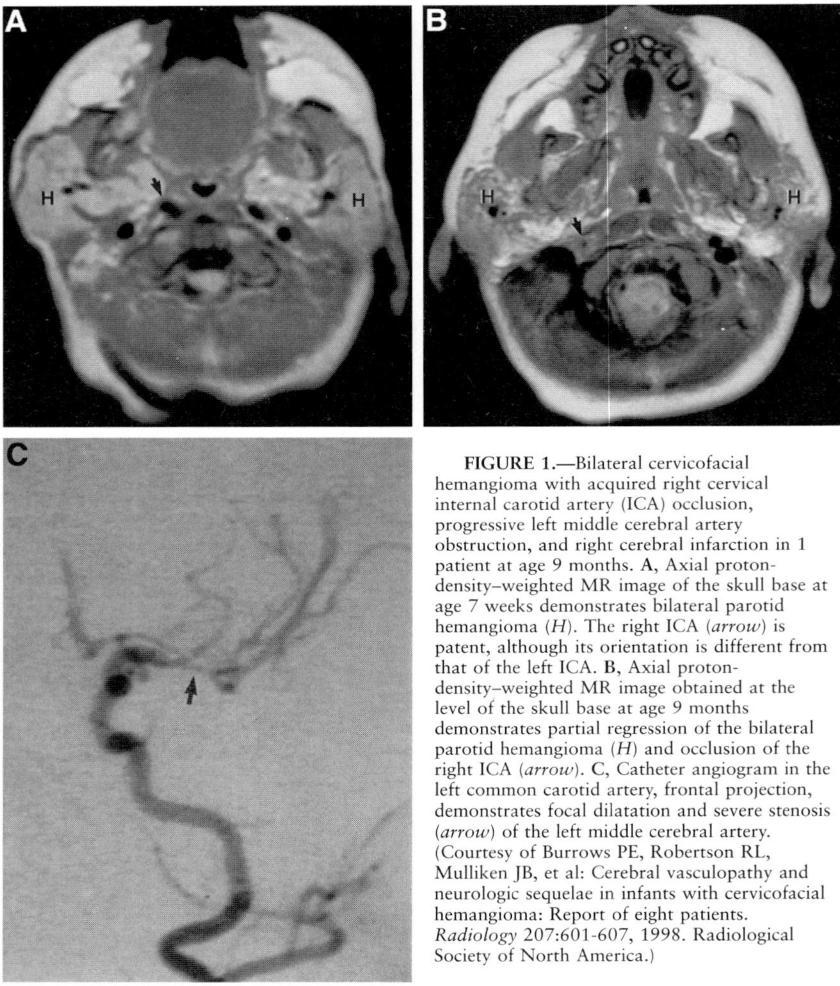

FIGURE 1.—Bilateral cervicofacial hemangioma with acquired right cervical internal carotid artery (ICA) occlusion, progressive left middle cerebral artery obstruction, and right cerebral infarction in 1 patient at age 9 months. **A**, Axial proton-density–weighted MR image of the skull base at age 7 weeks demonstrates bilateral parotid hemangioma (*H*). The right ICA (*arrow*) is patent, although its orientation is different from that of the left ICA. **B**, Axial proton-density–weighted MR image obtained at the level of the skull base at age 9 months demonstrates partial regression of the bilateral parotid hemangioma (*H*) and occlusion of the right ICA (*arrow*). C, Catheter angiogram in the left common carotid artery, frontal projection, demonstrates focal dilatation and severe stenosis (*arrow*) of the left middle cerebral artery. (Courtesy of Burrows PE, Robertson RL, Mulliken JB, et al: Cerebral vasculopathy and neurologic sequelae in infants with cervicofacial hemangioma: Report of eight patients. *Radiology* 207:601-607, 1998. Radiological Society of North America.)

Reference

1. Boukobza M, Enjolras O, Guichard JP, et al: Cerebral developmental venous anomalies associated with head and neck venous malformations. *AJNR* 17:987-994, 1996.

Clinical and Neuroradiologic Findings in Infants With Intracranial Ependymomas

Comi AM, and the Pediatric Oncology Group (State Univ of New York at Buffalo)

Pediatr Neurol 18:23-29, 1998 4–9

Background.—Ependymomas, responsible for about 10% of all brain tumors in children, are disproportionately common in young children. The clinical presentation and initial neuroradiologic findings of 40 children younger than 3 years with intracranial ependymomas were reported.

Patients and Findings.—Twenty-four boys and 16 girls, aged 3 to 35 months, whose condition was diagnosed between 1986 and 1990, were included. Common initial symptoms were vomiting, present in 70% of the children; ataxia, in 53%; headache, in 28%; lethargy, in 28%; increased head circumference, in 23%; and irritability, in 23%. Symptom duration before diagnosis ranged from 1 day to 11 months. Eighty-eight percent of the tumors were infratentorial. In the 23 patients undergoing noncontrast scans, the lesions were isodense to surrounding brain tissue in 57% and calcified in 57%. Ninety-seven percent of the contrast CT scans of 29

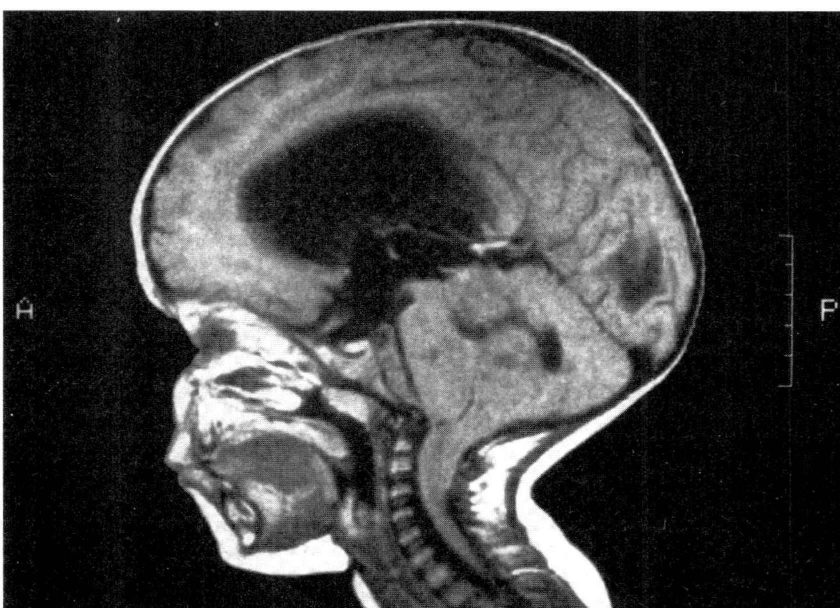

FIGURE 3.—Twelve-month-old female patient described in Figure 4. Sagittal T1-weighted MRI scan (repetition time = 500 ms; echo time = 40 ms) of a large lobular mass filling and expanding the fourth ventricle. The tumor is isosignal to gray matter and demonstrates the plasticity that is characteristic of infratentorial ependymomas. On this particular scan, the tumor is seen flowing out of the foramen of Magendie. (Reprinted by permission of the publisher from Comi AM, and the Pediatric Oncology Group: Clinical and neuroradiologic findings in infants with intracranial ependymomas. *Pediatr Neurol* 18:23-29, copyright 1998 by Elsevier Science Inc.)

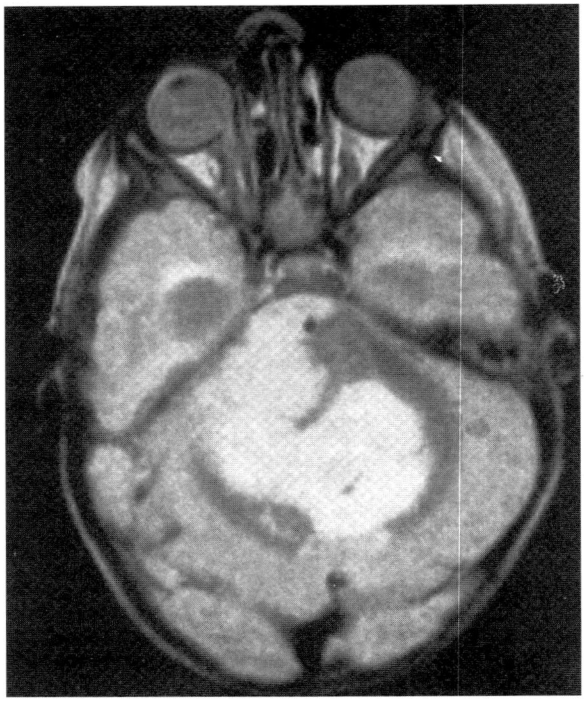

FIGURE 4.—Twelve-month-old female patient who presented with a head tilt and complaints of ataxia, vomiting, horizontal nystagmus, and increased head circumference. First ECHO of T2-weighted axial MRI scan (repetition time = 3,000 ms; echo time = 40 ms) revealed a large high-signal fourth-ventricular tumor spreading out of the right-sided foramen of Luschka. (Reprinted by permission of the publisher from Comi AM, and the Pediatric Oncology Group: Clinical and neuroradiologic findings in infants with intracranial ependymomas. *Pediatr Neurol* 18:23-29, copyright 1998 by Elsevier Science Inc.)

patients were enhanced. Sixty-seven percent of the 15 T1-weighted MR scans displayed low-signal intensity tumors, and 94% of the 16 T2-weighted scans showed high-signal tumors. Forty-three percent of the lesions were cystic. Blood was seen in only 2 tumors. Peritumoral edema was uncommon. Twenty-five percent of the ependymomas extended to the dura. Ninety-seven percent of the infratentorial tumors demonstrated characteristic plasticity. Eighty-five percent of the children had hydrocephalus (Figs 3 and 4).

Conclusion.—Most of the ependymomas in this series were isodense on noncontrast CT and enhanced with contrast, whereas they were low-signal on T1-weighted and high-signal on T2-weighted MR scans. The CT and MRI signal characteristics observed in this study were comparable to those reported previously in older children and adults.

► This article reports a series of children less than 3 years of age with ependymoma. The majority of ependymomas are infratentorial in location. Affected infants have a shorter duration of symptoms and a poorer prognosis than older children and adults. The tumors, in younger patients—usually larger in size at presentation—have anaplastic features and associated CNS metastases. Noteworthy is ependymomas plasticity demonstrated on sagittal MR images. Another recent article acknowledges the importance of neuroimaging in ependymoma, especially in a lateral posterior fossa location.[1]

T. Young Poussaint, M.D.
L.W. Young, M.D.

Reference

1. Nagib MG, O'Fallon MT: Posterior fossa lateral ependymoma in childhood. *Pediatr Neurosurg* 24:299-305, 1996.

MR Imaging in Idiopathic Growth Hormone Deficiency

Hamilton J, Blaser S, Daneman D (Univ of Toronto)

AJNR 19:1609-1615, 1998 4–10

Introduction.—Idiopathic growth hormone deficiency (GHD) may occur in isolation or be associated with several anterior pituitary hormone deficiencies. MRI findings of 1 or more of the following features have been indicated as sensitive and specific determinates of hypopituitarism: small anterior pituitary gland, attenuated or absent pituitary stalk, and ectopic posterior pituitary. It was hypothesized that these MRI findings are common in patients with idiopathic isolated GHD or multiple pituitary hormone deficiencies (MPHD) and may be of use in determining the severity of hypopituitarism. The usefulness of MRI findings was examined in patients with idiopathic GHD.

Methods.—Thirty-five patients with idiopathic GHD (20, isolated GHD and 15 MPHD) underwent MRI. Images were analyzed to define 1 or more of this triad of abnormalities: (1) small/absent anterior pituitary, (2) truncated/absent pituitary stalk, and (3) ectopic posterior pituitary, as well as other associated anomalies. These findings were correlated with clinical and biochemical characteristics.

Results.—Pituitary abnormalities were detected in 80% of patients with isolated GHD and 93% of patients with MPHD. There was a high frequency of midline CNS malformations, including optic nerve hypoplasia, Chiari type I malformations, and median deviation of the carotid arteries, in 9%, 20%, and 37% of patients, respectively (Fig 1). Breech delivery, neonatal hypoglycemia, jaundice, micropenis, and single central incisor were seen equally in patients with isolated GHD or MPHD. In 19 children whose peak growth hormone level was less than 3 µg/L, 90% had the MR triad, compared with a rate of 39% in 13 children with levels of 8 µg/L or greater ($P < .01$). Ninety-two percent of patients with ectopic posterior pituitary had anterior pituitary heights less than −2 standard deviations for age.

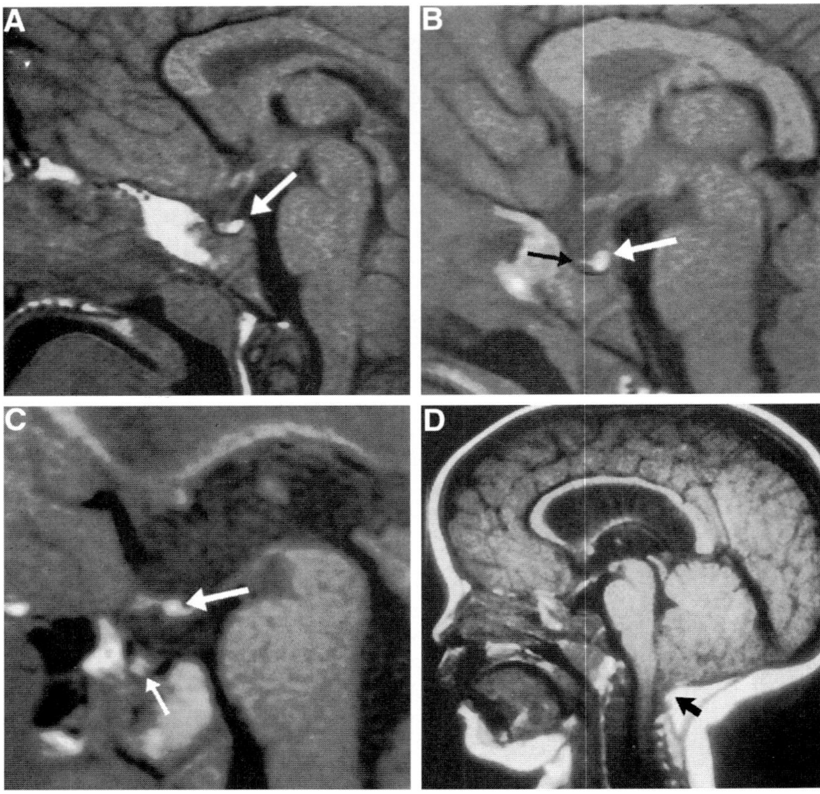

FIGURE 1.—Midsagittal T1-weighted (600/20/3) MRI findings. **A,** Five-year-old girl with idiopathic growth hormone deficiency (GHD) (isolated GHD; growth hormone peak level, 5.6 μg/L) and normal pituitary anatomy. Image shows the sella turcica, normal size anterior pituitary and bright spot of the posterior pituitary (*arrow*), and a well-defined pituitary stalk. **B,** Eight-year-old boy with idiopathic GHD (multiple pituitary hormone deficiencies [MPHD]; growth hormone peak level, 4 μg/L). Image shows a small anterior pituitary (*black arrow*) and the posterior pituitary in a normal position (*white arrow*). **C,** Seven-year-old boy with idiopathic GHD (isolated GHD; growth hormone peak level, 3.6 μg/L). Image shows small anterior pituitary (*small arrows*) and absent stalk and ectopic posterior pituitary at the base of the hypothalamus (*large arrow*). This patient also had asymptomatic hydrocephalus associated with a compression of the ectopic cerebellar tonsils in a small foramen magnum (not shown). **D,** Eighteen-month-old boy with idiopathic GHD (MPHD; growth hormone peak level, 1.2 μg/L). Image shows a small posterior fossa, cerebellar tonsils extending into and obstructing the foramen magnum (*arrow*), ventricular enlargement, a very small anterior pituitary and absent stalk, and an ectopic posterior pituitary. The posterior pituitary gland is not bright. (Courtesy of Hamilton J, Blaser S, Daneman D: MR imaging in idiopathic growth hormone deficiency. *AJNR* 19:1609-1615. Copyright 1998 by American Society of Neuroradiology.)

Conclusion.—Abnormal MRI findings were frequently detected in children with both isolated GHD and MPHD. These findings were closely related to peak growth hormone levels of less than 3 μg/L.

► This article confirms the high frequency of MRI pituitary abnormalities in children with idiopathic GHD, or MPHD. The information is useful for elucidating the types of MRI abnormalities in such patients. The data in this article and others do not support specific MRI findings as being reliable indicators of idiopathic GHD versus MPHD,[1-3] but in another recent article,[4] an absent pituitary stalk and adenohypophysis are demonstrated to be characteristic of MPHD.

T. Young Poussaint, M.D.

References

1. Hamilton J, Chitayat D, Blaser S, et al: Familial growth hormone deficiency associated with MRI abnormalities. *Am J Med Genet* 80:128-132, 1998.
2. Hellstrom A, Wiklund LM, Svensson E, et al: Midline brain lesions in children with hormone sufficiency indicate early prenatal damage. *Acta Paediatr* 87:528-536, 1998.
3. Nagel BH, Palmbach M, Petersen D, et al: Magnetic resonance images of 91 children with different causes of short stature: Pituitary size reflects growth hormone secretion. *Eur J Pediatr* 156:758-763, 1997.
4. Kornreich L, Horev G, Lazar L, et al: MR findings in hereditary isolated growth hormone deficiency. *AJNR* 18:1743-1747, 1997.

Cerebral Vasculopathy in Sickle Cell Anemia: Diagnostic Contribution of Positron Emission Tomography

Powars DR, Conti PS, Wong W-Y, et al (Univ of Southern California, Los Angeles; Long Beach Mem Hosp, Calif; Cedars Sinai Med Ctr, Los Angeles; et al)

Blood 93:71-79, 1999 4–11

Introduction.—Children with sickle cell anemia (SS) are at increased risk for cerebral vasculopathy with stroke (CVA) and cognitive impairment. The extent to which the addition of PET to MRI can improve detection of cerebral vasculopathy was evaluated in 49 children with SS.

Methods.—Of the 49 children with SS, 19 had clinically overt CVA, 20 had life-threatening hypoxic episodes or soft neurologic signs, and 10 were normal, as determined by neurologic history and examination.

Results.—Thirty (61%) and 36 (73%) had abnormal MRI findings and abnormal PET findings, respectively. Forty-four (90%) had either abnormal MRI or PET findings or both. Seventeen of 19 patients (89%) with overt CVA had abnormal MRI findings, 17 (89%) had abnormal PET findings, and 19 (100%) had either abnormal MRI or PET findings or both. Of 20 patients with soft neurologic signs, 10 (50%) had MRI abnormalities, 13 (65%) had PET abnormalities, and 17 (85%) had abnormal MRI or PET findings or both. Of 10 patients who were neurologically normal, 6 (60%) had abnormal PET findings. Twenty-five of 30 patients (83%) with no overt CVA had imaging abnormalities detected on either MRI, PET, or both (silent ischemia). There was an association between a lower-than-average full-scale intelligence quotient and either overt CVA or silent ischemic lesions. Four patients who received chronic red blood cell transfusions had improved metabolic and perfusion status, as determined by repeat PET scans. One 11-year-old patient who under-

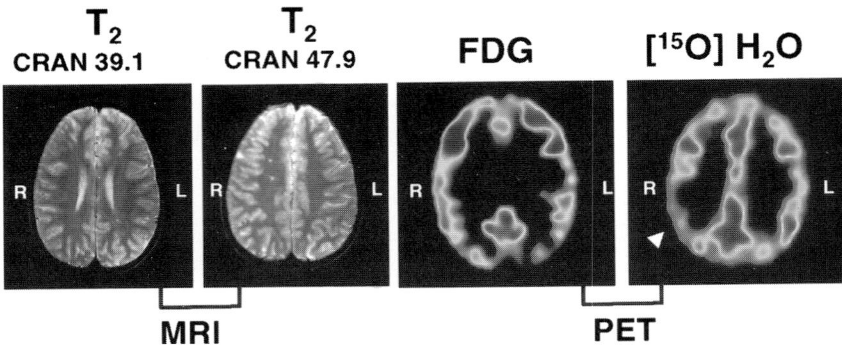

FIGURE 2.—*Abbreviation*: *FDG*, fluorodeoxyglucose. (Courtesy of Powars DR, Conti PS, Wong W-Y, et al: Cerebral vasculopathy in sickle cell anemia: Diagnostic contribution of positron emission tomography. *Blood* 93:71-79, 1999.)

went both MRI and PET died at 45 days post bone marrow transplant (Fig 2).

Conclusion.—A higher proportion of neuroimaging abnormalities were detected in children with SS when PET was added to MRI, especially in children with no history of overt neurologic events. The PET lesions were more extensive and often bihemispheric, compared with MRI abnormalities. Metabolic improvements after therapeutic interventions may be monitored by PET.

▶ This important prospective study shows the substantial contribution of PET to earlier identification of a greater proportion of SS children with neuroimaging abnormalities. The earlier assessment and treatment follow-up potential of PET combined with the advantages of transcranial Doppler and MR angiography need further correlation in future studies.[1,2]

L.W. Young, M.D.

References

1. Seibert JJ, Miller SF, Kirby RS, et al: Cerebrovascular disease in symptomatic and asymptomatic patients with sickle cell anemia: Screening with duplex transcranial Doppler US–correlation with MR imaging and MR angiography. *Radiology* 189:457, 1993.
2. Wang WC, Langston JW, Steen RG, et al: Abnormalities of the central nervous system in very young children with sickle cell anemia. *J Pediatr* 132:994-998, 1998.

Musculoskeletal

Diagnosis of Rett Syndrome: Can a Radiograph Help?

Glasson EJ, Bower C, Thomson MR, et al (Univ of Western Australia, Perth; Princess Margaret Hosp, Perth, Australia; Curtin Univ, Perth, Australia; et al)

Dev Med Child Neurol 40:737-742, 1998 4–12

Introduction.—Rett syndrome (RS) is a neurodevelopmental disorder that almost exclusively affects young females. It is associated with severe

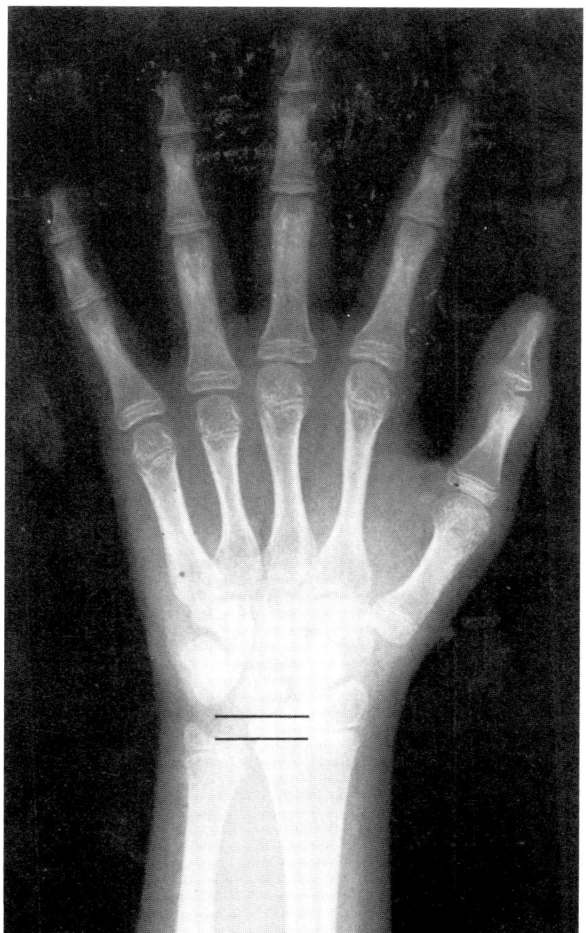

FIGURE 2.—Radiograph of the left wrist of a girl aged 9 years 11 months with classic Rett syndrome. The marked lines on the radiograph indicate a short ulna, defined by a distance of at least 5 mm between the distal articular surface of the ulna and the distal articular surface of the radius. (Courtesy of Glasson EJ, Bower C, Thomson MR, et al: Diagnosis of Rett syndrome: Can a radiograph help? *Dev Med Child Neurol* 40:737-742, 1998.)

intellectual and motor disability. A number of skeletal abnormalities reported in a series of patients with RS have not been systematically assessed in a large population. The abnormalities include short fourth metacarpals and metatarsals and a short ulna. A population-based radiologic examination was performed of the hands and feet of young females with RS.

Methods.—Radiographs of the hands and/or feet of 104 young females with RS from the Australian Rett Syndrome Study were matched with those of healthy controls for age, sex, and laterality. On radiographs, a tangent was drawn across the distal ends of the fifth and fourth metacarpal/metatarsal to ascertain the relative shortening of the fourth metacarpal or metatarsal. A "negative" sign was documented when the line was distal to the third metacarpal. A short ulna was determined as a minimum distance of 5 mm between the distal growth plate of the ulna and the distal growth plate of the radius (Fig 2).

Results.—A positive metacarpal sign was detected more frequently in young females with RA, compared with controls, in the right, but not the left, hand; it was seen in 1 or both hands in 35.7% of patients with RS. It was more common in subjects over age 5 years and in those with classic RS. A positive metatarsal sign was detected more frequently in both right and left feet in patients with RS, compared with controls. It was seen in 1 or both feet in nearly one third of children with RS. It was more common in subjects aged 5 years and older, and in those with classic RS. A short ulna was seen more often in patients with RS, compared with controls.

Conclusion.—Over half (56.6%) of females with RS over age 4 years had a negative ulnar variance in either wrist or a metatarsal sign in either foot. These radiographic findings offer a useful clinical tool for diagnosis of RS in adults and school-aged females.

► OK, add RS (but only for patients over 5 years of age) to the list of conditions with a frequently short fourth metacarpal or metatarsal. But be aware that the authors' control series of Australian girls also showed a 29% incidence of positive metacarpal sign (for shortness) in the left hand. RS is a "girls' health" neurodevelopmental affliction: It is seen almost only in female children. This large (94 hand and foot radiographs) study thus supports skeletal hints including ulna minus on radiographic imaging for suspecting this devastating neuromuscular disease, best recognized by its clinical pattern.[1,2]

A.E. Oestreich, M.D.

References

1. Hagberg B: Rett syndrome: Clinical peculiarities and biological mysteries. *Acta Paediatr* 84:971-976, 1995a.
2. Guerrini R, Bonanni P, Parmeggiani L, et al: Cortical reflex myoclonus in Rett syndrome. *Ann Neurol* 43:472-479, 1998.

Postnatal Development of the Human Sternum

O'Neal ML, Dwornik JJ, Ganey TM, et al (Shriners Hosp for Children, Tampa, Fla; Georgia Baptist Med Ctr, Atlanta)

J Pediatr Orthop 18:398-405, 1998 4–13

Background.—Postnatal development and maturation of the sternum vary greatly. Sternal development was further investigated.

Methods and Findings.—Fifty-six sterna from cadavers, ranging in age from neonate to 95 years, were obtained. Analysis indicated that endochondral ossification centers form in each cartilaginous segment of the sternum, with each center enveloped by a spherical growth plate. One or 2 ossification centers may be present in a cartilaginous center. Those with 2 centers retain and reflect the features of bilateral embryonic origin. In addition, malaligned bifid centers are associated with rib articulation asymmetry. Individual ossification center expansion progresses in the peripheral cartilaginous domains of the sternum. Sternebrae form between the costosternal articulations. Cartilage canals occur throughout unossified regions of the hyaline matrix, consistent with the biology of endochondral transition. Expanding ossification of adjacent sternebrae leads to the depletion of the common cartilaginous area between the 2 sternebrae

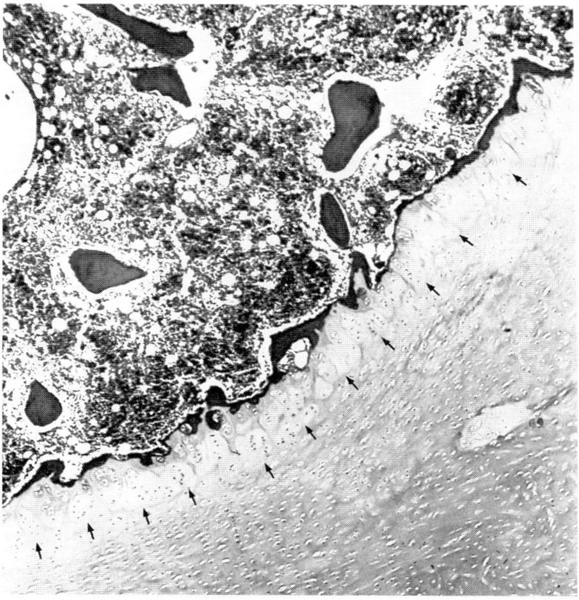

FIGURE 2.—The interface of the expanding ossification center with the surrounding matrix displayed a morphology similar to a secondary center of ossification. Adjacent to the mineralized bone were regions of basophilic staining matrix that were associated with cartilage mineralization. Peripheral to the area of chondrocyte hypertrophy were clusters of proliferating chondrocytes (*arrows*). (Courtesy of O'Neal ML, Dwornik JJ, Ganey TM, et al: Postnatal development of the human sternum. *J Pediatr Orthop* 18:398-405, 1998.)

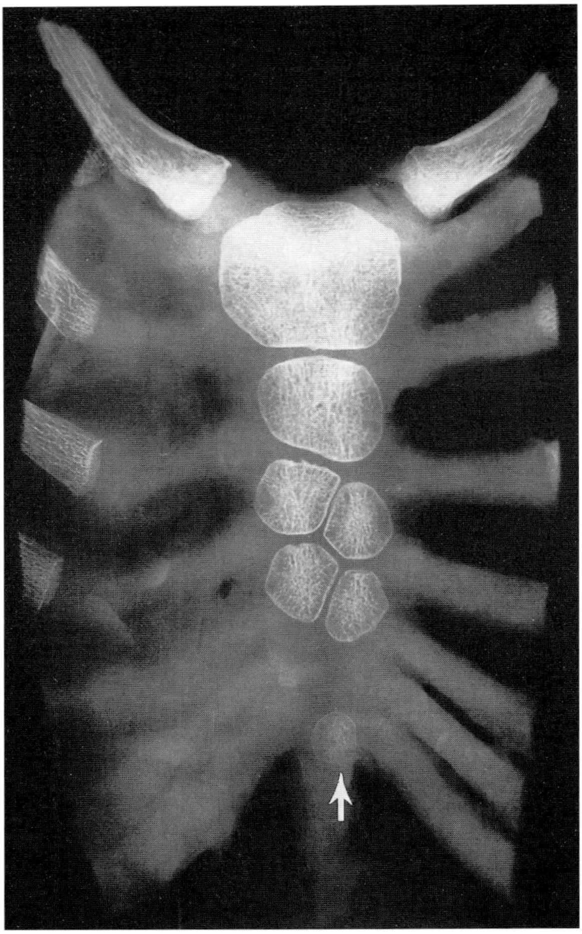

FIGURE 5.—Bilateral origin of the sternum is clearly evident in this sternum from a 9-year-old child. The separate centers of the third and fourth mesosternebrae, although paired, are not symmetrical along the long axis of the sternum. The second sternebra, although not demonstrating clear evidence of independent ossification sites, does retain a vestige of asymmetry along its caudal margin that seemingly attests to its dual origin. An ossification center for the xiphoid process is detectable, even though no ossification center for the fourth mesosternebra is apparent (*arrow*). (Courtesy of O'Neal ML, Dwornik JJ, Ganey TM, et al: Postnatal development of the human sternum. *J Pediatr Orthop* 18:398-405, 1998.)

and, eventually, physiologic epiphysiodesis. Mesosternebrae fusion reciprocates the initial pattern of sternebral ossification site–appearance in a caudal-to-cranial direction.

The union of adjacent sternebrea begins in a central osseous bridge and progresses through anterior, lateral, cephalocaudal, and posterior domains to achieve synostosis. Accessory and bifid centers of ossification in the same intercostal space coalesce before adjoining adjacent sternebrae. The presence of a fibrocartilaginous joint restricting ossification makes manubriosternal fusion rare. The xiphoid process is still connected to the most caudal mesosternum by a common zone of hyaline cartilage, which ossifies by middle-to-late adulthood (Figs 2 and 5).

Conclusion.—A more comprehensive knowledge of anatomical attributes of the developing human sternum may be used to differentiate pathologic conditions from normal variants.

► A worthwhile review and interpretation of ossification and union of ossification centers of the sternum from original anatomical and histologic investigation of cadaver material is displayed. In a word, ossification of the sternum centers is "enchondral" (see Fig 2). Also pertinent to practice are description and explanation of the multiple variations of sternal formation and topology seen by radiologists, for example, in several quoted references.[1,2,3] Radiologists should be grateful for the continuing pioneering anatomical-radiologic correlative work reported by orthopedist John Ogden (of this study) for over 20 years.

A.E. Oestreich, M.D.

References

1. Currarino G, Silverman N: Premature obliteration of the sternum sutures and pigeon breast deformity. *Radiology* 70:532-540, 1958.
2. Fischer KC, White RI Jr, Jordan CE, et al: Sternal abnormalities in patients with congenital heart disease. *Am J Roentgenol* 119:530-538, 1973.
3. Odita JC, Okolo AA, Omene JA: Sternal ossification in normal newborn infants. *Pediatr Radiol* 15:165-167, 1985.

Heterogeneity in Klippel-Feil Syndrome: A New Classification

Clarke RA, Catalan G, Diwan AD, et al (Univ of NSW, Kogarah, Australia; Murdoch Univ, Australia)

Pediatr Radiol 28:967-974, 1998 4–14

Backgound.—Klippel-Feil syndrome (KFS), characterized by congenital vertebral fusion of the cervical spine and other anomalies, is often considered to be sporatic. However, a number of families with KFS have been described, indicating heterogeneity complicated by a broad range of variable expression. An investigation was made of the differences and similarities in the postnatal appearance, morphology, position, and inheritance of vertebral fusions within and among families with KFS and a new KFS classification based on etiology was determined.

Methods.—Three families were assessed. Vertebral fusions were studied by spinal radiography. Chromosomal karyotypes were performed using routine cytogenetics.

Findings.—Variations in the developmental time of appearance and morphology of vertebral fusions, determined on radiographs, suggested different KFS causes. A new classification system, with KFS classes of 1 to 4, was developed. In KF1, C1 fusion is not dominant but is the most rostral

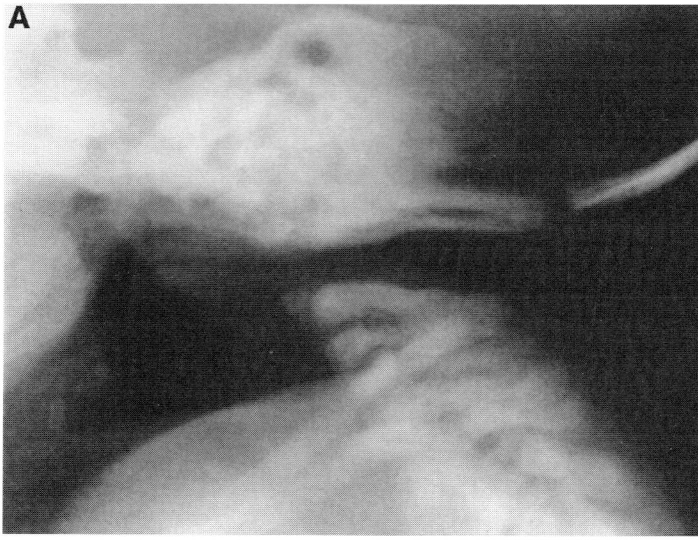

FIGURE 2.—A, Vertical fusions in the KF1-01 family. Lateral spinal radiographs of proband I. Cervical radiograph at 1 day of age showing malsegmentation of the cervical spine. Fusion of spinous processes extends caudal of C1. There is a clear interspace at C4-5 and fusion of C5-7 in association with a very short neck. (Courtesy of Clarke RA, Catalan G, Diwan AD, et al: Heterogeneity in Klippel-Feil syndrome: A new classification. *Pediatr Radiol* 28:967-974. Copyright 1998, Springer-Verlag.)

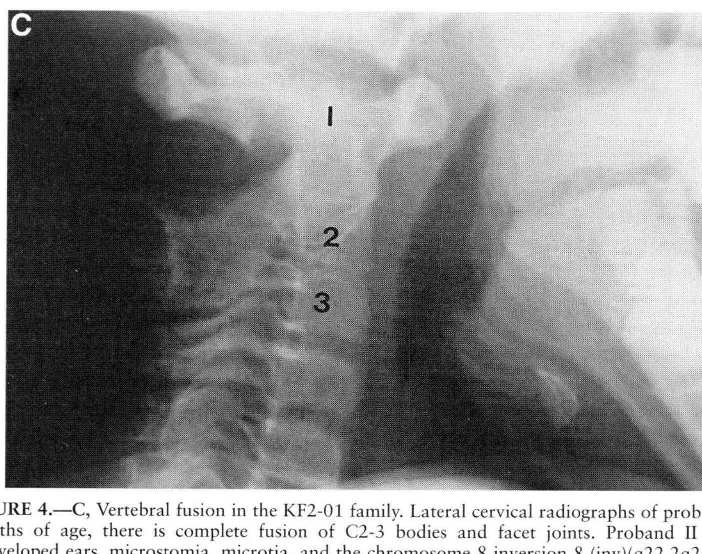

FIGURE 4.—C, Vertebral fusion in the KF2-01 family. Lateral cervical radiographs of proband II. At 48 months of age, there is complete fusion of C2-3 bodies and facet joints. Proband II also had underdeveloped ears, microstomia, microtia, and the chromosome 8 inversion 8 (inv)(q22.2q23.3) common to all other members of her family that display dominant expression of the C2-3 fusion. (Courtesy of Clarke RA, Catalan G, Diwan AD, et al: Heterogeneity in Klippel-Feil syndrome: A new classification. *Pediatr Radiol* 28:967-974. Copyright 1998, Springer-Verlag.)

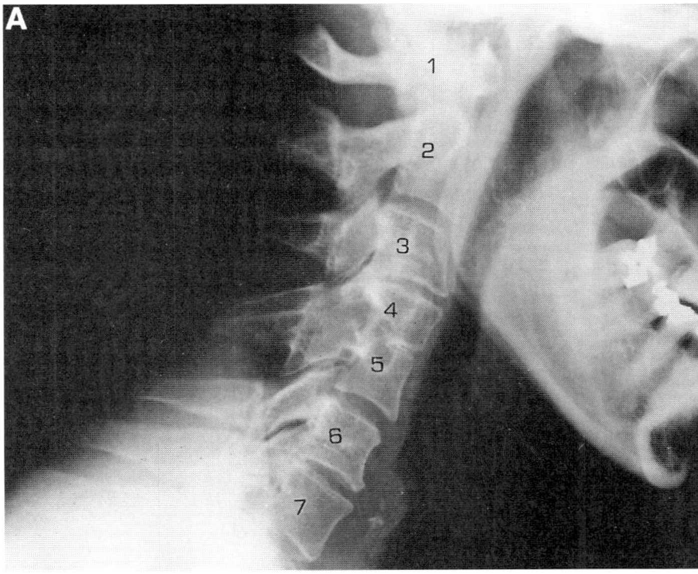

FIGURE 7.—A, Vertebral fusion in the KF3-01 family. Lateral cervical radiograph of proband III with congenital fusion of C4-5 with residual calcified disk. Fusion affects bodies, apophyseal joints, and spinous processes. Degenerative disk at C3-4 and C6-7. (Courtesy of Clarke RA, Catalan G, Diwan AD, et al: Heterogeneity in Klippel-Feil syndrome: A new classification. *Pediatr Radiol* 28:967-974. Copyright 1998, Springer-Verlag.)

fusion. Severe associated anomalies, including the very short neck, is common in this category, and fusion is obvious at birth. The mode of inheritance of KF1 is always recessive. In KF2, C2-3 fusion is dominant and always the most rostral fusion. Fusion is seen postnatally. The mode of inheritance of this form of KFS is dominant. In KF3, C3 fusion is not dominant but most rostral, and there is often a single isolated fusion. Reduced penetrance is the mode of inheritance. In KF4, vertebral fusion and ocular anomalies associated with Wildervanck syndrome are evident. The possible mode of inheritance of this form of KFS is X-linked (Figs 2 A, 4 C, and 7 A).

Conclusion.—This system defined 4 classes based on different vertebral fusion processes, morphologies, and positions; different associated anomalies; and different modes of inheritance. This new classification system is a useful clinical tool that will enable a better understanding of KFS etiology while providing a useful framework for localizing and characterizing the KFS genes.

► The position of the rostral fusion and mode of inheritance seem to justifiably warrant this new classification that recognizes the heterogeneity in KFS. This syndrome has associated anomalies of neurologic types that are not specifically addressed in this article but can be found in the recent literature.[1,2] Some of these are encompassed by this new classification.

L.W. Young, M.D

References

1. Ulmer JL, Elster AD, Ginsberg LE, et al: Klippel-Feil syndrome: CT and MR of acquired and congenital abnormalities of cervical spine and cord. *J Comput Assist Tomogr* 17:215-224, 1993.
2. McGaughran JM, Kuna P, Das V: Audiological abnormalities in the Klippel-Feil syndrome. *Arch Dis Child* 79:352-355, 1998.

Gadolinium-enhanced MR Imaging of Pediatric Patients After Reduction of Dysplastic Hips: Assessment of Femoral Head Position, Factors Impeding Reduction, and Femoral Head Ischemia

Jaramillo D, Villegas-Medina O, Laor T, et al (Harvard Med School, Boston)
AJR 170:1633-1637, 1998 4–15

Background.—CT examination is done in infants with developmental dysplasia of the hip to confirm the femoral head position after reduction and casting. However, CT provides little information about cartilaginous anatomy or perfusion of the femoral head, which is critical for determining the completeness and safety of the reduction. Gd-enhanced MRI of position and vascular enhancement of the femoral head in children who had reduction for hip dislocation was reported.

Methods.—Twenty-five Gd-enhanced MR images were obtained in 18 infants and young children with 23 dysplastic hips within 24 hours of hip reduction and spica casting. Closed reduction was done in all but 2 children. Intraoperative arthrograms were examined for obstacles to reduction and subsequent radiographs for avascular necrosis.

Findings.—On MRI, all femoral heads were in their respective acetabula, although several structures interfered with concentric reduction. Obstacles to reduction included a pulvinar, capsule infolding, labrum interposition, and a hypertrophied ligamentum teres and transverse ligament. All 50 femoral heads enhanced. Hips undergoing greater degrees of abduction showed decreased enhancement (Figs 2, A and F).

Conclusion.—Gd-enhanced MRI is useful for identifying abnormalities of hip position and proximal femoral epiphyseal and physeal vascularity that can occur after hip reduction. Enhancement abnormalities were more common in patients with greater femoral abduction.

► The theme of the 1998 Radiological Society of North America meeting, "Science into Practice," is nicely exemplified by this important article, applying clinically the MRI procedure previously investigated in piglets[1] by Dr. Jaramillo and his team. Structural obstructions to reduction of the congenitally subluxed hip were more frequently shown by MRI in their clinical cases when compared with arthrograms. The MRI method, as demonstrated, also

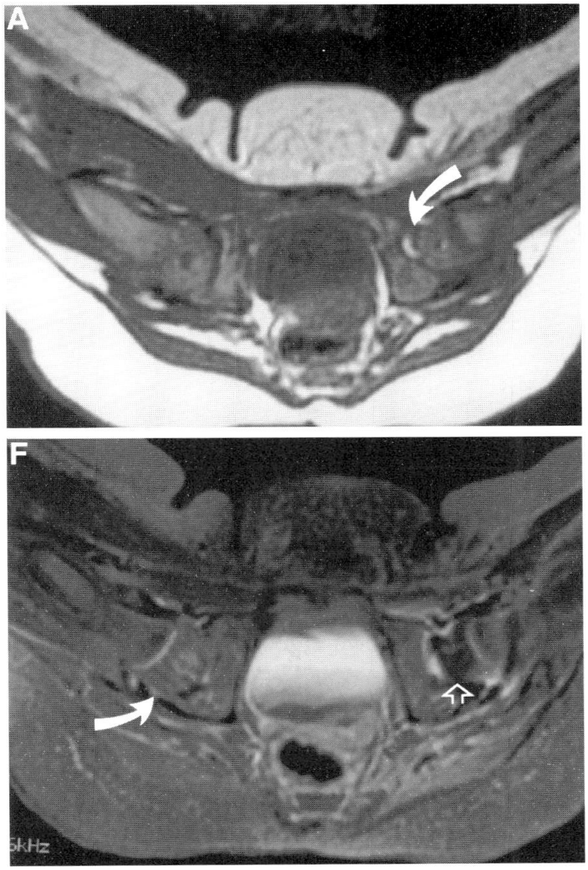

FIGURE 2.—Six-month-old girl who underwent closed reduction of left hip. Gd enhancement of T1-weighted MR images (repetition time/echo time, 300/20) shows focal areas of decreased enhancement (grade 3). **A**, Unenhanced MR image shows that reduction of hip can be clearly established. A pulvinar (*arrow*) is evident, and left femoral head is displaced laterally. **F**, 2 levels of axial fat-suppressed Gd-enhanced MR images obtained 4 minutes 30 seconds after contrast administration. Normal striped appearance of enhanced cartilaginous femoral head and normal articular relationships are evident on right side (*solid arrow*). On left, decreased enhancement in posterior (*open arrow*) and superior portions of femoral head are seen. (Courtesy of Jaramillo D, Villegas-Medina O, Laor T, et al: Gadolinium-enhanced MR imaging of pediatric patients after reduction of dysplastic hips: Assessment of femoral head position, factors impeding reduction, and femoral head ischemia. *AJR* 170:1633-1637, 1998.)

promises to allow identification of those reduced femoral heads whose vascularity is in jeopardy (those hips that showed decreased Gd enhancement in their reduced position had undergone greater degrees of abduction as demonstrated on MRI). As the infants were reasonably immobilized by the spica cast, formal sedation was not required—another useful insight.

A.E. Oestreich, M.D.

Reference

1. Jaramillo D, Villegas-Medina OL, Doty DK, et al: Gadolinium-enhanced MR imaging demonstrates abduction-caused hip ischemia and its reversal in piglets. *AJR* 166:879-887, 1996.

Sonography of Patellar Abnormalities in Children

Miller TT, Shapiro MA, Schultz E, et al (North Shore Univ Hosp, Manhasset, NY; North Shore Radiology, Great Neck, NY; Kernan Hosp, Baltimore, Md)
AJR 171:739-742, 1998 4–16

Introduction.—Sonography, with its ability to show cartilaginous structures, is widely used to examine the unossified hip in suspected developmental dysplasia. The use of US to examine the unossified patella and patellofemoral joint in 3 children with congenital abnormalities of the extensor mechanism of the knee was described.

Methods.—An HDI 3000 unit with a 10-5-MHz linear or compact linear probe was used for US. Scans were taken in both the longitudinal and transverse planes as the scan operator flexed and extended the patient's knee. The examination took less than 10 minutes to perform.

> *Case 1.*—Girl, 2 years, with proximal focal femoral deficiency, underwent scanning before multistage reconstruction and limb lengthening to determine whether a patella was present and if patellar tracking was normal. US demonstrated a skeletally immature patella, manifested by small size and absence of an ossific

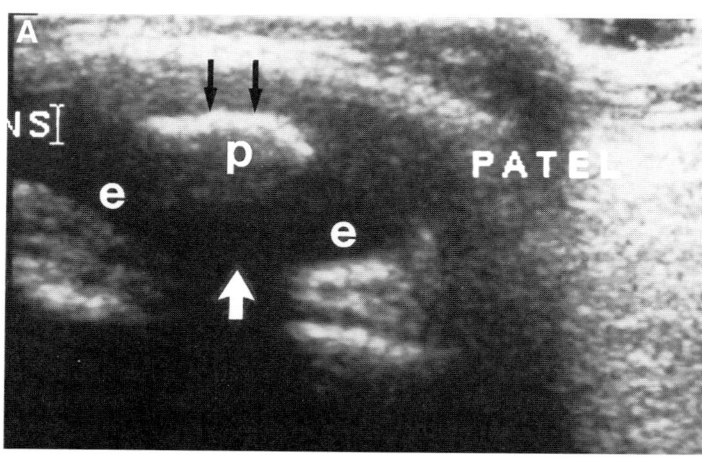

FIGURE 1.—Imaging in a 2-year-old girl with left-sided proximal focal femoral deficiency and lateral subluxation of left patella. **A**, Transverse sonogram of normal right knee shows patella (*P*) well centered in femoral sulcus (*white arrow*) and appropriately ossified for age (*black arrows*). *Abbreviation: E*, femoral epiphyseal cartilage. (Courtesy of Miller TT, Shapiro MA, Schultz E, et al: Sonography of patellar abnormalities in children. *AJR* 171:739-742, 1998.)

nucleus compared with the normal knee, and lateral patellar subluxation in both flexion and extension (Fig 1 A). The patient was doing well clinically at 17 months after initial limb lengthening and femoral valgus osteotomy and 7.5 months after patellar realignment, pelvic osteotomy, and soft-tissue releases.

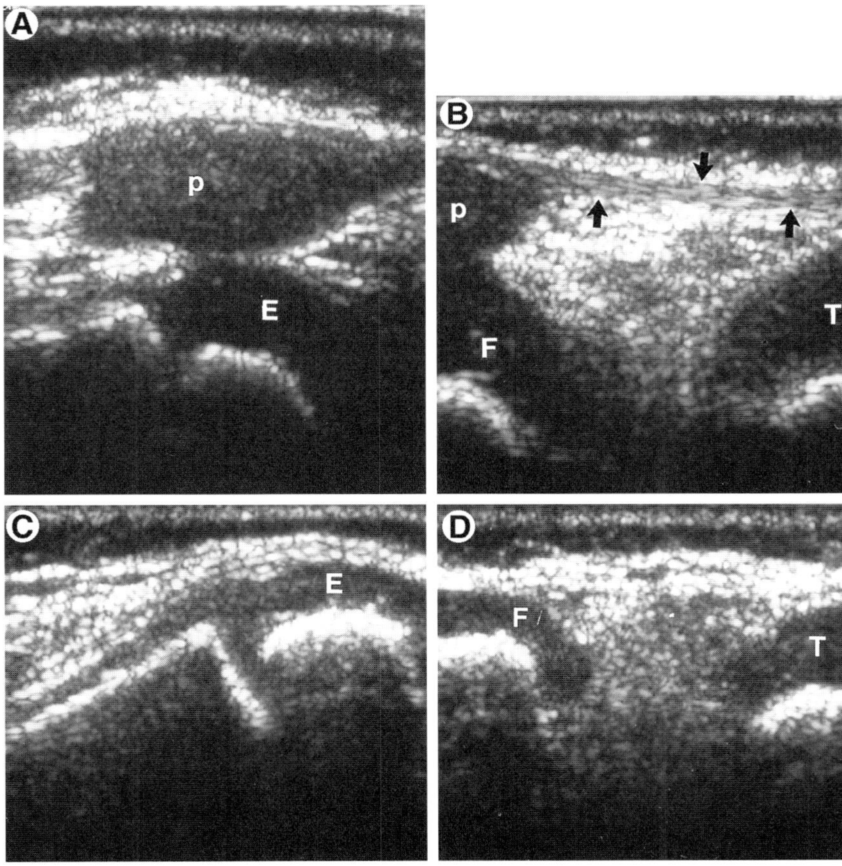

FIGURE 2.—Imaging in a 7-month-old girl with inability to actively extend right leg, depression over knee, and mass in thigh. **A**, Longitudinal sonogram of normal left knee at level of distal femur shows unossified patella (*P*) appropriately located anterior to cartilaginous portion of distal femoral epiphysis (*E*). **B**, Longitudinal sonogram of normal left knee at level of knee joint shows lower pole of patella (*p*), normal patellar tendon (*arrows*), and cartilaginous epiphyses of distal femur (*F*) and tibia (*T*). **C**, Longitudinal sonogram of affected right knee at level of distal femur shows distal femural epiphyses (*E*). Note lack of patella, unlike **A**. **D**, Longitudinal sonogram of affected right knee at level of joint shows cartilaginous epiphyses of distal femur (*F*) and tibia (*T*). Note lack of patellar tendon, unlike **B**. **E**, Longitudinal sonogram of affected right thigh at level of palpable mass shows unossified patella (*P*) located anterior to femoral shaft cortex (*white arrows*). Normal quadriceps tendon is present (*straight black arrows*), but patellar tendon is atretic (*curved arrow*). **F**, Postoperative longitudinal sonogram of affected right knee at level of distal femur and joint shows patella (*P*) appropriately located anterior to distal femoral epiphysis (*F*), neotendon (*arrows*), and proximal tibial epiphysis (*T*). (Courtesy of Miller TT, Shapiro MA, Schultz E, et al: Sonography of patellar abnormalities in children. *AJR* 171:739-742, 1998.)

(*Continued*)

FIGURE 2 (cont.)

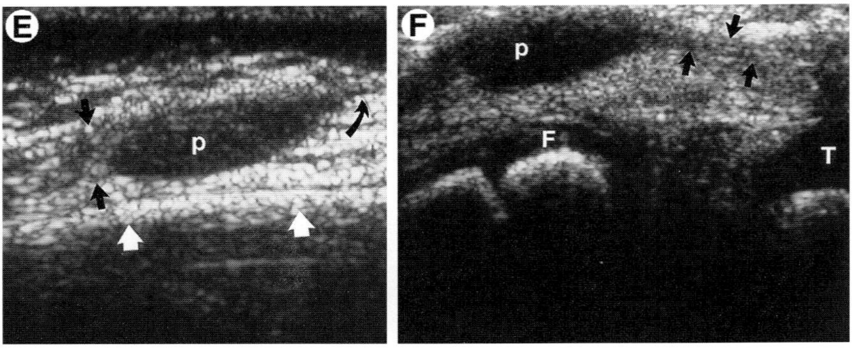

Case 2.—Girl, 7 months, was unable to actively extend the leg and had a depression over the anterior aspect of the knee joint and a palpable small mass over the anterior aspect of the distal thigh. US showed a normally developed patella. The patellar tendon was atretic and the patella had retracted into the thigh, which explained the depression over the knee and the mass in the thigh (Fig 2). These findings were confirmed at surgery. Follow-up sonographs 3 months after successful reconstruction of a patellar tendon revealed the neotendon and the corrected position of the patella with mild lateral subluxation. The patient was able to walk without support at 1 year after surgery.

Case 3.—Boy, 2 years 10 months, had a depression over both knees and a "toe out" gait. Abnormal thumbnails and absence of the patella were documented by MRI of both knees. Bilateral US revealed the normal position of the extensor tendons within the femoral sulci in both flexion and extension. Surgery was not considered.

Conclusion.—US is recommended as the imaging procedure of choice to determine the extensor mechanism and unossified patella in young children. The advantages of sonography over MRI include the following: no need for sedation, speed of examination and ability to compare with the contralateral knee, low cost, and the sonographer's ability to dynamically assess the extensor mechanism.

▶ This is a practical, well-illustrated article about the usefulness of US imaging in the young child with suspected abnormality of the extensor mechanism of the knee region. It should, by now, be well known that US can elegantly demonstrate the unossified patella, its tendons, and the nearby surfaces of the femur.[1,2] Because of the ease of dynamic sonographic imaging, exact clinical questions can be answered for such infants and toddlers, as nicely reported in this article regarding 3 children under 3 years of age.

A.E. Oestreich, M.D.

References

1. Oestreich AE: Imaging of the skeleton and soft tissue in children. *Curr Opin Radiol* 3:889-894, 1991.
2. Walker J, Rang M, Daneman A: Ultrasonography of the unossified patella in young children. *J Pediatr Orthop* 11:100-102, 1991.

US of the Painful Hip in Childhood: Diagnostic Value of Cartilage Thickening and Muscle Atrophy in the Detection of Perthes Disease

Robben SGF, Meradji M, Diepstraten AFM, et al (Univ Hosp, Rotterdam, The Netherlands; Erasmus Univ, Rotterdam, The Netherlands)

Radiology 208:35-42, 1998 4–17

Background.—US has been recommended as the examination of choice for painful hips. The combined use of several US criteria in the detection of Perthes' disease was described.

Methods.—One hundred forty-four consecutive children with a painful hip underwent US prospectively. The thicknesses of the anterior recess of the joint capsule, femoral head cartilage, and quadriceps muscle were evaluated. In addition, 68 asymptomatic children were studied for comparison.

Findings.—Final diagnoses were transient synovitis in 58 patients, Perthes' disease in 21, slipped capital femoral epiphysis in 5, and other in 6. Fifty-four patients had no abnormalities on US or radiography. These patients' symptoms disappeared during follow-up. In patients with transient synovitis, the anterior recess was significantly wider than that in other patients and control subjects. Patients with Perthes' disease had significant cartilage thickening in the symptomatic hip compared with the other patient and control groups. Those with Perthes' disease and with slipped capital femoral epiphysis had significant atrophy of the ipsilateral quadriceps muscle compared with all other groups. The use of these US criteria for diagnosing Perthes' disease had a sensitivity of 71%, a specificity of 99%, and positive and negative predictive values of 95% each (Fig 2).

Conclusion.—Combining several US criteria enhances the diagnostic value of US in the assessment of painful hip in patients with Perthes' disease. Regardless of symptom duration, Perthes disease should be suspected in patients with a painful hip who have ipsilateral cartilage thickening, muscle atrophy, or both on US.

► The first strong contribution here is a more elegant, somewhat oblique, US position (Fig 2) for measurement of femoral head cartilage thickness (as compared with using the sagittal position[1] used for detection of fluid by all of us). Secondly, the finding of 5 mm more femoral epiphyseal cartilage

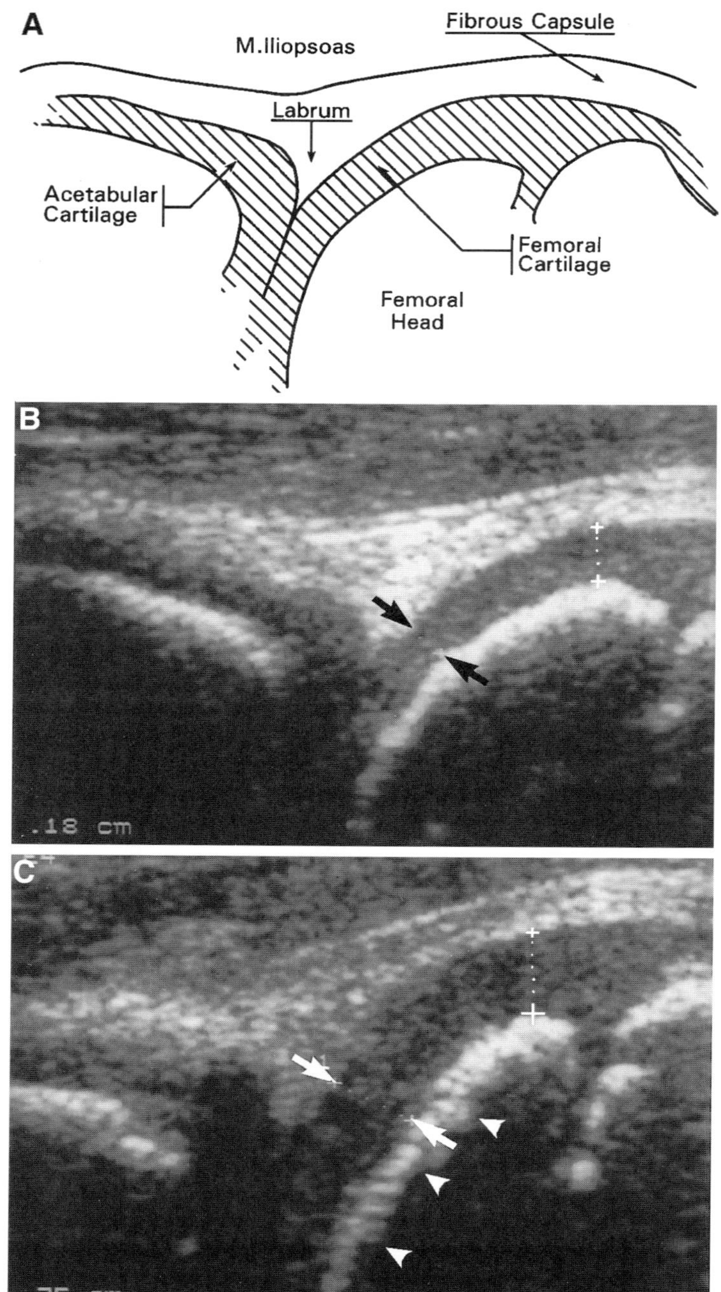

FIGURE 2.—A, Schematic shows a normal right hip. *Abbreviation: M*, musculus. B, C, Parasagittal US scans of the normal right hip (B) and the affected left hip (C) in a 5-year-old boy with Perthes' disease. The cartilage thickness (*arrows*) was 1.8 mm in B and 3.5 mm in C. Note the mild flattening of the osseous nucleus (*arrowheads*) in C. (Courtesy of Robben SGF, Meradji M, Diepstraten AFM, et al: US of the painful hip in childhood: Diagnostic value of cartilage thickening and muscle atrophy in the detection of Perthes disease. *Radiology* 208:35-42, 1998. Radiological Society of North America.)

in a Perthes'-diseased hip compared with an asymptomatic contralateral side is particularly helpful when US examination is the first imaging method for a child with unilateral hip pain. Because I favor the third explanation offered by the authors for the cartilage discrepancy (delayed bone maturation on the Perthes' disease side), I urge a term other than "thickening" of cartilage. A delayed commitment of epiphyseal cartilage to become bone in the femoral head, resulting from the decreased vascularity of the region, leaves more pre-existing cartilage compared with the normally matured contralateral side. A term that is theory neutral, such as "wider cartilage," would do just fine. Another recent article offers compelling information as to what constitutes the widening of the medial joint space from the MRI perspective.[2]

A.E. Oestreich, M.D.

References

1. Castriota-Scanderbeg A, Orsi E: Slipped capital femoral epiphysis: Ultrasonographic findings. *Skeletal Radiol* 22:191-193, 1993.
2. Song H-R, Lee S-H, Na J-B, et al: Comparison of MRI with subchondral fracture in the evaluation of extent of epiphyseal necrosis in the early stage of Legg-Calve-Perthes disease. *J Pediatr Orthop* 19:70-75, 1999.

Ultrasonography: Can It Differentiate Between Vasoocclusive Crisis and Acute Osteomyelitis in Sickle Cell Disease?

Sadat-Ahi M, Al-Umran K, Al-Habdan I, et al (King Fahd Hosp of the Univ, Al-Khobar, Saudi Arabia)

J Pediatr Orthop 18:552-554, 1998 4–18

Background.—Acute osteomyelitis (AO) and vaso-occlusive crisis (VOC) are common in patients with sickle-cell disease (SCD). The value of US in differentiating VOC from AO in patients with SCD was investigated.

Methods and Findings.—US was performed in 53 children, aged 1 to 14 years, with SCD and suspected of having VOC or AO. In 32% of the children, US changes suggested AO with a variety of findings including periosteal elevation, subperiosteal or intramedullary abscess, and cortical erosions. White cell counts ranged from 7,200/mm^3 to 9,900/mm^3 in uninfected patients. In 17 patients, the mean white cell count was 10,300/mm^3. In uninfected patients, the mean erythrocyte sedimentation rate was 32 mm for the first hour, compared with 43 mm in infected patients. Pus culture was positive in all infected patients. The infective organism was *Salmonella enteriitis* in 8, *Staphylococcus* species in 6, anaerobic streptococci in 2, and *Streptococcus pyogenes* in 1. Figures 1, B and C show changes seen in 1 patient on the third day of symptoms. All patients with VOC received analgesics and IV fluids, with no further treatment required. Patients with AO were treated with incision, drainage, bone drilling, and antibiotic therapy.

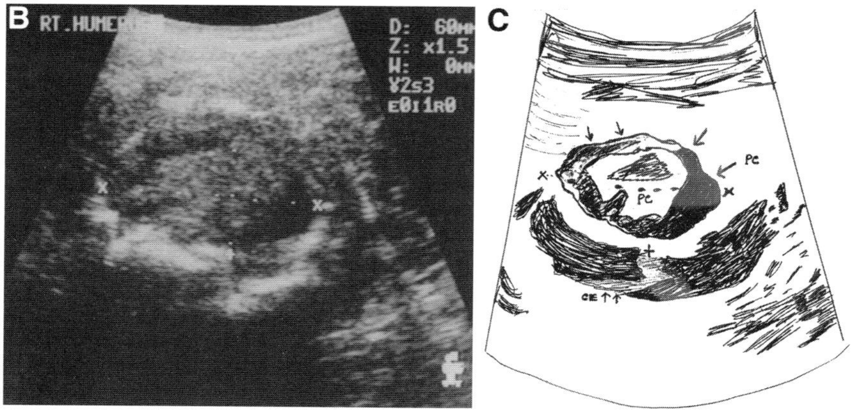

FIGURE 1.—B, US scan of the humerus showing cortical destruction and abscess formation. **C**, Schematic picture of **B**. Cortical destruction (*CE*) and subperiosteal collection (*PC*) are marked clearly. (Courtesy of Sadat-Ahi M, Al-Umran K, Al-Habdan I, et al: Ultrasonography: Can it differentiate between vasoocclusive crisis and acute osteomyelitis in sickle cell disease? *J Pediatr Orthop* 18:552-554, 1998.)

Conclusion.—US clearly differentiates AO from VOC in patients with SCD. With this modality as the first line of assessment, unnecessary surgery can be avoided.

► Although the results in this article seem too good to be true, the practical guidance of their recommendations should be helpful. The vexing question of infection versus infarction in SCD with limb symptoms has been one of the puzzlers of pediatric radiology. Dr. Sadat-Ali and colleagues report decisive differentiation using US imaging to detect or to deny subperiosteal (or cortical) abnormality. The more conservative conclusions of the Australian group[1] that US cannot be fully relied upon for the recognition of AO seem more reasonable. Nonetheless, when pus *is* seen by US, it can be diagnosed and drained. Or, as another recent article indicates, at least the US can confirm the presence of subperiosteal fluid as a guide to aspiration, which can distinguish between hematoma and abscess.[2]

A.E. Oestreich, M.D.

References

1. Mah ET, LeQuesne GW, Gent RJ, et al: Ultrasonic features of acute osteomyelitis in children. *J Bone Joint Surg Br* 76:969-974, 1994.
2. Rifai A, Nyman R: Scintigraphy and ultrasonography in differentiating osteomyelitis from bone infarction in sickle cell disease. *Acta Radiol* 38:139-143, 1997.

Use of Contrast-enhanced MR Imaging to Detect Sacroiliitis in Children

Bollow M, Braun J, Biedermann T, et al (Humboldt-Universität zu Berlin; Freie Universität Berlin; Krankenhaus Berlin Buch)

Skeletal Radiol 27:606-616, 1998 4–19

Background.—Previous research has shown that MRI demonstrates sacroiliitis as the key imaging finding of spondyloarthropathy (SpA) in its early stages in adults with negative radiographic findings. The diagnostic value of contrast-enhanced MRI compared with conventional radiography in the diagnosis of sacroiliitis in children was investigated.

Methods.—One hundred eighty-five children were studied. Three experienced radiologists, unaware of clinical data, independently assessed the radiographs based on the modified New York criteria. These radiologists then independently assessed the MR images, also without knowing the clinical data or radiographic findings.

Findings.—Radiography demonstrated sacroiliitis in 7.5% of the 53 children with undifferentiated spondyloarthropathy (group 1) and in 31% of the 45 patients with differentiated SpA (group 2). Radiography did not demonstrate sacroiliitis in the 39 children with no signs of SpA other than oligoarthritis (group 3), in 22 HLA-B27+ control subjects with various other non-SpA diagnoses (group 4), or in 26 histocompatability leukocyte antigen-B27 control subjects with various other non-SpA diagnoses (group 5). MR images showed acute and/or chronic sacroiliitis in 34% of group 1 children, 46.7% of group 2, 12.8% of group 3, and none of groups 4 or 5. MRI detected a significantly greater percentage of sacroiliitis cases than did radiography (Fig 5).

Conclusion.—Contrast-enhanced MRI is useful for identifying sacroiliitis in children. The advantages of contrast-enhanced MRI are its greater sensitivity because of its ability to document early and acute changes and the absence of radiation exposure.

▶ This excellent article and another current article thoroughly verify, in prospective study, the diagnostic value of contrast-enhanced MR imaging for the diagnosis of sacroiliitis in children.[1] The article's figures are well prepared and clearly show the superior MRI findings that provide for earlier diagnosis than can be achieved with radiographic imaging or with scintigraphy.[2] These authors have also recently published an article on normal MRI morphology of the sacroiliac joints in children.[3]

L.W. Young, M.D.

References

1. Bollow M, Biedermann T, Kannenberg J, et al: Use of dynamic magnetic resonance imaging to detect sacroiliitis in HLA-B27 positive and negative children with juvenile arthritides. *J Rheumatol* 25:556-564, 1998.
2. Blum U, Buitrago-Tellez C, Mundinger A, et al: Magnetic resonance imaging (MRI) for detection of active sacroiliitis: A prospective study comparing conventional radiography, scintigraphy, and contrast enhanced MRI. *J Rheumatol* 23:2107-2115, 1996.

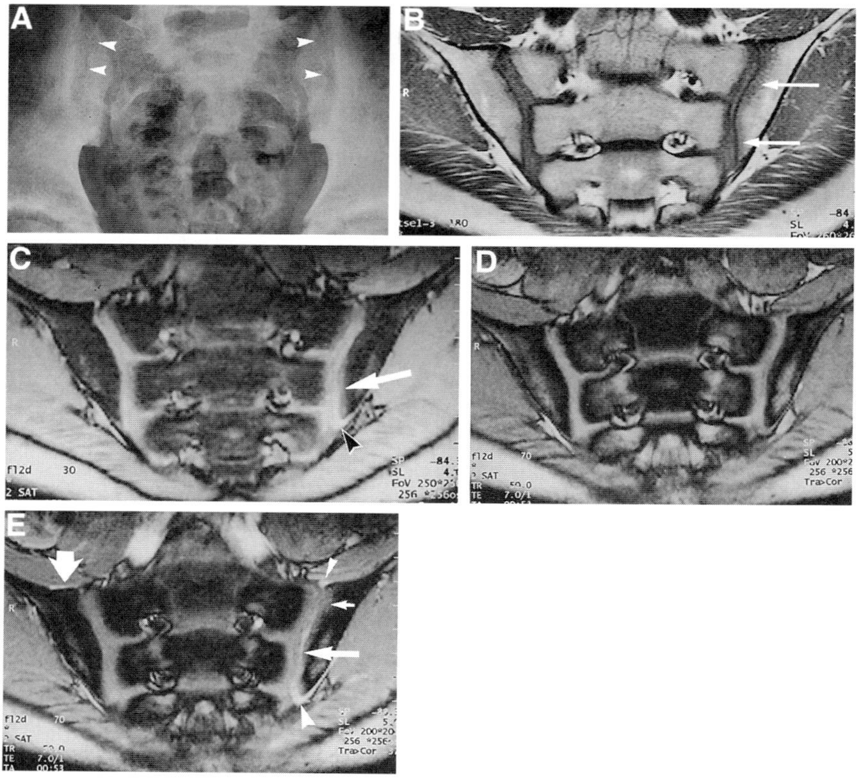

FIGURE 5.—Images obtained in a 13-year-old boy with histocompatability leukocyte antigen-B27–associated undifferentiated spondyloarthropathy (group 1: uSpA) and a duration of back pain of 8 weeks. The parents reported a severe iritis about 2 years previously and a positive family history of ankylosing spondylitis. **A**, The conventional radiograph of the pelvis depicted no pathologic changes of the sacroiliac joints. Bone margins were not sharply demarcated as the result of nonossified segmental apophyses of the sacral wings (*arrowheads*), **B**, An unenhanced longitudinal relaxation time–weighted turbo spin-echo sequence (583/12) depicted regularly delineated joint spaces, both sides with cartilage of intermediate signal intensity. The left iliac juxta-articular region showed blurred low-signal zones (*arrow*). **C**, On the unenhanced effective transverse relaxation time–weighted opposed-phase fast low-angle shot (FLASH) sequence (350/12, 30 degrees), obtained in the same section position as **B**, the left joint space appeared blurred and widened (8 mm) because of a hyperintense iliac subchondral zone (*arrow*), which was continuous with the dorsal joint capsule (*arrowhead*). **D**, Dynamic longitudinal relaxation time–weighted opposed-phase FLASH image (50/7,70 degrees) obtained before contrast enhancement. **E**, Same sequence as **D** 7 minutes after a bolus of Gd-DTPA. There is pronounced enhancement of the juxta-articular region (*medium arrow*: juxta-articular synovitis) and the dorsal joint capsule (*arrowhead*: capsulitis). Beyond it, there was moderate enhancement of the left iliac bone marrow (*small arrow*: periarticular osteitis). The ventral right joint capsule was visualized as linear zones of moderate enhancement (*large arrow*; physiologic capsule enhancement). In conclusion, the MR chronicity index was grade 0 on both sides with an activity index of grade X on the right and grade B on the left side. (Courtesy of Bollow M, Braun J, Biedermann T, et al: Use of contrast-enhanced MR imaging to detect sacroiliitis in children. *Skeletal Radiol* 27:606-616. Copyright 1998, Springer-Verlag.)

3. Bollow M, Braun J, Kannenberg J, et al: Normal morphology of sacroiliac joints in children: Magnetic resonance studies related to age and sex. *Skeletal Radiol* 26:697-704, 1997.

Contrast Enhanced Magnetic Resonance Imaging as a Method to Diagnose Early Inflammatory Changes in the Temporomandibular Joint in Children With Juvenile Chronic Arthritis

Küseler A, Pedersen TK, Herlin T, et al (Univ of Aarhus, Denmark)
J Rheumatol 25:1406-1412, 1998 4–20

Background.—Early diagnosis of temporomandibular joint (TMJ) involvement in children with juvenile chronic arthritis is important so that treatment can be initiated before condylar head destruction and growth changes occur. Although TMJ is often asymptomatic, studies with contrast-enhanced MRI of other joints have shown the possibility of detecting early inflammatory changes.

Methods.—Fifteen children, mean age of 12 years, with newly diagnosed juvenile chronic arthritis were studied. TMJs were examined clinically, radiographically, and with MRI enhanced with Gd-DTPA. Ten healthy children, mean age 11.5 years, were also assessed.

Findings.—In 87% of the patients, Gd-DTPA–enhanced MRI indicated inflammatory activity. Conventional MRI without contrast medium was not useful in the diagnosis of early inflammatory changes (Fig 2).

Conclusion.—Enhanced MRI is very effective for the diagnosis of early inflammatory changes of the TMJ. This modality is more sensitive than clinical examination and radiography.

► Juvenile chronic (in the United States, "rheumatoid") arthritis can have a major detrimental effect on jaw shape and function. The need (and hope) is to diagnose *early* TMJ inflammation reliably enough so that early enough preventive action[1] might be initiated. This article reports convincingly that MRI was effective in most of the authors' early patients (13 of 15), but *only* with the use of Gd-DTPA enhancement. Other recent articles[2,3] support this point.

A.E. Oestreich, M.D.

References

1. Pedersen TK, Gronhoj J, Melsen B, et al: Condylar condition and mandibular growth during early functional treatment of children with juvenile chronic arthritis. *Eur J Orthod* 17:385-394, 1995.
2. Sebag G, Herve-Somma C, Lallemand D: Imaging of joints in children. *Rev Prat* 44:2587-2591, 1994.
3. Murray JG, Ridley NT, Mitchell N, et al: Juvenile chronic arthritis of the hip: Value of contrast-enhanced MR imaging. *Clin Radiol* 51:99-102, 1996.

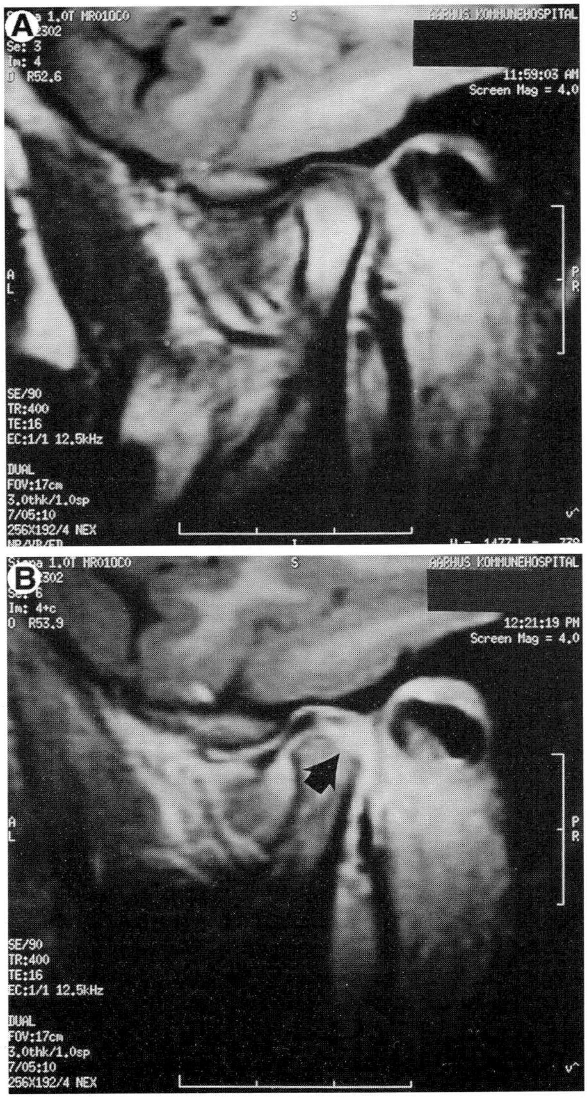

FIGURE 2.—A, Precontrast T1-weighted MR image of the temporomandibular joint in a child with juvenile chronic arthritis. **B**, Postcontrast T1-weighted image of the same patient. Note the enhancement of the synovial membrane (*arrow*). (Courtesy of Küseler A, Pedersen TK, Herlin T, et al: Contrast enhanced magnetic resonance imaging as a method to diagnose early inflammatory changes in the temporomandibular joint in children with juvenile chronic arthritis. *J Rheumatol* 25:1406-1412, 1998.)

Langerhans Cell Histiocytosis: Unusual Skeletal Manifestations Observed in Thirty-four Cases

Hindman BW, Thomas RD, Young LW, et al (Loma Linda Univ Med Ctr, Calif)

Skeletal Radiol 27:177-181, 1998 4–21

Introduction.—Langerhans' cell histiocytosis (LCH) consists of several diseases related by histiocytic proliferation and frequency of skeletal lesions. Skeletal manifestations of LCH vary by disease type. The frequency of unusual manifestations of LCH diseases was examined in 34 children.

Methods.—The average patient age was 4.4 years (range, 3 months to 16 years). Two hundred sixty-two skeletal lesions of biopsy-proven LCH were examined retrospectively. Unusual manifestations were defined as either atypical location of a skeletal lesion or an atypical radiographic appearance of a lesion.

Results.—There were 24 unusual lesions in this series. Findings included epiphyseal lesions, transphyseal lesions (Fig 5), extra-cranial "button" sequestra, posterior vertebral arch lesions, dural extension of vertebral lesions, and fluid-fluid levels. Radiographic literature has not previously described findings of fluid-fluid levels.

Conclusion.—A variety of unusual manifestations of LCH have been detected by radiography, CT, and MRI. Recognition of varied appearances

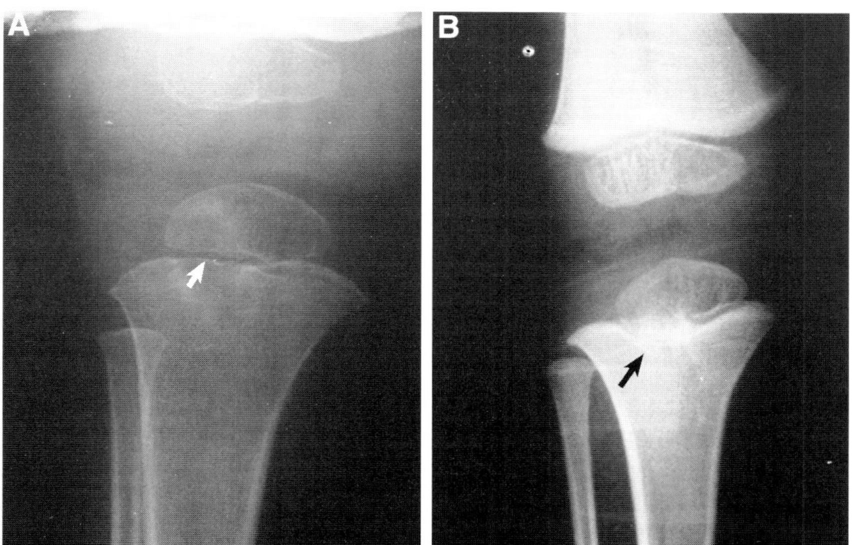

FIGURE 5.—Imaging in a 1-year-old boy with multiple lesions in the skull, pelvis, femur, and right tibia. The lesions were treated with vinblastine and prednisone and disappeared. **A**, Anteroposterior radiograph of the knee demonstrates transphyseal spread (*arrow*) of a lytic lesion. Sclerosis is identified proximal and distal to the lesion and represents a reparative process. **B**, Anteroposterior radiograph 10 months later reveals premature closure of the central physis (*arrow*) corresponding to the site of the original lesion. (Courtesy of Hindman BW, Thomas RD, Young LW, et al: Langerhans cell histiocytosis: Unusual skeletal manifestations observed in thirty-four cases. *Skeletal Radiol* 27:177-181. Copyright 1998, Springer-Verlag.)

of LCH can prevent confusion with the appearances of other pathologic processes.

► I am nostalgic for the old name "histiocytosis X," but sensitivity training would teach that children may not like being labeled with a disease containing "X" in its designation. Nonetheless, the cause and best treatment of these conditions that affect the dendritic cell system remain unknown.[1] One fascinating, unusual skeletal manifestation is the transphyseal lesion (see Fig 5), which may lead to a tether across that growth plate (why?). In our (Cincinnati Children's Hospital) patient with a proximal femoral transphyseal lesion, such a tether has not developed (yet).

After reading this article, we can add LCH (at least, of the skull) to the list of lesions that can show fluid-fluid levels. This article succinctly reminds us of some less common epiphyseal,[2] posterior vertebral arch, and other manifestations.[3]

A.E. Oestreich, M.D.

References

1. Egeler RM, D'Angio GJ: Langerhans cell histiocytosis. *J Pediatr* 127:1-11, 1995.
2. Leeson MC, Smith A, Carter JR, et al: Eosinophilic granuloma of bone in the growing epiphysis. *J Pediatr Orthop* 5:147-150, 1985.
3. Kilpatrick SE, Wenger DE, Gilchrist GS, et al: Langerhans' cell histiocytosis (histiocytosis X) of bone: A clinicopathologic analysis of 263 pediatric and adult cases. *Cancer* 76:2471-2484, 1995.

Appropriate Imaging in Children With Skull Fractures and Suspicion of Abuse

Mogbo KI, Slovis TL, Canady AI, et al (Children's Hosp of Michigan, Detroit; Wayne State Univ, Detroit)
Radiology 208:521-524, 1998 4–22

Introduction.—Screening radiography of the skull is performed in children with suspected abuse and a history of head trauma. When a skull fracture is detected, clinicians and radiologists are reluctant, however, to forego CT evaluation in those who are neurologically normal. The American College of Radiology specifically recommends that brain CT should be performed in children aged 2 years or younger with head trauma and no focal findings or neurologic abnormalities. Data supporting these head CT recommendations are lacking. The role of CT in children aged 2 years and younger with head trauma, suspected abuse, and normal neurologic findings were retrospectively examined.

Methods.—Between 1992 and 1995, 87 consecutive children with skull fractures visible on plain radiography were referred to child protective services for assessment of suspected abuse. Medical records were reviewed for skull radiographic findings, CT findings, clinical status on initial visit, neurologic findings, clinical outcome, and legal outcome (final placement

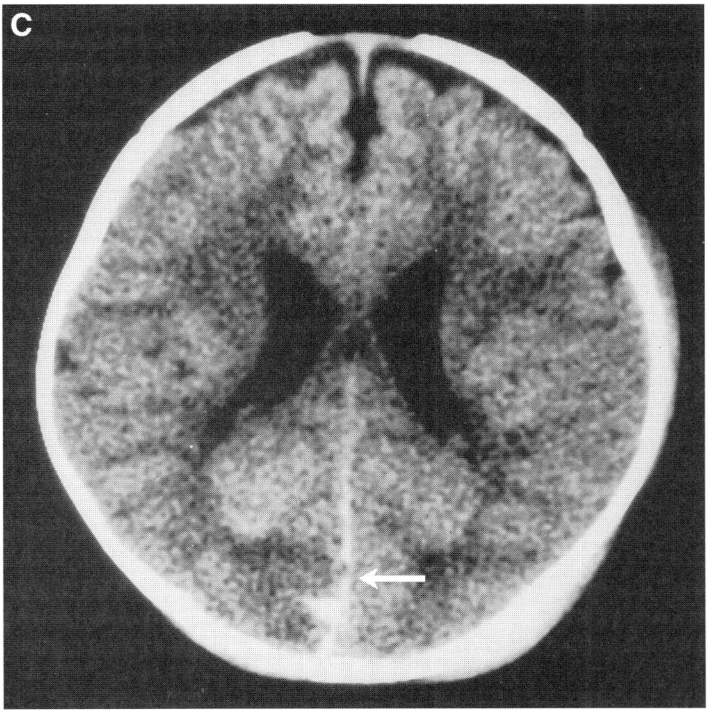

FIGURE 1.—Nonenhanced CT scan depicts findings associated with skull fractures in neurologically normal patients. C, Image obtained at the level of the atria reveals subarachnoid blood along the posterior falx (*arrow*) associated with a left parietal fracture. (Courtesy of Mogbo KI, Slovis TL, Canady AI, et al: Appropriate imaging in children with skull fractures and suspicion of abuse. *Radiology* 208:521-524, 1998. Radiological Society of North America.)

of the child). Only patients with skull fracture visible on plain radiography were included.

Results.—Of 87 children evaluated, 67 had normal neurologic findings. None of the children with normal findings needed further evaluation or intervention. Children referred for CT tended to have multiple or more complex skull fractures and additional injuries or illness. Of 32 patients (48%) in whom head CT was performed, only 6 (19%) had evidence of acute intracranial injury. This was in spite of the presence of minimal depression and stellate, multiple, and diastatic fractures (Fig 1 C). There were positive CT scans in 16 of 20 children (80%) with acute neurologic findings. Of these, 9 (45%) underwent neurosurgical intervention.

Conclusion.—Clinically important abnormalities were not detected at CT in any of the children with normal neurologic findings. Clinical management, clinical outcome, and legal outcome were not changed as a result of CT findings. Routine head CT of all children with skull fractures from abuse or suspected abuse may not be necessary.

► In general, the absence of skull fracture is not to be reassuring in children with head trauma. In the special situation of suspected child abuse, the presence of skull fracture alone may not support the suspicion, especially if no other fractures are detected elsewhere. This article further adds to the skull-fracture-in-suspected-abuse discussion[1-4] by providing support against the routine use of head CT in neurologically intact (and eyegrounds normal!) children thus examined. As the authors point out, cross-sectional imaging may, however, be relevant in the different situation of strong abuse suspicion but normal skeletal survey and grossly normal neurologic examination.

A.E. Oestreich, M.D.

References

1. Petitti N, Williams DW III: CT and MR imaging of nonaccidental pediatric head trauma. *Acad Radiol* 5:215-223, 1998.
2. Griscom NT: Imaging of nonaccidental head trauma in children (letter). *Acad Radiol* 6:81, 1999.
3. Zimmerman RA, Bilaniuk LT: Pediatric head trauma. *Neuroimaging Clin N Am* 4:349-366, 1994.
4. Ewing-Cobbs L, Kramer L, Prasad M, et al: Neuroimaging, physical, and developmental findings after inflicted and noninflicted traumatic brain injury in young children. *Pediatrics* 102:300-307, 1998.

Little Leaguer's Shoulder: A Report of 23 Cases

Carson WG Jr, Gasser SI (Sports Medicine Clinic of Tampa, Fla; Florida Orthopaedic Inst, Tampa)

Am J Sports Med 26:575-580, 1998 4–23

Introduction.—A total of 14 cases of Little Leaguer's shoulder have been reported in the literature by 8 different authors. The exact etiology is unknown. This clinical entity occurs in juvenile or adolescent baseball players with throwing-related pain localized to the proximal humerus, and the radiographic finding of widening of the proximal humeral physis. Other associated radiologic findings may include demineralization, sclerosis of the proximal humeral metaphysis, or fragmentation of the lateral aspect of the proximal humeral metaphysis. Described was a series of 23 patients with Little Leaguer's shoulder and recommendations for their diagnosis and treatment.

Findings.—The average patient age was 14 years (range, 11 to 16 years). All patients were male and had played continually for at least 6 months. Six players (26%) were playing on 2 different teams at the same time and 19 (83%) were pitchers. All complained of pain localized to the proximal humerus during the act of throwing, particularly hard throwing. All patients had radiographic widening of the proximal humeral physis of the throwing arm on internal and external rotation comparison anteroposte-

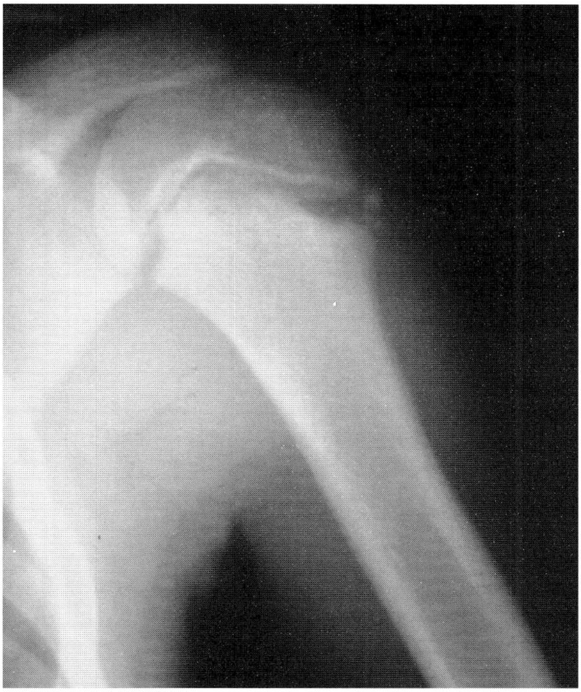

FIGURE 2.—Anteroposterior external rotation radiograph showing the commonly associated finding of lateral fragmentation over the lateral portion of the proximal humeral physis. (Courtesy of Carson WG Jr, Gasser SI: Little Leaguer's shoulder: A report of 23 cases. *Am J Sports Med* 26:575-580, 1998.)

rior radiographs of the shoulders. Twelve patients also had radiographic findings of lateral metaphyseal fragmentation (Fig 2). There was tenderness to palpation over the proximal humerus in 20 patients (87%). Sixteen (70%) had specific tenderness over the lateral aspect of the proximal humerus. Rest (average, 3 months) was prescribed for all patients. Of the 23 patients, 21 (91%) returned to playing baseball and were asymptomatic.

Conclusion.—Patients at risk for Little Leaguer's shoulder are adolescents around age 14 years who have played continually for several months. Patients usually experience localized pain at the proximal lateral humerus. Classic radiographic findings include widening of the proximal humeral physis with associated calcification or lateral fragmentation that is easily detected on bilateral anteroposterior internal and external rotation comparison radiographs of the proximal humerus. Players should be encouraged to report any throwing-related shoulder pain as soon as it occurs.

► A large enough series now makes "Little Leaguer's shoulder" a well established clinico-radiologic entity for baseball pitchers in the mid–second decade of life. Pediatric radiologists have become so familiar with the often bilateral "gymnast wrist"—irregular longitudinal widening of the distal radius (and ulna) physis[1]—that identifying a similar entity at the shoulder for pitchers should not be difficult. Indeed, a similar "gymnast shoulder" has been reported,[2] and we have seen the same pattern at the distal tibial physis in an adolescent gymnast.

A.E. Oestreich, M.D.

References

1. Shih C, Chang CY, Penn IW, et al: Chronically stressed wrists in adolescent gymnasts: MR imaging appearance. *Radiology* 195:855-859, 1995.
2. Dalldorf PG, Bryan WJ: Displaced Salter-Harris type I injury in a gymnast: A slipped capital humeral epiphysis? *Orthop Rev* 23:538-541, 1994.

Measurement of Vertebral Rotation in Adolescent Idiopathic Scoliosis Using Three-Dimensional Magnetic Resonance Imaging

Birchall D, Hughes DG, Hindle J, et al (Hope Hosp, Manchester, England)
Spine 22:2403-2407, 1997 4–24

Introduction.—Adolescent idiopathic scoliosis is a common spinal deformity characterized by complex vertebral distortion occurring in 3 planes. The severity of deformity in the coronal and sagittal plane is easily and reliably detected on plain radiographs. The degree of vertebral rotation in the axial plain is more challenging to determine. Described was the use of 3-dimensional MRI in the measurement of vertebral rotation in adolescent idiopathic scoliosis. The reproducibility and reliability of this technique was also examined.

Methods.—Ten patients (7 girls, 3 boys) between the ages of 12 and 17 years with adolescent idiopathic scoliosis underwent 3-dimensional volume imaging of the apical 5 vertebrae in the axial plane. This was processed through multiplanar reconstruction. Sections through the superior and inferior end plates of each vertebra were chosen in the sagittal and coronal planes, allowing axial reconstructions to be taken in the plane of each end plate. Vertebral rotation was calculated by identifying datum points on the inner surfaces and at the junction of the laminas. The angle subtended by these points was compared with a vertical drawn by the computer (Fig 2). Measurements were taken by the single scanning sequence on 2 occasions by 1 observer and on 1 occasion by a second observer. Interobserver and intraobserver error was calculated and correlated with readings taken from plain radiographs using Perdriolle's torsionmeter method.

Results.—Mean interobserver and intraobserver variations were a mean of 3.02 degrees and 2.56 degrees, respectively. The mean difference between measurements taken from MRI and plain film was 3.29 degrees.

Conclusion.—The degree of vertebral rotation may be accurately and reproducibly determined using 3-dimensional MRI. Measurements may be

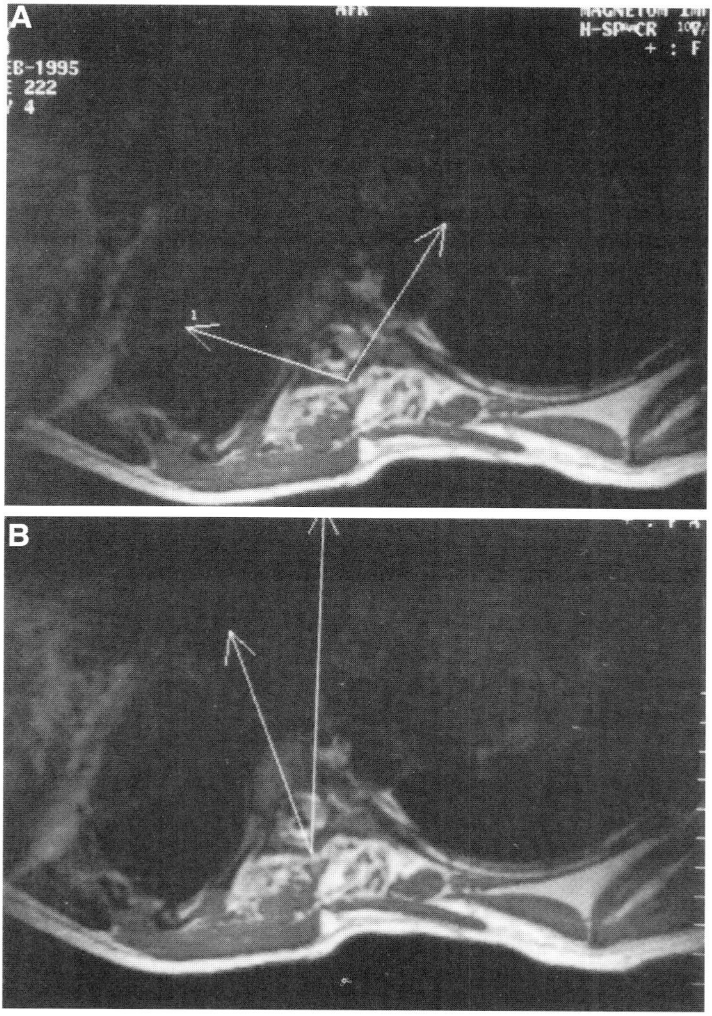

FIGURE 2.—A, Reconstructed image in the plane of the vertebral end plate indicating the angle subtended by datum points on the inner aspects and at the junction of the laminas. B, Reconstructed image in the plane of the vertebral end plate indicating measurement of the angle of axial rotation by comparison with a vertical drawn by the computer. (Courtesy of Birchall D, Hughes DG, Hindle J, et al: Measurement of vertebral rotation in adolescent idiopathic scoliosis using three-dimensional magnetic resonance imaging. *Spine* 22:2403-2407, 1997.)

made through individual end plates that allow evaluation of the relative amount of intervertebral and intravertebral deformity.

► This article complements Abstract 4–25. Use of MRI for measuring vertebral rotation is an important advance. The MRI method is based on the data points of Ho's preferred CT method.[1] MRI is attractive as a scoliosis pretreatment modality because the required repeated imaging is accomplished without ionizing radiation.

L.W. Young, M.D.

Reference

1. Ho EK, Upadhyay SS, Ferris L, et al: A comparative study of computed tomographic and plain radiographic methods to measure vertebral rotation in adolescent idiopathic scoliosis. *Spine* 17:771-774, 1992.

A Logical Coronal Pattern Classification of 2,000 Consecutive Idiopathic Scoliosis Cases Based on the Scoliosis Research Society-defined Apical Vertebra

Coonrad RW, Murrell GAC, Motley G, et al (Duke Univ, Durham, NC; St George Hosp, Sydney, Australia)
Spine 23:1380-1391, 1998 4–25

Introduction.—Classification systems are important in medicine for interobserver communication and identification. For scoliosis, classification is essential in the organization and consistency of treatment and its out-

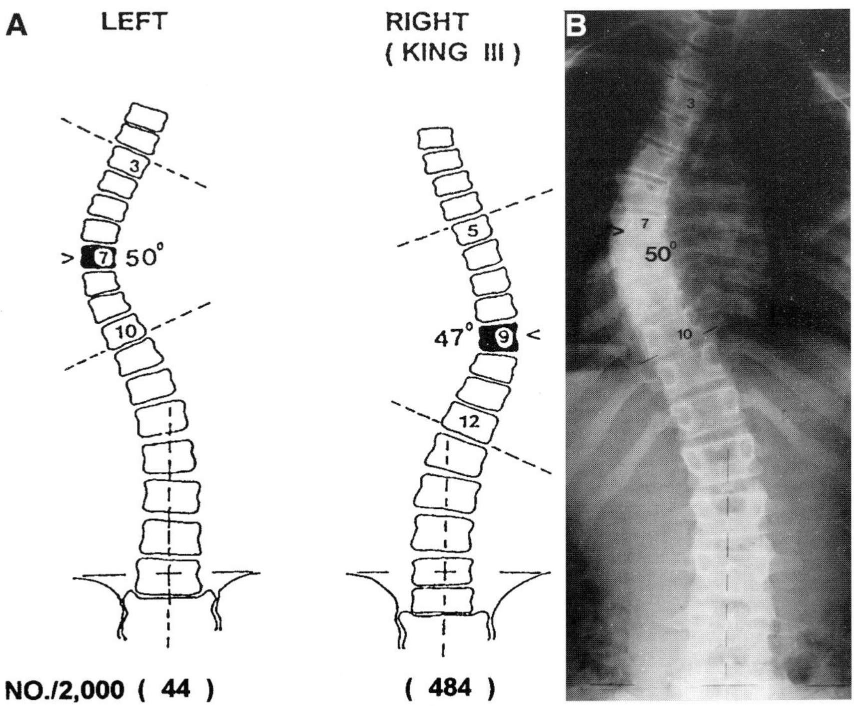

(*Continued*)

FIGURE 5 (cont.)

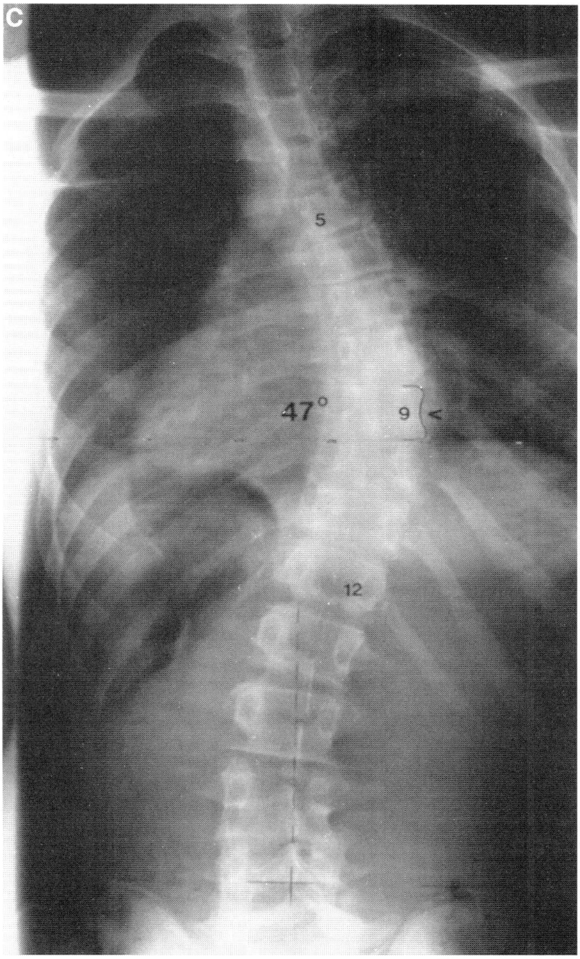

FIGURE 5.—A, Direct radiograph tracing example of type 3, right and left single thoracic curve patterns. B and C, Corresponding radiograph examples. (Courtesy of Coonrad RW, Murrell GAC, Motley G, et al: A logical coronal pattern classification of 2,000 consecutive idiopathic scoliosis cases based on the Scoliosis Research Society-defined apical vertebra. *Spine* 23:1380-1391, 1998.)

come. There is no comprehensive, data-based, and user-friendly coronal pattern classification of idiopathic scoliosis. A large sample of patients with idiopathic scoliosis was evaluated to identify and numerically pattern-type nomenclature for classification.

Methods.—Two thousand idiopathic curve patterns obtained from charts and radiographs were examined and the coronal patterns were categorized by the apical vertebra. The resulting classification then underwent interobserver and intraobserver reliability testing by 12 spinal surgeons and 6 orthopedic residents. Apical frequencies were tested for each pattern type.

Results.—There were 21 pattern categories, all of which were right or left mirror image patterns (except for a quadruple pattern) that allowed separation into 11 types as follows (the patterns incorporated the well-known 5 numbered King types; flexibility was determined by a supervised recumbent lateral bend film):

Type 1A (right or left); double structural thoracic and lumbar curve pattern, larger and/or less flexible lower curve, apex at or below the L1-L2 disk space.

Type 1B (right or left); double structural thoracic and thoracolumbar curve pattern, larger and/or less flexible lower curve, apex at T12, L1, or the interspace between.

Type 2A (right or left); double structural thoracic and lumbar curve pattern, larger and/or less flexible upper curve, apex of the lower curve at or below L1-L2 disk space.

Type 2B (right or left); double structural thoracic and thoracolumbar curve pattern, apex of the lower curve at T12, L1, or interspace between.

Type 3 (right or left); single structural thoracic curve, apex typically at T7, T8, or T9. A small number of high thoracic curves were detected, most commonly with left thoracic pattern (Fig 5).

Type 4 (right or left); single structural thoracic curve, usually with lower apex than type 3 at either T10 or T11, lower end vertebra usually at L2 or L3 and L4 always tilted into the curve.

Type 5 (right or left); double structural thoracic curve pattern (Moe type), T1 or T2 usually tilted into the upper curve, apices of both curves in the thoracic level.

Type 6 (right or left); single thoracolumbar curve pattern, apex always T12, L1, or in the interspace between.

Type 7 (right or left); single lumbar curve pattern, apex at or below L1-L2 disk space, to the level of the L4-L5 disk space.

Type 8 (right or left); triple curve pattern, laterality determined by size of largest of 3 curves.

Type 9; multiple curve pattern, quadruple being the largest curve pattern in this cohort, some curves in the pattern probably not structural and of small size. There was an interobserver reliability of 98.2%. The left single thoracic curve pattern was included as only 9 of 44 patients (20.4%) with left thoracic curves had intraspinal pathology.

Conclusion.—Eleven readily identifiable types that incorporating the 5 King types were created from 2,000 consecutive idiopathic curve patterns. This system should simplify identification and communication.

► Scoliosis is a subject with which we radiologists are often only peripherally involved concerning measurement details of vertebral curvature and rotation, but I think we need to know more about the dependence of its assessments on imaging.[1,2] The authors offer an important logical perspective on the radiographic coronal pattern classification of idiopathic scoliosis. The classification incorporates the frequently referenced King curve types and promises better interobserver and intraobserver reliability.[3,4] Full description of the scoliosis deformity must include sagittal and axial plane variables that are very well explored by radiography with the help of CT and MRI.[1,2] (See also Abstract 6–5.)

L.W. Young, M.D.

References

1. Oestreich AE, Young LW, Young-Poussaint T: Scoliosis circa 2000: Radiologic imaging perspective. I. Diagnosis and pretreatment evaluation. *Skeletal Radiol* 27:591-605, 1998.
2. Oestreich AE, Young LW, Young-Poussaint T: Scoliosis circa 2000: Radiologic imaging perspective. II. Treatment and follow-up. *Skeletal Radiol* 27:651-656, 1998.
3. Lenke LG, Betz RR, Bridwell KH, et al: Intraobserver and interobserver reliability of the classification of thoracic adolescent idiopathic scoliosis. *J Bone Joint Surg Am* 80-A:1097-1106, 1998.
4. Cummings RJ, Loveless EA, Campbell J, et al: Interobserver reliability and intraobserver reproducibility of the system of King et al. for the classification of adolescent idiopathic scoliosis. *J Bone Joint Surg Am* 80-A:1107-1111, 1998.

Respiratory/Vascular

Magnetic Resonance Imaging of a Left Circumflex Aortic Arch and Aberrant Right Subclavian Artery: The Other Vascular Ring

McLeary MS, Frye LL, Young LW (Loma Linda Univ Children's Hosp, Calif)
Pediatr Radiol 28:263-265, 1998 4–26

Background.—Left circumflex aortic arch (LCAA), a very rare anomaly, is characterized by an aorta that ascends to the left of the trachea, crosses posterior to the esophagus, and descends to the right of the spine. A 2-day-old girl with complex congenital heart disease in whom LCAA was diagnosed by MRI was described.

Case Report.—The infant, born vaginally at an estimated gestational age of 38 weeks, was initially cyanotic and hypotonic. Her 1- and 5-minute Apgar scores were 7 and 8, respectively. Eighty-six percent oxygen delivered through a hood was needed to maintain a 92% oxygen saturation. Chest radiographs demonstrated a right-sided descending aorta and tracheal deviation to the right and an elevation of the right hemidiaphragm and hypoplasia of the right lung (Fig 1). On echocardiography, the great arteries were transposed and there was a large atrial septal defect, a ventricular septal defect, a patent right-sided ductus arteriosus, trace mitral regurgitation, and hypoplasia of the right pulmonary artery. Two days later, MRI and MRA of the heart and great vessels verified these findings.

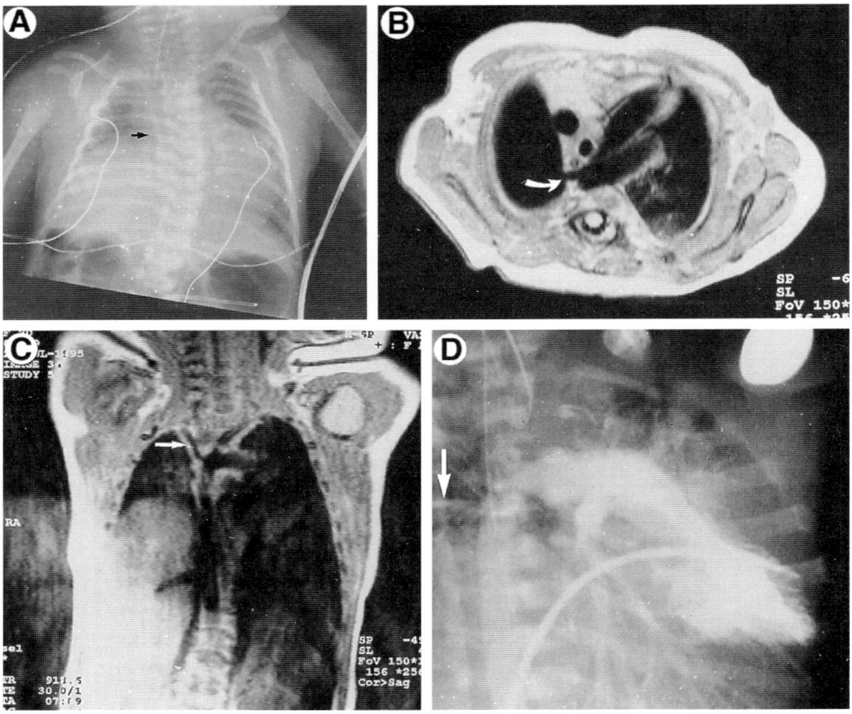

FIGURE 1.—Complex congenital heart disease in a 2-day-old girl. **A**, Chest radiograph shows hypoplasia of the right lung with elevation of the right hemidiaphragm and displacement of the trachea to the right. The descending aorta (*arrow*) is to the right of the spine. **B**, Cardiac gated T1-weighted axial image shows the anterior aortic arch coursing posterior to the trachea and esophagus. The aorta (*straight arrow*) is anterior to the pulmonary artery, which is diagnostic for transposition of the great vessels. The posterior, main pulmonary artery gives rise to a hypoplastic right pulmonary artery (*curved arrow*). **C**, Gated T1-weighted coronal image shows the aortic arch crossing midline to descend on the right, just anterior to the spine. The aberrant right subclavian artery is the last vessel off the aortic arch (*arrow*). A hypoplastic right lung with elevation of the right hemidiaphragm is also identified. **D**, Cine angiogram in RAO position demonstrates a left-sided aortic arch with a right-sided descending aorta. The retroesophageal course of the aorta is not radiographically evident. The pulmonary vasculature is seen secondary to the patent ductus arteriosus, and the hypoplastic right pulmonary artery is barely visible (*arrow*). The aortic root is visualized anterior to the pulmonary outflow tract, originating from the trabeculated right ventricle. (Courtesy of McLeary MS, Frye LL, Young LW: Magnetic resonanace imaging of a left circumflex aortic arch and aberrant right subclavian artery: The other vascular ring. *Pediatr Radiol* 28:263-265, 1998, copyright Springer-Verlag.)

Conclusions.—In this patient, MRI accurately demonstrated a left circumflex aortic arch, which was not apparent on conventional angiography or echocardiography. MR documentation of this anomaly is uncommon.

► The value of MRI is the demonstration of pertinent vascular ring anatomy without angiography.[1,2] This report of a rare circumflex aortic arch/aberrant right subclavian artery anomaly documents an example of the success of MRI in demonstrating vascular morphology better than angiography.

L.W. Young, M.D.

References

1. Azarow KS, Pearl RH, Hoffman MA, et al: Vascular ring: Does magnetic resonance imaging replace angiography? *Ann Thorac Surg* 53:882-885, 1992.
2. Van Son JA, Julsrud PR, Hagler DJ, et al: Imaging strategies for vascular rings. *Ann Thorac Surg* 57:604-610, 1994.

Braided Bronchus: A Previously Undescribed Airway Anomaly

Wheeler DS, Poss WB, Cocalis M, et al (Naval Med Ctr, San Diego, Calif; Univ of Virginia, Charlottesville)

Pediatr Pulmonol 25:348-351, 1998 4–27

Background.—Recurrent atelectasis is often seen in infants with congenital heart disease, which is associated with anomalous branching of the bronchial tree in many cases. The bridging bronchus, associated with left-sided obstructive lesions and a slinglike left pulmonary artery, has been well described. The "braided bronchus," a similar but distinct airway anomaly, was described in a report.

Case Report.—Girl, 12 days, born at term after an uncomplicated pregnancy, was brought for medical attention because of fever and respiratory distress. A chest radiograph showed consolidation adjacent to the right heart border and in the right upper lobe. Systemic antibiotic treatment was begun. Respiratory failure developed, necessitating mechanical ventilation. Echocardiography showed a coarctation of the aorta, prompting balloon angioplasty. After a 10-day course of antibiotics with negative cultures, the infant was discharged. When she was 2 months of age, balloon angioplasty was repeated for recurrent coarctation of the aorta. Chronic consolidation in the right anterior chest unresponsive to conventional chest physiotherapy and poor weight gain prompted further investigation at 6 months. Flexible bronchoscopy and cardiac catheterization were performed. The latter showed a proximal branch of the right pulmonary artery coursing to parts of the right lower lobe, then crossing the midline to divide to portions of the left lower lobe parenchyma; a wedge of right upper lobe parenchyma draining abnormally to the right atrium-superior vena cava junction; and the absence of a systemic arterial supply to the malformation. Bronchography, done with anteroposterior and lateral fluoroscopy in the cardiac catheterization laboratory, defined the distribution of the 4 branches of the right mainstem bronchus (Fig 2, B). Aggressive pulmonary toilet with bronchodilator treatment, chest percussion, and postural drainage was begun. Subsequently, the baby had normal growth and required no further hospitalization.

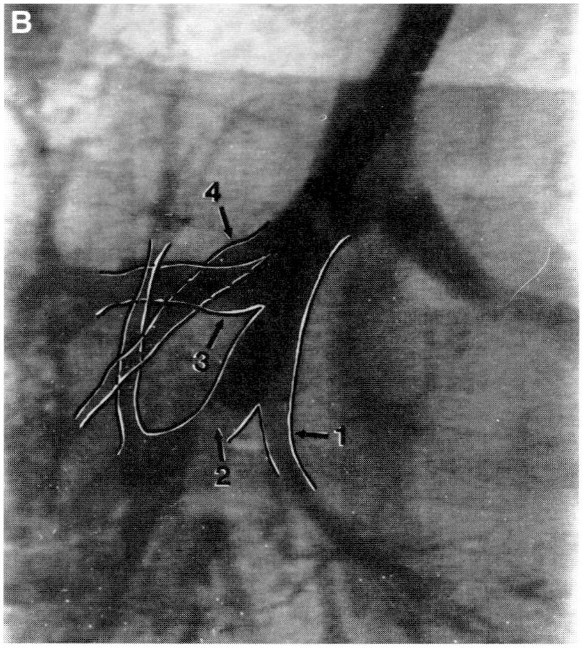

FIGURE 2.—B, the anomalous branching of the right mainstem bronchus was studied bronchographically. Bronchus No. 1 subtends a large retrocardiac lobe, which extends into the left chest. Bronchus No. 2 subtends additional right lower lung tissue. Bronchus No. 3 subtends the right lateral upper and middle lung fields. Bronchus No. 4 crosses beneath bronchus No. 3 on a path toward the region of the right heart border. The bronchial "braid" is formed by a subsegmental branch of bronchus No. 2, which travels posterior to bronchi No. 3 and No. 4 to supply the right lung apex. (Courtesy of Wheeler DS, Poss WB, Cocalis M, et al: Braided bronchus: A previously undescribed airway anomaly. *Pediatr Pulmonol* 25:348-351, 1998. Reprinted by permission of Wiley-Liss, Inc., a subsidiary of John Wiley & Sons, Inc.)

Conclusion.—In this patient, bronchography demonstrated therapeutically relevant anatomy that could not be defined endoscopically or by CT. A "braided bronchus"—a complex, previously unrecognized airway malinosculation—was defined. The braided bronchus in this infant was associated with bridging bronchus, partial anomalous venous return, and coarctation of the aorta.

► The braided bronchus merits recognition as a distinct airway anomaly associated with a bridging bronchus. The authors used bronchography as an effective imaging method for demonstrating the braided bronchus, and this emphasizes that in the demonstration of some entities, bronchography is still important. Another recent article on bridging bronchus is listed.[1]

L.W. Young, M.D.

Reference

1. Stokes JR, Heatley DG, Lusk RP, et al: The bridging bronchus. Successful diagnosis and repair. *Arch Otolaryngol Head Neck Surg* 123:1344-1347, 1997.

Congenital Thymic Cysts in Children: Mostly Misdiagnosed
Hendrickson M, Azarow K, Ein S, et al (Univ of Nevada, Las Vegas; Hosp For Sick Children, Toronto)
J Pediatr Surg 33:821-825, 1998 4–28

Background.—Congenital thymic cysts, rare lesions of the neck and mediastinum, are often not thought of as a differential possibility. Although these lesions are often considered inconsequential, they are frequently symptomatic. One experience was reported.

Patients and Findings.—Fourteen children, aged 2 weeks to 16 years, were seen at 1 center between 1984 and 1997. Seven children had cervical masses, 5 had mediastinal masses, and 2 had both. Seven children were symptomatic, with wheezing and upper respiratory infection. Cough and fever were the most common clinical features. Assessment included chest radiography, contrast esophagraphy, sonography, and CT (Figs 1, B and 3, B). Eight children had displacement of vital mediastinal or neck structures. In only 2 cases, correct diagnosis was made before surgery. All cysts were excised successfully and completely. The cysts ranged from 2 to 22 cm in diameter and were benign.

Conclusion.—Congenital thymic cysts are rare, benign, often symptomatic lesions that should be considered in the differential diagnosis of cervical and mediastinal masses in children aged 2 to 15 years of age. Differential diagnosis usually includes bronchial left cyst, lymphangioma and teratoma. In this series, all cysts were excised successfully.

► This important article brings attention to the congenital thymic cyst lesion that is frequently misdiagnosed, mainly because it usually isn't considered in differential diagnosis. In addition to radiography and CT, US and MRI may be used.[1] The congenital thymic cyst has pharyngeal pouch embryogenesis—

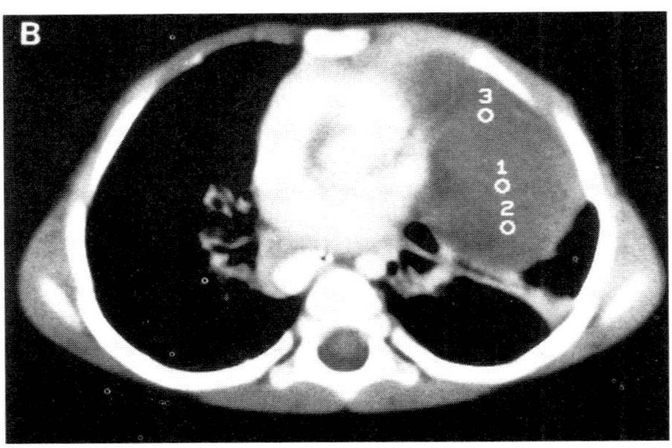

FIGURE 1.—B, CT scan shows a 7 × 6 × 5-cm cystic mass with atelectasis and distortion of a left peripheral bronchus. (Courtesy of Hendrickson M, Azarow K, Ein S, et al: Congenital thymic cysts in children: Mostly misdiagnosed. *J Pediatr Surg* 33:821-825, 1998.)

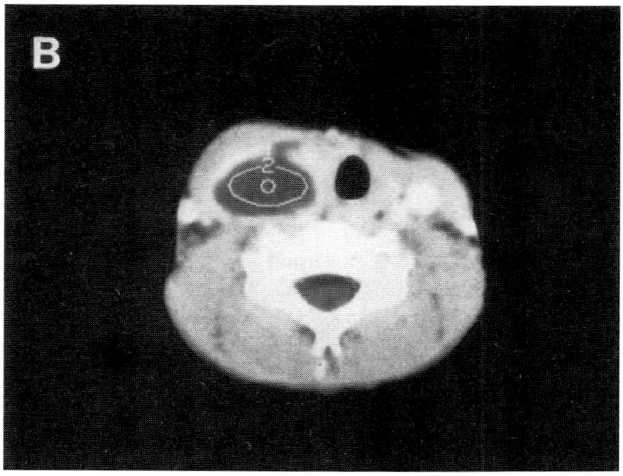

FIGURE 3.—B, CT scan shows the cystic nature of the mass with compression of the structures of the right cervical area and deviation of the trachea to the left. (Courtesy of Hendrickson M, Azarow K, Ein S, et al: Congenital thymic cysts in children: Mostly misdiagnosed. *J Pediatr Surg* 33:821-825, 1998.)

the third pharyngeal pouch. In a related recent article,[2] Mouri suggested the term pyriform sinus cysts for such lesions that drain into the pyriform sinus. Other recent related articles are listed.[3-5]

L.W. Young, M.D.

References

1. de Miguel Campos E, Casanova A, Urbano J, et al: Congenital thymic cyst: Prenatal sonographic and postnatal magnetic resonance findings. *J Ultrasound Med* 16:365-367, 1997.
2. Mouri N, Muraji T, Nishijima E, et al: Reappraisal of lateral cervical cysts in neonates: Pyriform sinus cysts as an anatomy-based nomenclature. *J Pediatr Surg* 33:1141-1144, 1998.
3. Vade A, Griffiths A, Hotaling A, et al: Thymopharyngeal duct cyst: MR imaging of a third branchial arch anomaly in a neonate. *J Magn Reson Imaging* 4:614-616, 1994.
4. Dano I, Dangoor E, Eliasher R, et al: Thymic cyst mimicking a branchial cleft cyst. *J Otolaryngol* 27:236-237, 1998.
5. Burton EM, Mercado-Deane MG, Howell CG, et al: Cervical thymic cysts: CT appearance of two cases including a persistent thymopharyngeal duct cyst. *Pediatr Radiol* 25:363-365, 1995.

Assessment of Adenoidal Obstruction in Children: Clinical Signs Versus Roentgenographic Findings

Paradise JL, Bernard BS, Colborn DK, et al (Univ of Pittsburgh, Pa; Children's Hosp of Pittsburgh, Pa)

Pediatrics 101:979-986, 1998 4–29

Introduction.—Chronic nasal obstruction attributable to large adenoids is a common condition of childhood. However, few children with nasal obstruction complain of difficulty in nasal breathing. Mouth breathing and hyponasal speech have been the classic physical signs considered indicative of adenoidal nasal obstruction. A study was conducted to determine whether the presence and degree of adenoidal nasal obstruction in children can be assessed satisfactorily by simple clinical means and whether these correlate with roentgenographic assessments.

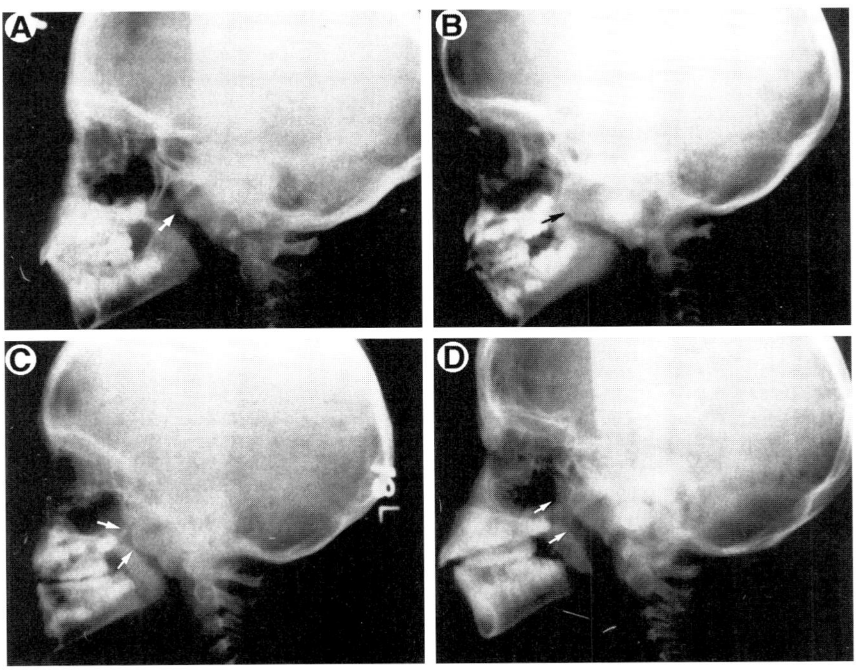

FIGURE 2.—In these lateral soft-tissue roentgenograms, the anterior nasopharyngeal airway is defined as the space between the anterior border of the adenoid and the posterior wall of the maxillary antrum. The inferior nasopharyngeal airway is defined as the space between the inferior border of the adenoid and the superior border of the soft palate. The *arrows* point to the salient findings. **A**, Normal-sized adenoid with ample anterior and inferior airways. **B**, Markedly enlarged adenoid with narrowed anterior and inferior airways. **C**, Large adenoid with ample anterior airway and narrowed inferior airway. **D**, Large adenoid with narrowed anterior airway and ample inferior airway. (Courtesy of Paradise JL, Bernard BS, Colborn DK, et al: Assessment of adenoidal obstruction in children: Clinical signs versus roentgenographic findings. *Pediatrics* 101:979-986, 1998. Reproduced by permission of PEDIATRICS.)

Methods.—A 4-point scale called the Nasal Obstruction Index, ranging from "none" to "marked," was used to rate the degree of children's mouth breathing and speech hyponasality. Classifications of lateral soft-tissue roentgenographs of the nasopharynx were based on assessment of adenoid size and of nasopharyngeal airway patency that showed either no obstruction, borderline obstruction, or obstruction (Fig 2). Levels of interobserver and intraobserver agreement concerning the classifications were also determined. Correlations in individual children between clinical rating and roentgenographic ratings of nasal/nasopharyngeal obstruction were determined. The roentgenographic ratings were used as the gold standard in the calculation of predictive values of clinical ratings.

Results.—Two hundred thirty-five children were measured for mouth breathing and 648 children were measured for speech hyponasality. Weighted κ values for interobserver agreement ranged from 0.84 to 0.91. Two hundred seven children were assessed roentgenographically, with a value for interobserver agreement in assessing nasopharyngeal airway status as 0.92, whereas the intraobserver agreement for 191 children was 0.88. For concordance between Nasal Obstruction Index values and roentgenographic ratings in 1,033 children, the Kendall's τ *b* value was 0.51. At the lower and upper extremes of 1.0 and 3.5 or more, the Nasal Obstruction Index values were highly predictive of concordant roentgenographic ratings.

Conclusion.—Reliable and reasonably valid assessment of the presence and degree of adenoidal obstruction of the nasopharyngeal airway can be provided by standardized clinical ratings of the degree of children's mouth breathing and speech hyponasality. At the extremes of either marked obstruction or no obstruction, these clinical assessments are particularly valid. To establish the presence of adenoidal obstruction, clinical assessment alone may be insufficient. However, when findings are unequivocally negative, clinical assessment can rule out adenoidal obstruction.

► Oh, how I remember this project!—from memorable years in Pittsburgh. Jack Paradise is to be commended for staying the course. I and others still consider the simple adenoidal-nasopharyngeal ratio an excellent and reliable measure of adenoidal size.[1-3] The effect of respiration on the method subsequently used in this article is probably still to be considered.[4] The bottom line is that the confirmatory roles of roentgenography and endoscopy have distinct value in simple but clinical assessment of adenoidal enlargement and obstruction.

L.W. Young, M.D.

References

1. Bartolome BM, Matos H-S: A radiological assessment of the nasopharynx in healthy children from the Madrid area. *An Esp Pediatr* 49:571-576, 1998.
2. Kemaloglu YK, Goksu N, Inal E, et al: Radiographic evaluation of children with nasopharyngeal obstruction due to the adenoid. *Ann Otol Rhinol Laryngol* 108:67-71, 1999.

3. Elwany S: The adenoidal-nasopharyngeal ratio (AN ratio): Its validity in selecting children for adenoidectomy. *J Laryngol Otol* 101:569-573, 1987.
4. Britton PD: Effect of respiration on nasopharyngeal radiographs when assessing adenoidal enlargement. *J Laryngol Otol* 103:71-73, 1989.

Cytomegalovirus Associated Neonatal Pneumonia and Wilson-Mikity Syndrome: A Causal Relationship?

Reiterer F, Dornbusch HJ, Urlesberger B, et al (Univ of Graz, Austria)
Eur Respir J 13:460-462, 1999 4–30

Background.—Wilson-Mikity syndrome (WMS), a chronic neonatal lung disorder, is characterized radiologically by alternating areas of cyst-like hyperaeration and infiltration developing within days or weeks after birth in the absence of preceding mechanical ventilation or high supplemental oxygen. Although the cause of this syndrome is uncertain, recent evidence strongly suggests that lung injury caused by intrauterine inflammation plays a role. The current case report supports this theory by suggesting a causative role of intrauterine cytomegalovirus (CMV) infection in WMS development.

Case Report.—Chronic lung disease consistent with WMS developed in a boy born at 33 weeks' gestational age. Diagnostic assessment was positive for CMV infection. High-resolution CT

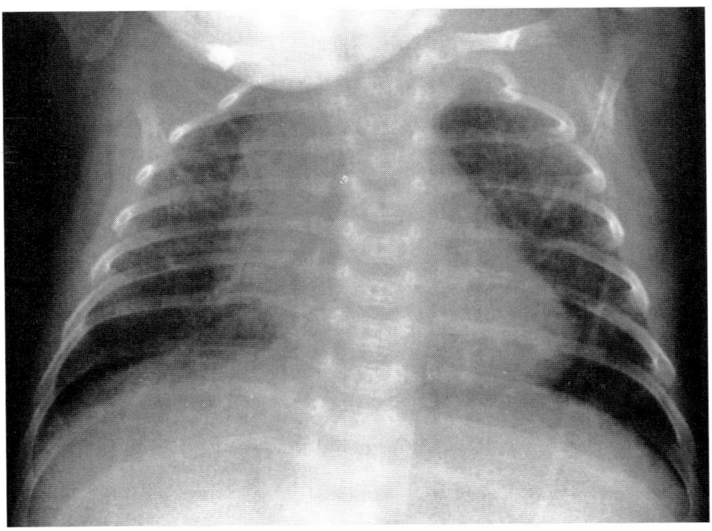

FIGURE 1.—Chest radiograph on the 15th day of life showing a reticulonodular pattern with areas of focal hyperaeration throughout both lungs and hyperaeration of the lower lobes. (Courtesy of Reiterer F, Dornbusch HJ, Urlesberger B, et al: Cytomegalovirus associated neonatal pneumonia and Wilson-Mikity syndrome: A causal relationship? *Eur Respir J* 13:460-462, 1999.)

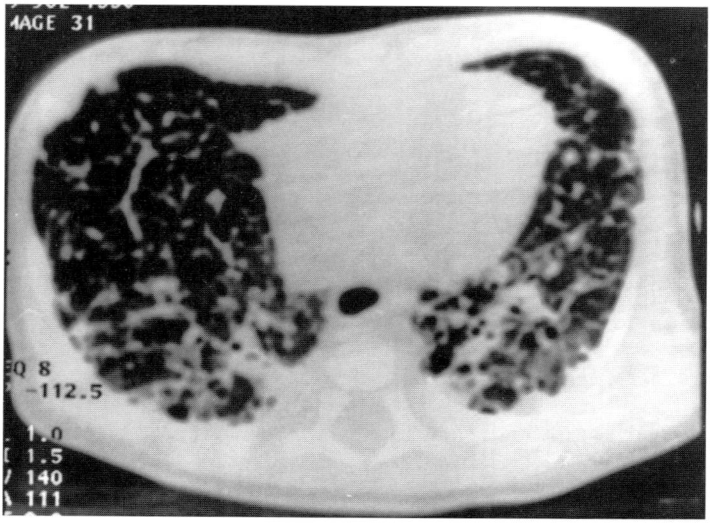

FIGURE 2.—Inspiratory high-resolution CT scan of lungs revealing hyperinflated cystlike areas surrounded by thickened peribronchovascular interstitium and interlobular septa. (Courtesy of Reiterer F, Dornbusch HJ, Urlesberger B, et al: Cytomegalovirus associated neonatal pneumonia and Wilson-Mikity syndrome: A causal relationship? *Eur Respir J* 13:460-462, 1999.)

scan and histologic findings in the lung showed typical features of WMS, associated with signs of interstitial pneumonia. Cytomegalovirus was identified in urine, breast milk, bronchoalveolar lavage material, and lung tissue from open lung biopsy. Ganciclovir and steroid therapy was initiated. Follow-up showed resolving lung disease at 6, 10, and 16 months of age, with lung function signs of mild obstruction (Figs 1 and 2).

Conclusions.—In this child, intrauterine CMV infection seems to have caused a pattern of lung injury consistent with WMS. The possible role of congenital infection in this syndrome should be investigated.

► A causal relationship between CMV neonatal pneumonia and WMS is provocative. In fact, in a separate publication,[1] the authors emphasized the high-resolution CT findings in this same case as being those of WMS. Nonetheless, in both articles, their impression was that "the relatively large amount of interstitial disease led to the suspicion of additional viral infection."[1] In the complete article abstracted here, the authors report supportive CMV evidence of positive in situ hybridization for CMV in portions of the lung tissue and CMV-early antigen in sputum. Imaging overlaps and contrasts of types of chronic lung disease of the very low birth weight infant[2]—including bronchopulmonary dysplasia, chronic neonatal pneumonia, and WMS—are well recognized. The fact that the cause of WMS is not known warrants continued pursuit by clinical, imaging, and laboratory means.

L.W. Young, M.D.

References

1. Reiterer P, Fotter R, Tillich M, et al: High-resolution CT findings in Wilson-Mikity syndrome: A case report. *Pediatr Radiol* 28:691-693, 1998.
2. Ogawa Y: Chronic lung disease of the very low birth weight infant—Is it preventable? *Turk J Pediatr* 40:35-44, 1998.

Ehrlichiosis: Findings on Chest Radiographs in Three Pediatric Patients

Fordham LA, Chung CJ, Specter BB, et al (Univ of North Carolina, Chapel Hill)

AJR 171:1421-1424, 1998 4–31

Background.—Ehrlichiosis, a newly recognized tick-borne infection that affects children and adults, is usually mild but can be fatal. The features of ehrlichiosis on the chest radiographs of 3 children were described.

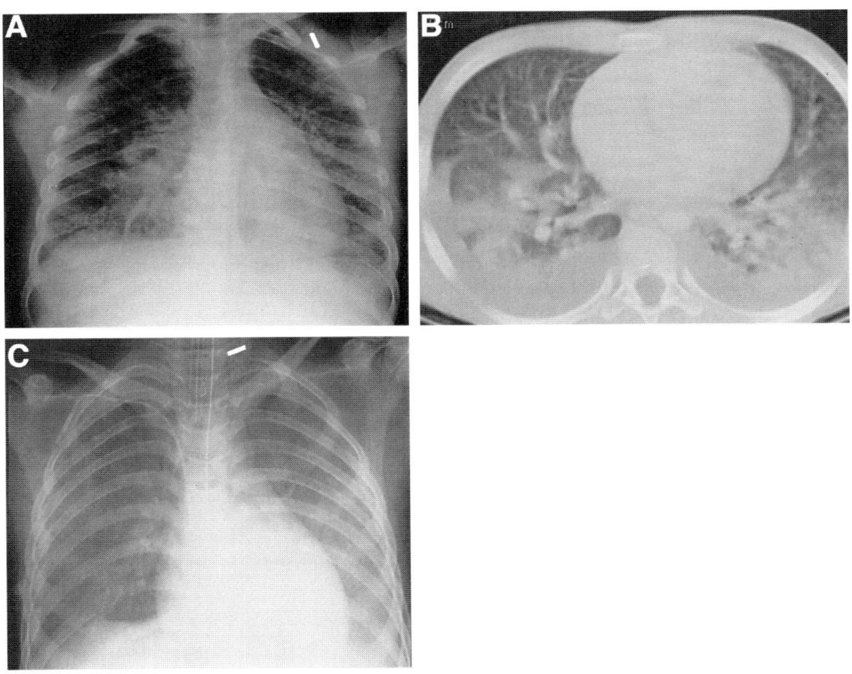

FIGURE 1.—Imaging in a 7-year-old girl with ehrlichiosis seen with fever, decreased appetite, mild cough, pancytopenia, and elevated values on liver function tests. Initial chest radiograph had normal findings. **A**, Posteroanterior chest radiograph on hospital day 3 shows bilateral alveolar opacities and pleural effusions. Heart size is slightly increased from that seen on admission radiograph. **B**, CT scan obtained 1 day after **A** reveals bilateral dependent airspace nodules. Note areas of consolidation and bilateral pleural effusions. **C**, Portable radiograph 1 day after **B** taken with smaller inspiratory volume reveals mild perihilar opacity consistent with pulmonary edema and bilateral pleural effusions. Radiographs had normal findings (not shown) 9 days later. (Courtesy of Fordham LA, Chung CJ, Specter BB, et al: Ehrlichiosis: Findings on chest radiographs in three pediatric patients. *AJR* 171:1421-1424, 1998.)

Patients and Findings.—The cases of 3 girls, aged 2, 7, and 13 years, were reviewed. All were acutely ill and had a history of possible tick exposure. In 2 patients, chest radiographs obtained on admission gave normal results. Chest radiography showed mild bilateral alveolar opacities in the 13-year-old girl, who died. In this patient, the opacities progressed to asymmetric alveolar infiltrates in the midlung and lower lung zones and small bilateral pleural effusions. In the first 2 patients, there was a pattern of progression from normal to alveolar opacities. In addition, pleural effusions were seen in the 2-year-old (Fig 1).

Conclusion.—Ehrlichiosis should be included in the differential diagnosis of acutely ill children with a history of possible tick exposure and characteristic radiographic patterns. Interstitial prominence, alveolar opacities, or consolidation that may be associated with pleural effusion should suggest the diagnosis in such patients.

► Ehrlichiosis, a newly recognized tick-borne infection, is well described in this article. Its role as a cause of acute pulmonary disease in 3 children is compelling. Although the respiratory tract is often not the main focus of this disease, several recent reports documented acute respiratory distress syndrome as a consequence of ehrlichiosis,[1-3] and 1 report indicated toxic shock syndrome in several patients, including children.[4]

L.W. Young, M.D.

References

1. Patel RG, Byrd MA: Near fatal acute respiratory distress syndrome in a patient with human ehrlichiosis. *South Med J* 92:333-335, 1999.
2. Weaver RA, Virella G, Weaver A: Ehrlichiosis with severe pulmonary manifestations despite early treatment. *South Med J* 92:336-339, 1999.
3. Vugia DJ, Holmberg E, Steffe EM: A human case of monocytic ehrlichiosis with adult respiratory distress syndrome in northern California. *West J Med* 164:525-528, 1996.
4. Fichtenbaum CJ, Peterson LR, Weil GJ: Ehrlichiosis presenting as a life-threatening illness with features of the toxic shock syndrome. *Am J Med* 95:351-357, 1993.

The Role of Ultrasound and Oesophagography in the Management of Acute Suppurative Thyroiditis in Children Associated With Congenital Pyriform Fossa Sinus

Ahuja AT, Griffiths JF, Roebuck DJ, et al (Prince of Wales Hosp, Shatin NT, Hong Kong)

Clin Radiol 53:209-211, 1998 4–32

Background.—Because the thyroid is very resistant to infection, pyriform fossa sinus (PFS) must be considered when an infection occurs, especially if it is recurrent and occurs on the left side. The clinical presentation and US and esophagographic appearances of PFS were described.

Methods and Findings.—During a 6-month period, 3 girls and 2 boys, aged 2 to 9 years, with acute suppurative thyroiditis and PFS were seen. In

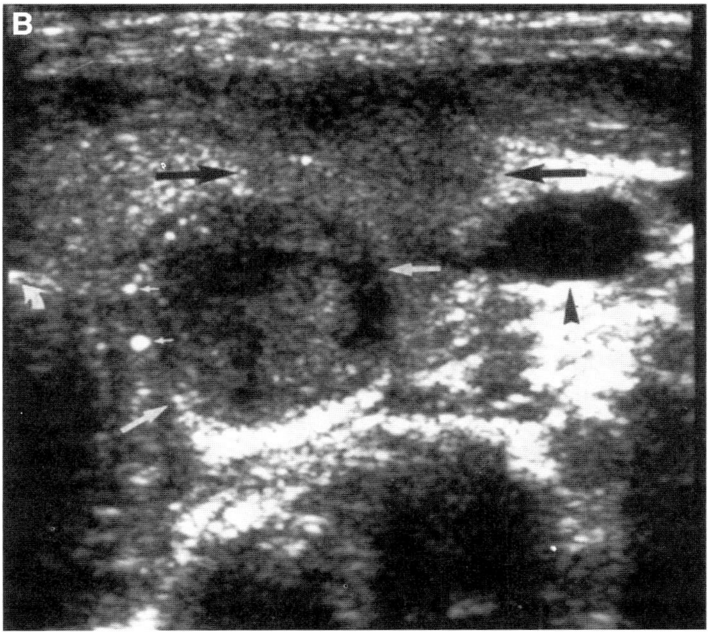

FIGURE 1.—B, Transverse sonogram shows a thyroid abscess (*large white arrows*) containing debris and gas (*small white arrows*). There is loss of fascial planes between the thyroid and adjacent soft tissues (*black arrows*). The *curved white arrows* indicates the trachea, and the *arrowhead* indicates the common carotid artery. (Courtesy of Ahuja AT, Griffiths JF, Roebuck DJ, et al: The role of ultrasound and oesophagography in the management of acute suppurative thyroiditis in children associated with congenital pyriform fossa sinus. *Clin Radiol* 53:209-211, 1998.)

4 children, US showed a thyroid abscess measuring 1 to 3 cm with internal debris and septa. One patient also had gas. The fascial planes were obliterated between the thyroid and adjacent tissue, which suggested extension. The fifth child had a hypoechoic, heterogeneous mass with internal debris anterior to the left lobe of the thyroid. A clear plane between it and the thyroid was evident, consistent with an extrathyroid abscess. In all children, a US-guided fine-needle aspiration confirmed an abscess. In the fifth patient, contrast-enhanced CT demonstrated a rim-enhancing mass with central low attenuation and surrounding edema, suggesting an abscess. The appearance of the thyroid was normal. On esophagography with barium sulfate suspension, performed in all children, the sinus was clearly seen in 4 children, on the left in 3 and on the right in 1. In all patients, the origin of the anomalous tract was at the apex of the pyriform fossa, with an anteroinferior course extending toward the thyroid. In the fifth child, only the origin of the fistula was seen (Figs 1 and 2).

Conclusions.—Findings on US and esophagography in 5 children with pyriform fossa sinus associated with suppurative thyroiditis were de-

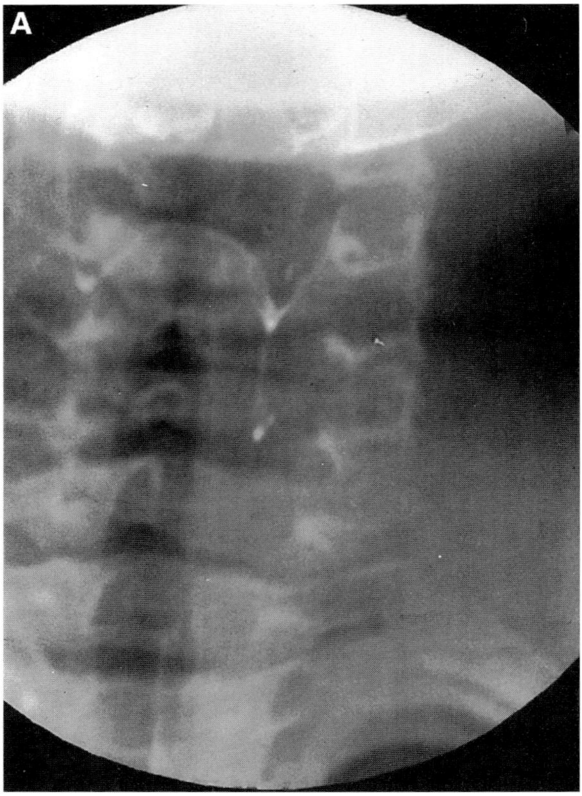

FIGURE 2.—A, Frontal esophagogram shows a sinus arising from the apex of the left pyriform fossa. (Courtesy of Ahuja AT, Griffiths JF, Roebuck DJ, et al: The role of ultrasound and oesophagography in the management of acute suppurative thyroiditis in children associated with congenital pyriform fossa sinus. *Clin Radiol* 53:209-211, 1998.)

scribed in the current paper. The abnormality was found on the left in 4 children and on the right in 1.

► The authors clearly demonstrate that US and pharyngography (esophagography) simply and uniquely are sufficient for the diagnosis of acute suppurative thyroiditis and congenital PFS. The big guns—CT, MRI and scintigraphy—were not needed. Other recent articles demonstrate the use of other imaging modality combinations or imaging and hypopharyngeal endoscopy to the same end result.[1,2]

L.W. Young, M.D.

References

1. Jordan JA, Graves JE, Manning SC, et al: Endoscopic cauterization for treatment of fourth branchial cleft sinuses. *Arch Otolaryngol Head Neck Surg* 124:1021-1024, 1998.
2. Mahomed A, Youngson G: Congenital lateral cervical cysts of infancy. *J Pediatr Surg* 33:1413-1415, 1998.
3. Hamoir M, Rombaux P, Cornu AS, et al: Congenital fistula of the fourth branchial pouch. *Eur Arch Otorhinolaryngol* 255:322-324, 1998.

Tracheal Schwannoma Presenting as Status Asthmaticus in a Sixteen-Year-Old Boy: Airway Considerations and Removal With the CO_2 Laser

Weiner DJ, Weatherly RA, DiPietro MA, et al (Univ of Michigan Med Ctr, Ann Arbor)

Pediatr Pulmonol 25:393-397, 1998 4–33

Background.—Tracheal tumors are uncommon, especially in children. The differential diagnosis includes squamous cell carcinoma, adenoid cystic carcinoma, and carcinoid, as well as benign tumors such as papilloma, hemangioma, hamartoma, and neurilemmomas and neurofibromas. A case of tracheal schwannoma manifesting with the clinical features of atypical asthma was described.

> *Case Report.*—Boy, 16, was admitted with cough, wheezing, and declining exercise tolerance since undergoing treatment for pneumonia 11 months earlier. One month before admission, spirometric results were consistent with severe obstructive airway disease. The initial radiograph demonstrated massive symmetrical hyperinflation and minimal peribronchial thickening but no infiltrates (Fig 1). Chest CT showed a lesion that appeared to be within the lumen of the trachea (Fig 3). In retrospect, this lesion could be seen as a round mass on the plain film. It was better visualized with magnified airway views and airway fluoroscopy (Fig 4).

Conclusions.—Spirometry showing the classic oval-shaped flow volume loops or radiologic studies may suggest the diagnosis of a fixed upper airway obstruction. The diagnosis is confirmed definitively by bronchoscopy. This case report illustrates the old adage "not all that wheezes is asthma."

► "Not all that wheezes is asthma." This report and the imaging findings confirm that the age-old adage rightfully lives on. The use of airway fluoroscopy is not to be forgotten, as it helped to confirm the intraluminal globular surface margins of this rare tracheal schwannoma. The differential diagnostic possibilities for the tracheal mass as well as other air-trapping entities

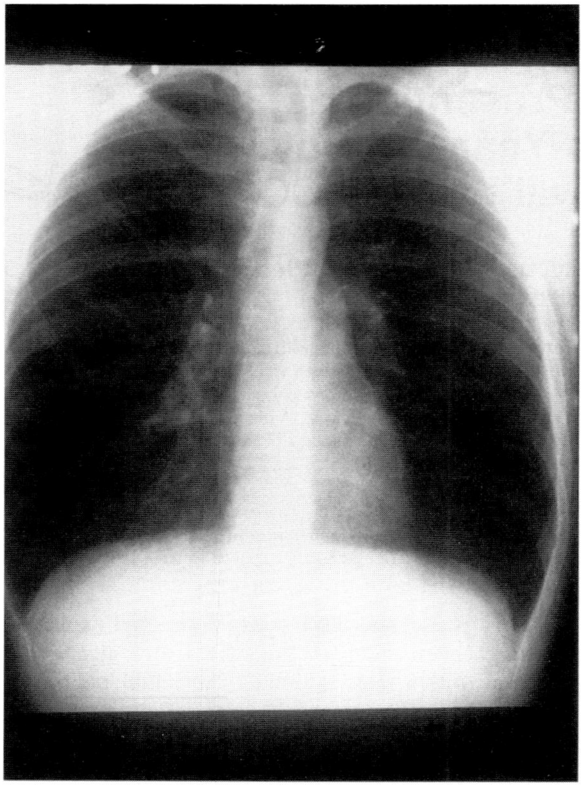

FIGURE 1.—Chest radiograph (posteroanterior view) at admission showing marked bilateral hyperinflation. (Courtesy of Weiner DJ, Weatherly RA, DiPietro MA, et al: Tracheal schwannoma presenting as status asthmaticus in a sixteen-year-old boy: Airway considerations and removal with the CO_2 laser. *Pediatr Pulmonol* 25:393-397, 1998. Reprinted by permission of Wiley-Liss, Inc., a subsidiary of John Wiley & Sons, Inc.)

such as asthma and bronchiolitis obliterans are appropriate. Recent literature addresses differential diagnoses quite well.[1,2] Also included is *follicular hyperplasia of bronchus-associated lymphoid tissue* as a cause of severe air trapping.[3]

L.W. Young, M.D.

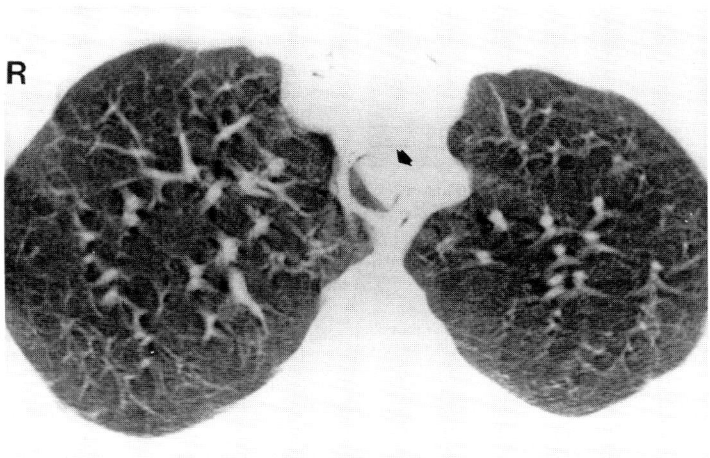

FIGURE 3.—Chest CT shows a soft-tissue mass within the lumen of the distal trachea (*arrow*). (Courtesy of Weiner DJ, Weatherly RA, DiPietro MA, et al: Tracheal schwannoma presenting as status asthmaticus in a sixteen-year-old boy: Airway considerations and removal with the CO_2 laser. *Pediatr Pulmonol* 25:393-397, 1998. Reprinted by permission of Wiley-Liss, Inc., a subsidiary of John Wiley & Sons, Inc.)

References

1. Holinger LD, Gonzalez-Crussi F: Tracheal neoplasms in children. *Ann Otol Rhinol Laryngol* 107:790-796, 1998.
2. Noda S, Sundaresan S, Mendeloff EN: Tracheal mucoepidermoid carcinoma in a 7-year-old child. *Ann Thorac Surg* 66:928-929, 1998.
3. Oh Y-W, Effman EL, Redding GJ, et al: Follicular hyperplasia of bronchus-associated lymphoid tissue causing severe air trapping. *AJR* 172:745-747, 1999.

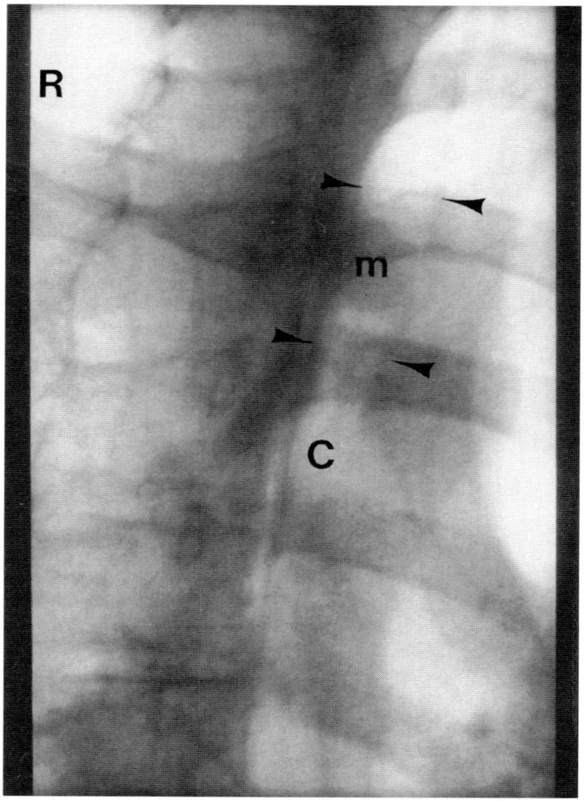

FIGURE 4.—Airway fluoroscopy reveals a mass (*m*) sitting in the distal airway (*outlined by arrows*) above the carina (*c*). (Courtesy of Weiner DJ, Weatherly RA, DiPietro MA, et al: Tracheal schwannoma presenting as status asthmaticus in a sixteen-year-old boy: Airway considerations and removal with the CO_2 laser. *Pediatr Pulmonol* 25:393-397, 1998. Reprinted by permission of Wiley-Liss, Inc., a subsidiary of John Wiley & Sons, Inc.)

MR Lymphangiography in Infants, Children, and Young Adults

Laor T, Hoffer FA, Burrows PE, et al (Children's Hosp, Boston)

AJR 171:1111-1117, 1998 — 4–34

Background.—Contrast-enhanced lymphangiography continues to be the most precise modality for defining conditions that primarily involve lymphatic channels, such as low-flow vascular malformations and chylothorax. However, current lymphangiographic methods have serious limitations. A preliminary study of MR lympangiography in infants, children, and young adults was reported.

Methods.—Twenty-nine patients with vascular malformations, other masses, soft-tissue swelling, gigantism, fluid accumulation, or pain underwent a total of 32 MR lymphangiographic evaluations. A heavily trans-

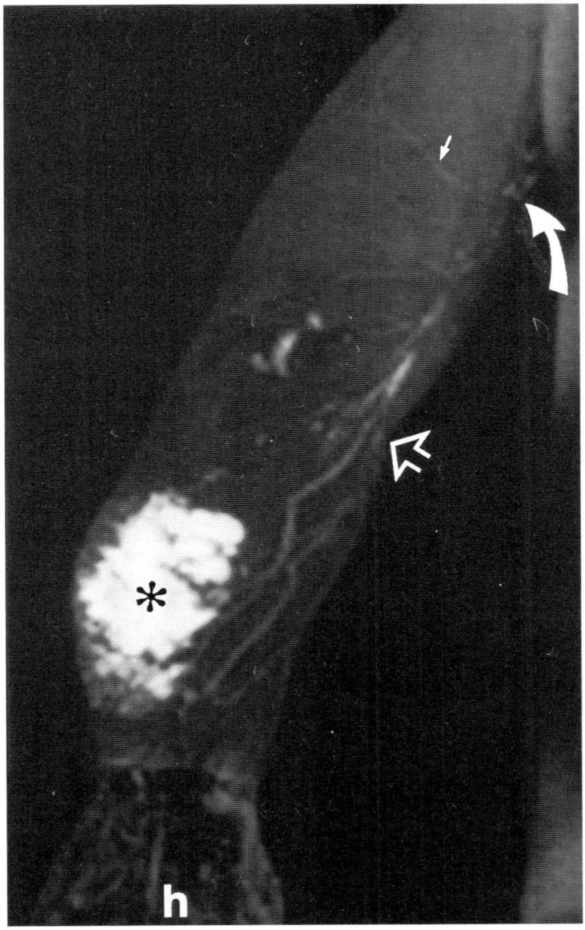

FIGURE 3.—Imaging in 14-month-old girl with localized macrocystic lymphatic malformation of right forearm. MR lymphangiogram shows well-demarcated high transverse relaxation time–weighted signal intensity of lymphatic malformation (*asterisk*). Although larger axial lymphatic channels of forearm follow course similar to that of superficial veins, off-axial channels (*small arrow*) are somewhat more horizontal in course than are superficial veins and drain toward small axillary lymph nodes (*curved arrow*). Small epitrochlear nodes are faintly seen (*open arrow*). *Abbreviation*: *h*, hand. (Courtesy of Laor T, Hoffer FA, Burrows PE, et al: MR lymphangiography in infants, children, and young adults. *AJR* 171:1111-1117, 1998.)

verse relaxation time–weighted fast spin-echo sequence was used with a maximum intensity projection algorithm. Axial and off-axial lymphatic channels were assessed in conjunction with MR venography to help distinguish veins from lymphatics.

Findings.—All studies showed presumed lymphatic channels, although 14 showed incomplete venous signal suppression. The appearance of the lymphatic channels was normal in 8 children as well as in 20 of the 21

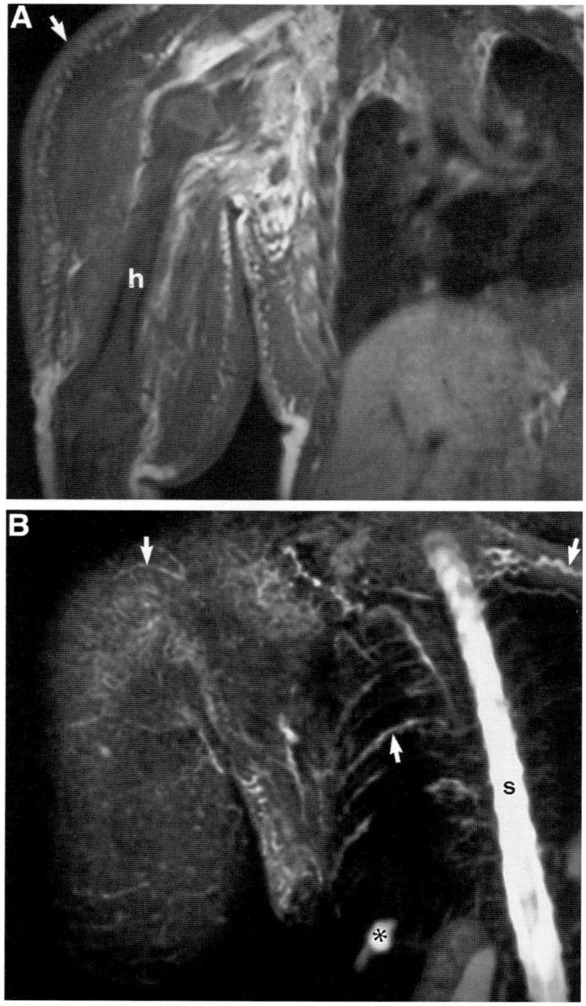

FIGURE 7.—Imaging in 1-year-old male infant with large Kaposiform hemangioendothelioma of right upper arm, axilla, and chest. **A**, Gd-enhanced longitudinal relaxation time–weighted MR image shows infiltration of soft tissues from lesion. Note hypointense soft tissue and hyperintense fatty elements. Also note enhancing thickened skin (*arrow*). Discrete vascular channels are not seen. **B**, MR lymphangiogram shows enlarged off-axial channels in soft tissues of upper arm, axilla, bilateral apices, and intercostal spaces (*arrows*). No axial lymphatic channels are seen in arm. Biopsy specimen (not shown) confirmed dilated lymphatic channels as described in Kaposiform hemangioendothelioma. *Asterisk* indicates gallbladder. *Abbreviations*: *s*, spinal canal; *h*, humerus. (Courtesy of Laor T, Hoffer FA, Burrows PE, et al: MR lymphangiography in infants, children, and young adults. *AJR* 171:1111-1117, 1998.)

asymptomatic contralateral limbs. In 10 children, the number and size of off-axial channels were increased. This group included 7 children with large, diffuse low-flow vascular malformations. Five children, including 4 with Klippel-Trénaunay syndrome, had enlarged axial and off-axial channels. Axial channels were absent or interrupted in 6 patients with an extensive hemangioendothelioma, Klippel-Trénaunay syndrome, Gorham syndrome, or unilateral body edema (Figs 3 and 7).

Conclusion.—Magnetic lymphangiography appears to be a useful, noninvasive modality for assessing superficial and deep lymphatic channels in children with local or diffuse vascular lesions or extremity swelling. This technique may provide further insight into the nature of vascular anomalies, help direct therapy, and predict the prognosis.

► The investigators have done it again! Their previous article[1] on MR venography documented that useful technique's applicability in demonstrating venous morphology of congenital vascular malformations of the extremities. This article on MR lymphangiography describes another noninvasive technique that examines superficial and deep lymphatic channels of vascular and lymphatic lesions of the extremities. Time will tell how effective these techniques will be for providing useful information in daily practice, but they seem to have substantial promise for use, alone or concurrently, based on the images included in the article.

L.W. Young, M.D.

Reference

1. Laor T, Burrows PE, Hoffer FA: Magnetic resonance venography of congenital vascular malformations of the extremities. *Pediatr Radiol* 26:371-380, 1996.

Gastrointestinal

Delayed Maturation of the Interstitial Cells of Cajal: A New Diagnosis for Transient Neonatal Pseudoobstruction: Report of Two Cases

Kenny SE, Vanderwinden JM, Rintala RJ, et al (Université Libre de Bruxelles, Brussels, Belgium; Univ of Liverpool, England)

J Pediatr Surg 33:94-98, 1998 4–35

Background.—Although the cause of gastrointestinal obstruction in neonates is usually known, some infants have a functional obstruction of unkown origin, meconium syndrome, or idiopathic neonatal pseudo-obstruction. Abnormalities of interstitial cells of Cajal, specialized type of cell responsible for maintaining gastrointestinal motility, may be involved in some cases of intestinal pseudo-obstruction. The cases of 2 infants with intestinal pseudo-obstruction requiring support with an ileostomy and total parental nutrition were reported.

Case 1.—Boy, born at 27 weeks' gestation, was shown on plain abdominal radiography to have features of small bowel obstruction with a single large loop of air-filled bowel in the right iliac fossa. Normal-caliber sigmoid and descending colon were seen on contrast enema, but the contrast agent did not pass the splenic flexure.

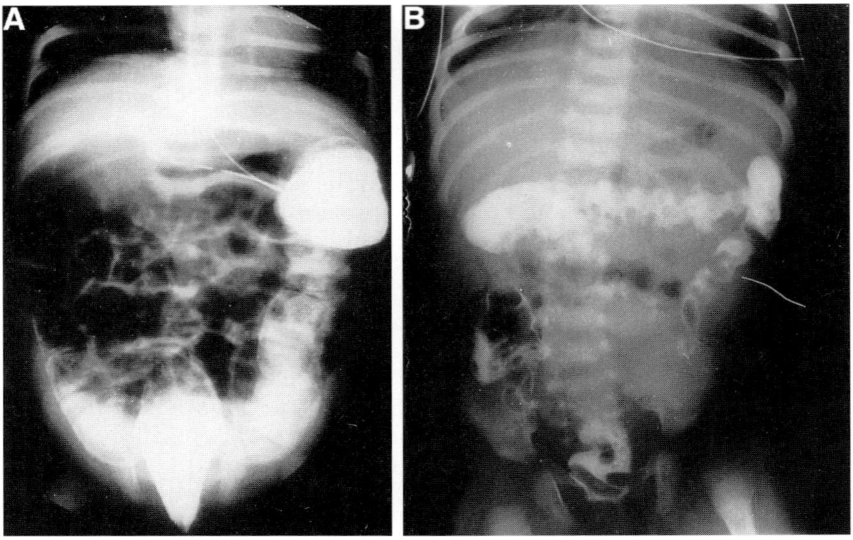

FIGURE 2.—Case 2. **A**, Enema with hydrosoluble contrast medium showing a normal rectum and absence of mechanical obstruction at the time of admission. **B**, Plain abdominal radiograph obtained 10 days later showing persistence of contrast medium in the colon and rectum. (Courtesy of Kenny SE, Vanderwinden JM, Rintala RJ, et al: Delayed maturation of the interstitial cells of Cajal: A new diagnosis for transient neonatal pseudoobstruction: Report of two cases. *J Pediatr Surg* 33:94-98, 1998.)

Ganglion cells were noted in biopsy specimens obtained from the terminal ileum during surgery.

Case 2.—Girl, born at term, was admitted at 19 days of age because of gross abdominal distension. Plain radiography suggested distal colonic obstruction (Fig 2), and Hirschsprung's disease was suspected. Subsequent plain radiographs showed an adynamic colon retaining the contrast agent for 10 days. Laparotomy was done at 1 month of age. The right and transverse colon were dilated, and the diameter of the left colon appeared normal. Strong propagated contractile activity occurred in the small intestine. Biopsy findings showed the presence of mature ganglion cells at all levels. A defunctioning ileostomy was created. Recovery was uneventful (Fig 4).

Conclusion.—Clinicians may consider the diagnosis of developmental delay of the interstitial cells of Cajal in the gastrointestinal tract in the assessment of neonates with pseudo-obstructive symptoms. Careful pathologic examination of multiple surgical biopsy specimens is needed to support the diagnosis.

► The correlation of delayed maturation of the interstitial cells of Cajal[1] with gut motility in neonates with pseudo-obstruction of the bowel is fascinating. Perhaps learning about the intricacies of intestinal *c*-kit pacemaker cells

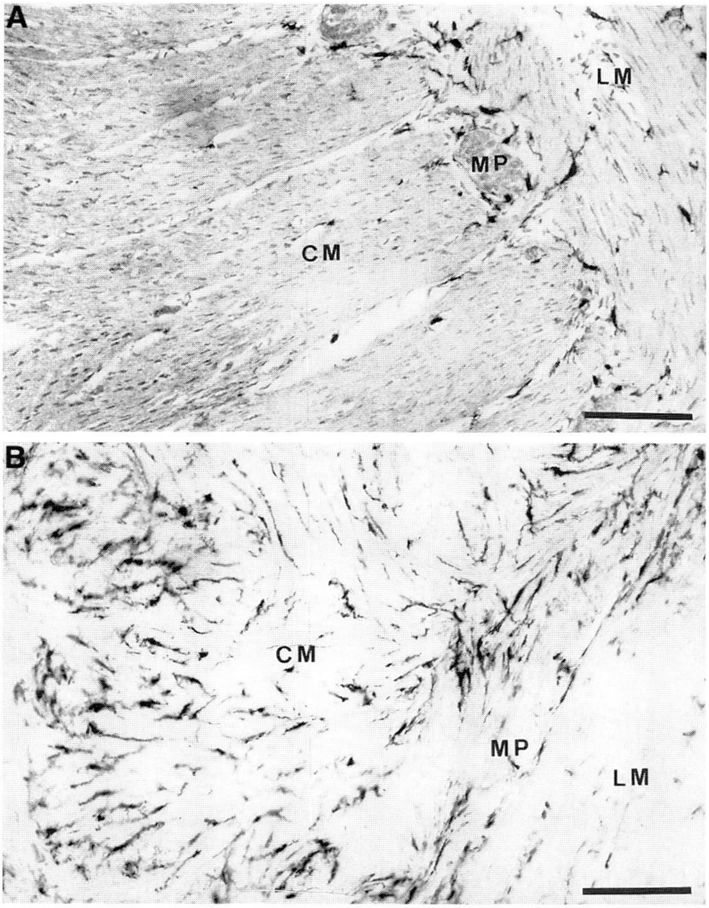

FIGURE 4.—Case 2. Micrographs of sections of descending colon show (**A**) the absence of *c*-kit immunoreactive interstitial cells of Cajal in the circular musculature at the time of first laparotomy (1 month of age) and (**B**) the presence of a normal pattern of *c*-kit immunoreactive interstitial cells of Cajal at the time of the second laparotomy (6 months of age). Scale bar: 100 μm. *Abbreviations: CM*, circular musculature; *LM*, longitudinal musculature; *MP*, myenteric plexus. (Courtesy of Kenny SE, Vanderwinden JM, Rintala RJ, et al: Delayed maturation of the interstitial cells of Cajal: A new diagnosis for transient neonatal pseudoobstruction: Report of two cases. *J Pediatr Surg* 33:94-98, 1998.)

(Cajal's interstitial cells) is a bit much for radiologists, but, at least, we need to know they exist. It is another apparently valid entity to add to our differential diagnosis list for suspected neonatal bowel obstruction. Another recent report of infantile bowel with delayed *c*-kit cell maturation is listed below.[2]

L.W. Young, M.D.

References

1. Thuneberg L, Rumessen JJ, Mikkelsen HG: Interstitial cells of Cajal: An intestinal impulse generation and conduction system? *Scand J Gastroenterol* (suppl) 72:143-144, 1982.
2. Yamataka A, Ohshiro K, Kobayashi H: Abnormal distribution of intestinal pacemaker (C-KIT-positive) cells in an infant with chronic idiopathic intestinal pseudoobstruction. *J Pediatr Surg* 33:859-862, 1998.

Gastric Cystic Duplication Communicating With a Bifid Pancreas: A Rare Cause of Recurrent Pancreatitis

Materne R, Clapuyt P, Saint-Martin C, et al (Université Catholique de Louvain, Brussels, Belgium; Centre Hospitalier de al Basse Sambre Reine Fabiola, Auvelais, Belgium)
J Pediatr Gastroenterol Nutr 27:102-105, 1998 4–36

Background.—Chronic pancreatitis is an uncommon cause of recurrent abdominal pain in children. Clinicians need to be aware that enteric duplications can cause recurrent pancreatitis. An unusual case of foregut anomaly, consisting of a gastric duplication cyst communicating with a pancreatic duplication, was reported in a child.

Case Report.—Girl, 11 years, had a 9-year history of recurrent abdominal pain that had required 2 previous hospitalizations. At the age of 9 years, she had an abdominal CT scan which revealed

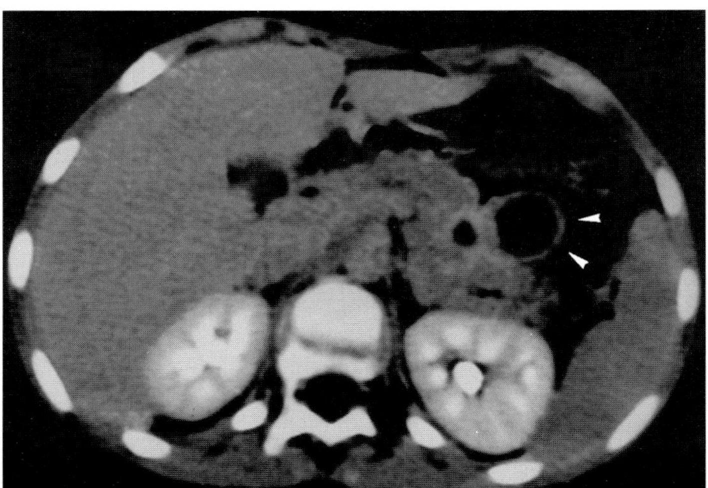

FIGURE 1.—Contrast-enhanced CT scan shows an enlarged pancreas with 2 cystic structures (*arrowheads*). (Courtesy of Materne R, Clapuyt P, Saint-Martin C, et al: Gastric cystic duplication communicating with a bifid pancreas: A rare cause of recurrent pancreatitis. *J Pediatr Gastroenterol Nutr* 27:102-105, 1998.)

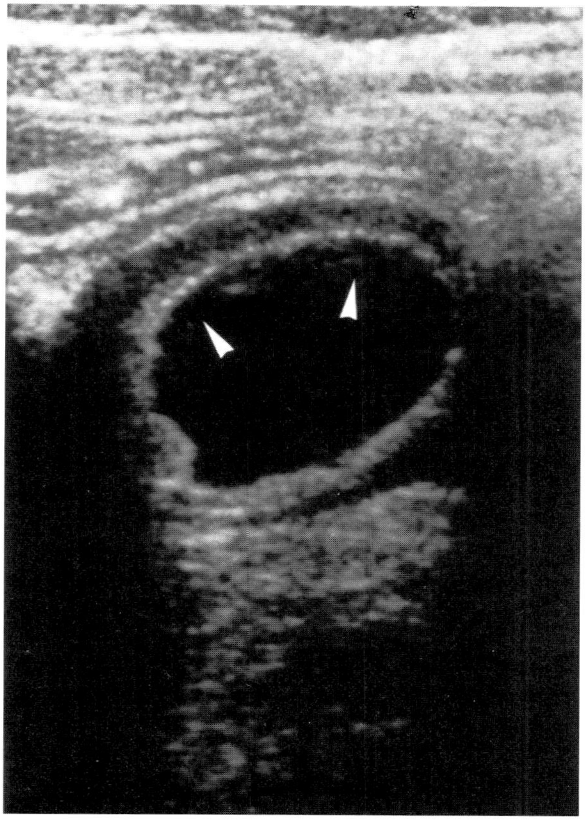

FIGURE 2.—Transverse sonogram of the extrapancreatic cystic structure shows an inner echogenic rim surrounded by a hypoechoic rim (*arrowheads*), suggestive of a cystic duplication. (Courtesy of Materne R, Clapuyt P, Saint-Martin C, et al: Gastric cystic duplication communicating with a bifid pancreas: A rare cause of recurrent pancreatitis. *J Pediatr Gastroenterol Nutr* 27:102-105, 1998.)

an enlarged pancreas with 2 cystic structures (Fig 1). An abdominal sonographic scan obtained at the latest assessment showed a heterogeneous pancreatic parenchyma with 2 cystic formations (Fig 2). Endoscopic retrograde cholangiopancreatography demonstrated a bifid main pancreatic duct with severe focal narrowing of the lower duct (Fig 3). A preoperative diagnosis of a gastric cystic duplication communicating with a bifid pancreas was confirmed intraoperatively.

Conclusion.—This patient had recurrent pancreatitis secondary to a gastric cystic duplication communicating with a bifid pancreas. The case report emphasizes the need to correctly diagnose the cause of this condition for effective treatment decision making.

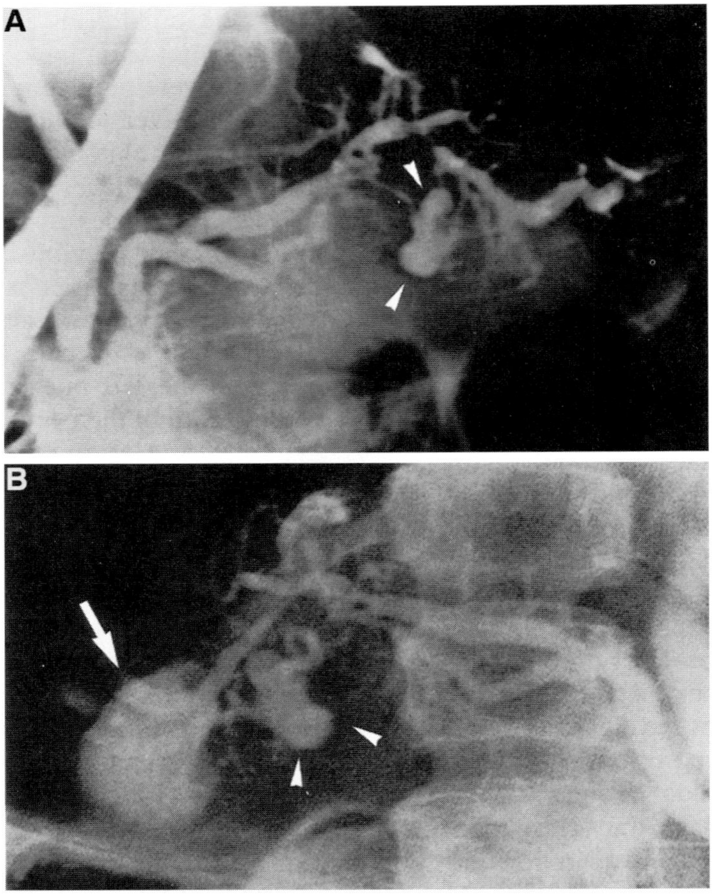

FIGURE 3.—Endoscopic retrograde cholangiopancreatogram shows duplication of the ductal system. The upper ductal system is normal. The lower ductal system reveals changes of chronic pancreatitis with filling of a cystic formation (**A**, supine; *arrowheads*), communicating lately with the extrapancreatic duplication (**B**, prone; *arrows*). (Courtesy of Materne R, Clapuyt P, Saint-Martin C, et al: Gastric cystic duplication communicating with a bifid pancreas: A rare cause of recurrent pancreatitis. *J Pediatr Gastroenterol Nutr* 27:102-105, 1998.)

► This case of gastric duplication cyst within a bifid pancreas is beautifully imaged—gut signature cysts by US, pancreatitis by CT, and bifid pancreatic ducts by endoscopic retrograde cholangiopancreatography. The well-written report briefly explains gastric duplication cyst/bifid pancreas embryogenesis and details its association with pancreatic ductal obstruction and chronic pancreatitis. The gastric duplication/bifid pancreas anomaly is but 1 of several pancreatic anomalies that may be predisposed to pancreatitis.[1] Although MR cholangiopancreatography was not used in this reported case, it is easier to do and should be more frequently used in place of endoscopic retrograde cholangiopancreatography in the future.[2-4]

L.W. Young, M.D.

References

1. Rizzo RJ, Szucs RA, Turner MA: Congenital abnormalities of the pancreas and biliary tree in adults. *Radiographics* 15:49-68; quiz 147-148, 1995.
2. Siddiqui AM, Shamberger RC, Filler RM, et al: Enteric duplications of the pancreatic head: Definitive management by local resection. *J Pediatr Surg* 33:1117-1121, 1998.
3. Chan Y, Yeung C, Lam WWM, et al: Magnetic resonance cholangiography: Feasibility and application in the paediatric population. *Pediatr Radiol* 28:307-311, 1998.
4. Hirohashi S, Hirohashi R, Uchida H, et al: Pancreatitis: Evaluation with MR cholangiopancreatography in children. *Radiology* 203:411-415, 1997.

Intestinal Rotational Abnormalities in Polysplenia and Asplenia Syndromes

Ditchfield MR, Hutson JM (Royal Children's Hosp, Parkville, Australia)

Pediatr Radiol 28:303-306, 1998 4–37

Background.—The asplenia and polysplenia syndromes are associated with intestinal malrotation and midgut volvulus. The anomalies of midgut intestinal rotation associated with these syndromes were characterized.

Methods.—Twenty-one children with asplenia and 6 with polysplenia were studied retrospectively. All had undergone upper gastrointestinal barium examinations between 1988 and 1996. Midgut intestinal rotation, determined by reviewing the barium exams, were classified as normal, incomplete rotation or nonrotation, reversed rotation, or reversed incomplete rotation or nonrotation. In 17 patients, findings were correlated with the results at laparotomy.

Findings.—Eleven percent of the children had normal midgut rotation; 19%, incomplete rotation or nonrotation; 19%, reversed rotation; and 52%, reversed incomplete rotation or nonrotation. In 2 of the 5 children with incomplete midgut rotation or nonrotation, midgut volvulus developed (Table 1).

TABLE 1.—Incidence of Rotational Abnormalities in Asplenia and Polysplenia Syndromes

	Normal	Reversed rotation	Non-Rotation	Reversed Non-rotation	Total
Asplenia	3	2*	12	12	21 (74%)
Polysplenia	0	3*	2	2	6 (26%)
Total	3 (11%)	5 (19%)	14 (52%)	14 (52%)	27

*Including 1 patient with midgut volvulus.

Conclusion.—Asplenia and polysplenia are often associated with midgut intestinal malrotation. All such children should undergo upper gastrointestinal barium examinations, as many will be at risk for midgut volvulus.

► This retrospective study documents the fact that midgut intestinal rotational abnormalities have high association with polysplenia and asplenia syndromes. An examination of the upper gastrointestinal tract with barium for demonstration of the midgut intestinal rotational status is appropriately recommended. Another recent article also makes this point.[1]

L.W. Young, M.D.

Reference

1. Nakada K, Kawaguchi F, Wakisaka M, et al: Digestive tract disorders associated with asplenia/polysplenia syndrome. *J Pediatr Surg* 32:91-94, 1997.

The Value of Sonography, CT and Air Enema for Detection of Complicated Meckel Diverticulum in Children With Nonspecific Clinical Presentation

Daneman A, Lobo E, Alton DJ, et al (Univ of Toronto)
Pediatr Radiol 28:928-932, 1998 4–38

Background.—Complicated Meckel diverticulum (MD) in children does not always manifest as painless rectal bleeding, which can create a diagnostic problem. In such patients, US, CT, or even air enema may be selected over the radionuclide Meckel scan (RNMS). The value of US, CT, and air enema in detecting complicated MD was investigated.

Methods and Findings.—Sixty-four children, aged 4 days to 14 years, with MD seen between 1990 and 1997 were included in the review. RNMS identified MD in 32 of 33 patients with rectal bleeding. Ten of these 32 patients underwent other imaging studies, all yielding negative findings. The remaining 31 patients had varied clinical presentations and did not undergo RNMS. Forty-four percent of this group, plus the 1 patient with a negative RNMS, had imaging features highly suggestive of MD on US. Air enema and CT findings strongly suggested MD in 3 patients and 1 patient, respectively (Figs 1 and 2 and Table 1).

Conclusion.—The inflamed hemorrhagic and inverted intussuscepted MDs have a spectrum of recognizable features on US, CT, and air enema. Some of these features are specific. Recognizing the features will facilitate the detection of complicated MD in more children who have symptoms in addition to those with painless rectal bleeding.

► Alan Daneman's interest in and contribution to pediatric gastrointestinal diagnostic imaging, including MD are again evident in this article.[1,2] Complicated MD may have a nonspecific clinical presentation. In such cases, the RNMS may not be obtained in the initial workup. The presence of sono-

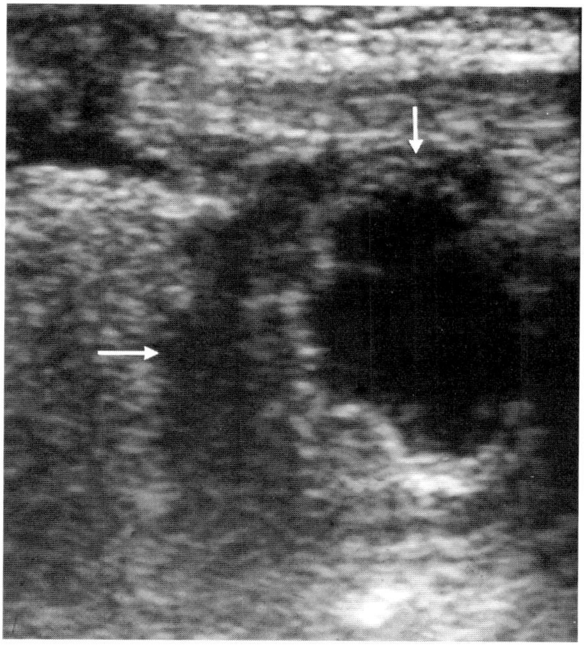

FIGURE 1.—Longitudinal sonogram of mid-abdomen in a 2½-year-old girl. The inflamed, hemorrhagic Meckel diverticulum appears as a thick-walled, irregular, cystic structure (*arrows*). The wall exhibits a gut signature. These appearances are similar to a gastrointestinal duplication cyst, but the wall is a little more irregular. (Courtesy of Daneman A, Lobo E, Alton DJ, et al: The value of sonography, CT and air enema for detection of complicated Meckel diverticulum in children with nonspecific clinical presentation. *Pediatr Radiol* 28:928-932. Copyright 1998, Springer-Verlag.)

graphic "gut signature" certainly helps in assessing the character of what may be a nonspecific mass of mixed echoes. The findings in this article and similar sonographic abnormalities found in another recent study are valuable for suspecting complicated MD.[3]

L.W. Young, M.D.

References

1. Kim G, Daneman A, Alton DJ, et al: The appearance of inverted Meckel diverticulum with intussusception on air enema. *Pediatr Radiol* 27:647-650, 1997.
2. Daneman A, Myers M, Shuckett B, et al: Sonographic appearances of inverted Meckel diverticulum with intussusception. *Pediatr Radiol* 27:295-298, 1997.
3. Gallego-Herrero C, del Pozo-Garcia G, Marin-Rodriguez C, et al: Torsion of a Meckel's diverticulum: Sonographic findings. *Pediatr Radiol* 28:599-601, 1998.

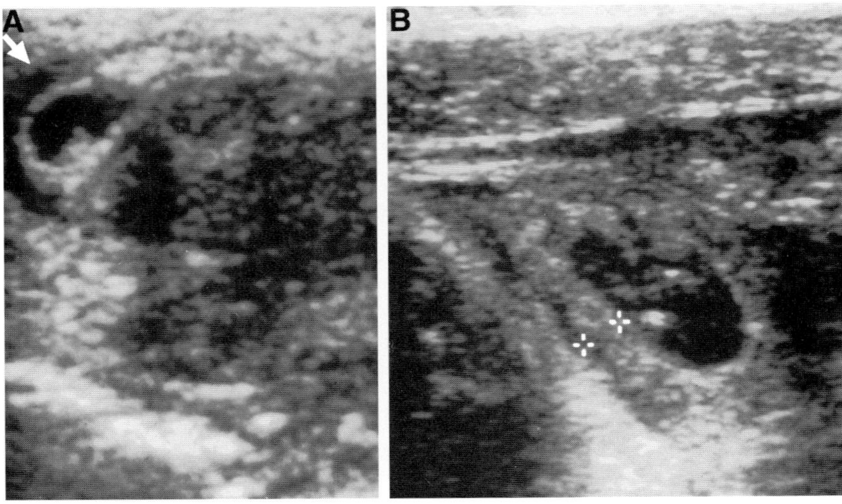

FIGURE 2.—Transverse sonograms of the lower abdomen in a 2-year-old girl (**A**) and a 4-month-old boy (**B**). The inflamed, hemorrhagic Meckel diverticulum appears as a thick-walled, teardrop-shaped structure. The wall exhibits a gut signature in **A** (*arrow*) and less so in **B** (*electronic cursors*). (Courtesy of Daneman A, Lobo E, Alton DJ, et al: The value of sonography, CT and air enema for detection of complicated Meckel diverticulum in children with nonspecific clinical presentation. *Pediatr Radiol* 28:928-932. Copyright 1998, Springer-Verlag.)

TABLE 1.—Utilization and Results of Imaging Modalities Other Than Radionuclide Meckel Scan in 41 of the 64 Symptomatic Children

Modality	# of Patients	# Negative	# Positive But Nonspecific	# Positive and Highly Suggestive for MD
Abdominal X-ray	31	7	24	—
Upper gastrointestinal series	13	10	3	—
Barium enema	16	9	6	1
Air enema	11	7	1	3
Sonography	21	2	5	14
Computed tomography	3	1	1	1

Abbreviation: MD, Meckel diverticulum.

(Courtesy of Daneman A, Lobo E, Alton DJ, et al: The value of sonograpy, CT and air enema for detection of complicated Meckel diverticulum in children with nonspecific clinical presentation. *Pediatr Radiol* 28:928-932. Copyright 1998, Springer-Verlag.)

Retropsoas Hernia as a Cause of Chronic Abdominal Pain: CT Diagnosis

Benson JE, Strauch ED (Johns Hopkins Hosp, Baltimore, Md)

Pediatr Radiol 28:312-314, 1998 4–39

Background.—Mobile bowel or omentum can herniate and sometimes strangulate in patients with congenital or acquired defects in the peritoneal lining of the abdominal wall or mesentery. The CT diagnosis of retropsoas hernia as a cause of abdominal pain was reported.

Case Report.—Girl, 15 years, with a 12-year history of recurrent abdominal pain and vomiting underwent elective upper gastrointestinal examination and small-bowel follow-through. A 6-cm mass effect compressing the small bowel in the left pelvis without obstruction was noted (Fig 1). The girl was admitted a few days

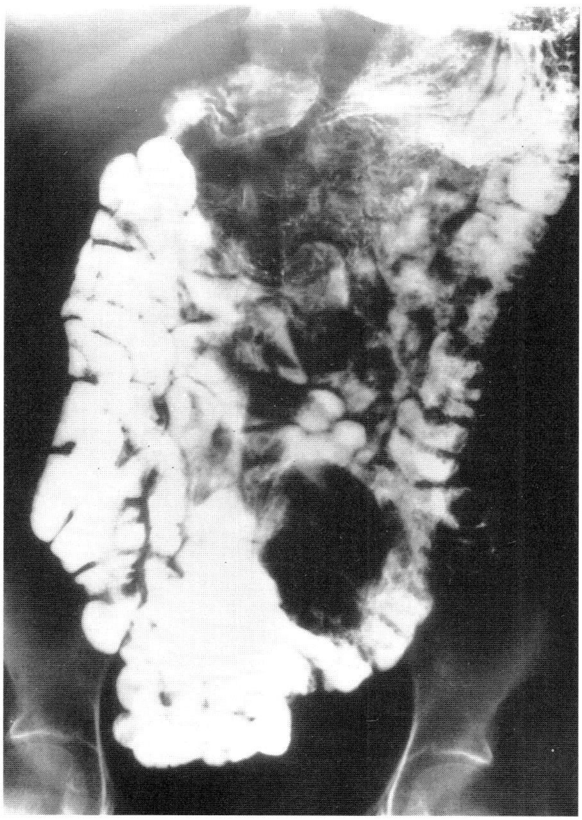

FIGURE 1.—Small-bowel follow-through, 45-minute film. Contrast opacifies the small bowel and the colon with no evidence of obstruction, despite the mass effect (*arrowheads*) on the left. (Courtesy of Benson JE, Strauch ED: Retropsoas hernia as a cause of chronic abdominal pain: CT diagnosis. *Pediatr Radiol* 28:312-314, copyright 1998, Springer-Verlag.)

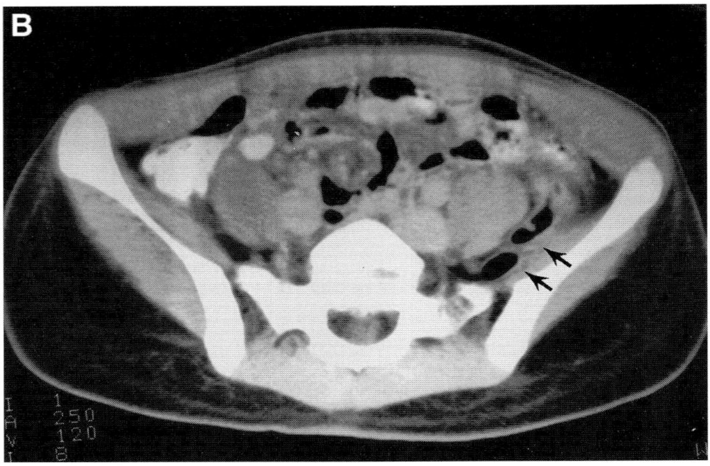

FIGURE 2.—Transverse CT scans of the abdomen, with oral and IV contrast. Small bowel (*arrow*) lies posterior to the left psoas muscle, medial to the contrast-filled descending colon. **B**, Scan is 2 cm inferior to the left iliac crest, showing the distribution of the hernia. This suggests that the "mass" seen on the small-bowel follow-through was actually the left psoas muscle. (Courtesy of Benson JE, Strauch ED: Retropsoas hernia as a cause of chronic abdominal pain: CT diagnosis. *Pediatr Radiol* 28:312-314, copyright 1998, Springer-Verlag.)

later because of coffee-ground emesis. On CT scan, herniation of a loop of small bowel lateral and posterior to the left psoas muscle was noted at the level of L4, extending into the pelvis (Fig 2, B). No strangulation, obstruction, or other mass was observed. Surgery revealed a true peritoneal defect 2.5 cm long along the lateral border of the psoas muscle just superior to the iliac crest, with small bowel herniating through this defect to a depth of 4 cm. The bowel was moved back to the peritoneal cavity. Recovery was uneventful. At the 1-year follow-up, the patient reported no recurrence of symptoms.

Conclusion.—In this patient, congenital retropsoas small bowel herniation was found to be the cause of long-standing recurrent abdominal pain. This entity should be considered in the differential diagnosis of abdominal pain, mass, or retroperitoneal gas and fluid. Clinicians also need to be aware of this entity to avoid complications of percutaneous renal interventions.

► Appreciation of the variant anatomy of the peritoneal attachments is highlighted by this diagnostic imaging analysis. The authors merit commendation for imaging recognition by CT of the unique retropsoas hernia.

L.W. Young, M.D.

References

1. Meyers MA: *Dynamic Radiology of the Abdomen.* New York, Springer, 1988, pp 179-278.
2. Meyers MA: *Dynamic Radiology of the Abdomen*: New York, Springer, 1988, pp 300-317.

MR Imaging in Children With Nonperforated Acute Appendicitis: Value of Unenhanced MR Imaging in Sonographically Selected Cases

Hörmann M, Paya K, Eibenberger K, et al (Univ of Vienna)

AJR 171:467-470, 1998 4–40

Background.—Although acute appendicitis is a common cause of abdominal pain, only 1 study of MRI in the detection of acute appendicitis has been published. The MR appearance of acute appendicitis was described, and its value in diagnosing acute appendicitis in children was investigated.

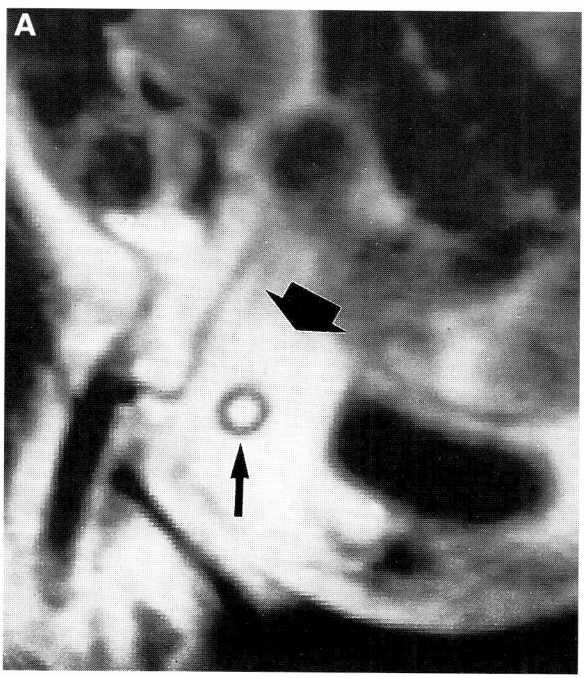

FIGURE 2.—A 12-year-old boy with paraumbilical pain and clinically suspected acute appendicitis. **A,** T2-weighted ultra turbo spin-echo sequence in coronal plane shows target sign with fluid-filled appendix and thickened wall of appendix (*thin arrow*). Also notice hyperintense periappendiceal inflamed fat (*thick arrow*). (Courtesy of Hörmann M, Paya K, Eibenberger K, et al: MR imaging in children with nonperforated acute appendicitis: Value of unenhanced MR imaging in sonographically selected cases. *AJR* 171:467-470, 1998.)

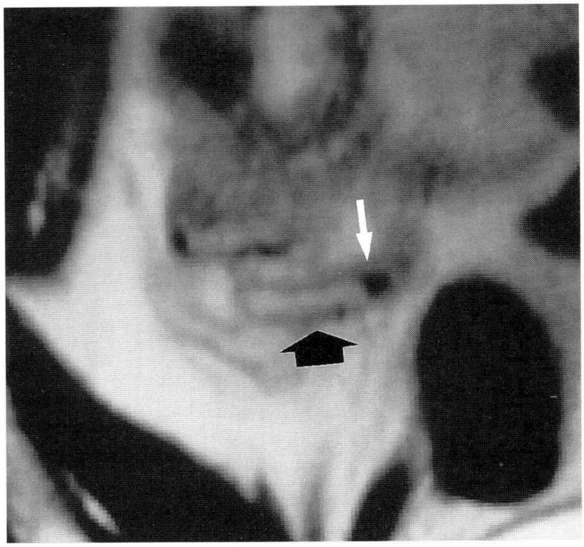

FIGURE 3.—A 14-year-old girl with acute appendicitis. Coronal T2-weighted ultra turbo spin-echo sequence shows rounded intraluminal structure without signal intensity caused by calcification, surgically proven as appendicolith (*white arrow*). Also notice thickened fluid-filled appendix coursing medially from cecum (*black arrow*). (Courtesy of Hörmann M, Paya K, Eibenberger K, et al: MR imaging in children with nonperforated acute appendicitis: Value of unenhanced MR imaging in sonographically selected cases. *AJR* 171:467-470, 1998.)

Methods.—Forty-five children, aged 7 to 16 years, were studied. All had clinically diagnosed acute appendicitis and underwent compression sonography, interpreted independently by 2 radiologists. Axial T1-weighted turbo spin-echo sequences, T2-weighted turbo spin-echo sequences in the axial and coronal planes, and fat-suppressed short inversion time inversion recovery turbo spin-echo sequences in the axial plane were also obtained and assessed independently by 2 radiologists.

Findings.—Both radiologists interpreted MR images as showing appendicitis in all cases. Acute appendicitis appeared with a markedly hyperintense center, slightly hyperintense thickened wall, and markedly hyperintense periappendiceal tissue on T2-weighted ultra turbo spin-echo images. The most sensitive sequence was unenhanced axial T2-weighted spin-echo imaging (Figs 2, A and 3).

Conclusion.—MRI appears to be useful for assessing children with acute appendicits. In this MRI application, it is not necessary to administer either MRI or CT contrast media, which is especially advantageous in children.

► MRI is a worthwhile technique in childhood nonperforated acute appendicitis, as shown in this prospective study on sonographically selected cases. The authors make a case for favoring unenhanced MRI over Gd-enhanced MR, also recently advocated,[1] for the diagnosis of nonperforated acute appendicitis.

L.W. Young, M.D.

Reference

1. Inescu L, Coskun A, Selcuk MG, et al: Acute appendicitis: MR imaging and sonographic correlation. *AJR* 249:53-58, 1997.

Dynamic Gadolinium-enhanced MR Findings in Infantile Hepatic Hemangioendothelioma

Mortele KJ, Mergo PJ, Urrutia M, et al (Univ of Florida, Gainesville)
J Comput Assist Tomogr 22:714-717, 1998 4–41

Background.—The most common primary mesenchymal tumor in the first year of life is infantile hemangioendothelioma (IHE) of the liver. To date, the dynamic Gd-enhanced MR characteristics of this tumor have not

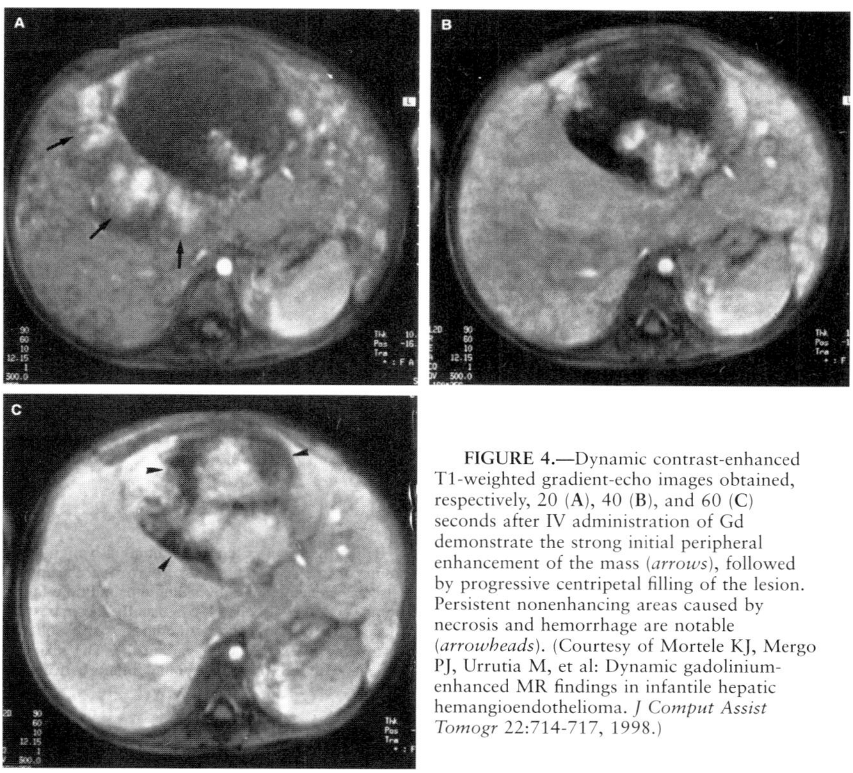

FIGURE 4.—Dynamic contrast-enhanced T1-weighted gradient-echo images obtained, respectively, 20 (**A**), 40 (**B**), and 60 (**C**) seconds after IV administration of Gd demonstrate the strong initial peripheral enhancement of the mass (*arrows*), followed by progressive centripetal filling of the lesion. Persistent nonenhancing areas caused by necrosis and hemorrhage are notable (*arrowheads*). (Courtesy of Mortele KJ, Mergo PJ, Urrutia M, et al: Dynamic gadolinium-enhanced MR findings in infantile hepatic hemangioendothelioma. *J Comput Assist Tomogr* 22:714-717, 1998.)

been described. An unusual case of IHE in a child whose condition was diagnosed with the use of a dynamic GD-enhanced MRI was reported.

Case Report.—Girl, 2½ years, was brought for medical care because of a 2-day history of fever, nonbilious vomiting, and abdominal pain. Her family history included renal failure and diabetes mellitus. MRI was performed with 8-mm–thick axial and coronal longitudinal relaxation time (T1)–weighted, 10-mm–thick axial transverse relaxation time–weighted spin-echo images, and 8-mm–thick axial dynamic T1-weighted gradient-echo images 20, 40, and 60 seconds, respectively, after the administration of gadopentetate. On T1-weighted images, the liver mass was mostly hypointense. Peripheral regions of hyperintensity were evident in the largest lesion, corresponding to presumed regions of hemorrhage. The largest mass was heterogeneously hyperintense on transverse relaxation time–weighted images. After Gd administration with subsequent dynamic scanning, centripetal tumor enhancement occurred with initial peripheral enhancement, eventually followed by more uniform enhancement (Fig 4).

Conclusion.—Despite this patient's unusual age at presentation, IHE was diagnosed with the aid of dynamic Gd-enhanced MR. The findings of this modality were highly specific for the diagnosis of IHE because of its characteristic enhancement pattern.

► CT does an excellent job of demonstrating IHE. It is not surprising—although it is of considerable interest—that dynamic Gd-enhanced MR findings have a similar centripetal imaging pattern. Our recent IHE case in a neonate was imaged by MRI. MRI has the usual advantages of excellent resolution, superb vascular delineation, multiplanar capability, and lack of ionizing radiation. Another recent article emphasizes management strategy for IHE, including hepatic artery embolization.[1]

L.W. Young, M.D.

Reference

1. Daller JA, Bueno J, Gutierrez J, et al: Hepatic hemangioendothelioma: Clinical experience and management strategy. *J Pediatr Surg* 34:99-106, 1999.

Genitourinary

Ureteral-Sciatic Hernia in a Child Demonstrated by Voiding Cystography

Arat A, Haliloglu M (Hacettepe Univ, Ankara, Turkey)

J Urol 160:157-158, 1998 4–42

Background.—Since 1994, several cases of herniation of the ureter through the sciatic foramen, an extremely uncommon condition, have been reported. In the case reported here ureteral-sciatic hernia was demonstrated by voiding cystography.

Case Report.—Girl, 3 months, given a diagnosis of Down's syndrome shortly after birth, was referred for a urinary tract infection. Abdominal US showed bilateral hydronephrosis. Bilateral grade V vesicoureteral reflux was seen on voiding cystourethrography. On fluoroscopy, a portion of the tortuous left ureter was seen herniating into the sciatic foramen, demonstrated by ureteral curling when the baby cried (Fig 1). Both ureters were otherwise normal.

Conclusion.—Ureteral-sciatic herniation associated with Down's syndrome has not been reported previously. This case report also shows that

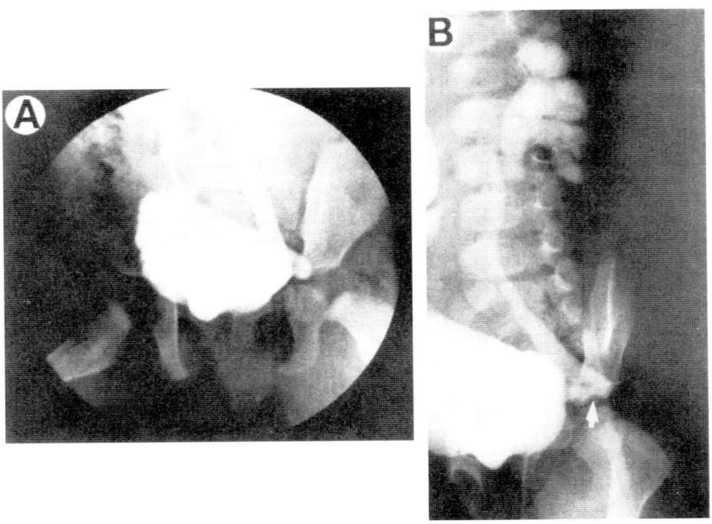

FIGURE 1.—Voiding cystourethrogram. **A**, Anteroposterior view reveals curling ureter and inferolateral axis of curl. **B**, Oblique view shows curling ureter better with hairpin turn where ureter exits from hernial sac (*arrow*). (Courtesy of Arat A, Haliloglu M: Ureteral-sciatic hernia in a child demonstrated by voiding cystography. *J Urol* 160:157-158, 1998.)

clinicians can learn more from voiding cystourethrography than simply whether reflux is present.

▶ The ureteral-sciatic hernia has been previously recognized by excretory urography, but, apparently, this is the first demonstration by voiding cystourethrography. The value of the fluoroscopic part of the examination is appropriately emphasized. The herniation is probably a dynamic of the tortuous left ureter. Another recent article on this subject is listed.[1]

L.W. Young, M.D.

Reference

1. Ritschel S, Heimbach D, Schoeneich G: Ureterosciatic hernia. *Scand J Urol Nephrol* 30:423-424, 1996.

Cystic Dysplasia of the Testis Associated With Multicystic Dysplasia of the Kidney

Robson WLM, Thomason MA, Minette LJ (Children's Hosp, Greenville, SC; Univ of South Carolina, Greenville)

Urology 51:477-479, 1998 4–43

Background.—Cystic dysplasia of the testis (CDT), a rare cause of testicular mass in boys, usually appears as 1 or more cysts on US imaging. This paper reports the case of a child with atypical CDT, in whom US showed a solid lesion, with cystic changes in the epididymis and ipsilateral multicystic dysplasia of the kidney (MCDK).

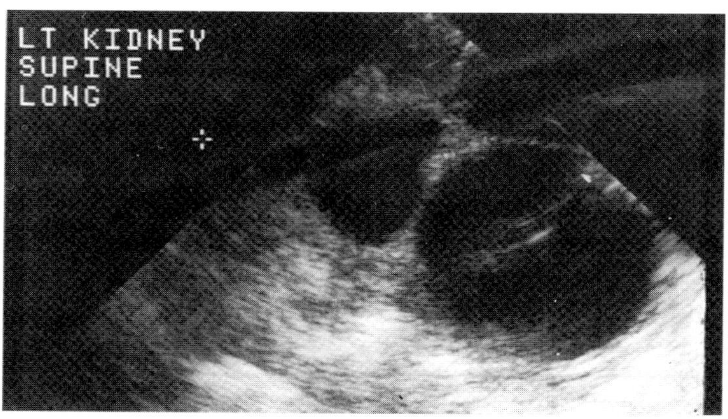

FIGURE 1.—Longitudinal image of the left kidney showing multiple noncommunicating cysts consistent with a multicystic dysplasia of the kidney. (Reprinted from *Urology* courtesy of Robson WLM, Thomason MA, Minette LJ: Cystic dysplasia of the testis associated with multicystic dysplasia of the kidney. *Urology* 51:477-479. Copyright 1998 with permission from Elsevier Science.)

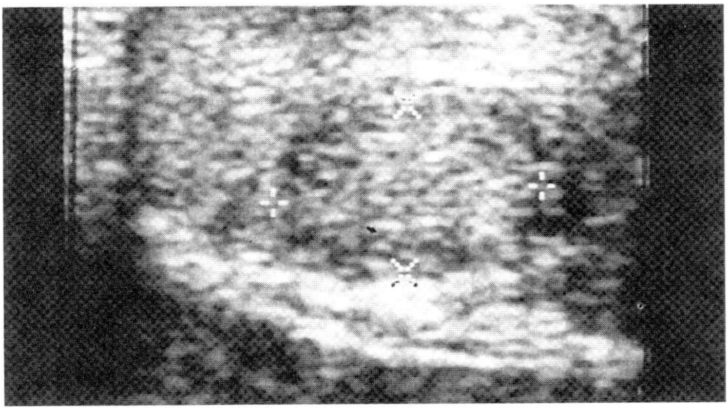

FIGURE 2.—Longitudinal image of left testis showing the mass (surrounded by *white markers*) as solid and hypoechoic compared with the rest of the testis. (Reprinted from *Urology* courtesy of Robson WLM, Thomason MA, Minette LJ: Cystic dysplasia of the testis associated with multicystic dysplasia of the kidney. *Urology* 51:477-479. Copyright 1998 with permission from Elsevier Science.)

Case Report.—Prenatally, MCDK was found on a routine US examination. US assessment postnatally confirmed the presence of a left MCDK and a normal contralateral kidney (Fig 1). At 4 months, US imaging continued to show an MCDK, but by 3 years of age, there was no evidence of MCDK in the affected kidney and compensatory hypertrophy of the right kidney. However, after a bicycle accident at age 3 years, the boy's mother noticed bruising

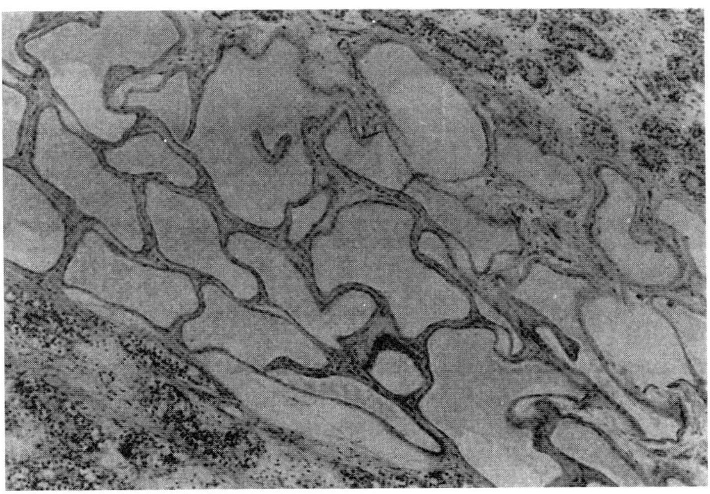

FIGURE 3.—Left testis. The center shows cystically dilated tubules. The upper right and lower left show focal residual immature tubules; hematoxylin-eosin; original magnification ×100. (Reprinted from *Urology* courtesy of Robson WLM, Thomason MA, Minette LJ: Cystic dysplasia of the testis associated with multicystic dysplasia of the kidney. *Urology* 51:477-479. Copyright 1998 with permission from Elsevier Science.)

and enlargement of the left testis. Testicular US showed an enlarged left testis and a smaller, solid, hypoechoic area in the left postero-inferior aspect of the testis. Images acquired with B-color mapping accentuated the differences in echogenicity (Fig 2). The left testis was removed surgically along with the cord structures. Histologically, elongated lobular areas of anastomosing microcystic tubules were noted in the testis proper (Fig 3). Cystic dysplasia of the testis and epididymis was diagnosed.

Conclusion.—Typically, CDT is associated with unilateral renal agenesis or MCDK and appears as a solid lesion ultrasonographically. Cystic changes in the epididymis may be associated with CDT more commonly than previously reported.

► This well-written case report including literature review gives the essentials on the association of CDT and MCDK. The frequent involution of MCDK to renal agenesis is also noteworthy.[1,2] In another recent publication,[3] the sonographic differentiation between CDT and testicular microlithiasis was emphasized.

L.W. Young, M.D.

References

1. Ngai RL, Yeung BK, Tsui WM, et al: Cystic dysplasia of the testis associated with ipsilateral renal agenesis and high anorectal anomalies. *J Pediatr Surg* 33:787-788, 1998.
2. Bonnet JP, Aigrain Y, Ferkadji L: Cystic dysplasia of the testis with ipsilateral renal agenesis: A case report and review of the literature. *Eur J Pediatr Surg* 7:57-59, 1997.
3. Levin TL, Kogan SJ: Cystic dysplasia of the testis: Sonographic diagnosis and differentiation from testicular microlithiasis. *Pediatr Radiol* 28:955-957, 1998.

Acute Scrotal Symptoms in Boys With an Indeterminate Clinical Presentation: Comparison of Color Doppler Sonography and Scintigraphy

Paltiel HJ, Connolly LP, Atala A, et al (Harvard Med School, Boston; Yale Univ, New Haven, Conn)

Radiology 207:223-231, 1998 4–44

Background.—Scrotal scintigraphy and color Doppler US have been reported to be very accurate in detecting testicular perfusion. To date, these 2 modalities have not been compared in a pediatric population. A comparison was made of color Doppler US and scintigraphy in the assessment of testicular perfusion in boys with equivocal clinical findings.

Methods.—Forty-one boys underwent Doppler US and scintigraphy. Findings were classified retrospectively as consistent with torsion or nontorsion or as indeterminate.

TABLE 5.—Results of Treating Indeterminate Studies as Positive for Torsion

Parameter	Original Color Doppler US Diagnosis	Original Scintigraphic Diagnosis
Sensitivity	11/11 (100)	11/11 (100)
Specificity	23/30 (77)	29/30 (97)

Note: Numbers in parentheses are percentages.

(Courtesy of Paltiel HJ, Connolly LP, Atala A, et al: Acute scrotal symptoms in boys with an indeterminate clinical presentation: Comparison of color Doppler sonography and scintigraphy. *Radiology* 207:223-231, 1998. Radiological Society of North America.)

Findings.—Color Doppler US demonstrated 9 of 11 cases of torsion and 23 of 30 cases of nontorsion. Eight Doppler US studies were indeterminate, and 1 was false positive. Scintigraphy demonstrated 10 of 11 cases of torsion and 29 of 30 cases of nontorsion. Two scintigraphic studies were indeterminate, both in boys with inguinal testis. When indeterminate findings were considered positive for torsion, scintigraphy and color Doppler US had specificities of 77% and 97%, respectively. No other significant differences between sensitivies and specificities were noted (Tables 5 and 6).

Conclusion.—Scintigraphy and color Doppler US are comparable in their ability to demonstrate testicular torsion in boys with acute scrotal symptoms and indeterminate clinical presentations. Because of its high specificity, scintigraphy may help prevent unnecessary surgery when color Doppler US shows equivocal flow.

► The roles of color Doppler sonography and scintigraphy are complimentary in assessing testicular perfusion but are not definitive, especially in prepubertal boys. Scintigraphy, however, is still probably the imaging modality of choice because of its better specificity when indeterminate results, as in this study, were treated as positive. However, there is no faulting of some who prefer power and color Doppler sonography for the imaging of acute scrotal symptoms in boys.[1] Other pertinent references are listed.[2,3]

L.W. Young, M.D.

TABLE 6.—Results of Treating Indeterminate Studies as Negative for Torsion

Parameter	Original Color Doppler US Diagnosis	Original Scintigraphic Diagnosis
Sensitivity	9/11 (82)	10/11 (91)
Specificity	29/30 (97)	30/30 (100)

Note: Numbers in parentheses are percentages.

(Courtesy of Paltiel HJ, Connolly LP, Atala A, et al: Acute scrotal symptoms in boys with an indeterminate clinical presentation: Comparison of color Doppler sonography and scintigraphy. *Radiology* 207:223-231, 1998. Radiological Society of North America.)

References

1. Albrecht T, Lotzof K, Hussain HK, et al: Power Doppler US of the normal prepubertal testis: Does it live up to its promises? *Radiology* 203:227-231, 1997.
2. Bader TR, Kammerhuber F, Herneth AD: Testicular blood flow in boys as assessed at color Doppler and power Doppler sonography. *Radiology* 202:559-564, 1993.
3. Kass EJ, Lundak B: The acute scrotum. *Pediatr Clin North Am* 44:1251-1266, 1997.

Reflux in Young Patients: Comparison of Voiding US of the Bladder and Retrovesical Space With Echo Enhancement Versus Voiding Cystourethrography for Diagnosis

Darge K, Troeger J, Duetting T, et al (Heidelberg Univ Hosp, Germany)
Radiology 210:201-207, 1999 4–45

Background.—The main diagnostic procedure for assessing vesicoureteral reflux (VUR) is fluoroscopic voiding cystourethrography (VCUG). Digital fluoroscopy has enabled a decrease in radiation dose. Radionuclide cystography, which involves markedly less radiation, appears to be a sensitive alternative method for detecting VUR, but it lacks spatial resolution. The utility of voiding US of the bladder and retrovesical space with echo enhancement was compared with that of VCUG for the diagnosis of VUR.

Methods.—One hundred eighty-eight patients, aged 5 days to 20 years, underwent voiding US with echo enhancement for assessment of VUR. In 110 patients, this procedure was followed by VCUG. After renal tract US,

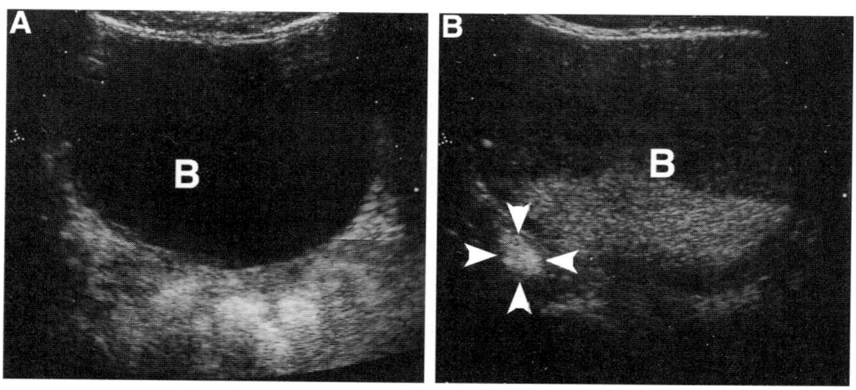

FIGURE 2.—Transverse US scans of the bladder (**B**). **A**, Scan obtained before the administration of the echo-enhancing agent SH U 508 A. Note the absence of any visibly dilated ureter in the retrovesical space. **B**, After the intravesical administration of SH U 508 A, an oval-shaped, strongly hyperechogenic spot (*arrowheads*) caused by the regurgitating microbubbles can be identified on the right side. During real-time US, one can also visualize the constant movement of these microbubbles and thus make a definite diagnosis of reflux on the right side. No vesicoureteral reflux is depicted on the left side. (Courtesy of Darge K, Troeger J, Duetting T, et al: Reflux in young patients: Comparison of voiding US of the bladder and retrovesical space with echo enhancement versus voiding cystourethrography for diagnosis. *Radiology* 210:201-207, 1999. Radiological Society of North America.)

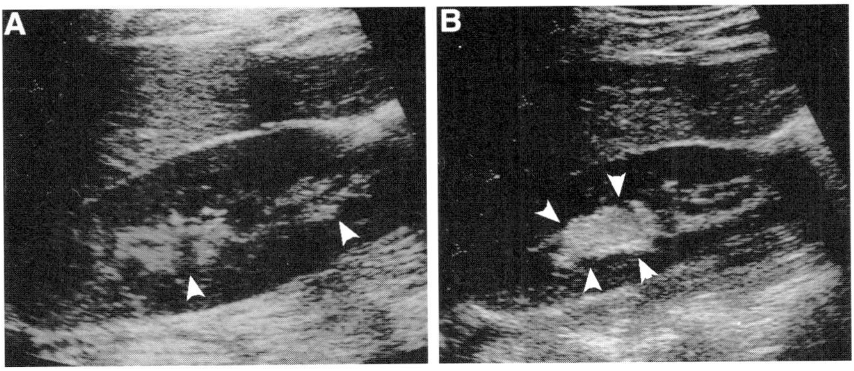

FIGURE 3.—Longitudinal US scans of the ventral region of the right kidney in an 11-year-old girl seen with recurrent urinary tract infection. Note the 2 renal pelves (*arrowheads*) in the kidney with renal duplication (**A**) before and (**B**) after the administration of the echo enhancer into the bladder. There is reflux of microbubbles in the upper pole (*arrowheads*) of the kidney. (Courtesy of Darge K, Troeger J, Duetting T, et al: Reflux in young patients: Comparison of voiding US of the bladder and retrovesical space with echo enhancement versus voiding cystourethrography for diagnosis. *Radiology* 210:201-207, 1999. Radiological Society of North America.)

the bladder was filled with normal saline solution, and a galactose-based, microbubble-containing, echo-enhancing agent (SH U 508 A) was administered. Microbubbles appearing in the ureter or pelvicalyceal system indicated the diagnosis of reflux.

Findings.—One or both methods demonstrated VUR in 80 of the 226 kidney-ureter units assessed. All reflux grades were seen. Reflux diagnosed on voiding US was not shown on VCUG in 15 units, and the reverse was seen in 3 units. The 2 methods concurred on the diagnosis or exclusion of VUR in 92% of the kidney-ureter units. Patients tolerated the echo-enhancing agent well (Figs 2 and 3).

Conclusion.—Voiding US enhanced with SH U 508 A is as efficient as VCUG in detecting or excluding VUR. The use of this procedure will reduce the number of children exposed to ionizing radiation.

▶ This excellent article beautifully shows that echo enhancement voiding sonography is an alternative to cystourethrography or radionuclide cystography for the demonstration of VUR. It is as definitive as VCUG for establishing reflux, but no attempt at grading of reflux was made in this study. Reduction in exposure to ionizing radiation is a worthy goal in stimulating additional refinements in this sonographic advance, which is coming of age. Several other investigators and authors have recently contributed their experiences with this technique.[1,2]

L.W. Young, M.D.

References

1. Bosio M: Cystosonography with echocontrast: A new imaging modality to detect vesicoureteric reflux in children. *Pediatr Radiol* 28:250-255, 1998.
2. Atala A, Ellsworth P, Share J, et al: Comparison of sonicated albumin enhanced sonography to fluoroscopic and radionuclide voiding cystography for detecting vesicoureteral reflux. *J Urol* 160:1820-1822, 1998.

Childhood Pyelonephritis: Comparison of Gadolinium-enhanced MR Imaging and Renal Cortical Scintigraphy for Diagnosis

Lonergan GJ, Pennington DJ, Morrison JC, et al (Willford Hall Med Ctr, Lackland Air Force Base, San Antonio, Tex; Uniformed Services Univ of the Health Sciences, Bethesda, Md; Armed Forces Inst of Pathology, Washington, DC)

Radiology 207:377-384, 1998 4–46

Introduction.—Children with suspected pyelonephritis are usually evaluated by renal cortical scintigraphy (RCS) with ^{99m}Tc dimercaptosuccinic acid (DMSA). Radiologically evident scarring from the disease process can be detected in up to 64% of pediatric kidneys using scintigraphy. As with RCS, Gd-enhanced inversion-recovery MRI of pyelonephritis depends on diminished delivery and concentration of contrast material to make areas of infection visible. Gd-enhanced inversion-recovery MRI and RCS were compared in the diagnosis of childhood pyelonephritis in 37 children with fever-producing urinary tract infection.

Methods.—All patients underwent Gd-enhanced inversion-recovery MRI and RCS that was read in double-blind fashion by 2 pediatric radiologists. Each kidney was divided into 3 zones and studies were graded as positive, equivocal, or negative for pyelonephritis.

Results.—Two-hundred ten zones of 70 kidneys were evaluated. Of these, 26 kidneys (54 zones) had evidence of pyelonephritis on both MRI and RCS. Both study results were negative for pyelonephritis in 24 kidneys (100 zones). There were 12 kidneys (42 zones) that were positive for pyelonephritis on MRI and negative on RCS (Fig 2); 4 kidneys (7 zones) were negative for pyelonephritis on MRI and positive on RCS. The proportion of positive agreement between readers for presence of pyelonephritis was 0.85 for MRI and 0.57 for RCS. The proportion of negative agreement was 0.88 for MRI and 0.80 for RCS.

Conclusion.—The MRI images were read as positive for pyelonephritis in more renal zones than was true for RCS. Pyelonephritis was shown in 29 of 37 patients (78%) using MRI, compared with 25 patients (68%) with RCS. Discrimination of the scar from pyelonephritis may be easier to detect on MRI than on RCS because MRI allows direct visualization of the parenchyma. Interobserver agreement was superior with MRI, compared with RCS.

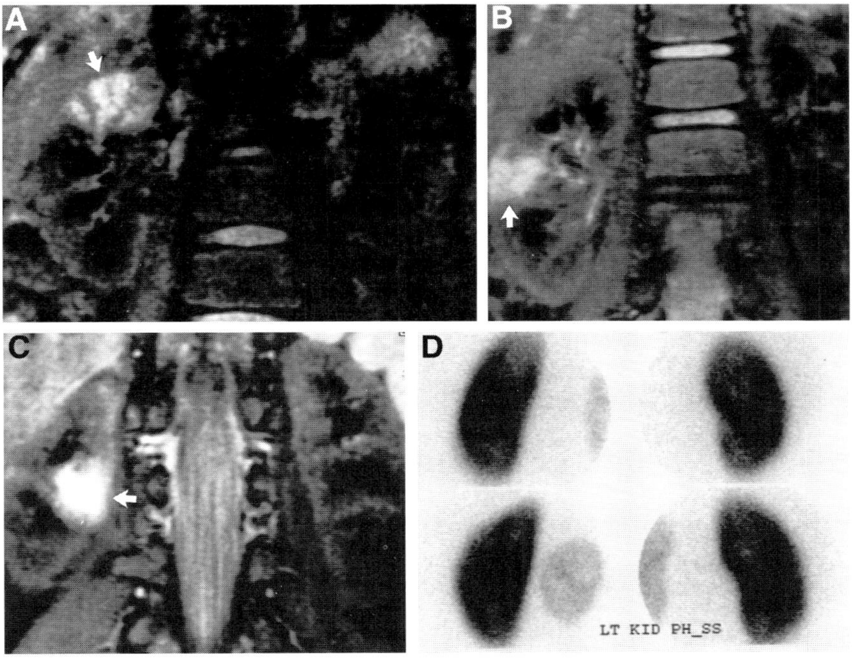

FIGURE 2.—Pyelonephritis overlooked at RCS. (**A-C**) Coronal Gd-enhanced inversion-recovery MR images (2,000/16/160, 90 degree flip angle) show foci of high signal intensity (*arrow*), consistent with multifocal pyelonephritis in the right kidney; the left kidney appears normal. (**D**) On ^{99m}Tc dimercaptosuccinic acid renal cortical scintigraphy scans in the same patient, both kidneys appear normal. *Abbreviations*: *KID*, kidney; *LT*, left; *PH-SS* pinhole. (Courtesy of Lonergan GJ, Pennington DJ, Morrison JC, et al: Childhood pyelonephritis: Comparison of gadolinium-enhanced MR imaging and renal cortical scintigraphy for diagnosis. *Radiology* 207:377-384, 1998. Radiological Society of North America.)

► This is an important article for its demonstration of another excellent method for the diagnosis of childhood pyelonephritis. It may not replace the accepted "gold standard" of ^{99m}Tc RCS,[1,2] but these results should stimulate additional reports to further test their validity. SPECT imaging was not used in this study, and it might make a difference.

L.W. Young, M.D.

References

1. Lavocat MP, Granjon D, Allard D, et al: Imaging of pyelonephritis. *Pediatr Radiol* 27:159-165, 1997.
2. Stokland E, Hellstrom M, Jacobsson B, et al: Evaluation of DMSA scintigraphy and urography in assessing both acute and permanent renal damage in children. *Acta Radiol* 39:447-452, 1998.

US, CT and MR Imaging Characteristics of Nephroblastomatosis

Rohrschneider WK, Weirich A, Rieden K, et al (Univ of Heidelberg, Germany; Univ of Homburg/Saar, Germany)

Pediatr Radiol 28:435-443, 1998 4–47

Background.—Nephroblastoma is an embryonal renal tumor thought to originate from renal histogenesis abnormalities. Abnormal foci consisting of persistent embryonal cells, called nephrogenic rests (NR), are considered precursor lesions. The location of NRs can be in the lobar periphery or anywhere in the renal lobe. They may occur in a unifocal, multifocal, or diffuse pattern of distribution. NRs are associated with 99% multicentric or bilateral Wilms' tumors (WTs). The presence of multiple or diffuse NR is termed nephroblastomatosis is. The imaging features of nephroblastomatosis on US, CT, and MRI were described, and the differentiation between NR and WT was discussed.

Methods.—The US, CT, and MR images of 29 patients with histopathologically confirmed nephroblastomatosis were reviewed. There were 17 kidneys with NR, 6 with WT, and 32 with both.

Findings.—The most common presentation of NR was as multinodular, peripheral, cortical lesions. The diffuse form of distribution was less common. Foci were homogeneous, with low echogenicity, density, or signal intensity. The lesions were seen most clearly on contrast-enhanced CT and T1-weighted MR images. US rarely visualized lesions smaller than 1 cm.

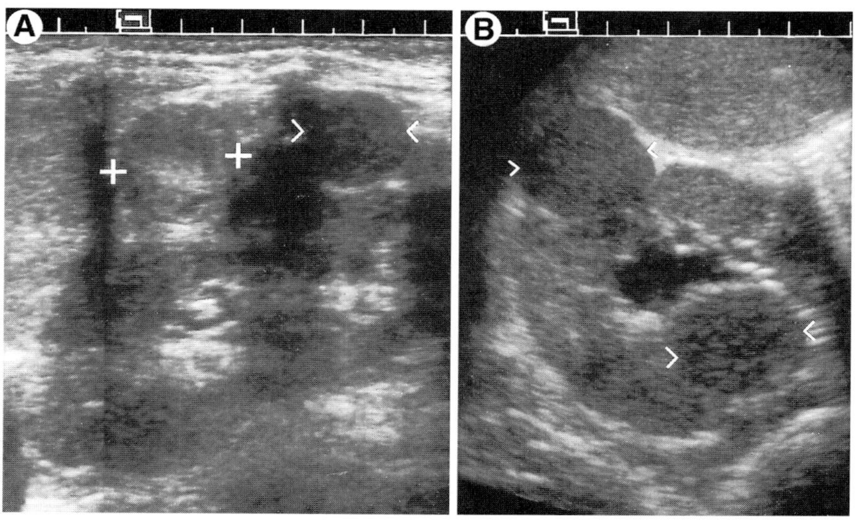

FIGURE 6.—Predominance of multifocal nephroblastomatosis with additional Wilms' tumor. Longitudinal US scan of the left kidney (**A**) and, transverse scan of the right kidney (**B**) clearly demonstrate 3 homogeneous hypoechoic nephrogenic rests (*arrowheads*). A further focus in the left kidney which is more echogenic and markedly inhomogeneous (+) proved to be a Wilms' tumor. Note that all lesions are of the same size and are spherical. (Courtesy of Rohrschneider WK, Weirich A, Rieden K, et al: US, CT and MR imaging characteristics of nephroblastomatosis. *Pediatr Radiol* 28:435-443, copyright 1998, Springer-Verlag.)

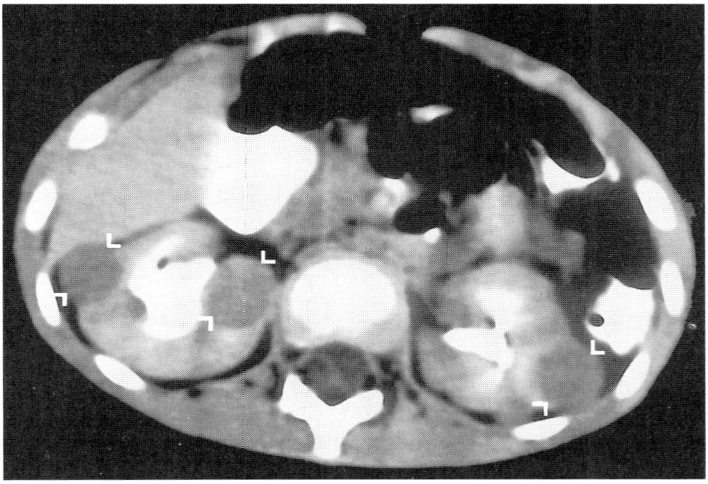

FIGURE 7.—Contrast-enhanced CT of the same patient as in Figure 6. The nephrogenic rests are homogeneously hypodense (*arrowheads*), whereas the Wilms' tumor in the left kidney (+) is of somewhat higher density with an inhomogeneous area. (Courtesy of Rohrschneider WK, Weirich A, Rieden K, et al: US, CT and MR imaging characteristics of nephroblastomatosis. *Pediatr Radiol* 28:435-443, copyright 1998, Springer-Verlag.)

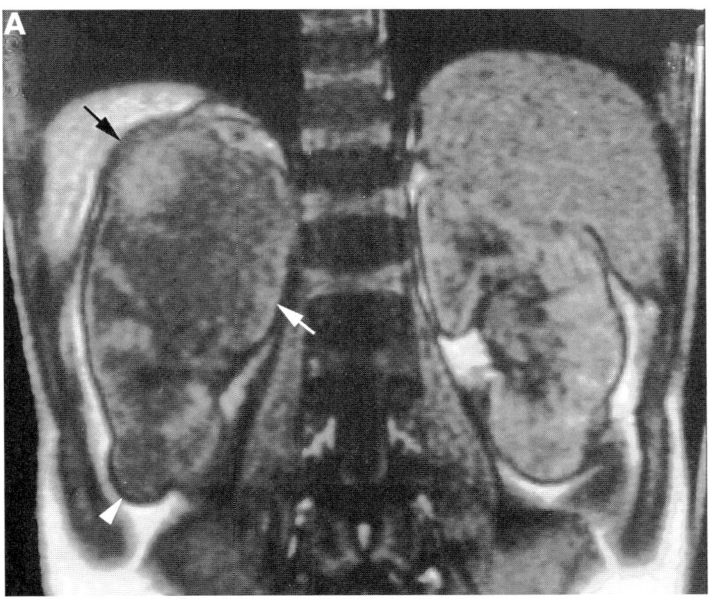

FIGURE 8.—**A**, a large Wilms' tumor with additional nephrogenic rests. **A**, T2-weighted coronal MR image shows a typical Wilms' tumor on the upper pole of the right kidney (*arrows*). A small nephrogenic rest depicted on the lower pole is homogeneously hypointense to renal cortex (*arrowhead*). This appearance compares well with the gross pathologic specimen of another patient. (Courtesy of Rohrschneider WK, Weirich A, Rieden K, et al: US, CT and MR imaging characteristics of nephroblastomatosis. *Pediatr Radiol* 28:435-443, copyright 1998, Springer-Verlag.)

Homogeneity was the most reliable criterion for differentiating NR from WT (Figs 6, 7, and 8, A).

Conclusion.—Contrast-enhanced CT and T1-weighted MR images are comparable in value and superior to US in the diagnosis of nephroblastomatosis. Because serial CT is associated with a significant dose of radiation, MRI should be the method of choice when available. The cost effectiveness and availability of US make it ideal for monitoring known lesions.

► This is an excellent demonstration of the utility of sonography and MRI for demonstration and follow-up of nephroblastomatosis—usually homogeneous in image texture, even in the presence of Wilms' tumor—usually in homogeneous in image texture. CT with contrast enhancement is of equal value to MRI for diagnosis and is superior to US, but has a disadvantage of ionizing radiation as a follow-up mode. A case with atypical sonographic imaging features of nephroblastomatosis was also recently published.[1]

L.W. Young, M.D.

Reference

1. Santiago J, Bouvier R, Pouillaude JM, et al: Unusual presentation of nephroblastomatosis. *Arch Pediatr* 5:627-632, 1998.

Simultaneous Adrenocortical Carcinoma and Ganglioneuroblastoma in a Child With Turner Syndrome and Germline p53 Mutation

Pivnick EK, Furman WL, Velagaleti GVN, et al (Univ of Tennessee, Memphis; St Jude Children's Research Hosp, Memphis, Tenn; Pediatric Cardiology, Memphis, Tenn)

J Med Genet 35:328-332, 1998 4–48

Background.—Li-Fraumeni syndrome (LFS), a rare autosomal dominant condition with incomplete penetrance, increases the patient's risk of any of a variety of tumors. This predisposition to malignant neoplasms is associated with germline mutations of the tumor suppressor gene p53. Second malignant neoplasms in children with p53 mutations have been reported previously. The current study described the synchronous occurrence of 2 embryologically different tumors in a child with Turner's syndrome and germline p53 mutation.

Case Report.—Girl, born after 35 weeks' gestation to healthy parents, was seen at 4 months of age with failure to thrive and congestive heart failure from a high-flow ventricular septal defect (VSD), an abnormal nonstenotic mitral valve, and normal blood pressure, with an irregular but not obstructive aortic isthmus. The family history included colon and prostate cancer in 3 generations on the maternal side and a benign brain tumor on the paternal side.

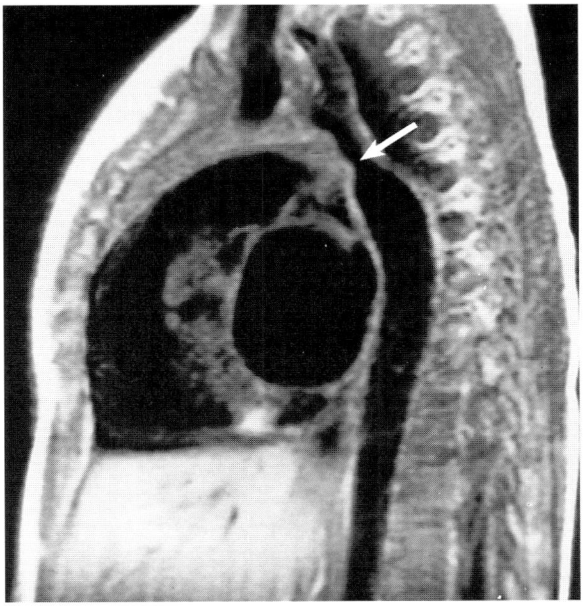

FIGURE 3.—Magnetic resonance image of the chest with *arrow* showing coarctation of the aorta. (Courtesy of Pivnick EK, Furman WL, Velagaleti GVN, et al: Simultaneous adrenocortical carcinoma and ganglioneuroblastoma in a child with Turner syndrome and germline p53 mutation. *J Med Genet* 35:328-332, 1998.)

By 18 months, the child had differential pulses and sweating on exertion, consistent with progressive coarctation and a VSD shunt. She had no history of paroxysmal sweating or flushing. However, after injection of contrast material at cardiac catheterization for mild Shone's complex and VSD, such a paroxysm did occur. This prompted investigation for hypertension excessive for contrast or coarctation. Renal US demonstrated a probable right adrenal mass. Chest and abdominal CT and MRI showed a right pulmonary nodule and a right adrenal mass (Figs 3, 4, and 5). Findings on CT scans of the head, neck, and pelvis as well as a bone scan were normal. Laparotomy followed by thoracotomy resulted in complete tumor resection. Two histologically distinct right adrenal tumors—an adrenocortical carcinoma and a ganglioneuroblastoma—were found; the former metastasizing to the lung.

Conclusions.—This child had 2 constitutional genetic abnormalities—Turner's syndrome and a germline mutation of the p53 gene. She also had 2 simultaneous but different tumors—a localized ganglioneuroblastoma and a metastatic nonfunctioning adrenocortical carcinoma. The effect that

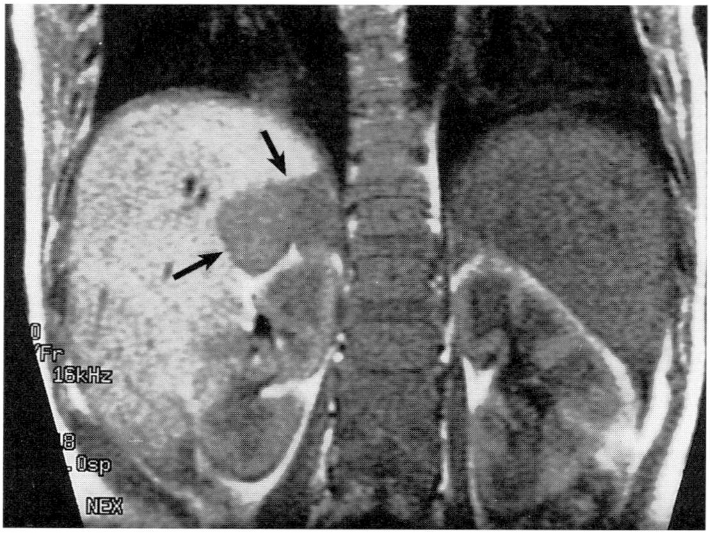

FIGURE 4.—Selected MRI of the abdomen with *arrows* showing two well-defined, low-density masses in the right suprarenal region. The larger was approximately 1.8 cm in maximum diameter and had no internal calcifications. The second measured approximately 1.5 cm and had flecks of calcium within it. (Courtesy of Pivnick EK, Furman WL, Velagaleti GVN, et al: Simultaneous adrenocortical carcinoma and ganglioneuroblastoma in a child with Turner syndrome and germline p53 mutation. *J Med Genet* 35:328-332, 1998.)

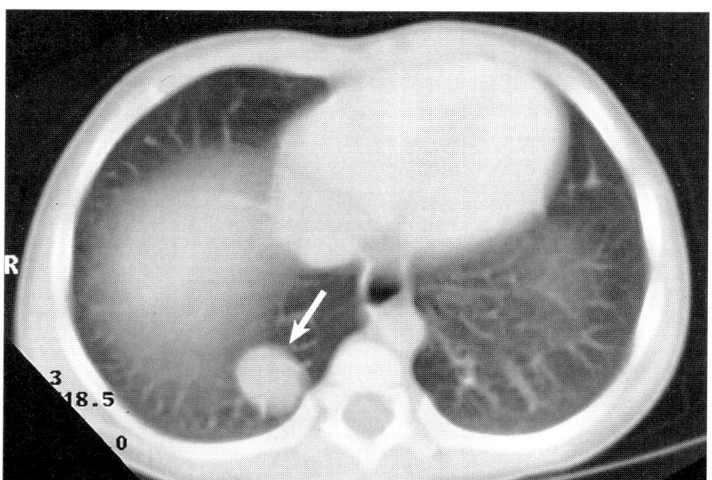

FIGURE 5.—Selected CT image of the chest with *arrow* showing a well-defined, round intermediate density in the right lower lobe measuring approximately 2 cm in diameter. (Courtesy of Pivnick EK, Furman WL, Velagaleti GVN, et al: Simultaneous adrenocortical carcinoma and ganglioneuroblastoma in a child with Turner syndrome and germline p53 mutation. *J Med Genet* 35:328-332, 1998.)

the 45,X chromosomal complement may have on the expression of neoplasms in patients with p53 germline mutations remains to be determined.

▶ This article is included to bring attention to concurrent tumors and second malignant neoplasms that, by their mass effect, are demonstrable with diagnostic imaging. Thus, the dominantly inherited neoplasms of Li-Fraumeni syndrome,[1-3] associated with germline mutation of the tumor suppressor gene p53, are a part of the articles revealing discussion. The case presented is that of a child with Turner's syndrome who was afflicted with simultaneous adrenocortical carcinoma and ganglioneuroblastoma. The article's imaging figures are excellent. Another child afflicted with the same two neoplasms was recently reported.[4]

L.W. Young, M.D.

References

1. Frebourg T, Barbier N, Yan YX, et al: Germ-line p53 mutations in 15 families with Li-Fraumeni syndrome. *Am J Hum Genet* 56:308-315, 1995.
2. Wagner J, Portwine C, Rabin K, et al: High frequency of germline p53 mutations in childhood adrenocortical cancer. *J Natl Cancer Inst* 26:1707-1710, 1994.
3. Grayson GH, Moore S, Schneider BG, et al: Novel germline mutation of the p53 tumor suppressor gene in a child with incidentally discovered adrenal cortical carcinoma. *Am J Pediatr Hematol Oncol* 26:341-347, 1994.
4. Smets A, Mortele K, De Wever N, et al: Coexistence of an adrenocortical carcinoma with an abdominal ganglioneuroma in a child. *Pediatr Radiol* 28:329-331, 1998.

5 Economics, Education, and Quality

Introduction

This section of the YEAR BOOK OF DIAGNOSTIC RADIOLOGY concentrates on subjects that do not fit neatly into the organ system orientation of the publication. Instead, it is highly reflective of what's going on in the minds of radiology leaders and related to administrative activities of both academic and private practice departments. This year's top areas of interest address the following questions. How will radiology "weather" the next millennium? Will digital radiology, particularly "filmless" radiology, actually prove successful, both from the standpoint of patient care delivery and that of cost-effectiveness? What will be the role of research training in our residency programs, and how should radiology respond to the need for an increased involvement by radiologists in the development and execution of appropriate, meaningful clinical trials? Are we really correct in our estimate of future needs for diagnostic radiologists? Are we training too many? Too few? Turf. How does organized radiology deal with constant invasion by other specialists of territory we fervently believe is ours? What important trends in radiologic practice are occurring as a result of the ever-changing health care scene, and how can we adapt to be successful?

Three articles in this section (Abstracts 5–1 through 5–3) deal primarily with the future of radiology in the next millennium. Both the American College of Radiology and the Society of Chairmen of Academic Radiology Departments have tried to maintain a weather eye on the job market for diagnostic radiologists. In general, both groups have done a good job of letting medical students know that the future outlook for jobs is very positive. The time is past when medical students were so concerned about jobs in radiology that applications to diagnostic radiology residency programs were decreasing. Attracting the best and brightest students into radiology is a goal that cannot be compromised if we are to maintain the quality of radiologists needed to function in this highly technical, rapidly changing field.

Radiologists are being asked, in academic departments as well as in private practice groups, to increase the number of studies performed per year. This demand is directly related to decreased reimbursement per study by all payers. Anything that could increase efficiency of operations is now being evaluated, from the impact of PACS and teleradiology to the use of computer-based speech recognition systems. Although the trend toward heavier workloads is apparent and the need to become more efficient is obvious, the time will inevitably come when no futher gains can be achieved. When that occurs, either radiologists will accept lower compensation or patient care will suffer. If third-party payers (particularly Medicare because it sets the trend) continue to decrease what they are willing to pay per study, the appointed time is not far off!

Turf continues to be a major issue for all radiologists. From US in the emergency department to interventional vascular procedures in a hospital setting, other specialists see our procedures as a method to help allay their decreased funding. David Levin has been an outspoken leader in showing radiologists how to counter these intrusions. However, every institution, every city, every state is unique in some aspects, and therefore generalizations are difficult to make. Unfortunately, there seems to be no respite in sight.

In spite of the challenges that radiology is currently experiencing—decreased reimbursement, turf issues, and many others—our field continues to experience major advances. Thrall (Abstract 5–1), Rothenberg, et al., (Abstract 5–2), and Holden (Abstract 5–3) provide insightful views of the future from multiple perspectives. Thrall, the chair of a major radiology department, Rothenberg, a medical physicist, and Holden, a radiology chair turned medical school dean, offer their visions from very different perspectives, but all three predict an exciting future with continued technological advances in the context of vast changes in our health care environment. At no time in the history of radiology has it been more important for radiologists to clearly establish their positions in the health care delivery system. How we can contribute the most to patient care and how we position our specialty to respond to the needs of a reengineered system of delivery and reimbursement will be extremely important to the next generation of radiologists.

Digital radiology continues to make advances in clinical practice. With the advent of direct digital capture devices, the tools necessary for the full-scaled deployment of picture archiving and communication systems are now available. It will be up to those in the field to ensure that these advances in technology benefit the health care system both by providing improved patient care and by reducing costs. It is important for radiology to demonstrate the value of improved technology in the evolution of the most cost-effective health care system. Proper management of information is a key to decreasing the cost of patient care, and radiologists, by virtue of their training and experience in dealing with massive amounts of information, are in a great position to take a leadership role in this revolution.

How to increase research activity as well as strengthen research training within our academic radiology programs, continues to plague our field. To take advantage of the increased funding by the National Institutes of Health and the growing need to participate in meaningful clinical research, we need a "call to arms" by radiology department chairs. Research by radiologists will be extremely important as we move into the next millennium to claim our position among other medical disciplines. Research by radiologists may well determine our success at guaranteeing radiology by radiologists in the future.

Manpower issues continue to be a major topic of conversation among academic breakthroughs in technology, from virtual reality applications for PET. Radiology remains an exciting, dynamic, adaptable specialty that continues to provide more accurate diagnoses and more versatile, less-invasive interventional procedures. Radiology is still the place to be!

C. Douglas Maynard, M.D.

Radiology in the Next Millennium

Directions in Radiology for the Next Millennium
Thrall JH (Harvard Med School, Boston)
AJR 171:1459-1462, 1998 5–1

Background.—Radiology will enter its second century as the new millennium begins. Directions in radiology for the next millennium were discussed in a lecture presented by James H. Thrall.

Discussion.—Three major revolutions in medical science will affect the direction of radiology in the 21st century. These revolutions are occurring in molecular biology and genetics; neurobiology and explorations of the brain, mind, and behavior; and electronics and computer technology (Fig 1). Radiology has a unique role to play in each of these trends (Fig 2). The new radiology practice paradigm for the 21st century will include filmless, electronic image acquisition and viewing; earlier, better diagnosis through

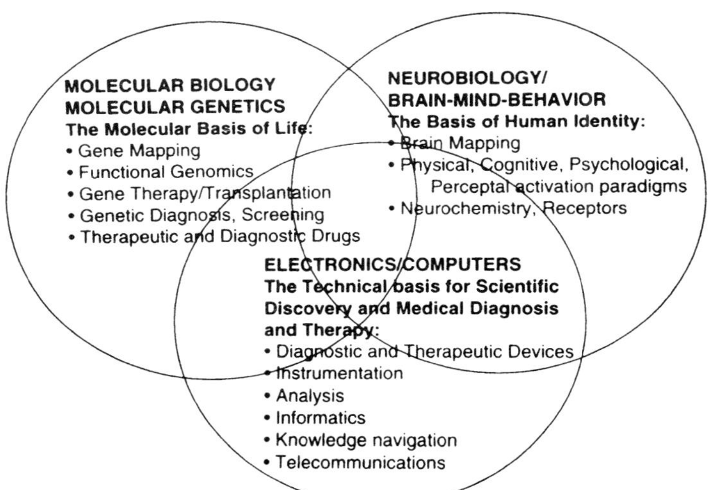

FIGURE 1.—Venn diagram shows 3 major trends or revolutions that are shaping medical science and practice for the 21st century. Note that each of these contributes to the other 2. (Courtesy of Thrall JH: Directions in radiology for the next millennium. *AJR* 171:1459-1462, 1998.)

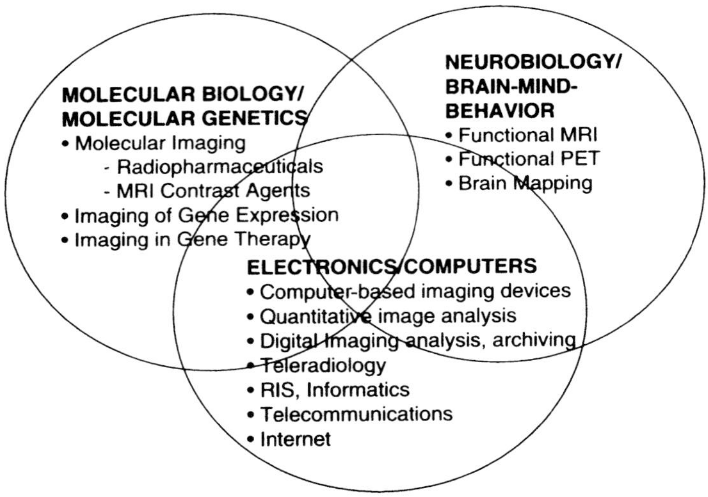

FIGURE 2.—Venn diagram shows implications for radiology of 3 overarching trends found in Fig. 1. Note that radiology has a strong role to play and will benefit significantly from all 3. *Abbreviation*: *RIS*, radiology information system. (Courtesy of Thrall JH: Directions in radiology for the next millennium. *AJR* 171:1459-1462, 1998.)

quantitative and functional imaging; and tissue-specific contrast enhancement and improved treatments through image guidance. An increasing percentage of the total medical care delivered to patients is radiologic, a trend fueled by the enhanced diagnostic value of new imaging techniques and the shift from invasive surgical methods to image-guided, minimally invasive procedures.

The leading radiology departments in the next century will be able to exploit the new opportunities offered by advances in medical sciences as well as in the science of radiology. At the same time, they will reshape their practices to address the rapidly changing expectations and needs that arise from the increasing cost and time pressures that affect the more highly developed health care systems worldwide.

► The Aubrey O. Hampton Lecture, presented at Massachusetts General Hospital gives an enlightened view of the field of radiology into the next millennium. James H. Thrall, M.D., chairman of the Department of Radiology at Massachusetts General Hospital, is one of the most thoughtful, insightful, and forward-looking individuals in our field today. His ideas concerning the emphasis on radiology that will be needed in the future are worth considering. Many will prove true.

C.D. Maynard, M.D.

A Perspective on the New Millennium

Rothenberg LN, Nath R, Price RR, et al (Mem Sloan-Kettering Cancer Ctr, New York; Yale Univ, New Haven, Conn; Vanderbilt Med Ctr, Nashville, Tenn; et al)

Radiology 209:600-603, 1998 5–2

Purpose.—The continued development of digital technology will have a major impact on the future of diagnostic imaging. Furthermore, advances in image receptor technology and image data reduction are ongoing within each modality. A report from the American Association of Physicists in Medicine outlined future developments in the various imaging modalities.

Radiography and Fluoroscopy.—Two technologies likely to have a major impact on radiography are the use of amorphous silicon detectors with a scintillator and amorphous selenium with an amorphous silicon electronic panel readout. It remains to be seen which of these technologies will prove most advantageous, but they offer new approaches to the limited dynamic range and contrast capabilities of the screen-film combination. In fluoroscopy, new interventional procedures requiring lengthy fluoroscopic times necessitate new approaches to reducing radiation dose to the patient. Flat-panel technology has the potential to meet this objective while eliminating geometric distortion and improving contrast, although the transition from image intensifiers will require a major investment. Direct digital acquisition promises to overcome many of the limitations of radiography and fluoroscopy; however, this technology is still in its infancy, with new techniques still under development.

CT and MRI.—In CT scanning, continued developments are needed in solid-state detectors, signal acquisition electronics, artifact suppression using reconstruction software, and 3-dimensional reconstruction work stations. All of these new developments must be validated in well-designed studies. Areas of ongoing research in MRI scanning include "open" magnet systems and new advancements in high-field–strength MRI, interventional and functional MRI, and contrast agents.

Nuclear Medicine and US.—Nuclear medicine has benefited from ongoing improvements in camera design, with continued rapid advances expected in the near future. These include the development of a semiconductor camera based on cadmium zinc and telluride, which should find applications in cardiac and general nuclear medicine. Many new avenues of progress have been opened in the use of US scanning, including advances in transducer array technology, harmonic imaging, and a new technique called elastography, described as a "high-tech" form of palpation.

Summary.—The new century will see continued major advances in the classic fields of diagnostic imaging. This article reviews some of the ongoing and expected developments in each field, contributed by experts in their respective disciplines.

► Physics has always been a very important partner to radiology throughout the development of our field since the discovery of the x-ray more than 100 years ago. It is imperative that radiologists follow activities of our physicist colleagues closely, as these activities are very likely to affect us in the future. This report constitutes a view into the future, as espoused by the leadership of the American Association of Physicists in Medicine. As such, it clearly presents the advances that will potentially have a profound effect on the field of radiology during the next 20 years. It is "must" reading for radiologists who wish to get a vision of what likely will change in our practice of radiology.

C.D. Maynard, M.D.

Dream No Small Dreams

Holden RW (Indiana Univ, Indianapolis)

AJR 171:547-551, 1998 5–3

Background.—Like other areas of medicine, radiology is going through a period of dramatic change. In this lecture, delivered as the Eugene W. Caldwell Lecture at the 1988 annual meeting of the American Roentgen Ray Society, Dr. Robert W. Holden urges radiologists to respond to the dramatic opportunities presented by change.

Discussion.—Ongoing changes in the health care system stem from issues related to health care reimbursement and to the physician workforce. Health care spending continues to rise, to the point where employees making minimum wage cannot afford health insurance. At the same time, society has come to view health care is a right, not a privilege. In terms of workforce, the number of specialist physicians has increased dramatically in past decades, while the number of generalists has increased much more slowly. Because of its very high physician reimbursement rate, the United States has significantly higher health care costs than other developed countries, yet infant mortality and life expectancy are poor compared with other countries. Thus, the current reimbursement system is not producing the best possible health care. The aging and expanding pluralism of American society are further confounding factors. In a country where one-fourth of Americans may soon be unable to afford health care, a national initiative is needed to promote universal care and to deal with the high cost of care.

The author believes that a focus on productivity and efficiency, similar to that followed by American business in the 1980s, is needed to produce an integrated health care system with affordable, high-quality care. The current system, with its emphasis on turf protection, is inefficient. Health care must be viewed as the global phenomenon it is. The author calls for a compatible system of primary and tertiary care providers. The current managed care system is simply taking the easy profits, and cannot succeed in the long term. Physician-led organizations are needed that can respond to the marketplace and compete in terms of service, cost, and quality. Radiologists recognize the advantages of the team approach to delivering quality service. They understand the value of technology to support change, and should take the initiative to facilitate change as soon as possible. Healthcare leaders take the lead in developing more cost-effective systems, thus avoiding a more intrusive governmental role. The necessity for change has important implications for the team approach to medicine, the promises of medical research, and medical education.

Summary.—Dr. Holden challenges medical leadership to recognize the absolute necessity for change in the health care system. Physicians are challenged to exercise the values, vision, and courage needed to follow the correct strategies to empower a successful future for the medical profession.

► The words of Robert W. Holden, M.D., chair turned dean, of the University of Indiana are definitely worthy of our attention. He brings a fresh perspective to the future of our field. This is highly recommended reading!

C.D. Maynard, M.D.

Images of the Imager: The Essential Role of Ethics in the Future of Radiology

Gunderman RB (Indiana Univ Med Ctr, Indianapolis)

Acad Radiol 6:148-155, 1999 5–4

Background.—The radiology literature has paid little attention to ethics. However, a number of ethical liabilities are associated with medical imaging. These liabilities were discussed.

Ethics in Radiology.—Because radiologists study images that are separate and exportable from the patient, they do not enter into a personal relationship with patients the way that other clinicians do. Thus, radiologists may create the impression that they regard their professional responsibility as limited to the contents of the image, with no reference to or interest in the welfare of an individual patient. In addition, radiologists make diagnoses, figuratively speaking, by analyzing their patients into their component parts and searching for abnormalities in those parts. Also separating the radiologist from the patient is the elaborate technology of image making and analysis.

An excellent radiologist would possess excellence not only in technical skill but in character. Patients and colleagues would feel comfortable approaching that radiologist with problems and leave feeling that the radiologist had done his or her best for them.

► Dr. Gunderman offers a very provocative look at our specialty. The author's clear view as to the direction our specialty should take makes this article well worth reading. It will make you think!

C.D. Maynard, M.D.

Digital Radiology

Principles of Digital Radiography With Large-area, Electronically Readable Detectors: A Review of the Basics

Chotas HG, Dobbins JT III, Ravin CE (Duke Univ Med Ctr, Durham, NC)
Radiology 210:595-599, 1999 5–5

Background.—The rapid proliferation of electronically readable x-ray detectors is bringing about dramatic changes in the practice of digital radiographic imaging. An overview of digital electronic x-ray detectors, including 2 broad classes of detectors based on thin-film transistor arrays and the older, charged-coupled device (CCD)-based designs, was presented.

Overview.—The 2 classes of electronic x-ray detectors are those that use direct methods to convert x-rays into an electric charge and those that use indirect methods (Fig 1). "Direct conversion" is not synonymous with "direct readout," a capability of all electronic detectors. Direct-conversion detectors include an x-ray photoconductor that directly converts x-ray photons into an electric charge. Amorphous selenium is an example of such a photoconductor. On the other hand, indirect-conversion detectors use a 2-step process for x-ray detection. The primary material for x-ray

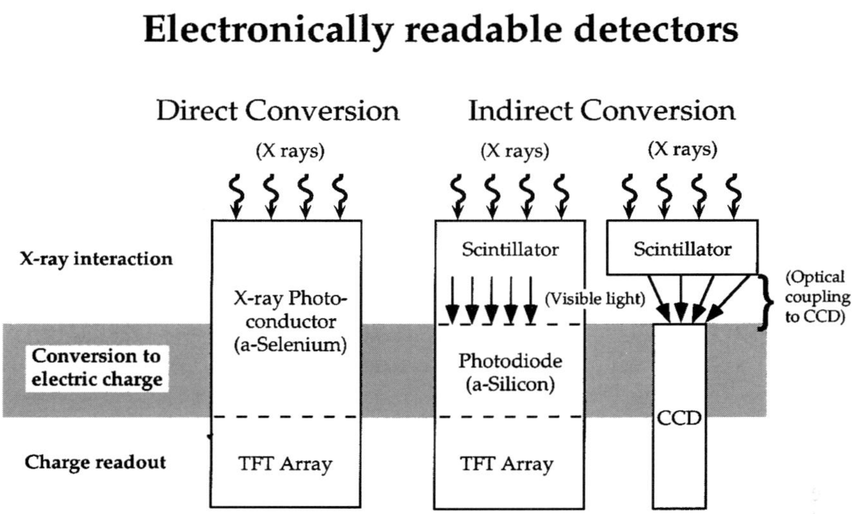

FIGURE 1.—Direct-readout electronic x-ray detectors use either a direct technique or an indirect technique for converting x-rays into an electric charge. Direct-conversion detectors have an x-ray photoconductor, such as amorphous selenium, that converts x-ray photons into an electric charge directly, with no intermediate stage. Indirect-conversion devices have a scintillator that first converts x-rays into visible light. That light is then converted into an electric charge by using an amorphous silicon photodiode array or a charged-coupled device (CCD). Thin-film transistor (TFT) arrays may be used in both direct-conversion and indirect-conversion detectors. (Courtesy of Chotas HG, Dobbins JT III, Ravin CE: Principles of digital radiography with large-area, electronically readable detectors: A review of the basics. *Radiology* 210:595-599, 1999. Radiological Society of North America.)

interaction is a scintillator. When x-rays strike the scintillator, the x-ray energy is converted into visible light. That light is then converted into an electric charge by photodetectors, such as amorphous silicon photodiode arrays or CCDs. The electric charge pattern that remains after x-ray exposure in both direct- and indirect-conversion detectors is sensed by an electronic readout mechanism. Analogue-to-digital conversion is then performed to generate the digital image.

Conclusions.—Electronically readable, large-area x-ray detectors promise rapid access to images, improved image quality, decreased patient examination time, a reduction in consumable agents, and the possibility of reduced patient exposure. However, radiologists must understand that these new self-scanning digital radiographic systems are not interchangeable and can produce images with very different image quality.

► As we progress toward a filmless radiology environment, we recognize the need for a reliable, reasonably priced direct-readout digital device capable of handling all the plain-film needs of a department. Many such devices are currently under development. This article is an excellent primer for radiologists who want to understand the basis underlying these techniques, inasmuch as they do not use the same technology. All of us need to understand the differences in the basic technology behind the various systems, as well as the advantages and limitations they offer. These systems are here to stay and are vital to the further implementation of picture archiving and communication systems.

C.D. Maynard, M.D.

Reporting Requirements for Skeletal Digital Radiography: Comparison of Soft-Copy and Hard-Copy Presentation

O'Connor PJ, Davies AG, Fowler RC, et al (Gen Infirmary at Leeds, England)

Radiology 207:249-254, 1998 5–6

Background.—The diagnostic accuracies between different computed radiography (CR) formats and reader preferences during radiography of the hand were compared.

Methods.—One hundred fifteen hands were imaged with a photostimulable-phosphor CR system. Hard-copy reports were enhanced with the algorithm that comes with the CR system; the authors created a similar algorithm to enhance the soft-copy reports. Radiographic signs of hyperparathyroidism were confirmed by 2 readers, then 4 readers graded pathologic changes and reported their image preferences on 3 different formats: a hard-copy report, a soft-copy report at resolution 1,000 × 1,000 ($1K^2$), and a soft-copy report at resolution 2,000 × 2,000 ($2K^2$). Receiver operating characteristic analysis was used to determine the diagnostic performance of each format.

Findings.—Diagnostic performance and reader preferences were significantly higher for both soft-copy formats compared with the hard-copy

TABLE 5.—Summary of Receiver Operating Characteristic Results

Formats	Critical Ratio	*P* Value
SC2K vs CRHC	4.29	<.001
SC1K vs CRHC	4.07	<.001
SC2K vs SC1K	0.221	.588

Abbreviation: CRHC, computed radiology hard copy.
(Courtesy of O'Connor PJ, Davies AG, Fowler RC, et al. Reporting requirements for skeletal digital radiography: Comparison of soft-copy and hard-copy presentation. *Radiology* 207:249-254, 1998. Radiological Society of North America.)

report (Table 5). Accuracies of the 2 soft-copy formats were similar. However, reader preference was significantly higher for the $2K^2$ images.

Conclusion.—Even at a modest resolution, soft-copy images provided a superior diagnostic performance. The $1K^2$ monitors are 5 times less expensive than the $2K^2$ monitors, yet provide similar accuracy. However, readers preferred the latter.

► As we move toward making primary interpretations from soft copy, we must gain confidence that the quality of these interpretations is comparable to those based on film. Articles of this type reassure us that we are on the right track in our quest for a filmless environment.

C.D. Maynard, M.D.

Effect of Film-based Versus Filmless Operation on the Productivity of CT Technologists

Reiner BI, Siegel EL, Hooper FJ, et al (Univ of Maryland, Baltimore; VA Maryland Health Care System, Baltimore; American Radiology Services, Baltimore, Md)
Radiology 207:481-485, 1998 5–7

Background.—Although industry-wide productivity norms have been established for film-based radiologic examinations, there are currently none for filmless operation. The relative time needed for a technologist to perform CT in a filmless compared with a film-based setting was determined.

Methods.—Time-motion studies of 204 consecutive CT assessments were done. Images from 96 examinations were transferred electronically to a picture archiving and communication system without being printed to film. One hundred eight were printed to film.

Findings.—The time needed to complete a CT examination with direct image transfer was 45% less than that needed in the film-based mode. The elimination of a number of steps in the filming process, such as the printing at multiple window or level settings, enabled this reduction.

Conclusion.—The use of a picture archiving and communication system can eliminate many time-intensive tasks for the CT technologist, thereby substantially decreasing examination time. The result will be increased productivity and greater cost effectiveness.

► This excellent article adds another dimension to the advantages of picture archiving and communication systems. As these systems become more widely deployed, savings to hospitals like the 1 described will become apparent, and the installations will be further justified.

C.D. Maynard, M.D.

Radiology Report Times: Impact of Picture Archiving and Communication Systems

Bryan S, Weatherburn G, Watkins J, et al (Brunel Univ, Uxbridge, Middlesex, England; Univ of Birmingham, England; Hammersmith Hosp, London)

AJR 170:1153-1159, 1998 5–8

Background.—Substantial resources are devoted to radiology department reporting services. The current study determined the effect on radiologist reporting time of changing from conventional film to hard-copy computerized radiography and a subsequent shift to soft-copy images on picture archiving and communication system (PACS) workstations.

Methods and Findings.—Data on 5,568 report observations were collected on a total of 4 different occasions: 2 for conventional film; 1, hard-copy computerized radiography; and 1, soft-copy PACS images. Report time in the PACS data collection period did not differ significantly from that in the computerized radiography hard-copy period. Reporting with the PACS resulted in significantly increased viewing of previously obtained images of the same patient.

Conclusions.—The introduction of the PACS apparently does not increase report time. In addition, the PACS increased viewing of historical images, which is a positive change in reporting practice.

► Opinions about whether a filmless environment slows down or speeds up the reporting process conflict considerably. In all likelihood, many more years will pass before the answer is in. Even then, results will vary from 1 department to another and even among individual radiologists. Such inconsistencies should be no surprise, as variations in reporting times are also common between departments and individual radiologists in the film environment. Factors that influence how rapidly a case is reported include file room personnel, use of film alternators, availability of comparison films, interruptions for teaching and providing consultations, and general room environment. Furthermore, some radiologists are just more efficient than others. Reporting times should not be the governing factor in acceptance of PACS; patient care should be. PACS will unquestionably improve patient care. Rapid access to images old and new, no lost studies, and availability from remote sites are only a few reasons why PACS will enhance the quality of radiologic practice.

C.D. Maynard, M.D.

Economic and Clinical Impact of Filmless Operation in a Multifacility Environment

Siegel EL (Univ of Maryland, Baltimore)
J Digit Imaging 11(suppl 2):42-47, 1998 5–9

Background.—In 1993, the Baltimore Veterans Affairs (VA) Medical Center began operating a picture archiving and communication system (PACS) for diagnostic imaging and other visual studies. Two years later, the PACS was expanded to include the multifacility VA Maryland Health Care System. The clinical and economic benefits of this move to a "virtual" radiology and nuclear medicine department were described.

Methods.—The PACS uses computed radiography to acquire the image, which is stored on a central server and routed to individual work stations on demand. Hospital and departmental records were examined before and after the institution of the filmless environment to determine the impact of the PACS on volume, costs, and other operating measures.

Findings.—With the PACS, the annual volume of reports almost doubled (from 34,000 to 60,000), yet only 1 additional radiologist was hired (from 4.5 to 5.5 attending radiologists), mainly to perform MRI and mammography. "Unread" imaging studies were virtually eliminated (from 8% pre-PACS to 0.3% in 1996), in large part because the computer can be used to identify unread reports. The image retake rate has dropped dramatically, also, by 84% (from 5% to 0.8%). Furthermore, reports that used to take an average of 24 hours to interpret, now take 2 hours. Given these advantages, 98% of clinicians say that the PACS helps them make more efficient use of their time, and they have indicated a strong preference for the PACS (92%). The main costs of the PACS are the depreciation of equipment (the PACS infrastructure cost $7.8 million dollars in 1991) and the service contract (about $5,000,000 annually). However, annual film costs are less than $10,000, and the need for film folders and chemicals has been reduced to about $15,000. Furthermore, office space that would have been taken up by film files can now be recovered for other purposes (ie, new equipment), which avoids more than $307,000/year in space costs. Finally, fewer personnel are needed with the PACS, including film room clerks, resulting in annual savings of $100,000. Overall, the costs of the PACS in the radiology and nuclear medicine departments exceed the generated savings, but only slightly. However, across the hospital, the economics of the PACS (quicker physician access to reports, fewer lost studies) greatly outweighs its costs. And the economic benefits for the VA Maryland Health Care System as a whole further support the cost effectiveness of the PACS.

Conclusion.—The future is likely to see more sharing of radiology services and digital imaging equipment, both within and among government health care organizations. These changes will certainly affect the future practice of radiology and nuclear medicine, and the efficiency and effectiveness of clinical care.

► Everyone who is interested in committing to a PACS should read this article. Eliot Siegel is a pioneer in the field and has implemented a major PACS at the Baltimore VA Medical Center. He has endured the trials and tribulations of installing one of the early true PACS, and his experience is invaluable. Even if this article does not answer all of your questions, you can always give him a call. I do!

C.D. Maynard, M.D.

Radiology Training—Emphasis on Research

Research in Radiology Residency Programs: A Survey

McGuire CW, Herberman HB (Univ of Kansas, Wichita)

Acad Radiol 5:698-700, 1998 5–10

Background.—The Accreditation Council for Graduate Medical Education (ACGME) has not set specific requirements for research by diagnostic

TABLE.—Radiology Research Survey

Survey Question	University (n = 47)	Private Practice (n = 45)	Total (n = 92)
Independent research required?			
Yes	10 (10.9)	8 (8.7)	18 (19.6)
No	37 (40.2)	37 (40.2)	74 (80.4)
Is assistance or faculty research required?			
Yes	17 (18.5)	13 (14.1)	30 (32.6)
No	30 (32.6)	32 (34.8)	62 (67.4)
Is time off allowed for research?			
Yes	4 (4.3)	2 (2.2)	6 (6.5)
No	31 (33.7)	34 (37.0)	65 (70.7)
By request	12 (13.0)	9 (9.8)	21 (22.8)
Is an elective research rotation available?			
Yes	10 (10.9)	3 (3.3)	13 (14.1)
No	37 (40.2)	41 (44.6)	78 (84.8)
By request	0 (0)	1 (1.1)	1 (1.1)
If research is required, how many publications are required?			
0	38 (41.3)	33 (35.9)	71 (77.2)
1	8 (8.7)	9 (9.8)	17 (18.5)
2	1 (1.1)	0 (0)	1 (1.1)
How many presentations are required?			
0	28 (30.4)	29 (31.5)	57 (61.9)
1	19 (20.7)	14 (15.2)	33 (35.9)
2	0 (0)	0 (0)	0 (0)
3	0 (0)	2 (2.2)	2 (2.2)

(Courtesy of McGuire CW, Herberman HB: Research in radiology residency programs: A survey. *Acad Radiol* 5:698-700, 1998.)

radiology residents. The research requirements of individual United States diagnostic radiology residency programs were assessed.

Methods.—A survey was mailed to all 203 diagnostic radiology residency programs accredited by the ACGME. The requirements and criteria for independent research, residents' support from faculty (including elective research rotations), and whether residents were allowed time off for doing research, were explored.

Findings.—Responses were received from 92 programs (45%). Independent research is required by 18 of the programs (20%) (Table), and another 30 programs (33%) require residents to participate in research projects with faculty. However, only 6 programs (7%) routinely set aside time for research in the curriculum. Furthermore, most programs do not require publications (77%) or presentations (62%); some programs accept case reports, resident conferences, and lectures as meeting the requirement for research. Only about one third of programs (62, or 67%) requires faculty to participate in residency research training, and only about one fifth of programs (21, or 23%) allow residents time off for research (by request). Finally, only 13 programs (14%) offer an elective research rotation.

Conclusion.—About half of the programs surveyed (53%) expect some type of research from diagnostic radiology residents. However, there was no consensus among programs as to what specific activities were required to meet the ACGME guidelines. A proposal has been made to the ACGME's Radiology Residence Review Committee to set specific standards for diagnostic radiology residents' participation in research projects. This survey indicates that, were the ACGME to set specific standards, most radiology programs would have to modify their training.

Radiology Residents' Research in Canada: Status of Infrastructure

Karlik SJ, Sauerbrei E (Univ of Western Ontario, London, Canada; Queen's Univ, Kingston, Ont, Canada)

Can Assoc Radiol J 49:314-319, 1998 5–11

Background.—Anecdotal evidence suggests that the extent of critical inquiry and research training available to Canadian radiology residents varies greatly depending on the program. All 16 radiology programs in that country were surveyed to assess the research infrastructure available to residents.

Methods.—A 40-item questionnaire was sent to each of the 16 radiology residency training programs in Canada. The questionnaire was designed to assess whether the school had a training program in critical inquiry, its organization, components, and support, and the type of critical inquiry or research projects.

Findings.—All but 2 of the 16 schools (88%) have a program in critical inquiry and research. However, only about half (9, or 56%) have personnel available to run the research program, and only one third (5, or 31%)

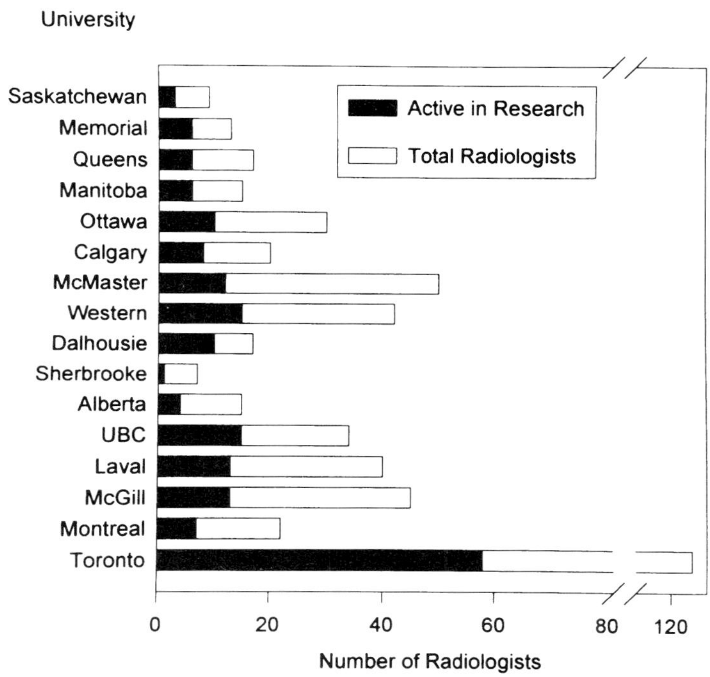

FIGURE 6.—Total number of radiologists (*entire bar*) and radiologists who participated in research (*black portion*) in Canadian radiology training programs. (Reprinted by permission of the publisher, Canadian Association of Radiologists, from Karlik SJ, Sauerbrei E: Radiology residents' reseach in Canada. Status of infrastructue. *Can Assoc Radiol J* 49: 314-319, 1998.)

allocate funds to the research program. The most commonly taught skills were ethics (81%), critical appraisal (75%), quality assurance (75%), and study design (69%). Only half of the schools (50%) taught biostatistics, and only 44% taught the assessment of diagnostic tests. The mean time allotted for teaching the research program was 18 hours per year but varied considerably depending on the school (range, 4 to 50 hours). The mean time allocated to residents for these programs ranged from 0 to 250 days (median, 1 month). Nationwide, between 14% and 46% of academic radiologists participated in research (Fig 6) (mean, 39%). Whereas all but 1 of the programs required residents to present the results of their research at an annual residents' day, only 19% required that the resident prepare a manuscript for journal submission.

Conclusion.—Critical inquiry and research training varies considerably across the different Canadian schools, but it appears that mentors and residents dedicate a substantial amount of time to these endeavors.

► It can be stated emphatically that radiology residents and fellows do not receive adequate training in research or research methodology. In a 1998 survey of directors of radiology residency programs that I conducted in preparation for a presentation to the Radiology 1998 Intersociety Summer Conference in Beaver Creek, Colorado, only 8 of 100 program directors believed their residents or fellows were adequately prepared for research careers in academic radiology. This lack of preparation does not bode well for the future of our field, because it is important for radiologists to be active participants in the advances in such areas as molecular imaging, functional MR imaging, and PET, as well as in interventional vascular procedures.

To allow physicians in other disciplines to assume the lead roles in these imaging research arenas is fraught with danger. To do so could clearly lead to the loss of these areas to other disciplines. Recognition of the inadequacy of our research training is clear in these articles, 1 from the United States and the other from Canada. It is high time for organized radiology to attack this deficiency directly though the American Board of Radiology and the Accreditation Council for Graduate Medical Education.

C.D. Maynard, M.D.

The RSNA-AUR-ARRS Introduction to Research Program for 2nd Year Radiology Residents: Effect on Career Choice and Early Academic Performance

Hillman BJ, Nash KD, Witzke DB, et al (Univ of Virginia, Charlottesville; Radiological Society of North America, Oak Brook, Ill; Univ of Kentucky, Lexington)

Radiology 209:323-326, 1998 5–12

Background.—In 1990, the Radiological Society of North America (RSNA), the Association of University Radiologists (AUR), and the American Roentgen Ray Society (ARRS) began a collaborative program called "Introduction to Research" in response to the perceived lack of quality clinician researchers in radiology. The graduates of the first 5 years of this program were evaluated to determine whether they entered and demonstrated early success in academic careers more often than did nonparticipants.

Methods and Findings.—All 396 program participants between 1990 and 1995 and 2,047 nonparticipants in the same residencies as the participants during the same period were surveyed. Eighty-one percent of program participants and 56% of nonparticipants responded to the survey. More than one third of the program participants said the program strongly affected their initial career decisions. Forty-one percent of program participants who completed training currently worked in academia, compared with 26% of nonparticipants. Thirty-five percent of the program participants who responded to the survey said they planned to spend most of their careers in academia, and 15% thought that research would be their primary focus, compared with 19% and 8%, respectively, of program nonparticipants. Academic achievement levels were higher earlier in the careers of the participants than of the nonparticipants (Table 1).

TABLE 1.—Comparison of Research Experiences and Accomplishments Between Participants in the Program and Nonparticipants

Item	Participants (n = 321)	Nonparticipants (n = 1,153)	Significance
Percentage with research time during residency	32	25	$\chi^2 = 8.10$, $df = 2$, $P = 0.17$
Mean residency research time (mo)*	3.6	2.6	$t = 3.69$, $P = .001$
Percentage with research time during fellowship	40	29	$\chi^2 = 15.05$, $df = 2$, $P = .01$
Mean fellowship research time (mo)*	2.9	3.0	$t = 0.35$, $P = .73$
Percentage with a research mentor	52	37	$\chi^2 = 24.81$, $df = 2$, $P < .001$
Mean no. of publications	3.6	2.3	$t = 4.19$, $P < .001$
Mean no. of first-authored publications	1.8	1.2	$t = 4.07$, $P < .001$
Principal investigator on grant application	16	9	$\chi^2 = 12.69$, $df = 2$, $P = .002$
Percentage who received intramural grant	13	5	$\chi^2 = 27.11$, $df = 2$, $P < .001$
Percentage who received extramural grant	11	6	$\chi^2 = 9.28$, $df = 2$, $P = .01$

*Among those having any research time.

(Courtesy of Hillman BJ, Nash KD, Witzke DB, et al: The RSNA-AUR-ARRS introduction to research program for 2nd year radiology residents: Effect on career choice and early academic performance. *Radiology* 209:323-326, 1998. Radiological Society of North America.)

Conclusion.—The "Introduction to Research" program appears to encourage the development of successful research careers. The findings may be influenced by the participants' preexisting orientation toward research.

► This special report describes an experiment undertaken by the RSNA, AUR, and the ARRS to encourage young radiology residents to consider research careers in radiology as a viable option. Although still in its early years, the program could be of future significance to our field if it can help to prepare our trainees to take advantage of recent increases in congressional funding for the National Institutes of Health. Only time will allow us to measure its success, but the joint program is certainly a step in the right direction.

C.D. Maynard, M.D.

Effect of Health Care Financing Administration Regulation on Radiology Fellowship Training

Smith JJ, Gay SB, Maurer EJ, et al (Univ of Virginia Health Sciences Ctr, Charlottesville)

Acad Radiol 6:126-131, 1999 5–13

Background.—Recent changes in the Health Care Financing Administration (HCFA) Part B reimbursement regulations for teaching hospitals require attending physicians to be present for key portions of the procedures for which they seek payment. The effects of these policies were assessed.

Methods.—Surveys were mailed to 157 fellowship program directors in body imaging and vascular/interventional radiology. Data were elicited on program accreditation status, faculty supervision of fellows, and changes in faculty supervision of fellows in response to the HCFA's revised plan for Medicare Part B reimbursement. The response rate was 51%.

Findings.—Thirty-seven percent of the respondents indicated that fellow supervision had changed after implementation of the new HCFA rules in 1996. Forty-nine percent of the vascular/interventional program directors and 17% of the body imaging program directors had changed their practice. Ninety-seven percent of the respondents who reported a change had increased supervision. Thirty-three percent of the respondents said that faculty supervision was more than necessary for patient care and house staff education. Seventy-eight percent of these respondents said that the new HCFA regulations were responsible for this change. Many program directors were concerned that the HCFA regulations may prevent fellows from getting enough experience to become independent clinical decision makers.

Conclusions.—The change in the Medicare Part B reimbursement policy may have the unintended effect of changing radiology fellow training, prompting physicians to engage in close supervision and direct decision-making to avoid difficulty in obtaining reimbursement. This may adversely affect fellows' ability to make meaningful clinical decisions in a reasonably supervised environment.

► This is an informative article about the effect of regulation by the HCFA on radiology training programs. Without a doubt, the training of radiologists is influenced by the HCFA. In recent years, the regulations have generally served to restrict the activities that can be performed by residents and fellows without supervision by the faculty. Although such restrictions seem like a good idea, and in general they probably are in the overall scheme of training a qualified radiologist, this undoubtedly is not a positive approach. At some point in their training, residents and fellows must make decisions on their own and deal with the consequences of these decisions, just as they will be expected to do after they complete the training program. A more orderly transition between trainee and practitioner is needed, and at the moment the HCFA does not allow this transition to occur. The ugly duckling may transform into a swan overnight, but radiology fellows do not gain the necessary skills to become independent radiologists on July 1 each year. I understand both the need to protect the patient from poorly trained physicians and the need to prevent the abuse of trainees by training programs; however, we need to find that middle ground that is best for everyone. We should seek this goal with the HCFA's help. After all, they pay the bill!

C.D. Maynard, M.D.

Current Status of Musculoskeletal Radiology Fellowships in the United States

De Smet AA, Resnik CS (Univ of Wisconsin, Madison; Univ of Maryland, Baltimore)

Acad Radiol 5:509-512, 1998 5–14

Background.—The Education Committee of the American Society of Musculoskeletal Radiology recently met to discuss accreditation for musculoskeletal radiology fellowships. The committee surveyed all program directors to determine the status of training and supervision during musculoskeletal fellowships.

Methods and Findings.—Forty-eight of the 50 fellowship directors returned the survey. Six of these programs had discontinued their fellowships in musculoskeletal radiology since 1994. Of the remaining 42 programs, 34 had fellowships for the 1997-1998 academic year. Twenty-five programs had 1 fellow, 8 had 2, and 1 had 4. The programs varied substantially in their fellow supervision (Table 1). Faculty members reportedly review fellows' interpretations of nearly all MRI studies. However, 15% of 41 programs reported supervision of 60% or fewer of the procedures performed by fellows, and 29% supervised 60% or fewer of the fellows' interpretations of plain radiographs. Breadth of training also varied markedly among programs. All provided experience with MRI of the extremities, and 93% trained fellows in biopsy procedures. About half of the programs trained their fellows to perform facet joint injections. Thirty-one percent of the programs did not provide training in spinal CT interpretation, and 43% did not train fellows in spinal MRI interpretation. Few programs provided training in musculoskeletal US, diskography, or epidural steroid injections.

Conclusions.—The rapid increase in the number of musculoskeletal radiology training programs in the past decade has resulted in a marked variation in the degree of supervision of the fellows and in the breadth of training. These current findings should be useful for musculoskeletal fellowship directors in the assessment of their programs.

► The establishment of fellowships in musculoskeletal radiology is an interesting phenomenon to watch. These fellowships have existed in some form for a number of years, but they are rapidly gaining stature and generating interest among diagnostic residents seeking further training. Why is that? First, musculoskeletal fellowship programs can now obtain accreditation from the Accreditation Council for Graduate Medical Education. Second, and probably more important, jobs for radiologists trained in this subspecialty are becoming more abundant outside medical schools, in large practice groups. Until recently, job opportunities for these individuals were confined mainly to institutions with diagnostic radiology training programs. Are fellowship programs in thoracic, gastrointestinal, and genitourinary radiology

TABLE 1.—Supervision of Fellows Provided by 42 Musculoskeletal Fellowship Programs

Training Area	No. of Programs with Varying Degrees of Supervision						
	0%-20% Supervised	21%-40% Supervised	41%-60% Supervised	61%-80% Supervised	81%-95% Supervised	96%-100% Supervised	Total
Skeletal radiography	6	2	4	5	6	18	41
Musculoskeletal MR imaging	0	0	0	0	5	36	41
Musculoskeletal procedures	1	1	4	3	5	27	41

Note: Of the 42 survey responses, one did not include these percentages.
(Courtesy of De Smet AA, Resnik CS: Current status of musculoskeletal radiology fellowships in the United States. *Acad Radiol* 5:509-512, 1998.)

next in line for recognition by the Accreditation Council for Graduate Medical Education? I think so!

C.D. Maynard, M.D.

Executive Summary

Ascher SM, Shtern F (US Public Health Service, Washington, DC)
Acad Radiol 6(suppl 1):S3-S7, 1999 5–15

Background.—Most previous evaluations of radiologic modalities have consisted mainly of retrospective or prospective analyses of their sensitivity and specificity. In most studies, sensitivity and specificity data have not been linked to clinical decisions, patient outcomes, or cost effectiveness. A workshop called "Methodological Issues in Diagnostic Clinical Trials: Health Services and Outcomes Research in Radiology," was held in 1998 to review state-of-the-art methodologic issues in diagnostic clinical trials, with an emphasis on breast cancer; to develop a research agenda focused on the design and modeling of clinical research for analysis of patient outcomes and cost effectiveness; and to create a document to help guide program development. Recommendations from each of the 8 workshop sessions are reported.

Summary of Sessions.—The first session, a critical review of past outcomes research in radiology, identified several limitations in past research together with several key areas needing further development for advancing and disseminating health services and outcomes research in radiology. They included methods for diagnostic randomized clinical trials, radiology-specific health status measures, and validation of intermediate outcomes and decision analysis modeling. Barriers to conducting outcomes research in medical imaging in the past were discussed in the second session, as well as ways to overcome these barriers. In the third session, on assessing the appropriateness of diagnostic tests, a research agenda was developed, with the recognition that appropriateness criteria are used for a variety of purposes. The fourth session focused on intermediate outcomes, which are critical for rapidly and efficiently assessing new technologies. Traditional health outcomes in the evaluation of diagnostic tests were discussed in the fifth session, and health profiles and quality of life were discussed in the sixth. In session 7, on measuring and incorporating patient preferences and utilities in the assessment of diagnostic technology, reasearch areas were proposed. In the final session, estimating costs and cost effectiveness for diagnostic technologies were discussed.

Conclusion.—By the end of the conference, 6 needs essential to the advancement of diagnostic radiologic clinical trials emerged. These included (1) a multidisciplinary approach to health services and outcomes research; (2) intermediate outcomes to facilitate assessment and implementation of new imaging technologies; (3) a new generation of models to facilitate research synthesis studies, attend to preferences, optimize or alter traditional randomized clinical trial design, and assess appropriateness; (4)

measures of quality of life and preferences to determine the therapeutic value of diagnostic radiologic tests; (5) improved shared clinical databases and a common lexicon that are easy to access; and (6) better education in fundamental methods early in postgraduate radiology training programs.

► This article is excellent for those interested in a detailed synopsis of the current issues associated with clinical trials in diagnostic radiology. It derives from the background material that was provided to those attending a workshop titled "Methodological Issues in Diagnostic Clinical Trials: Health Services and Outcomes Research in Radiology," sponsored jointly by the United States Public Health Service's Office on Women's Health, the National Cancer Institute, and the American College of Radiology's Commission on Research and Technology Assessment, and held in Washington, D.C. in 1998. Because measurement of outcomes is so important in managed care, radiologists must become conversant with this topic.

C.D. Maynard, M.D.

Manpower Issues

Initial Employment Experience of 1996 Graduates of Diagnostic Radiology and Radiation Oncology Training Programs

Lalman D, Porter S, Sunshine JH, et al (Univ of Maryland, College Park; American College of Radiology, Reston, Va; Rhode Island Hosp, Providence; et al)

AJR 171:301-310, 1998 5–16

Background.—The American College of Radiology (ACR) surveyed 1996 graduates in diagnostic radiology and radiation oncology about their employment situations and analyzed factors that influenced outcomes.

Methods.—All summer 1996 graduates of diagnostic radiology or radiation oncology training programs were sent a survey; 69% responded by mid-January 1997. The survey asked about employment shortly after graduation and at the time of the survey and factors associated with their employment situation (such as geographic constraints, etc.).

Findings.—Shortly after graduation, 3% to 7% of diagnostic radiology graduates and 10% of oncology residents were working as a locum tenens, working outside their field, or unemployed (Table 2). However, by the time of the survey, 2% or less of respondents were doing so. Half the respondents not working were women (11 of 21), although only 27% of respondents were women. Graduates who needed to find a job in the same locality as their spouse typically had poorer job outcomes, as did graduates who reported that a major aspect of their training was inadequate. Median starting salaries in 1996 were the same as in 1995 for oncology residents but significantly lower for diagnostic residents and fellows.

Conclusion.—Less than 1% of these graduates are working outside their field. However, the poorer employment outcomes for women are worrisome, and it appears that salaries are not keeping up with inflation.

TABLE 2.—Employment Outcomes for Graduates

Employment Outcomes	Type of Graduate: Diagnostic Radiology Resident*	Diagnostic Radiology Fellow†	Radiation Oncology Resident‡	Radiation Oncology Fellow§
Difficulties after graduation				
Spent time as locum tenens, working outside radiology or radiation oncology, or unemployed	3%	7%	10%	2 of 9
Worked as locum tenens	2%	4%	5%	1 of 9
Average weeks working as locum tenens	10	11	9	4
Actually unemployed	2%	5%	9%	1 of 9
Average weeks unemployed	12	10	13	20
Status 3.5-6.5 months after graduation				
Fellowship	74%	1%	14%	0
Academic position	2%	28%	24%	5 of 9
Private radiology or radiation oncology group	14%	57%	52%	3 of 9
Other radiology or radiation oncology (multispecialty group, government, etc.)	8%	11%	7%	0
Working outside radiology or radiation oncology	<0.5%	<0.5%	1%	0
Not working at all	1%	2%	2%	1 of 9
Deliberately	0.1%	0.6%	0.7%	0 of 1
Involuntarily unemployed	0.7%	1.7%	1.3%	1 of 1
General view of employment				
Reasonably matches training and job goals	88%	80%	88%	8 of 8
"Holding-pattern" employment while seeking something better or more permanent	36%	24%	24%	0 of 7

Note: Numbers of respondents and entire study exclude persons who did not complete the training program in the summer of 1996. Details may not add to totals because of rouding.

*689 respondents.

†549 respondents.

‡101 respondents.

§9 respondents.

(Courtesy of Lalman D, Porter S, Sunshine JH, et al: Initial employment experience of 1996 graduates of diagnostic radiology and radiation oncology training programs. *AJR* 171:301-310, 1998.)

The Situation of Diagnostic Radiology Training Programs and Their Graduates in 1997

Crewson PE, Sunshine JH, Schepps B (American College of Radiology, Reston, Va; Brown Univ, Providence; Rhode Island)

AJR 171:919-922, 1998 5–17

Background.—The American College of Radiology surveyed diagnostic radiology residency directors regarding the employment situations of their 1997 graduates and about their programs.

Methods.—Directors of 111 of the 221 United States diagnostic radiology residency programs answered a survey regarding the number of 1997 graduates who had a committed position upon graduation and the types of position. The directors also answered questions about their perception of the employment outlook, any plans for changes in program size, and how many training positions were filled.

Findings.—Within 6 months of graduation, diagnostic radiology residents and fellows who wanted to be employed, were employed. The directors believed most of the graduates (95%) were in positions that

TABLE 2.—Program Directors' Perceptions of the Job Market and Plans for Changing Program Size

Perceptions or Plan	Residency Programs			Fellowship Programs		
	1995	1996	1997	1995	1996	1997
Difficulty of finding jobs compared with recent years*						
Much easier (%)	1	0	2	0	2	4
Somewhat easier (%)	0	5	10	0	2	14
About the same (%)	24	36	50	9	31	31
Somewhat more difficult (%)	35	32	29	39	37	36
Much more difficult (%)	27	20	9	37	21	15
Most difficult in many years (%)	14	7	0	16	6	0
Expecting change in size of program (%)	29	48	47†	44	54	33‡
Changing size of program§						
Old size			7.4			11.3
New size			5.9‖			8.3‖

*Percentage of responses weighted by size of program.
†No statistical significance of difference between 1996 and 1997; 2-tailed probabilities, $P > 0.05$.
‡Statistical significance of difference between 1996 and 1997; 2-tailed probabilities, $P \leq$ to 0.05.
§Average total number of positions in incoming class.
‖Statistical significance of difference between old size and new size; 2-tailed probabilities, $P \leq$ to 0.05.
(Courtesy of Crewson PE, Sunshine JH, Schepps B: The situation of diagnostic radiology training programs and their graduates in 1997. *AJR* 171:919-922, 1998.)

matched their training and personal employment goals. Directors were more optimistic than in past years about the difficulty graduates have in finding jobs (Table 2). Overall, the average program size is changing from 7.4 to 5.9 for residency positions and from 11.3 to 8.3 for fellowship positions. By mid-May 1997, 93% of slots for first-year residents were filled.

Conclusion.—Unemployment rates for 1997 graduates were low and directors' optimism about outlooks was high. Changes in program size will result in about a 13% reduction in the number of graduates each year.

► The job market for diagnostic radiology residents remains very good. The ACR has taken on the task of surveying graduates and training program directors to monitor the job market. The ACR has done an excellent job. Clearly the "scare" that affected the field 2 or 3 years ago, when many believed that the job market had been saturated, has proven to be unfounded. With the downsizing of some training programs and the failure of other programs to fill, we could actually experience a shortage of qualified diagnostic radiologists in early 2000!

C.D. Maynard, M.D.

Hiring of Diagnostic Radiologists in 1997

Elliott SD, Sunshine JH, Busheé GR, et al (Elliott Research, Vienna, Va; American College of Radiology, Reston, Va; Brown Univ, Providence, RI; et al)

AJR 172:885-892, 1999 5–18

Background.—The American College of Radiology (ACR) has been monitoring employment opportunities for diagnostic radiologists and radiation oncologists since 1991. The results of the fifth survey, conducted in the fall of 1997, were reported.

Methods.—The survey was mailed to a stratified, random sample of 589 physician groups. The response rate was 76%. Responses were weighted to represent all practices in the United States with more than one radiologist.

Findings.—In the year preceding the survey, groups sought to hire 1,909 diagnostic radiologists. Almost half of these jobs were new positions. Groups did not seek to replace 366 diagnostic radiologists who had left the practice in the preceding year. Groups successfully hired 1,488 diagnostic radiologists. In general, the percentage of available positions successfully filled did not differ among subspecialty fields. A greater perceived effect of managed care on a group was associated with fewer expansion positions and a lower likelihood that positions were offered on a partnership-track basis. Otherwise, this perceived effect was not related to hiring activity. Eighty-one percent of the positions available were in groups that preferred recently trained radiologists to those with 10 to 20 years of experience. Twenty-eight percent of the full-time positions in private nonacademic groups were not partnership track (Figs 1 and 2; Tables 1 and 2).

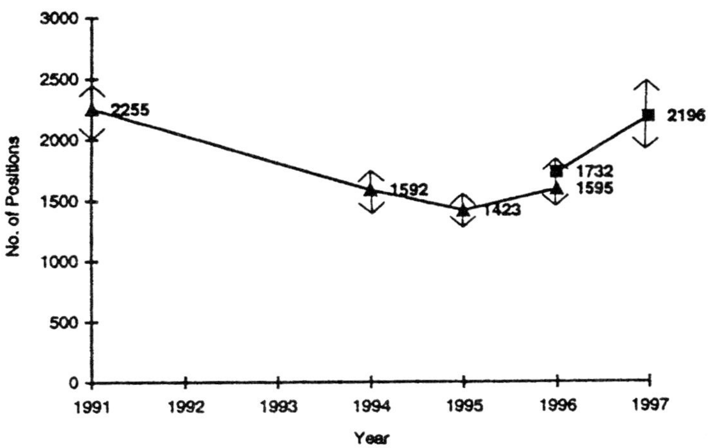

FIGURE 1.—Graph shows number of diagnostic radiology and radiation oncology positions that groups sought to fill in 1991 and 1994-1996 on year-to-date basis (*triangle*) and in 1996 and 1997 for 12 months preceding survey date (*square*). *Error bars* represent standard error of estimation. (Courtesy of Elliott SD, Sunshine JH, Bushee GR, et al: Hiring of diagnostic radiologists in 1997. *AJR* 172:885-892, 1999.)

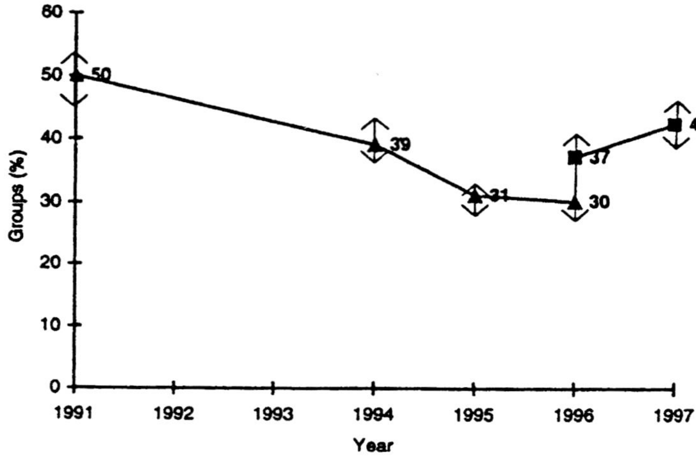

FIGURE 2.—Graph shows percentage of groups that were actively recruiting diagnostic radiologists or radiation oncologists in 1991 and 1994-1996 on year-to-date basis (*triangle*) and in 1996 and 1997 on 12-month basis (*square*). *Error bars* represent standard error of estimation. (Courtesy of Elliott SD, Sunshine JH, Busheé GR, et al: Hiring of diagnostic radiologists in 1997. *AJR* 172:885-892, 1999.)

TABLE 1.—Recruitment of Diagnostic Radiologists in the Most Recent 12 Months

Recruitment Variable	No. of Positions (±SE)	% of Total Openings
All openings	1909 ± 111	100
Hired	1488 ± 92	78
Departures with no replacement	366 ± 57	NA
Openings for fellowship-trained	1458 ± 96	76
Expansion positions	888 ± 77	47
Replacement positions for those who left radiology	648 ± 67	34
Replacements for those who moved	373 ± 49	20
Hired with fellowship training	1211 ± 80	63
Interviews conducted	6041 ± 447	NA
Offers made	2007 ± 137	NA
Recruitment Ratios	Ratio Values	
Interviews to openings	3.2	
Interviews to hires	4.1	
Offers to openings	1.1	
Offers to hires	1.3	
Effect of Managed Care on Group	% of Groups Reporting This Effect (±SE)	
None	3 ± 1	
A little	33 ± 3	
Moderate	37 ± 3	
Significant	19 ± 2	
Great	8 ± 2	

Note: Data are weighted to reflect the answers that would have been given had all of the approximately 3,286 radiology groups in the United States responded to the survey.

Abbreviations: NA, not applicable; *SE*, standard error of the mean.

TABLE 2. Groups Actively Recruiting in the Most Recent 12 Months

Group Characteristic	%
All groups	44
Group type*	
Academic	77
Private multispecialty	36
Government	54
Private radiology or radiation oncology	44
Group size*	
Two radiologists	22
Three or four radiologists	31
Five to seven radiologists	42
Eight to 10 radiologists	57
Eleven or more radiologists	76
Urbanization of location*	
Main city, area pop. > 1 million	62
Suburbs, area pop. > 1 million	64
Main city, area pop. 100,000-1 million	54
Suburbs, area pop. 100,000-1 million	24
Area pop. < 100,000	38
Geographic region	
Northeast	34
Midwest	52
South	45
West	47
Employed part-time radiologists	
No	40
Yes	49
Employed locum tenens radiologists	
No	40
Yes	53
Effect of managed care on group	
None	32
A little	46
Moderate	42
Significant	43
Great	51

Note: Data are weighted to reflect the answers that would have been given had all of the approximately 3,286 radiology groups in the United States responded to the survey.
Abbreviation: pop, population.
*The percentage differences for this characteristic had at least one significant, pairwise difference.
(Courtesy of Elliott SD, Sunshine JH, Busheé GR, et al: Hiring of diagnostic radiologists in 1997. *AJR* 172:885-892, 1999.)

Conclusions.—The decline in hiring that was observed between 1991 and 1995 has been reversed. In 1997, for the first time in recent years, the number of positions available exceeded the number of radiologists to fill them. The excess was about 278.

► As many of us suspected, the fear that there were going to be too many radiologists was not well founded. Ironically, we may now be faced with a more serious problem: too few radiologists. On a positive note, however, the number of unfilled positions in diagnostic radiology residency programs was lower at the end of the 1999 match than in the previous 2 years. We can hope that this development indicates a sea change and that medical students no longer perceive the opportunities in our field to be limited.

C.D. Maynard, M.D.

Employment in Radiology Is Even Higher in 1998

Dunnick NR (Univ of Michigan, Ann Arbor)

Acad Radiol 5:868-869, 1998 5–19

Background.—Employment opportunities markedly affect medical students' choice of a career in radiology. A job survey of graduating residents and fellows in 1996, 1997, and 1998, conducted by the Society of Chairmen of Academic Radiology Departments (SCARDs), was reported.

Methods and Results.—Surveys were sent to 135 active SCARD members. The response rate was 75%. The absolute numbers and percentages of residents and fellows who had and had not found jobs were tabulated (Table 2). In 1998, most radiology residents who graduated continued their training as fellows. About 20% went into the military or accepted a permanent job. Most graduating residents who did not have a job had not looked for personal reasons. When these residents were excluded from the analysis, only 0.3% had no position at the completion of their residency.

Conclusion.—Employment for fellows completing their training in 1998 was even higher than for those finishing in 1997 and 1996. Very few fellows did not have jobs after finishing training.

► SCARD should be complimented for addressing this issue in a timely fashion. The job market has such a strong effect on the recruitment of medical students into our field that we rely on accurate data, concerning the

TABLE 2.—Society of Chairmen of Academic Radiology Departments Survey of Fellowship Graduates

Question	1996	1997	1998
How many fellows do you have who are finishing this academic year?	535 (100)	507 (100)	567 (100)
How many of them have found jobs?			
Academic	141 (26.4)	143 (28.2)	148 (26.1)
Private	351 (65.6)	338 (66.7)	378 (66.7)
Military	12 (2.2)	11 (2.2)	6 (1.1)
Residency/fellowship	6 (1.1)	0 (0)	24 (4.2)
Total	510 (95.3)	492 (97.0)	556 (98.1)
If they do not have jobs, why not?			
Did not look	6 (1.1)	5 (1.0)	3 (0.5)
Nothing in right geographic area	6 (1.1)	2 (0.4)	2 (0.4)
Nothing in same area as spouse requirement	3 (0.6)	4 (0.8)	2 (0.4)
Nothing in area of specialty training	2 (0.4)	0 (0)	0 (0)
Dissatisfied with terms of contract	5 (0.9)	1 (0.2)	1 (0.2)
No job offers at all	3 (0.6)	1 (0.2)	0 (0)
Other	0 (0)	2 (0.4)	3 (0.5)
Total	25 (4.7)	15 (3.0)	11 (1.9)

Note: Numbers in parentheses are percentages.

(Courtesy of Dunnick NR: Employment in radiology is even higher in 1998. *Acad Radiol* 5:868-869, 1998.)

success of residents and fellows in obtaining desirable jobs each year, to continue to attract highly qualified trainees into our programs. Although the American College of Radiology also plays a major role in tracking the availability of jobs in radiology, their data may be a year or 2 behind the data available to radiology department chairs. In a volatile job market, the more current the data, the more valuable the information.

C.D. Maynard, M.D.

Practice

U.S. Radiologists' Workload in 1995-1996 and Trends Since 1991-1992

Sunshine JH, Busheé GR, Mallick R (American College of Radiology, Reston, Va; PraCon, Reston, Va)

Radiology 208:19-24, 1998 5–20

Background.—What is a diagnostic radiologist's typical workload? This study answered this question based on surveys of the American College of Radiology in 1995-1996, with a comparison to 1991-1992 data.

Methods.—In 1996, 608 United States diagnostic radiology groups completed questionnaires regarding workload and the procedures performed for Medicare patients (who represent about one third of the total workload of United States physicians). Responses were weighted to project what the responses would be if all 3,286 United States radiology groups had responded. Also, weights were multiplied by the number of radiologists in each group so that data reflected the radiologist, not the group.

Findings.—The average workload per full-time equivalent diagnostic radiologist increased by 5% between 1991 and 1992 (11,100 ± 200 procedures) and 1995 and 1996 (11,600 ± 200 procedures) (Table 1). Workloads increased significantly in practices with 2 to 4 radiologists (by 20%), in hospital-based practices (by 18%), and in nonacademic radiology-only private groups (by 8%). In 1995-1996, the number of procedures ranged from 10,300 ± 300 in groups with 11 or more radiologists, to 13,200 ± 500 in groups of 4 or less.

Conclusion.—Workloads varied considerably, and these data should not be taken to represent what workload is "right." What they do indicate is that radiologists are working harder despite the concerns that there is a surplus of radiologists.

► Not surprisingly, the workload for radiologists is increasing. Any radiologist you ask would probably substantiate that fact! As price per unit declines in response to pressures from HMOs, commercial insurers, and Medicare, radiologists are inclined to increase their productivity as the only way to maintain incomes. In nonacademic radiology practices, this means working harder or giving up free time. In the academic world, it means working harder and it also results in less time for teaching and research. Somewhere along the way, however, quality in each of these areas will decline, and

TABLE 1.—Annual Workload Per Full-Time Equivalent Radiologist: 1995-1996 and 1991-1992

	1995-1996					
		Percentile				
Group Characteristic	Mean*	25th	50th	75th	1991-1992 Mean*	Difference Between 1995-1996 and 1991-1992 Means
	Diagnostic-only Groups (n = 457)†					
All groups	11.6 (0.2)	9.2	11.6	14.7	11.1 (0.2)	0.5
No. of radiologists in group						
Two to four	13.2 (0.5)	9.6	12.9	16.0	11.2 (0.5)	2.0‡
Five to seven	12.6 (0.4)	9.4	11.5	14.4	12.0 (0.4)	0.6
Eight to 10	11.7 (0.5)	9.4	11.5	14.4	11.8 (0.7)	−0.1
11 or more	10.3 (0.3)	8.5	10.8	13.3	10.0 (0.4)	0.3
Practice type						
Primarily academic	8.0 (0.8)	6.2	7.8	9.7	7.8 (0.6)	0.2
Nonacademic multispecialty	10.6 (0.8)	8.6	11.0	13.8	11.8 (0.7)	−1.2
Nonacademic private, radiology only	12.3 (0.2)	9.9	12.0	15.0	11.5 (0.3)	0.8§
Practice location						
Hospital	12.9 (0.4)	10.0	12.5	15.0	11.1 (0.3)	1.8‡
Office or imaging center	9.6 (0.9)	7.8	10.0	11.2	7.4 (0.9)	2.2
Region‖						
Midwest	13.5 (0.5)	11.7	13.3	15.9	13.4 (1.1)	0.1
Northeast	10.9 (0.5)	8.9	11.0	13.1	11.6 (0.4)	−0.7
South	13.4 (0.5)	10.3	13.2	16.0	12.8 (0.7)	0.7
West	10.8 (0.5)	8.3	10.5	14.4	10.9 (0.5)	−0.1
	Oncology-only Groups (n = 52)					
No. of new patients	209 (9)	183	211	250	188 (11)	21

*Number in parentheses is the standard error.
†Data are thousands of procedures.
‡Difference between 1995-1996 data and 1991-1992 data was significant ($P < 0.01$).
§Difference between 1995-1996 data and 1991-1992 data was significant ($P < 0.05$).
‖Data are for private, nonacademic, nonmultispecialty groups with both hospital and office or imaging center activity.
(Courtesy of Sunshine JH, Busheé GR, Mallick R. U.S. radiologists' workload in 1995-1996 and trends since 1991-1992. *Radiology* 208:19-24, 1998. Radiological Society of North America.)

additional radiologists must be hired. The result will be lower pay but more jobs.

C.D. Maynard, M.D.

Trends in the Use of Radiology With Inpatients: What Has Changed in a Decade?

Khorasani R, Goel PK, Ma'luf NM, et al (Harvard Med School, Boston)
AJR 170:859-861, 1998 5–21

Background.—Have the new imaging technologies made an impact on the diagnostic workup of inpatients? These authors examined 10 years of data at their institution regarding the utilization of both new and conventional radiologic methods to address this question.

Methods.—Retrospective analysis of the billing database of Brigham and Women's Hospital between 1984 and 1993 identified all inpatients for whom radiologic studies were performed. The studies of interest included plain films, fluoroscopy, CT, MRI, US, and nuclear medicine. Because disease severity varied, the number of annual admissions was multiplied by the average case mix severity index of admissions in that year (i.e., case mix–adjusted admissions [CMAs]). Changes in the radiology workload were estimated based on relative value units.

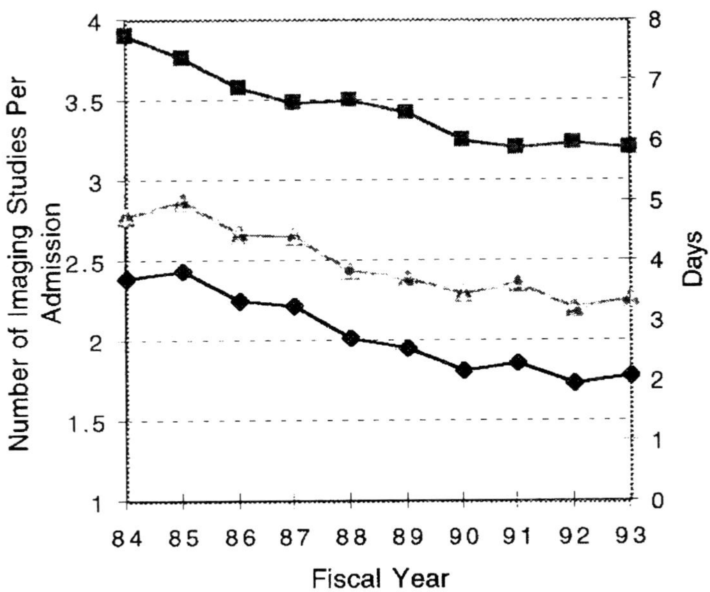

FIGURE 2.—Graph shows average length of stay (*squares*), number of imaging studies (*triangles*), and number of conventional studies per admission (*diamonds*), adjusted for severity of disease, per year. Note significant decrease in all categories over time. (Courtesy of Khorasani R, Goel PK, Ma'luf NM, et al: Trends in the use of radiology with inpatients: What has changed in a decade? *AJR* 170:859-861, 1998.)

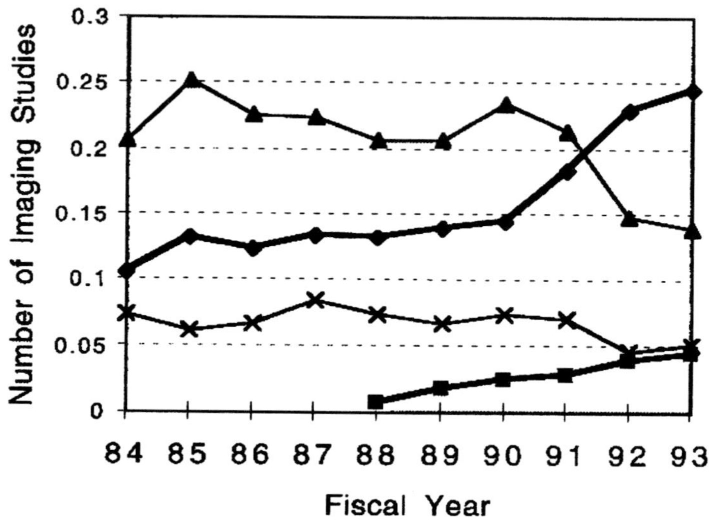

FIGURE 4.—Graph shows number of studies per admission per year for each imaging technique adjusted for severity of disease. Note significant increase in CT (*diamonds*) and MR imaging studies (*squares*), decrease in sonography (*triangles*), and lack of change for nuclear medicine studies (*crosses*). (Courtesy of Khorasani R, Goel PK, Ma'luf NM, et al: Trends in the use of radiology with inpatients: What has changed in a decade? *AJR* 170:859-861, 1998.)

Findings.—Over the study period, the number of imaging studies per CMA decreased significantly (Fig 2), mainly because of significant decreases in the utilization of conventional studies and sonograms (Fig 4). The utilization of CT and MRI studies increased, however, by 200% and 600%, respectively. In the latter half of the study period, global, professional, and technical relative value units per CMA increased significantly.

Conclusion.—The concomitant increase in CT and MRI and decrease in plain films and fluoroscopy suggest that the older studies are being replaced by the new methodologies.

► This study is of particular interest in that it depicts a clear increase in the use of somewhat sophisticated imaging studies such as MR imaging and CT in the workup of inpatients. In an era when much attention is directed toward decreasing the length of hospital stay, judicious use of more expensive, but also more informative, studies may actually be cost effective.

C.D. Maynard, M.D.

Effect of Real-Time Teleradiology on the Practice of the Emergency Department Physician in a Rural Setting: Initial Experience

Lee JKT, Renner JB, Saunders BF, et al (Univ of North Carolina, Chapel Hill; Chatham Hosp, Siler City, NC)

Acad Radiol 5:533-538, 1998 5–22

Background.—The effect of online teleradiology with high-speed transmission on the practice of emergency department (ED) physicians has not been reported previously. The feasibility and utility of online teleradiology consultation for ED physicians in a rural hospital were reported.

Methods.—Electronic linkage was established by a fiberoptic network between the ED department of a rural hospital and a university medical center. The ED physicians at the remote site graded their satisfaction and comfort levels with the system on a scale of 1 to 7, with 7 being the highest. Online soft-copy interpretation was compared with a later interpretation of the original hard copy.

Findings.—One hundred twenty-three separate studies with a total of 460 radiographs were transmitted successfully in 90 discrete teleradiology events. Teleradiology consultations had a mean turnaround time of 1.3 hours. These consultations resulted in changes to the initial diagnosis in 30% of the patients and in treatment changes in 26%. The mean satisfaction score was 5.4, and the mean comfort level score was 5.6. There were no discrepancies between soft- and hard-copy interpretations (Fig 2).

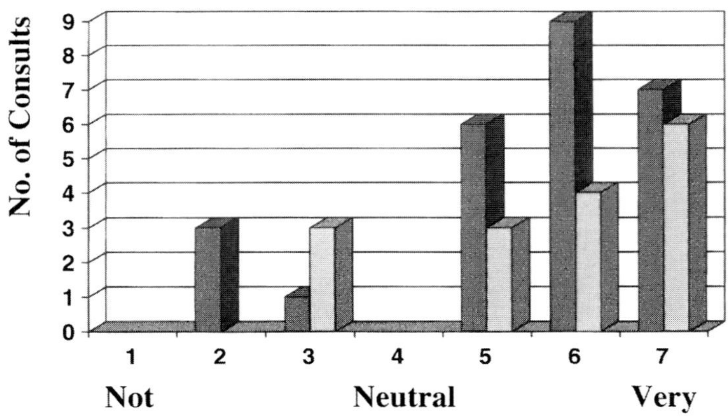

FIGURE 2.—Bar graph of levels of physician satisfaction and comfort with teleradiology consultations (N = 26). *Dark gray bars* indicate satisfaction; *light gray bars* indicate comfort level. (Courtesy of Lee JKT, Renner JB, Saunders BF, et al: Effect of real-time teleradiology on the practice of the emergency department physician in a rural setting: Initial experience. *Acad Radiol* 5:533-538, 1998.)

Conclusion.—Online real-time teleradiology consultation is feasible with current technology. The role of high-speed image transmission and the cost-benefit ratio of this practice need to be further defined.

► Without a doubt, teleradiology will ultimately play a large role in the delivery of high-quality interpretations in the emergency department environment. As the transition toward a digital environment continues during the next 10 years, transmission of images acquired in emergency departments, both large and small, will make expert consultations easier to obtain. Large group practices are already employing teleradiology for on-call purposes, and only a slightly greater leap will be needed to develop networks of cooperating radiology practices to cover many emergency departments from a single distant site. Teleradiology offers a sure way to provide patients with the best care and at the same time protect "turf" for radiology.

C.D. Maynard, M.D.

Consultation Skills in Radiology: A Qualitative Study

Dacher J-N, Charlin B, Bergeron D, et al (Hôpital Charles Nicolle, Rouen, France; Université de Sherbrooke, Quebec)
Can Assoc Radiol J 49:167-171, 1998 5–23

Background.—Because consultation is such an important part of radiologic practice, consultation skills need to be addressed adequately in radiologist training programs. To improve the instruction and assessment of radiology trainees, a qualitative study was conducted to specify the consultation skills expected from a trainee by the end of residency.

Methods.—Three focus groups were held with professors of radiology, residents in radiology, and referring physicians, respectively. Participants were asked to identify the various competencies needed by radiologist consultants. These data were elicited spontaneously and by use of a previously generated list and common clinical problems in radiology.

Findings.—The consultation skills identified were organized into a framework consisting of 2 groups: observable skills and standards of practice. Observable skills consisted of 5 problem-setting skills and 6 results-management skills. The standards of practice rubric included 7 qualities and attitudes (Table 1).

Conclusions.—In this study, consultation abilities and competencies required by radiologists were specified through a consensus process. Such an approach should permit the teaching of these skills and their assessment through objective, structured examinations.

► The subject of the radiology Intersociety Summer Conference, held in 1998 in Beaver Creek, Colorado, was "Are Today's Residents Ready for (Tomorrow's) Practice?" The consensus at the retreat was that our residents are extremely well trained in interpretive skills but need help in 3 areas: handling volume, recognizing normal variants, and developing communica-

TABLE 1.—A Framework of Consultation Skills in Radiology

Group 1: observable skills
Problem-setting
The consultant
1. identifies and clarifies the problem
2. takes into account the referring physician
3. looks for additional pertinent information
4. takes into account the human and technical environment
5. identifies urgent requisitions

Results-management
The consultant
1. adapts communication to the referring physician
2. uses relevant means of communication
3. does not overstep the bounds of radiology
4. reports on the right issues
5. describes pertinent technical points, limitations and intellectual process
6. concludes reports and synthesizes

Group 2: standards of practice
The consultant
1. is patient-centered
2. acts in accordance with ethical principles
3. acts in accordance with general health care policies
4. is responsible and conscious of his or her limits
5. is committed to continuous medical education
6. is capable of self-criticism
7. is available and friendly

(Reprinted from Dacher J-N, Charlin B, Bergeron D, et al: Consultation skills in radiology: A qualitative study, by permission of the publisher, *Can Assoc Radiol J* 1998; 49:167-171.)

tive skills. These Canadian authors address the area of communication, and they present a framework on which to build a teaching program for our residents. This area is one that could easily be addressed by the Residency Review Committee in Diagnostic Radiology and incorporated into the basic framework of our training programs. Communication is such a vital part of our practices that it should not be left to the residents to acquire the appropriate skills entirely on their own. Establishment of a more formal process seems advisable. This article is a good beginning for such a course.

C.D. Maynard, M.D.

Voice Recognition—An Emerging Necessity Within Radiology: Experiences of the Massachusetts General Hospital

Mehta A, Dreyer KJ, Schweitzer A, et al (Harvard Med School, Boston)
J Digit Imaging 11(suppl 2):20-23, 1998 5–24

Objective.—With continued technologic advances, computer voice recognition (VR) systems have become a practical reality. These systems have obvious applications in radiology, where dictation of reports has always been a time-consuming and expensive process. Experience with implementation of a VR system in the radiology department is discussed.

The VR System in the Radiology Department.—The department uses the IBM Medspeak/Radiology package, which offers a 25,000-word vocabulary and an average accuracy rate of more than 95% for native English speakers. The software requires no special "training," although a short enrollment process helps the system to detect and store individual voice nuances. Key features include an open interface between the radiology and hospital information systems. Prestored reports can be stored for recall with a single command (eg, a "normal chest" report), and customized templates can be used to create standardized report formats. The system is flexible enough to permit additional information to be added to a "final" report, or to input other additional information. A barcode interface and system security features are also included.

The radiology department, which performs more than 400,000 radiologic studies annually, was a test site for development of the VR system. On the basis of initial experience, a multiphase rollout was started at the beginning of 1997. By mid-1998, 35 workstations were producing more than 400 reports per day, accounting for 40% of reports generated. Continued improvement in technology is expected; use of microphones with noise-cancellation technology is particularly important. Problems with user acceptance arise because it takes longer at first to produce reports using the VR system. Management and technical support are key to overcoming objections. Initial evaluations suggest that the VR system has reduced reporting times, from the end of the study to the final report, by 90%. Through phase III of a scheduled 5-phase implementation, the system has saved $350,000 over 2 years. The VR system also improves accuracy, because the radiologists can finalize reports immediately after dictating them.

Discussion.—VR systems are a technology ready for implementation in radiology reporting. The challenges of implementing such a system are justified by the technical and financial benefits that accrue. The improved turnaround times and decreased operating costs possible with VR will become increasingly important in the changing health care environment.

► Voice recognition technology has been around for some time, and clearly it is here to stay. Newer systems now make voice recognition transcription in radiology practice a viable reality. As departments deal with diminishing financial resources, moving to direct voice recognition transcription would result in major savings. There is 1 caveat, however: at the moment, voice recognition technology transfers the job of transcription partially to the dictating radiologists. Still, the advantages of these systems—immediate turnaround of dictated reports, being able to attach a report to the digital images within the picture archiving and communication systems before sending it to a referring physician, and reducing the cost of transcription—will lead to their wide acceptance. This is definitely the way to go!

C.D. Maynard, M.D.

Computer-based Speech Recognition as a Replacement for Medical Transcription
Rosenthal DI, Chew FS, Dupuy DE, et al (Harvard Med School, Boston)
AJR 170:23-25, 1998 5–25

Background.—The use of computerized speech recognition technology in radiology has been limited by computer systems' inability to recognize continuous speech and the less-than-perfect accuracy. However, recent advances have led to improvements in the computer's ability to recognize large vocabularies. The implementation of computerized speech recognition using a new commercial software system in a high-volume clinical setting was described.

Methods.—The performance of MedSpeak was compared with that of conventional transcription during a 1-week trial, followed by 3 months of routine clinical use. MedSpeak was used for 97% of the cases during the trial week and for 87% of the cases during the subsequent months.

Findings.—The length of reports did not change after the computerized system was introduced. The mix of cases was similar. The use of MedSpeak reduced the time to report availability by 99%, resulting in a substantial savings in transcription costs.

Conclusion.—Computerized speech recognition has become a feasible alternative to medical transcription in high-volume clinical radiology practices. The system used in the current study was practical and fast enough to replace conventional transcription.

► Without a doubt, computerized speech recognition as a replacement for traditional medical transcription is a reality. The advantages for patient care, resulting from the rapid turnaround time for reports and increased accuracy, are self-evident coupled with the cost savings realized. These advantages will make it difficult for any radiology department chair to resist implementation of speech recognition technology.

C.D. Maynard, M.D.

Turf

Turf Battles in Radiology: How Individual Radiologists Can Respond to the Challenge
Levin DC, Rao VM, Bree RL, et al (Thomas Jefferson Univ, Philadelphia; Univ of Michigan, Ann Arbor; Western Pennsylvania Hosp, Pittsburgh)
Radiology 209:330-334, 1998 5–26

Introduction.—"Turf battles" in which nonradiologists attempt to gain control of imaging examinations or image-guided interventions are a growing phenomenon in radiology. The radiologists view these encroachments as financially or politically motivated, while the nonradiologists may claim convenience or greater familiarity or expertise with the patient and his condition. Strategies that radiologists can follow in dealing with turf battles in their own hospitals are discussed.

Strategies for Dealing with Turf Battles.—The results may be poor when physicians perform examinations or procedures for which they have no formal training. To protect their expertise, radiologists should be aware of studies concerning the consequences of having nonradiologists perform diagnostic imaging tests. Such studies suggest that nonradiologists are not only prone to make errors of interpretation, but that the quality of the studies themselves may be inferior. Radiologists facing turf battles may also document the errors committed by nonradiologists performing imaging studies in the hospital. Another strategy is to challenge the nonradiologist to a test, using side-by-side comparisons of preselected sets of images. Another key argument to bring up is the nonradiologists' lack of formal training in interpretation of diagnostic images. This has important implications for the safety of percutaneous peripheral vascular interventions performed by vascular surgeons and cardiologists. If such a specialist claims to have received formal training for interventional procedures elsewhere, his or her credentials may be challenged.

Nonradiologists may be offered training in a particular area of diagnostic imaging. However, the radiologist should insist that the rigor of the training should approach that required for radiology residents. Radiologists should recognize the potential for overuse, and associated high costs, when self-referral for imaging studies is permitted. Another effective strategy is to promote collaborative relationships with other departments for the purpose of performing diagnostic imaging or image-guided procedures. Such agreements ensure that the radiologist will play a role in the provision of services, while avoiding the conflict associated with a full-scale turf war. Keeping up with radiologic research and becoming involved in medical staff affairs and hospital administrative functions are also effective strategies.

Discussion.—These strategies will be of assistance to hospital radiologists facing encroachment on their scope of practice from nonradiologists. Their success will depend on the underlying strength of the radiology group. The most effective strategy is to make the point that radiologists are almost always the physicians most competent to perform diagnostic imaging studies and image-guided interventions.

▶ David Levin, chairman of radiology at Thomas Jefferson University Hospital, has for years been a leader in analyzing turf issues in our field. Every radiologist, whether in private practice or in an academic environment, faces the complexities of dealing with turf issues every day. In fact, these concerns are among our most time-consuming, distressing, and challenging. What is fair to you and your colleagues in other fields? What is in the best interests of the patient? When should you compromise? When should you "go to the mattress"? When are joint ventures the answer? This article addresses such issues intelligently and certainly deserves your consideration.

C.D. Maynard, M.D.

Impact of Emergency Medicine Resident Training in Ultrasonography on Ultrasound Utilization

Heller M, Melanson S, Patterson J, et al (St Luke's Hosp, Bethlehem, Pa)
Am J Emerg Med 17:21-22, 1999 5–27

Background.—Many radiologists are resistant to the idea of training emergency physicians in bedside US, partly because of concern that this practice would reduce the number of radiology-interpreted studies ordered from the emergency department (ED). The impact of an ED training program in US on the ordering of formal studies from a department of radiology was investigated in a retrospective, computer-assisted review.

Methods and Findings.—All abdominal sonograms ordered from the ED of a community hospital 3 years before the implementation of a US training program (1992-1994) were compared with those ordered in the 2 years after program's implementation. The number of formal studies increased significantly after the training program was implemented. The absolute number of examinations increased from 102 in the year before US training to 197 in the year after implementation. In addition, the percentage of all outpatient US studies rose from 5.1% to 9.8% (Fig 1).

Conclusions.—Implementing a bedside US training progrm in the ED of this hospital resulted in a significant increase in the number of formal US examinations ordered by ED physicians. Both the absolute numbers and the percentage of all outpatient sonograms ordered increased.

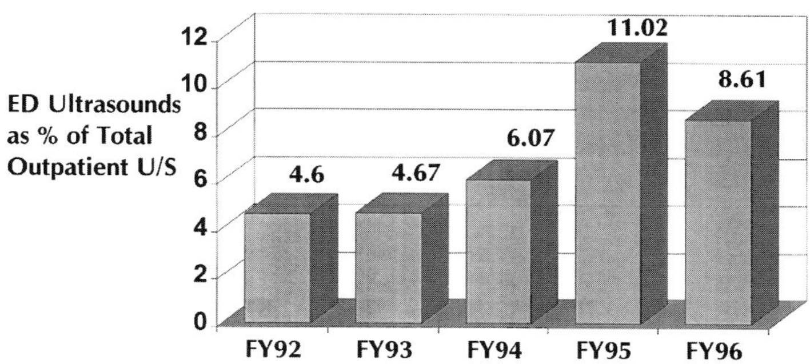

Ordered by ED	93	90	102	197	164
Yearly total	2020	1929	1681	1788	1904

FIGURE 1.—Percentage of ultrasonograms ordered by emergency medicine physicians. (Courtesy of Heller M, Melanson S, Patterson J, et al: Impact of emergency medicine resident training in ultrasonography on ultrasound utilization. *Am J Emerg Med* 17:21-22, 1999.)

Do Gastroenterologists Want To Be Trained in Ultrasound? A National Survey of Trainees in Gastroenterology

Jamieson CP, Denton ERE, Burnham WR (Royal London Hosp; Guy's Hosp, London; Oldchurch Hosp, Romford, England)

Gut 44:123-126, 1999 5–28

Background.—Currently, many radiology departments in the United Kingdom have a significant waiting list for abdominal US assessments. Whether gastroenterologists wish to train in abdominal US and whether the US workload generated by gastroenterologists differ from that generated by other clinicians were determined.

Methods.—A questionnaire was mailed to all 278 gastroenterology trainees. The response rate was 82%. The indications and findings of 100 consecutive scans requested by gastroenterologists were compared with 100 scans requested sequentially by other clinicians through a teaching hospital radiology department.

Findings.—Seventy-seven percent of the trainees said they wished to train in abdominal US. Sixty-eight percent were prepared to train according to the Royal College of Radiologists guidelines. However, 86% preferred not to assess renal or pelvic abnormalities but to limit diagnoses to hepatobiliary abnormalities only. Seventy-three percent of the trainees did not anticipate needing a further scan by a radiologist. Comparison of gastroenterology scans with those requested by other clinicians showed a relative excess of hepatobiliary indications and findings, with a notable lack of renal and pelvic diagnoses in gastroenterology practice.

Conclusions.—In general, these gastroenterology trainees were interested in US training and accepted the guideline document. However, most trainees favored training limited to hepatobiliary disease. Thus, a more focused US training for gastroenterologists should be considered.

Institutional Learning Curve of Surgeon-performed Trauma Ultrasound

Smith RS, Kern SJ, Fry WR, et al (Univ of Kansas, Wichita; Penrose-St Francis Hosp, Colorado Springs, Colo)

Arch Surg 133:530-536, 1998 5–29

Background.—Although US now the primary method for initially assessing abdominal injury in many trauma centers, the rate at which nonradiologists become proficient in this modality has not been established. The learning curve for surgeon-performed trauma US at 1 center was determined.

Methods.—Senior surgical residents underwent 11.5 hours of hands-on and didactic instruction in focused US examination for trauma. US then became a standard component of the assessment of injured patients. Subsequent groups of senior residents underwent 8 hours of instruction at the beginning of the new academic year, 6 and 18 months after the initial course.

Findings.—Nine hundred two sonographic assessments were performed during the 24-month study period. When any 6-month period was compared with other 6-month periods or with values calculated for the entire study, there were no significant differences in sensitivity, specificity, accuracy, positive predictive value, or negative predictive value.

Conclusions.—Senior surgical residents can perform focused US examination for trauma with a high level of skill after a concise introductory course. In this study, no learning curve was evident.

► US is permeating more and more specialty groups. It is almost as if the US machine is becoming the new stethoscope of the clinician. Articles such as those by Heller et al (Abstract 5–27), Jamieson et al (Abstract 5–28), and Smith et al (Abstract 5–29), which describe the training of nonradiologists in clinical applications of US, are appearing with increasing frequency in nonradiology journals. This has become a definite trend, not only in the United States but throughout the rest of the world as well. Almost inevitably, radiology will have a difficult time maintaining its dominance in this field as US equipment becomes less expensive and easier to operate and as clinicians recognize the advantages of incorporating the technique into their clinical practices. I guess we can't win them all! We must, however, try to ensure that the highest standards are maintained, regardless of who performs and interprets the studies.

C.D. Maynard, M.D.

Can Academic Radiology Departments Become More Efficient and Cost Less?

Seltzer SE, Saini S, Bramson RT, et al (Harvard Med School, Boston; Massachusetts Gen Hosp, Boston; Integral, Cambridge, Mass)

Radiology 209:405-410, 1998 5–30

Background.—Academic radiology departments are feeling the crunch for improving efficiency and reducing costs. The outcomes of efforts at Brigham and Women's Hospital (BWH) and Massachusetts General Hospital (MGH) to meet these imperatives were examined.

Methods.—Two cost and productivity measures—cost per relative value unit (RVU) and RVU per full-time–equivalent employee (FTE)—were used to assess the technical operations at BWH and MGH over a 5-year period (1992 through 1996). Data were collected on the billed charges, operating costs, number of examinations performed, technical RVUs, and number of FTEs.

Findings.—Both hospitals kept the costs per examination to a 10% or less increase over the 5 years studied. Both hospitals did this while simultaneously significantly decreasing their cost per RVU: a decrease of 19.0% at BWH and a decrease of 28.8% at MGH (Figs 1 and 2). The RVU of FTEs increased significantly over this period also, with an increase of 46% at BWH and 55.8% at MGH.

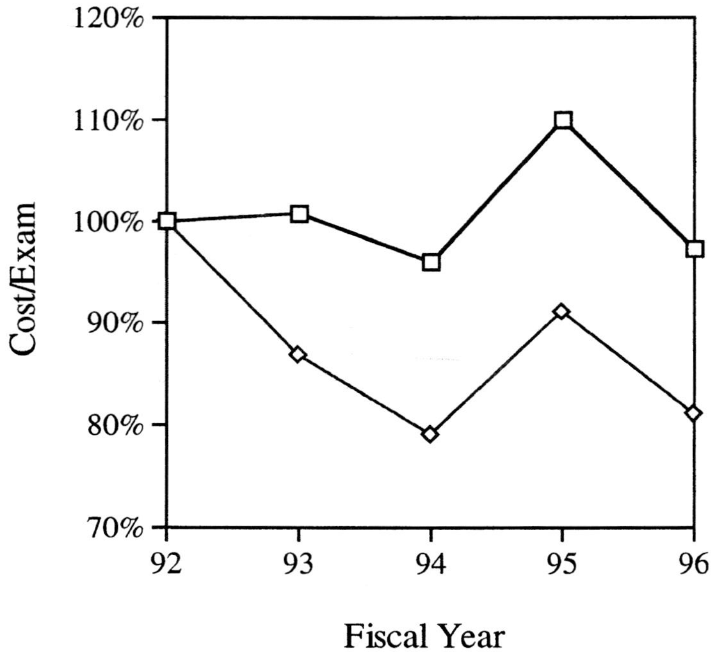

FIGURE 1.—Graph of the changes in cost per examination (*squares*) and cost per relative value unit (*diamonds*) at Brigham and Women's Hospital for fiscal years 1992-1996. Costs are normalized to fiscal year 1992 (i.e., 1992 values are set to 100%) to facilitate the temporal pattern of percentage changes. Note the general stability in cost per examination but the statistically significant declines in cost per relative value unit. (Courtesy of Seltzer SE, Saini S, Bramson RT, et al. Can academic radiology departments become more efficient and cost less? *Radiology* 209:405-410, 1998. Radiological Society of North America.)

Conclusion.—These 2 academic radiology departments have been able to respond to market forces and have steadily become less expensive and more productive over the past 5 years.

► Every academic radiology department in the United States is undergoing some form of reengineering. As academic medical centers cope with decreasing reimbursements for clinical work, as well as decreases in indirect and direct payments for graduate medical education, the scramble is on! How to maintain an environment that fosters education and research while

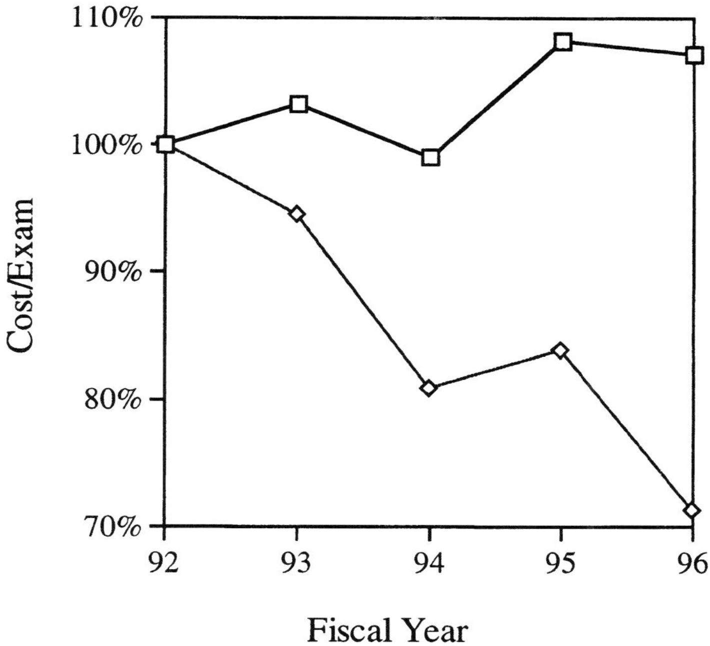

FIGURE 2.—Graph of the changes in cost per examination (*squares*) and cost per relative value unit (*diamonds*) at Massachusetts General Hospital for fiscal years 1992-1996. Costs are normalized to fiscal year 1992. Note the general stability of slight increases in cost per examination but the statistically significant declines in cost per relative value unit. (Courtesy of Seltzer SE, Saini S, Bramson RT, et al. Can academic radiology departments become more efficient and cost less? *Radiology* 209:405-410, 1998. Radiological Society of North America.)

competing clinically with departments that have no other obligation but to provide clinical care is clearly a challenge. The answers for each department vary greatly because of major differences in how the departments are funded (ie, private vs public). However, sharing experiences as to successful strategies can be very useful. Department chairs can then adapt those changes that have the best chance of success in their own institutions. The radiology departments at Brigham and Women's Hospital and Massachusetts General Hospital in Boston share their experiences as they attempt to become more efficient and cost effective.

C.D. Maynard, M.D.

6 Vascular and Interventional Radiology

Introduction

As I mentioned last year, one of the hottest topics in interventional radiology is uterine fibroid embolization.[1] In 1998, the news was how effective the procedure was. That opinion has been fortified with the article by Worthington-Kirsch (Abstract 6–6), the headlines are about how well the procedure is accepted, even demanded, by women. Part of this rapid dissemination takes place through traditional means—newspaper and magazine articles, television news, word of mouth, etc. Of great interest, in our practice at least, is how many women learn of the procedure on the Internet. And that may be the real story—how information about an innovative elective procedure is spread through the Web and how people rapidly access this medium for information about medical advances.

Several articles were published this year about venous thrombolysis. Chronic venous insufficiency is a very disabling condition, though out of site from many interventional radiologists. Any advance in its prevention is significant and venous thrombolysis holds such promise. The Venous Registry does seem to establish that regional thrombolysis is safe. Whether or not it prevents postthrombotic syndrome remains to be seen.

CT and MR pulmonary angiography hold great promise because they are quick and safe. Well, no grass grows under the feet of vascular radiologists. Two articles this year substantiate the accuracy of digital subtraction compared with screen film angiography (Abstracts 6–3 and 6–4). This permits catheter angiography to be performed much faster (cut-film pulmonary angiography may have been definitive, precise, even aesthetic, but no one ever said it was fast).

I am a big fan of outcomes research, clinical economics, health services research, or whatever you want to call it. Hence the inclusion of articles by Kazmers (Abstract 6–1) and Murphy (Abstract 6–21). Both challenge the fundamental tenet of peripheral vascular therapy that only medical management is needed for patients with claudication. Why? Because claudication is not that bad and only a small number of afflicted progress to limb-threatening ischemia. In reality, claudication is very debilitating and significantly diminishes the quality of a patient's life. So a blanket exclusion of operative/interventional alternatives, long the gospel in this condition, may be shortchanging a lot of patients.

Finally, editorship duties with the YEAR BOOK permit a review of journals far afield from mainstream radiology. Contributions about vascular radiotherapy, hemobilia, nitric oxide and radiation exposure are but a few examples of such meanderings through the literature of other fields.

Michael J. Pentecost, M.D.

Reference

1. 1998 YEAR BOOK OF DIAGNOSTIC RADIOLOGY, p 425.

Health Status in Veterans Undergoing Noninvasive Lower Extremity Arterial Evaluation

Kazmers A, Striplin D, Jacobs LA, et al (Wayne State Univ, Detroit; Univ of Michigan, Ann Arbor)

J Surg Res 81:2-5, 1999 6–1

Introduction.—Functional status of patients with lower extremity arterial disease is clinically and therapeutically important in determining the need for revascularization. Functional limitation is typically determined by walking distance. These patients have also been found to have profound reduction in health status, as determined by the SF-36 Health Survey. The health status of 299 outpatients undergoing lower extremity arterial Doppler studies (LES) in a Veterans Affairs Medical Center-based vascular laboratory between September 1995 and June 1996 was assessed by means of the SF-36 Health Survey.

Methods.—The health status of the veteran outpatients was compared with national norms to determine whether Doppler-derived ankle-brachial indices (ABI) are associated with the 8 health concepts measured by the SF-36 Health Survey: physical functioning (PF), role limitations by physical illness (RP), bodily pain (BP), general health (GH), vitality (VT), social functioning (SF), role limitations by emotional illness (RE), and mental health (MH). These measures were significantly more impaired in the veterans group, when compared with national norms for men age 65 years and older. Each of the health measures was below the 25th percentile of national norms for the veterans group. Physical functioning was the only SF-36 health measure that correlated with the lowest ABI. Veterans who underwent only carotid duplex scans were compared with those who underwent only LES. In the LES group, PF, RP, BP, GH, VT, SF, and RE were significantly more impaired than in those who underwent carotid duplex scans.

Conclusion.—Broad-based and profound impairment in health status was observed in veteran outpatients referred to a vascular laboratory. Only physical functioning was associated with ABI, as determined by the SF-36.

► This very important article raises questions about the traditionally nonoperative approach to patients with intermittent claudication. This particular group is a Veterans Hospital population in which the SF-36 Health Survey was applied to men with lower extremity arterial disease. The study shows that claudication is more than simply an annoyance. It is a serious limitation to individuals' enjoyment of life. The SF-36 survey quantifies this impairment and lends credibility to a more aggressive approach to the treatment of peripheral vascular disease and hence has a powerful positive impact on the patients' lives.

M.J. Pentecost, M.D.

Treatment of Thromboangiitis Obliterans (Buerger's Disease) by Intramuscular Gene Transfer of Vascular Endothelial Growth Factor: Preliminary Clinical Results

Isner JM, Baumgartner I, Rauh G, et al (Tufts Univ, Boston)
J Vasc Surg 28:964-975, 1998 6–2

Background.—Buerger's disease, also called thromboangiitis obliterans (TAO), is a peripheral artery occlusive disease affecting young smokers (Fig 2). Once critical limb ischemia with ulceration or gangrene has occurred, the course of TAO is relentlessly progressive, even if the patient quits smoking. Initial results with intramuscular (IM) gene transfer therapy with vascular endothelial growth factor for TAO are reported.

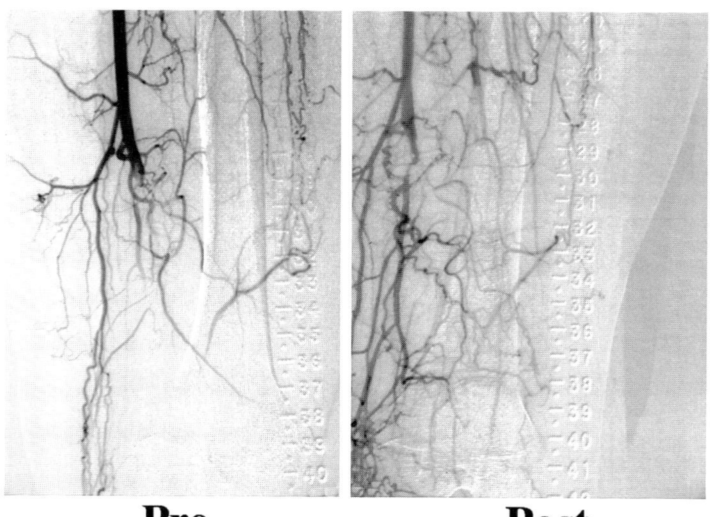

FIGURE 2.—Digital subtraction angiogram from a patient before gene therapy showing typical findings of Buerger's disease at distal popliteal and tibial levels with normal femoral vessel proximally. Angiogram after gene therapy at 8 weeks shows significant increase in collateral formation. (Courtesy of Isner JM, Baumgartner I, Rauh G, et al: Treatment of thromboangiitis obliterans (Buerger's disease) by intramuscular gene transfer of vascular endothelial growth factor: Preliminary clinical results. *J Vasc Surg* 28:964-975, 1998.)

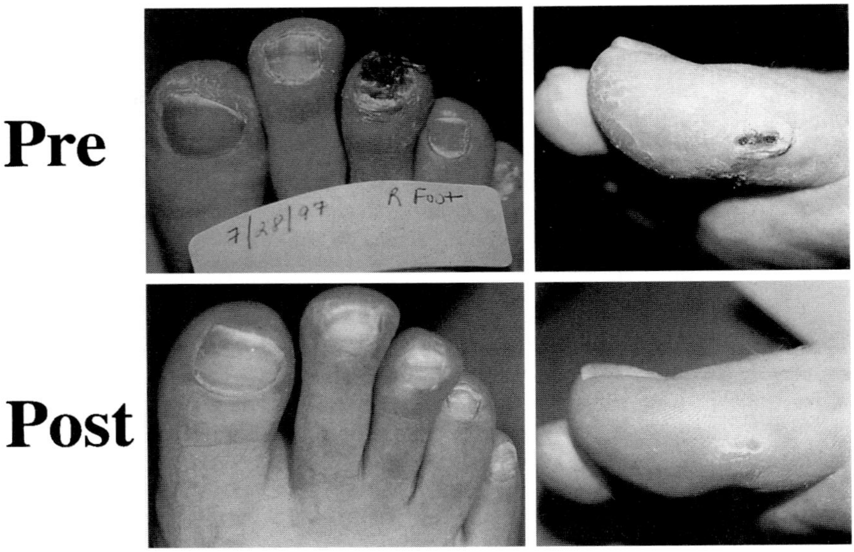

FIGURE 4.—Photograph of feet of 2 patients showing healing of necrotic lesions of toes 6 to 8 weeks after initiation of gene therapy with phVEGF$_{165}$. (Courtesy of Isner JM, Baumgartner I, Rauh G, et al: Treatment of thromboangiitis obliterans (Buerger's disease) by intramuscular gene transfer of vascular endothelial growth factor: Preliminary clinical results. *J Vasc Surg* 28:964-975, 1998.)

Methods.—The phase I clinical trial included 6 patients with critical limb ischemia associated with TAO. There were 3 men and 3 women, mean age 33 years. The patients received 2 treatments with naked plasmid DNA-encoding vascular endothelial growth factor (phVEGF$_{165}$). The treatments, given 4 weeks apart, consisted of direct IM injection at 4 arbitrary sites in the ischemic extremity. Peripheral blood samples were taken for enzyme-linked immunosorbent assay to measure gene expression.

Results.—In 3 of 5 limbs with ulcers that had failed to heal for longer than 1 month, complete ulcer healing occurred after gene therapy (Fig 4). In the other 2 patients, gene therapy relieved nocturnal rest pain, though symptoms of claudication continued. Various modalities demonstrated improved perfusion to the distal portion of the ischemic limb, including a greater than 0.1 increase in ankle brachial index in 3 limbs, improved flow on MRI in all 7 limbs, and new collateral vessels on contrast arteriography in 7 limbs. Three patients had temporary ankle or calf edema; this was the only adverse effect of gene therapy. Even with improved perfusion, however, 2 patients required below-knee amputation because of distal forefoot gangrene. Histologic examination of the surgical specimens confirmed the presence of TAO.

Conclusions.—Encouraging early results with phVEGF$_{165}$ gene transfer therapy for advanced TAO are reported. This form of therapeutic angiogenesis may offer a new approach for patients with TAO that does not respond to conventional medical or surgical treatments. To be successful, gene therapy must be initiated before the onset of forefoot gangrene.

► VEGF has shown considerable early promise in the treatment of coronary and peripheral vascular disease. Buerger's disease is an especially vexing condition. These initial results with VEGF in the treatment of thromboangiitis obliterans are encouraging.

M.J. Pentecost, M.D.

Possible Pulmonary Embolus: Evaluation With Digital Subtraction Versus Cut-film Angiography—Prospective Study in 80 Patients

Johnson MS, Stine SB, Shah H, et al (Indiana Univ, Indianapolis)

Radiology 207:131-138, 1998 6–3

Introduction.—Rapid and certain diagnosis of pulmonary embolism (PE) would allow appropriate and timely treatment and potentially decrease morbidity. The standard imaging test for diagnosing PE is cut-film (film hard-copy) angiography (CFA). It has been suggested that digital subtraction angiography (DSA) could be used to facilitate reliable diagnosis of PE, but there is no report of a large series comparing CFA and DSA. Patients with suspected PE underwent CFA and DSA in a prospective, blinded investigation to determine whether DSA is as diagnostically accurate as CFA.

Methods.—Both CFA and DSA images were taken in identical posteroanterior and oblique projections in 1 lung in 80 patients undergoing pulmonary angiography. The CFA and DSA images were interpreted separately and independently in blinded fashion by 3 vascular radiologists. No patient histories were provided. These diagnoses were compared with those made by a physician who performed a physical examination and was able to compare both CFA and DSA images. When there was disparity between CFA and DSA diagnosis among the 3 blinded reviewers, CFA and DSA findings were reviewed concurrently by all 3 reviewers.

Results.—Thirteen of 80 patients (16%) had PE. Two hundred thirty-six (98.3%) of DSA diagnoses (80 patients × 3 examiners) and 231 (96.3%) of 240 CFA diagnoses were accurate. The sensitivity of DSA was 92% and of CFA was 69% in patients in whom identification of emboli was correct by all 3 reviewers. There were no significant differences in specificities of either modality. The reviewers' confidence in their DSA diagnoses was significantly higher.

Conclusions.—All emboli were accurately detected by all 3 reviewers in 7 of 13 patients with PE. DSA provides more confident identification of PE than CFA does, with no loss in diagnostic accuracy.

Pulmonary Embolism: Comparison of Cut-Film and Digital Pulmonary Angiography

Hagspiel KD, Polak JF, Grassi CJ, et al (Harvard Med School, Boston)
Radiology 207:139-145, 1998 6–4

Introduction.—Selective "cut-film" (film hard-copy) angiography (CFA) is regarded as the standard in the examination of patients with suspected pulmonary embolism (PE). These are time-consuming techniques. Digital pulmonary angiography (DPA) decreases imaging time by shortening all steps of the task. The diagnostic performance and image quality of CFA and DPA were compared in 36 adult patients (39 lungs) with suspected PE.

Methods.—The examination was performed in 1 patient before pulmonectomy for emphysema. Both lungs were evaluated in all patients with findings negative for PE and in patients with findings positive for acute PE when renal function was normal. The projection that best portrayed the areas of abnormality on lung scan was repeated by means of CFA with the same catheter position, projection, amount of contrast material, and injection rate. Digital and cut-film images were reviewed in blinded fashion by 3 vascular radiologists who ranked the likelihood of the presence of PE on a 5-point scale. The 2 modalities were compared by means of receiving

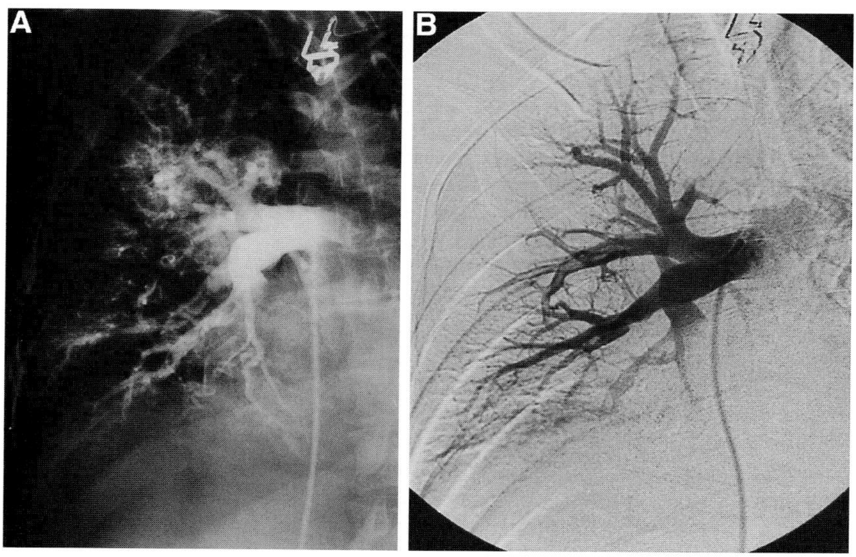

FIGURE 1.—Images of the right lung in a 47-year-old woman with a massive PE in the lower and upper lobes. **a,** CFA image shows the cutoff sign (*arrow*) in the lower-lobe segmental artery as well as filling defects (*arrowheads*) in the segmental arteries of the lower and upper lobes. **b,** digital pulmonary angiographic image reveals similar cutoff sign (*arrow*) and filling defects (*arrowheads*), but the filling defects in the upper lobe are more easily recognized because of the higher contrast between the pulmonary artery and the filling defect. The mean score on the 5-point scale for the presence of PE was 5 for both modalities. (Courtesy of Hagspiel KD, Polak JF, Grassi CJ: Pulmonary embolism: Comparison of cut-film and digital pulmonary arteriography. *Radiology* 207:139-145, 1998. Radiological Society of North America.)

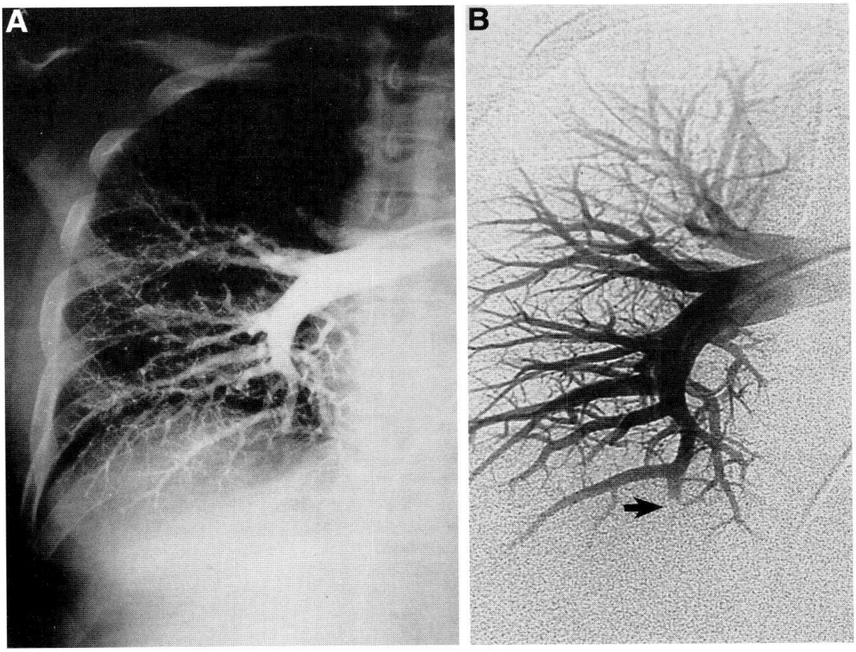

FIGURE 2.—Images of the right lung in a 54-year-old woman with a PE in the posterobasal segmental artery. Both the CFA image (**a**) and the digital pulmonary angiographic image (**b**) show a cutoff sign (*arrow*), which was missed by 2 observers on CFA but was seen by all observers on DPA. The mean score on the 5-point scale for the presence of PE was 2 for CFA and 5 for DPA. (Courtesy of Hagspiel KD, Polak JF, Grassi CJ: Pulmonary embolism: Comparison of cut-film and digital pulmonary arteriography. *Radiology* 207:139-145, 1998. Radiological Society of North America.)

operator characteristics (ROC) analysis. A 3-point scale was used to rate image quality. The highest-order pulmonary artery branch observed on each study was documented.

Results.—The ROC curve analyses for the 3 operators revealed similar diagnostic performance for both DPA and CFA. One operator had better performance with digital subtraction angiography (DSA) , than with CFA. In the evaluation of final diagnosis, single-plane digital pulmonary angiography had greater sensitivity for distinguishing PE than CFA. Specificity was 100% for both examinations. The mean score in patients with positive PE findings was significantly higher in the DPA group, than in the CFA group (Figs 1 and 2). Both procedures produced similar findings in the smallest detectable subsegmental branch or in the average estimate of image quality.

Conclusion.—Selective digital pulmonary angiography and CFA provide similar diagnostic performance and image quality. For diagnosis of PE, DPA is a reasonable alternative to CFA.

► CFA is a wonderful way to image vascular disease. The trouble is that it takes forever and, the less we use it, the longer it takes to perform. The last thing that most patients with suspected PE need is a delay in diagnosis or treatment. Thus, the validation of DPA with its attendant ease and rapidity is a significant advance in the diagnosis of pulmonary thromboemboli.

M.J. Pentecost, M.D.

Clinically Occult Pelvic-Vein Thrombosis in Cryptogenic Stroke

Cramer SC, Rordorf G, Kaufman JA, et al (Univ of Washington, Seattle; Harvard Med School, Boston; Clinical Investigator Training Program, Boston)

Lancet 351:1927-1928, 1998 6–5

Introduction.—Cryptogenic strokes are those in which there is no apparent etiology. Many of these strokes are associated with a patent foramen ovale. Some reports have suggested that paradoxical embolism may play a pathogenetic role in cryptogenic stroke, but a venous source is rarely demonstrated in patients with a patent foramen ovale. The pelvic vein may be the source of embolism, but this is difficult to identify on US or venography. MR venography evaluated the presence of pelvic vein thrombosis in patients with cryptogenic stroke.

Methods.—The study included 16 patients with ischemic stroke of no identifiable cause. In each case, echocardiography demonstrated interarterial communication. (ie, a patent foramen ovale or atrial septal defect). The patients had no US or clinical evidence of venous thrombosis. Each patient underwent MR venography, from the inferior vena cava to the midthigh, a median of 7 days after stroke. The scans were graded for the presence of venous thrombosis, by a vascular radiologist, in masked fashion.

Results.—The scans showed thrombosis in 4 patients, located in the pelvis in 3 patients and the proximal thigh in 1. Seven patients had suspicious results on MR venography. In 1 patient in this group, the presence of pelvic vein thrombosis was confirmed by contrast venography with selective cannulation.

Discussion.—In this study, 5 of 16 cases of cryptogenic thrombosis were associated with venous thrombosis, most often of the pelvic vein. It is unknown how many cryptogenic strokes may be explained by paradoxical embolism. The pathogenetic role and treatment implications of pelvic vein thrombosis warrant further study.

► Vena cava filters are an accepted treatment of pulmonary thromboemboli. But in patients who have only internal iliac vein thrombus, the attendant risks of caval inclusion and chronic venous insufficiency may represent a large price to pay. If only the internal iliac veins could be occluded (with coil embolization), patients could be spared the small but discrete morbidity of vena cava filter placement.

M.J. Pentecost, M.D.

Uterine Arterial Embolization for the Management of Leiomyomas: Quality-of-Life Assessment and Clinical Response

Worthington-Kirsch RL, Popky GL, Hutchins FL Jr (Philadelphia College of Osteopathic Medicine; Delaware Valley Imaging, Bala Cynwyd, Pa; Allegheny Univ, Philadelphia; et al)

Radiology 208:625-629, 1998 6–6

Introduction.—Uterine arterial embolization is safe and effective in the treatment of uterine hemorrhage. It has recently been described as effective in managing symptoms caused by uterine myomas. The effectiveness of uterine arterial embolization as a primary therapy in the management of symptomatic leiomyomas was examined in 53 patients.

Methods.—Patients ranged in age from 33 to 58 years. Symptoms caused by leiomyomas were menometrorrhagia and bulk-related symptoms, including frequency of urination, sensation of pressure, and sensation of mass. All patients underwent arteriography before the embolization procedure (Fig 1). Patient acceptance of treatment was determined by interviews 3 months after surgical intervention.

Results.—Fifty-two of 53 patients (98%) underwent technically successful procedures. The patient in whom the procedure was not successful had a very small right uterine artery; embolization of the left uterine artery was successful. Collateral vessels were used to reconstitute the vascular bed of the right uterine artery. The patient experienced no clinical benefit from the procedure. Forty-six patients (88%) reported a marked decrease in symptoms of abnormal bleeding. Of 31 patients with bulk-related symptoms, 29 (94%) had marked improvement in symptoms. Follow-up ultrasonography revealed a mean 46% decrease in uterine volume. Three patients had complications; 2 were rehospitalized for pain control because of postembolization syndrome, so severe in 1 patient that hysterectomy was performed on postembolization day 12. One patient had severe nausea and vomiting several hours after the procedure and experienced a self-limiting episode of hematemesis. Forty-one patients (79%) reported that they would consider this procedure again; 3 (6%) reported that they would choose another treatment option.

Conclusion.—Uterine embolization is effective in the management of symptomatic leiomyomas. It may be a useful alternative to myomectomy, hysterectomy, or other operative procedures.

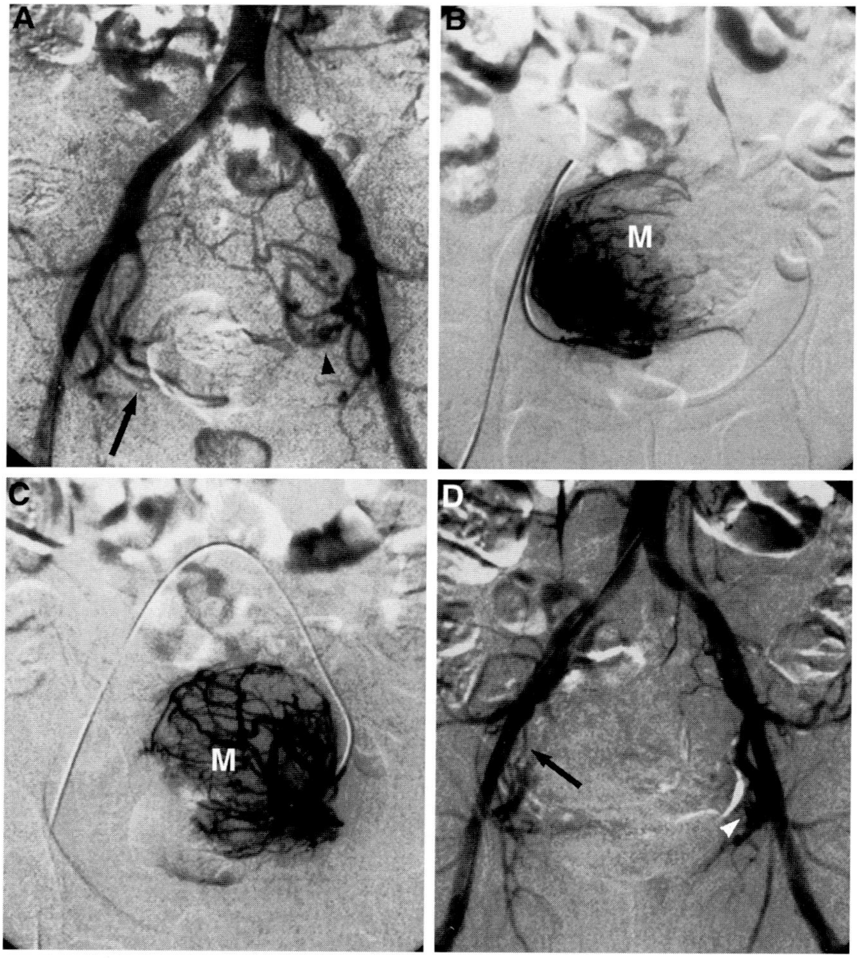

FIGURE 1.—A, Mapping arteriographic image obtained after aortic injection of contrast material shows bilateral enlarged and tortuous right (*arrow*) and left (*arrowhead*) uterine arteries. B, arteriographic image obtained after selective injection of contrast material into the right uterine artery shows marked hypervascularity of the myomatous uterus. The hypervascular mass (*M*) in the center is the leiomyoma. C, arteriographic image obtained after selective injection of contrast material into the left uterine artery shows marked hypervascularity of the myomatous uterus. The hypervascular mass (*M*) in the center is the leiomyoma. D, postprocedural arteriographic image obtained after aortic injection of contrast material shows no visible flow into either uterine artery. The origins of the right (*arrow*) and left (*arrowhead*) uterine arteries are marked. (Courtesy of Worthington-Kirsch RL, Popky GL, Hutchins FL: Uterine arterial embolization for the management of leiomyomas: Quality-of-life assessment and clinical response. *Radiology* 208:625-629, 1998, Radiological Society of North America.)

Transcatheter Uterine Artery Embolisation to Treat Large Uterine Fibroids

Bradley EA, Reidy JF, Forman RG, et al (Guy's and St Thomas' Hosp Trust, London)

Br J Obstet Gynaecol 105:235-240, 1998 6–7

Introduction.—The management of symptomatic uterine fibroids is especially challenging in women who have had an earlier myomectomy, in those whose religious faith does not allow blood transfusions, and in women who do not wish to undergo hysterectomy. Bilateral uterine artery embolization was performed in a pilot investigation of 8 women with symptomatic large fibroids that required treatment.

Methods.—Uterine volume was quantitatively determined by MRI. All patients underwent arteriography and embolization by the percutaneous right femoral artery approach. Patients were examined at regular intervals and were asked to complete a patient satisfaction questionnaire 3 months after the procedure.

Results.—The median patient age was 37½ (range, 31 to 48 years). Seven patients were of Afro-Caribbean origin, and 1 was white. Both uterine arteries were effectively occluded in all patients. Procedure length varied between 1.25 and 2.25 hours. The procedure was well tolerated; 6 women experienced pain (severe in 3 cases) as the second artery was embolized. After embolization, some patients experienced intermittent vaginal discharge and pain. None of the patients experienced significant complications. Six of 7 patients had improved symptoms, and 1 conceived during follow-up. Uterine volume at 3-month follow-up was less than 350 cm^3.

Conclusion.—Embolization seems to be an effective alternative to surgical intervention. Long-term follow-up is needed to evaluate the effects of transcatheter uterine artery embolization in the treatment of large uterine fibroids and to determine the patients for whom the procedure is most suitable.

► Without doubt, uterine fibroid embolization (UFE) is the hottest topic in interventional radiology. Nearly 200,000 women undergo hysterectomy annually. If UFE can be effectively used in half, a fourth, or even a tenth of these women, this procedure has the possibility of having the biggest public health impact of interventional radiology since angioplasty. Worthington-Kirsch et al, validate the earlier, smaller experience from UCLA by Goodwin et al, and set the stage for a multicenter trial to further evaluate this promising new treatment.

M.J. Pentecost, M.D.

Noninvasive In Vivo High-Resolution Magnetic Resonance Imaging of Atherosclerotic Lesions in Genetically Engineered Mice

Fayad ZA, Fallon JT, Shinnar M, et al (Mount Sinai School of Medicine, New York; Children's Hosp of Philadelphia; Rockefeller Univ, New York)

Circulation 98:1541-1547, 1998 6–8

Introduction.—The pathogenesis of atherosclerosis is currently being examined in genetically engineered small animals, particularly mice. It would be advantageous to have an in vivo procedure with which to follow the time course of developing disease or responses to therapy in vivo in the same animal vs. multiple experimental groups with larger numbers of animals killed at different time points. A noninvasive magnetic resonance (MR) microscopy technique was developed and used to evaluate in vivo atherosclerotic lesions without a priori knowledge of lesion location or lesion type in live apolipoprotein E-knockout (apoE-KO) mice.

Methods.—Wild-type and apoE-KO mice underwent MR microscopy of the abdominal aorta and the common iliac arteries. Raw data of MR images were transferred to a computer and reconstructed by means of a custom program. Mice were killed and histopathologic cross sections were correlated with MR images. Manual tracing of the lumen and outer wall boundaries was performed, and cross-sectional areas of the outer boundary and lumen of the vessel were measured on both MR images and histopathologic sections in 58 animals. Lesion type was graded by MR by morphological appearance/severity and by histopathology according to the AHA classification system.

Results.—The spatial resolution was 0.0012 to 0.005 mm^3 and the lumen and wall of the abdominal and iliac arteries were visualized on all images in both apoE-KO and wild-type mice. MR microscopy accurately illustrated wall area in comparison with histopathologic in examination (Fig 1). Atherosclerotic lesions could be characterized by MR microscopy in terms of lesion shape and type. Agreement was excellent between MR and histopathologic examination in the grading of lesion shape and type.

Conclusion.—The use of high-resolution MR microscopy and genetically engineered animals is an important tool for serial and noninvasive examination of the progression and regression of atherosclerotic lesions in vivo.

► Many of the efforts in applying MRI to the coronary circulation have been concentrated on primary detection or screening. Fayad and colleagues present very interesting findings in a mouse model by examining the vulnerable plaque—those atheromatous areas likely to rupture and cause myocardial infarct. Conversely, one could imagine the same technology being used to monitor the regression of atherosclerosis with appropriate medical therapy.

M.J. Pentecost, M.D.

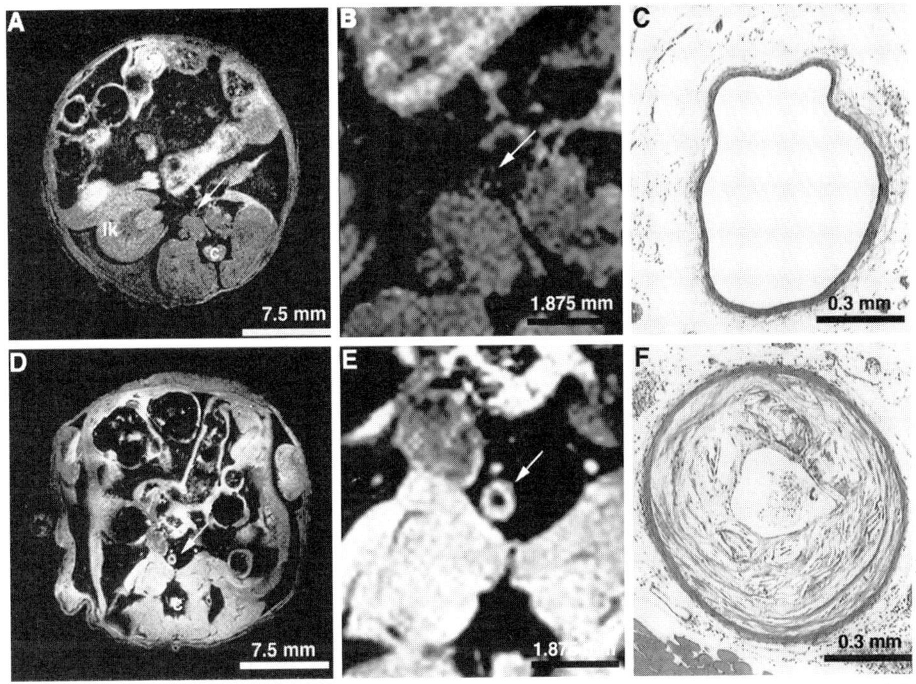

FIGURE 1.—MR images (proton density–weighted) of abdominal aorta (*arrows*) in normal mouse and apoE-KO mouse showing differences between normal and atherosclerotic arteries. On all MR images, lumen is dark. Normal abdominal aorta wall thickness is approximately 50 μm and was not clearly visible at spatial in-plane resolution of 97 μm. Wild-type mice were free of atherosclerotic lesions as shown on MR image in **A** and **B** (magnified, see scale) and histopathologic section (**C**), as shown by hematoxylin-eosin staining; magnification ×40. Large atherosclerotic lesion (*arrow*) that encircles abdominal aorta of 12-month-old apoE-KO mouse is shown on MR images in **D** and **E** (magnified). These findings correlated with histopathologic findings as shown in **F** (hematoxylin-eosin stain; magnification ×40). All MR images have pixel size of 97 × 97 × 500 μm^3. Left kidney and spinal cord are used as anatomic landmarks to facilitate comparison between MR images and histopathologic sections. (Courtesy of Fayad ZA, Fallon JT, Shinnar M: Noninvasive in vivo high-resolution magnetic resonance imaging of atherosclerotic lesions in genetically engineered mice. *Circulation* 98:1541-1547, 1998.)

Selective Salpingography and Fallopian Tubal Occlusion With *n*-Butyl-2-Cyanoacrylate: Report of Two Cases

Pelage J-P, Herbreteau D, Paillon J-F, et al (Hôpital René Dubos, Pontoise, France; Hôpital Lariboisière, Paris Cedex)
Radiology 207:809-812, 1998 6–9

Introduction.—Surgical ligation of the fallopian tubes is the most frequently used method of female sterilization. Transcervical fluoroscopically guided tubal sterilization has recently been performed in an animal model. No ideal occluding agent has been found. Preliminary experience with selective tubal occlusion with *n*-butyl-2-cyanoacrylate (NBCA), a cyanoacrylic glue, in 2 women in whom no other method of sterilization was feasible is reported.

Case 1.—Women 41 years, had severe heart failure and thrombotic disease. A new pregnancy was considered potentially dangerous. She was gravida 3, para 2. Oral contraceptives and laparoscopic and celioscopic sterilization procedures under general anesthesia were contraindicated. Vaginal tubal ligation was not possible because of major obesity. The patient did not wish to use male contraception because of personal convictions.

Case 2.—Woman 42 years, had severe asthma and arterial hypertension. She was gravida 7, para 6. A new pregnancy was considered potentially dangerous because of multiple uterine scars. Other forms of contraception were contraindicated. Vaginal tubal ligation was not successful. The patient refused male contraception for religious reasons.

Results.—Bilateral occlusion of the fallopian tubes was achieved with NBCA during an occlusion procedure in which hysterosalpingographic images were used. Patients experienced only mild pain. No peritoneal or uterine extravasation of the NBCA was detected. Average duration of the procedure was 30 minutes. At 4-year follow-up, neither patient had become pregnant, despite normal sexual activity. Persistent tubal occlusion was determined on a yearly basis by means of repeated hysterosalpingography.

Conclusion.—Tubal occlusion with NBCA is a safe, effective, and inexpensive method of sterilization. It provides long-term occlusion of fallopian tubes.

► A number of agents have been used in animals to occlude the fallopian tubes for sterilization. In this very small series, Pelage et al use *n*-butyl-2-cyanoacrylate in women who, because of severe cardiovascular and pulmonary disease, could not undergo even laparoscopic sterilization. The results are impressive and may lead to a wider application of this technique.

M.J. Pentecost, M.D.

Catheter-directed Thrombolysis for Lower Extremity Deep Venous Thrombosis: Report of a National Multicenter Registry

Mewissen MW, Seabrook GR, Meissner MH, et al (Froedtert Mem Lutheran Hosp, Milwaukee, Wis; Univ of Washington Harborview Med Ctr, Seattle; Montefiore Med Ctr, Bronx, NY; et al)

Radiology 211:39-49, 1999 6–10

Background.—Deep venous thrombosis of the lower extremity can cause pulmonary embolism and postthrombotic syndrome. Anticoagulation can prevent pulmonary embolism and recurrent deep venous thrombosis, but does not protect patients from postthrombotic syndrome, which can occur months or years after an acute episode of deep venous thrombosis. Lytic therapy can help to restore the lumen and to remove the thrombus lining of the venous valves.

Methods.—The results of 312 urokinase infusions in 303 limbs of 287 patients with deep venous thrombosis were analyzed. There were 137 men and 150 women, with a mean patient age of 47.5 years. A history of deep venous thrombosis was recorded in 31% of patients. Symptoms of deep venous thrombosis were acute in 66% of patients, chronic in 16% of patients, and acute and chronic in 19% of patients. Venographic results were used to determine lysis grade.

Results.—Iliofemoral and femoral-popliteal deep venous thrombosis were treated with urokinase infusions for 53.4 hours. After thrombolysis, 1 inferior vena cava, 5 femoral vein, and 99 iliac lesions were treated with stents. Lysis was calculated as grade III in 31% of infusions, grade II in 52% of infusions, and grade I in 17% of infusions. Grade III lysis was achieved in 34% of cases of acute thrombosis and in 19% of cases of chronic thrombosis. About 11% of patients had major bleeding complications, occurring mainly at the puncture site. Pulmonary emboli developed in 1% of patients. Two patients died as a result of pulmonary embolism and intracranial hemorrhage. At 1 year, primary patency was 60%. Lysis grade predicted 1-year patency.

Discussion.—Catheter-directed thrombolysis is safe and effective. This information may help clinicians to select patients for catheter-directed thrombolysis.

Safety and Efficacy of Catheter-directed Thrombolysis for Iliofemoral Venous Thrombosis

Grossman C, McPherson S (Univ of Mississippi Med Ctr, Jackson; St Dominic Hosp, Jackson, Miss)

AJR 172:667-672, 1999 6–11

Background.—Catheter-directed thrombolysis for iliofemoral venous thrombosis can significantly reduce clot burden, sometimes salvaging valve function. Many studies have reported the results of catheter-directed thrombolysis for patients with deep venous thrombosis of the lower extremities involving the inferior vena cava (IVC), the iliac veins, or the femoral veins; patients with limited popliteal vein involvement have generally been excluded. The findings of 15 published studies of catheter-directed thrombolysis for iliofemoral venous thrombosis were reviewed.

Discussion.—The technique of catheter-directed thrombolysis and the data from 15 reported studies involving 263 patients are summarized. The review addresses the adjunctive procedures performed, the short-term results, and the prophylactic use of IVC filters. The available data suggest that the technique can safely and effectively restore venous system patency and relieve acute symptoms in most patients. Urokinase is the usual agent of choice. The combined success rate in the studies reviewed is 84%. The major complications are bleeding and pulmonary embolism, with rates of 5% and less than 1% (2 of 263), respectively. These risks appear to be lower than in patients treated with systemic heparin or systemic thrombolysis alone. The success rate may be improved through the use of adjunctive angioplasty, stent placement, or thrombectomy. Because of the low rate of pulmonary embolism, the benefits of IVC filters are questionable. The success rate may be higher for patients with acute rather than chronic iliofemoral venous clots. Catheter-directed thrombolysis shortens treatment time and allows faster discharge from the hospital than does systemic heparinization. There are few data on the long-term results, including the risk of postthrombotic syndrome.

Summary.—Catheter-directed thrombolysis appears to be a safe and effective treatment for iliofemoral venous thrombosis. Success rates are high, complication rate is lower, and hospital stay is shorter than with conservative therapy. Data from a U.S. venous registry will help in ascertaining the long-term benefits and costs of this intervention.

► This large multicenter (63 institutions) trial substantiates the earlier work of Semba and Dake.[1] Eighty-three percent of these patients experienced marked dissolution of thrombus with venous thrombolysis and the primary patency was 60% at 1 year. Most investigators believe that rapid resolution of thrombosis (whatever the means) leads to less valvular damage and, correspondingly, less chronic venous insufficiency.

M.J. Pentecost, M.D.

Reference

1. Semba CP, Dake MD,: Iliofemoral deep venous thrombosis: aggressive therapy With catheter-directed thrombolysis. *JVIR*: 191:487-494, 1994.

Transcatheter Coil Embolotherapy: A Safe and Effective Option for Major Colonic Haemorrhage

Nicholson AA, Ettles DF, Hartley JE, et al (Hull Royal Infirmary, East Yorkshire, England; Univ of Hull, East Yorkshire, England)

Gut 43:79-84, 1998 6–12

Background.—Treatment of major colonic bleeding is difficult. Emergency surgery is associated with high morbidity and mortality. Percutaneous embolotherapy may be an alternative treatment option for patients requiring surgery.

Methods.—The safety and efficacy of transcatheter coil embolotherapy for life-threatening colonic hemorrhage were evaluated in 38 patients with colorectal bleeding. All patients were actively bleeding and had been referred for surgery because conservative treatment had failed. Angiography showed a bleeding site or vascular abnormality in 14 patients. A coaxial catheter was introduced into the most distal bleeding artery, which was embolized with platinum coils.

Results.—In 14 patients, bleeding sites or vascular abnormalities were detected and embolized. Immediate and sustained hemodynamic improvement occurred in 12 patients, although 2 patients continued to bleed and had emergency hemicolectomy. Ischemic complications developed in 3 patients, who were managed conservatively. At 30 days, mortality was 7.1% in patients who had had embolotherapy and 10.5% in the 38 patients overall.

Discussion.—Transcatheter embolotherapy with platinum microcoils for life-threatening colonic hemorrhage was effective and relatively safe. The incidence of major complications was low. The use of this procedure requires the identification of a focal bleeding point or vascular abnormality in patients who are hemodynamically stable at the time of angiography.

► At the 1997 Society of Cardiovascular and Interventional Radiology Mortality and Morbidity Conference, a huge ruckus erupted over the proper interventional treatment of colonic bleeding. The difference of opinion among experts was amazing but, in retrospect, reflected the relative paucity of published data about the best embolic agent (some physicians even advocated pitression infusion ... imagine that!). This article substantiates the safety and efficacy of coil embolization (the appropriate treatment all along).

M.J. Pentecost, M.D.

Anastomotic Intimal Hyperplasia: A Comparison Between Conventional and Endovascular Stent Graft Techniques

Ohki T, Marin ML, Veith FJ, et al (Jikei Univ, Tokyo; Mount Sinai School of Medicine, New York; Montefiore Med Ctr, New York)
J Surg Res 69:255-267, 1997 6–13

Background.—Endovascular grafting is a new procedure for treating vascular disease, although its long-term efficacy is not known.

Methods.—In 7 dogs, an endovascular graft was placed in 1 iliac artery and a conventional bypass graft was placed in the other. Polytetrafluoroethylene grafts 5 mm × 4 cm were used. The percentage of stenosis at the distal anastomosis was determined by intravascular ultrasound. The thickness of distal anastomic intimal hyperplasia was determined by light microscopic analysis, and the percentage of endothelial coverage of the graft was determined by scanning electron microscopic analysis.

Results.—The percentage of stenosis at the distal anastomosis was significantly greater in endovascular grafts than in conventional grafts, because of intimal hyperplasia. The percentage of area covered by endothelial cells was also greater in endovascular grafts than in conventional grafts. Intraluminal location improved endothelialization of the polytetrafluoroethylene grafts, but also caused greater anastomic intimal hyperplasia.

Discussion.—Further refinement of devices, including stent design, and better understanding of the healing mechanisms of endovascular grafts may improve the efficacy of endovascular grafting.

► As if the biomechanical mismatches with stent grafts weren't causing enough problems, now we have to worry about increased intimal hyperplasia also! In a canine model, Ohki and colleagues found a marked difference in intimal hyperplasia between iliac limbs with a surgically placed Gortex graft and limbs with the contralateral iliac stent graft. Back to the drawing board!

M.J. Pentecost, M.D.

Spontaneous Tibial Artery Thrombosis Associated With Varicella Pneumonia and Free Protein S Deficiency

Peyton BD, Cutler BS, Stewart FM (Univ of Massachusetts, Worcester)
J Vasc Surg 27:563-567, 1998 6–14

Background.—The incidence of varicella infection in individuals older than 20 years is increasing. Pneumonia is a common complication of varicella infection in adults. Various thrombotic complications have been reported in children with varicella, but not in adults. Congenital deficiency of protein C, S, or both is also associated with thrombotic complications. Two cases of varicella pneumonia and significant ischemia of the lower extremity, caused by thrombosis of the profunda femoris and tibial arteries, are described.

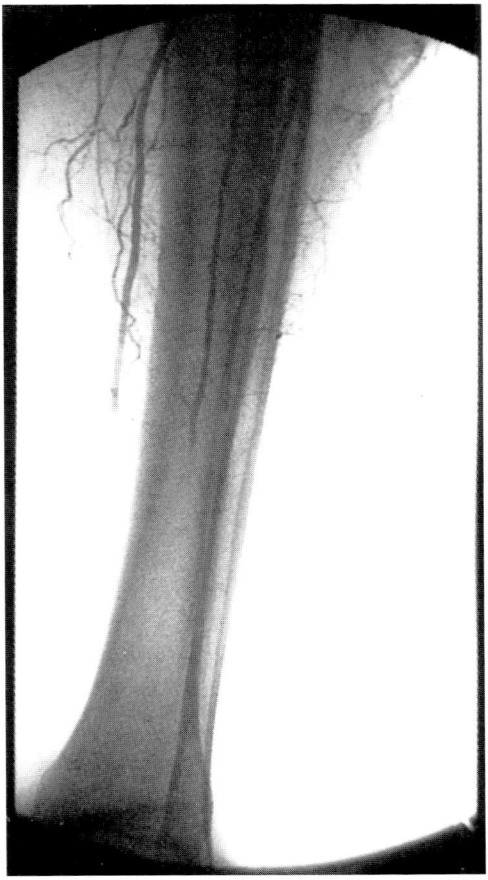

FIGURE 1.—Patient 1. After 12 hours of intra-arterial urokinase, thrombolysis has occurred from trifurcation to midcalf. Note complete absence of flow distally caused by thrombosis of all collateral vessels. (Courtesy of Peyton BD, Cutler BS, Stewart FM: Spontaneous tibial artery thrombosis associated with varicella pneumonia and free protein S deficiency. *J Vasc Surg* 27:563-567, 1998.)

Case 1.—Man, 47, had a 1-day history of confusion, dyspnea, and fever of 40° C after a 5-day history of myalgia, rhinorrhea, nonproductive cough, and a characteristic pustular varicella rash. A child at home was recuperating from chickenpox. Three days after admission, the man had severe ischemia of both legs below the knees. Bilateral occlusion of all 3 tibial vessels just below their origins was seen with transfemoral aortography with bilateral run-off arteriography (Fig 1). Treatment with urokinase resulted in lysis of clot in the popliteal and tibial vessels. Progressive hypoxia and hemodynamic collapse developed, the family requested supportive care only, and the patient died.

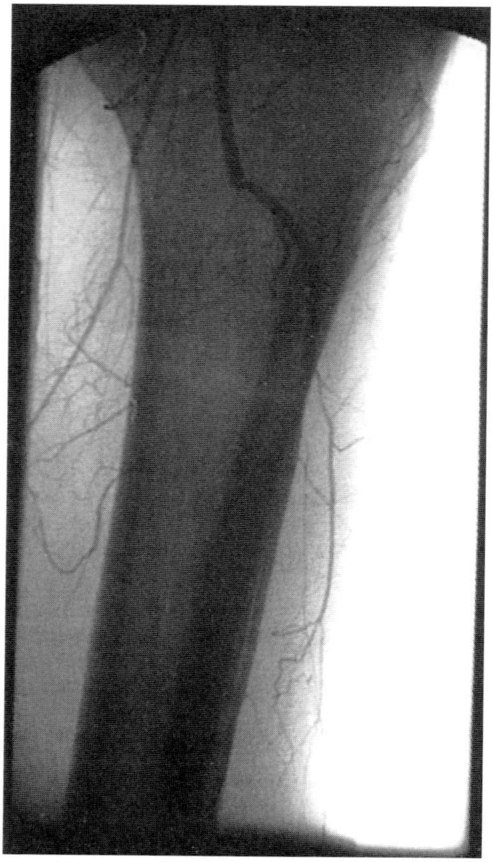

FIGURE 2.—Patient 2. Initial arteriogram demonstrating thrombosis of left tibioperoneal trunk. (Courtesy of Peyton BD, Cutler BS, Stewart FM: Spontaneous tibial artery thrombosis associated with varicella pneumonia and free protein S deficiency. *J Vasc Surg* 27:563-567, 1998.)

Case 2.—Man, 37, had a 9-hour history of dyspnea and pain and numbness in his left foot after a 5-day history of fever and characteristic pustular varicella rash. Two weeks earlier, he had been exposed to chickenpox. The patient had an ischemic left foot with no Doppler signal below the left popliteal artery. Thrombosis of the left tibioperoneal trunk was seen by arteriography (Fig 2). Treatment with urokinase resulted in lysis of the thrombus in the tibial and profunda vessels and restored palpable pulses in the foot by 48 hours (Fig 3). No amputation was needed and the patient regained normal function of his foot. He required long-term anticoagulation because of persistent antiphospholipid antibodies.

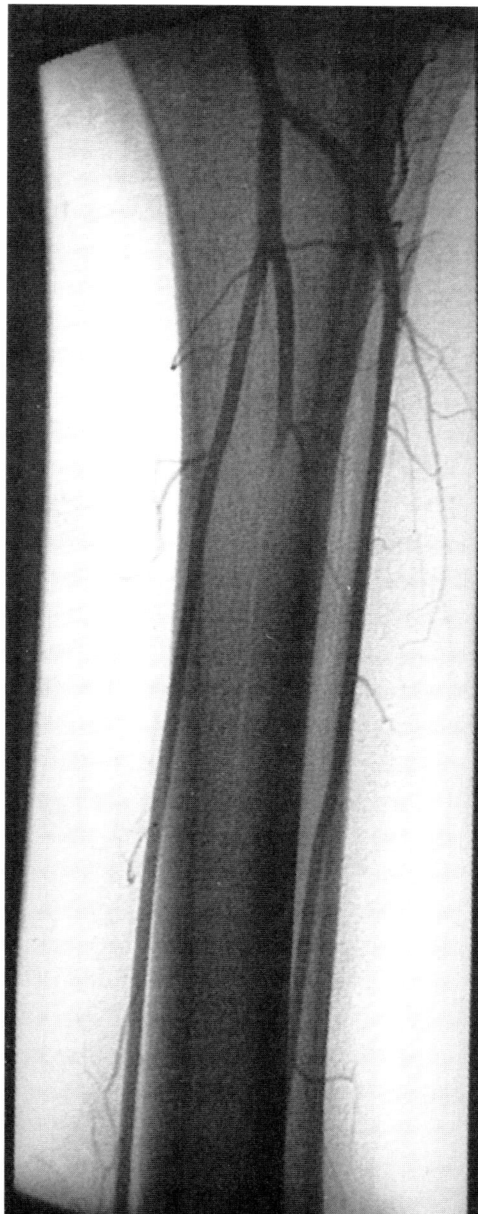

FIGURE 3.—Patient 2. After 48 hours of intra-arterial urokinase, posterior tibial artery patency and foot viability have been restored. (Courtesy of Peyton BD, Cutler BS, Stewart FM: Spontaneous tibial artery thrombosis associated with varicella pneumonia and free protein S deficiency. *J Vasc Surg* 27:563-567, 1998.)

Discussion.—Both of these patients had vascular thrombosis and free protein S deficiency associated with varicella pneumonia, without obvious evidence of disseminated intravascular coagulation or purpura fulminans. This form of acquired free protein S deficiency may be caused by an acquired protein S antibody associated with varicella infection. Antiphospholipid and anticardiolipin antibodies and lupus anticoagulant were also seen in these patients. Thrombotic complications can respond dramatically to anticoagulation and intra-arterial thrombolysis with urokinase.

▶ The hypercoagulable syndromes are of increasing interest to interventional radiologists, because of both the need for thrombolytic treatment and their proclivity for thrombotic complications during angiography. Although the cerebral complications of varicella pneumonia are well known, the involvement of the peripheral circulation is much less common. As pointed out by the authors, thrombolysis may be indicated, depending on the clinical status of the extremity.

M.J. Pentecost, M.D.

Survival Following Pancreaticoduodenectomy With Resection of the Superior Mesenteric-Portal Vein Confluence for Adenocarcinoma of the Pancreatic Head

Leach SD, Lee JE, Charnsangavej C, et al (Univ of Texas, Houston)
Br J Surg 85:611-617, 1998 6–15

Purpose.—Survival in patients who underwent pancreaticoduodenectomy with *en bloc* resection of the superior mesenteric-portal vein confluence for adenocarcinoma of the pancreatic head was compared with survival in patients who underwent pancreaticoduodenectomy without resection.

Methods.—Patients eligible for surgery had to have CT scans showing absence of extrapancreatic disease, no evidence of tumor extension to the superior mesenteric artery or coeliac axis, and a patent superior mesenteric-portal vein confluence. During surgery, tumor adherence to the superior mesenteric vein or superior mesenteric-portal vein confluence was evaluated and *en bloc* venous resection was performed, when necessary, to completely remove the tumor.

Results.—Pancreaticoduodenectomy was performed in 75 consecutive patients, 42 men and 33 women, with a mean patient age of 65 years. Pancreaticoduodenectomy was performed without venous resection in 44 patients and with *en bloc* resection of the superior mesenteric-portal vein confluence in 31 patients. There were no perioperative deaths. The deaths of 2 patients were related to late occlusion of the reconstructed superior mesenteric-portal vein confluence. Median survival was 22 months in the 31 patients who had venous resection during pancreaticoduodenectomy and 20 months in the 44 patients who had pancreaticoduodenectomy without venous resection.

Discussion.—Survival was similar in patients who had standard pancreaticoduodenectomy and patients who had venous resection during pancreaticoduodenectomy for isolated tumor extension to the superior mesenteric vein or superior mesenteric-portal vein confluence. Venous involvement appears to be a function of tumor location rather than an indicator of aggressive disease.

► A great deal of time and energy is expended assessing the superior mesenteric vein and artery prior to pancreaticoduodenectomy for adenocarcinoma of the pancreas. Leach et al establish that for patients who undergo resection of the superior mesenteric vein or superior mesenteric vein-portal vein confluence, the prognosis is similar to that for patients who undergo pancreaticoduodenectomy alone.

M.J. Pentecost, M.D.

Percutaneous Drainage of Fluid Collections in the Extremities
Wu HP, Vesely TM (Washington Univ, St Louis)
Radiology 208:159-165, 1998 6–16

Background.—The insertion of drainage catheters into abscesses for temporization or cure is an alternative to open-incision drainage. There have been several reports of the efficacy of percutaneous drainage of intra-abdominal fluid collection, but less information about percutaneous drainage of fluid collection in the extremities is available.

Methods.—Between 1990 and 1997, 28 patients had percutaneous drainage of 33 fluid collections in the extremities. The patients were 14 to 90 years old. Fluid collection was in the hip-groin area in 16 patients, in the thigh in 6 patients, buttocks in 6 patients, knee in 3 patients, calf in 1 patient, and axilla in 1 patient. There were 2 intra-articular collections. Prior procedures were surgical drainage in 8 patients, needle aspiration in 10 patients, and surgical débridement in 1 patient. US localization and fluoroscopy were the most common guidance methods.

Results.—Drainage was maintained for 1 to 93 days. Cavity size was estimated at 4 cm^3 to 733 cm^3. Purulent fluid was found in 13 patients. Lymphoceles were found in 9 patients, 5 of whom had sclerotherapy. The most common organism was *Staphylococcus aureus* (9 patients). Two patients had 2 complications each; 1 complication was major. Failure occurred in 16% of 25 patients; 2 of these patients had repeat drainage for recurrence and 2 had surgery. Three patients were lost to follow-up.

Discussion.—Percutaneous drainage of fluid collection in the extremities was an effective alternative to open-incision drainage. Percutaneous drainage may be appropriate for inpatient and outpatient settings. It can relieve local symptoms and normalize indices of infection, which make it ideal for palliation or temporization in debilitated patients.

► Remarkably little attention has been paid to the percutaneous drainage of fluid collections of the extremities, despite the widespread acceptance of such procedures in the abdomen and chest. Wu details the Mallinckrodt experience in an eclectic group of cases, including cancerous and benign, sterile and infected, and upper and lower extremity. This will be a tougher sell because the alternative surgical methods aren't invasive either. That said, an 84% success rate is encouraging, and the area is deserving of more attention and refinement.

M.J. Pentecost, M.D.

Life-threatening Primary Postpartum Hemorrhage: Treatment With Emergency Selective Arterial Embolization

Pelage J-P, Le Dref O, Mateo J, et al (Hôpital Lariboisière, Paris)
Radiology 208:359-362, 1998 6–17

Purpose.—The safety and efficacy of emergency arterial embolization in women with intractable primary postpartum hemorrhage were determined.

Methods.—Uterine embolization was performed in 27 consecutive women with life-threatening primary postpartum hemorrhage. All patients had intractable hemorrhage that could not be controlled by vaginal packing or uterotonic drugs. Before embolization, the mean hemoglobin level was 7.48 g/dL. In 2 patients, hysterectomy performed before embolization did not stop the bleeding.

Results.—Angiography showed extravasation in 9 women and spasm of the internal iliac artery branches in 5 women. Procedures included embolization of 46 uterine arteries, 5 vaginal arteries, and 2 ovarian arteries, and anterior division of 8 internal iliac arteries. External bleeding disappeared immediately or decreased significantly in all patients. Two women had repeat embolization the next day. There were no major complications related to embolization. Delayed hysterectomy was performed in 1 patient with placenta accreta. After embolization, normal menstruation resumed in all women who did not have hysterectomy, and 1 woman became pregnant.

Discussion.—Emergency selective arterial embolization is safe and effective for treating intractable primary postpartum hemorrhage. With arterial embolization, high-risk surgery can be avoided and the patient's reproductive ability can be maintained.

► Pelage and colleagues report by far the largest experience to date of transcatheter embolization in the treatment of postpartum hemorrhage. Despite the seemingly ideal nature of gelfoam as an embolic agent in this setting, the authors substituted polyvinyl alcohol in some patients because of the fear of transmitting Creutzfeldt-Jakob disease with the former. Yikes!

M.J. Pentecost, M.D.

Percutaneous Thrombolysis and Stent Placement for the Treatment of Portal Vein Thrombosis After Liver Transplantation: Long-term Follow-Up

Cherukuri R, Haskai ZJ, Naji A, et al (Univ of Pennsylvania, Philadelphia)

Transplantation 65:1124-1126, 1998 6–18

Purpose.—The rate of portal vein thrombosis (PVT) after liver transplantation is 1% to 2%. A wide range of treatment options have been described, but there have been few reports of local thrombolytic therapy with metallic stent placement. Two cases of posttransplant PVT managed with this minimally invasive approach are reported, and the long-term results are described.

Patients.—The patients were 2 women, aged 40 and 45, one undergoing secondary liver transplantation. Within 1 month after transplant, graft dysfunction developed, manifested by elevated liver enzymes or marked ascites. The diagnosis of PVT was confirmed by sonography and angiography. Both patients were managed with percutaneous thrombolysis. To reach the occluded portal vein, transjugular transhepatic puncture was performed in 1 patient and direct transhepatic catheterization in the other. Intraportal infusion of urokinase was performed for thrombolysis (Fig 1). One patient underwent balloon angioplasty to clear residual thrombus (Fig 2). Palmaz stents or Wallstents were then placed to restore brisk portal flow (Fig 3). There were no complications. At 2½ and 4½ years' follow-up, both patients had continued portal vein and stent patency and good graft function.

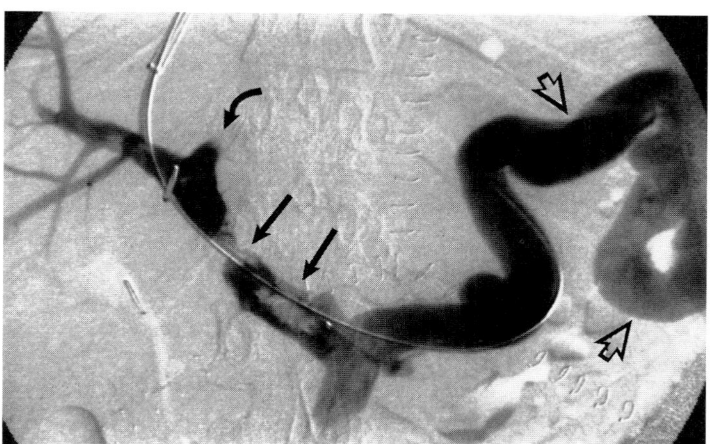

FIGURE 1.—After partial thrombolysis, the stenotic anastomosis is visible. A residual clot remains within the main portal vein, at the anastomosis (*arrows*) and within the occluded left portal vein (*curved arrow*). A large competitive native splenorenal shunt is present (*open arrows*). (Courtesy of Cherukuri R, Haskai ZJ, Naji A, et al: Percutaneous thrombolysis and stent placement for the treatment of portal vein thrombosis after liver transplantation: long-term follow-up. *Transplantation* 65:1124-1126, 1998.)

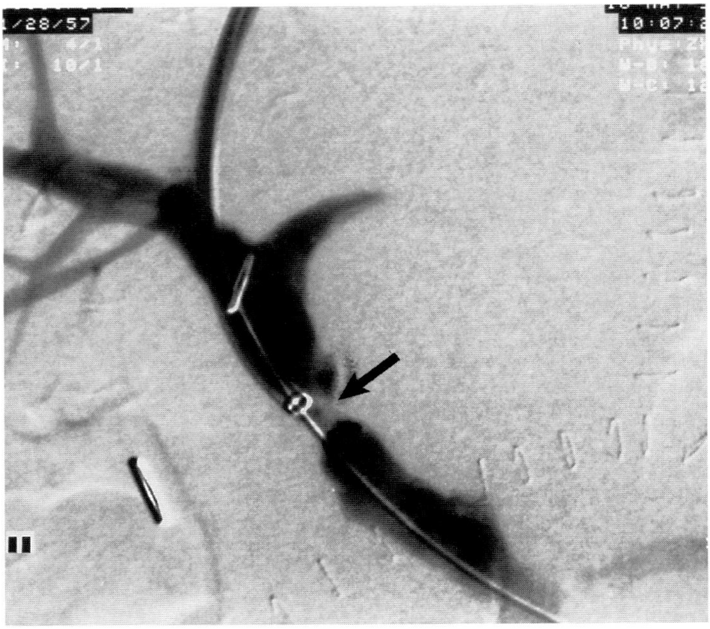

FIGURE 2.—Postangioplasty appearance of portal anastomosis demonstrates significant residual stenosis (*arrow*). (Courtesy of Cherukuri R, Haskai ZJ, Naji A, et al: Percutaneous thrombolysis and stent placement for the treatment of portal vein thrombosis after liver transplantation: Long-term follow-up. *Transplantation* 65:1124-1126, 1998.)

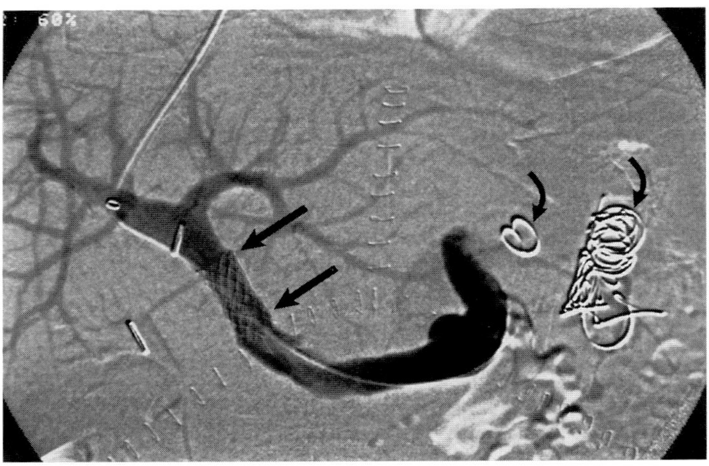

FIGURE 3.—The final image demonstrates full restoration of patency to the intrahepatic and extrahepatic portal vein. The main portal vein stent is seen (*arrows*). Embolization coils within the splenorenal shunt are present (*curved arrows*). (Courtesy of Cherukuri R, Haskai ZJ, Naji A, et al: Percutaneous thrombolysis and stent placement for the treatment of portal vein thrombosis after liver transplantation: Long-term follow-up. *Transplantation* 65:1124-1126, 1998.)

Discussion.—This experience demonstrates the safety and effectiveness of percutaneous thrombolysis and stent placement for patients with PVT after liver transplantation. The intervention restores brisk portal flow, thus providing good long-term patency. Percutaneous thrombolysis is safe, even in the perioperative period. A transjugular intrahepatic portosystemic shunt-type approach may reduce the risk of bleeding from the transhepatic puncture site.

► Percutaneous interventions have been a boon to the field of liver transplantation—most notably TIPS as a temporizing measure before surgery. This report chronicles a similar technique but *after* transplantation in the patient in whom stenosis develops at the venous anastomosis. Also, the report dispels some of the appropriate concerns about the durability of metal stents within the portal venous circulation.

M.J. Pentecost, M.D.

Aneurysms of the Mid Axillary Artery in Major League Baseball Pitchers—A Report of Two Cases

Todd GJ, Benvenisty AI, Hershon S, et al (Columbia Univ, New York)
J Vasc Surg 28:702-707, 1998 6–19

Introduction.—True aneurysms of the axillary artery and its branches are rarely detected. Recent successful repairs of symptomatic aneurysms of the axillary arteries at the origin of the circumflex humeral arteries in 2 major league baseball pitchers are described.

Case Report 1.—Man, 33, a right-handed pitcher, was seen with recent history of numbness, cyanosis, and reduced temperature of the fingers of his right hand. Symptoms were intensified after pitching and in cold weather. He had no history of pain in the arm or shoulder. All pulses of the arm and hand were palpable and there were no bruits or abnormal pulsations of the neck, chest wall, supraclavicular fossa, or right upper extremity. There were no neurological deficits and no cervical ribs. There were punctate areas of digital ischemia consistent with embolic events on the right second, third, and fourth fingers. A duplex ultrasound scan did not show any evidence of aneurysmal or occlusive disease in the subclavian, axillary, or brachial arteries. Plethysmographic studies of the digital arteries revealed markedly flattened curves in the right second, third, and fourth fingers, with normal tracings of the first and fifth fingers and all fingers of the left hand. An incomplete palmar arch and partial occlusion of the digital arteries of the second, third, and fourth fingers, consistent with emboli, were detected on conventional contrast arteriogram (Fig 1) and an aneurysm was seen at the junction of the right axillary, anterior circumflex humeral, and posterior circumflex humeral arteries (Fig 2).

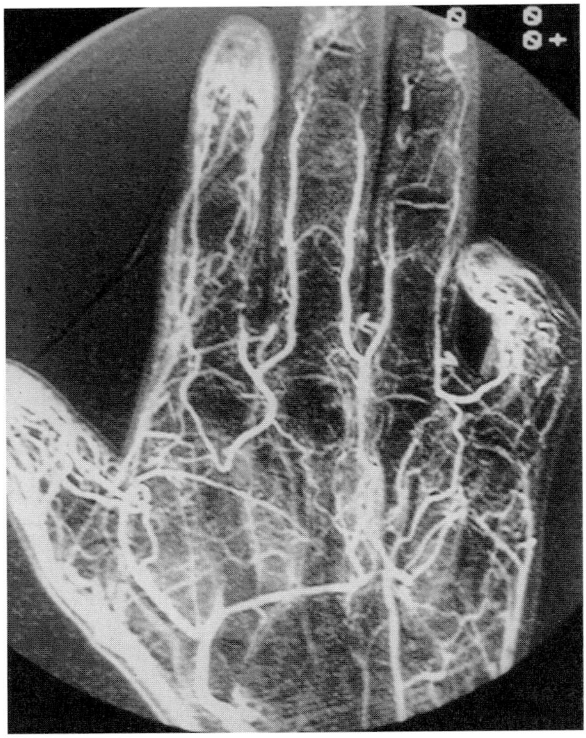

FIGURE 1.—Case 1. Arteriogram shows partial occlusion of digital arteries of second, third, and fourth fingers of right hand. (Courtesy of Todd GJ, Benvenisty AI, Hershon S: Aneurysms of mid axillary artery in major league baseball pitchers—A report of two cases. *J Vasc Surg* 289:702-707, 1998.)

Intra-arterial urokinase was infused for 36 hours. The patient had subjective improvement and improved color and temperature of the hand. He underwent surgical repair and had an uneventful recovery. He won the pivotal game of the World Series 5.5 months after aneurysm repair.

Case Report 2.—Man 27, a right-handed pitcher, was seen for numbness and cyanosis of the right second finger. His medical history was unremarkable and he had no history of pain in the arm or shoulder. All pulses of the arm and hand were normal and there were no abnormal pulsations or bruits. Angiography revealed an aneurysm of the right axillary artery at its junction with the anterior and posterior circumflex humeral arteries. He underwent repair of the aneurysm and was doing well, in a rehabilitation program, at 6-week follow-up.

Conclusion.—Aneurysm of the mid-axillary artery should be suspected in all athletes with hand pain, numbness, or signs of digital ischemia.

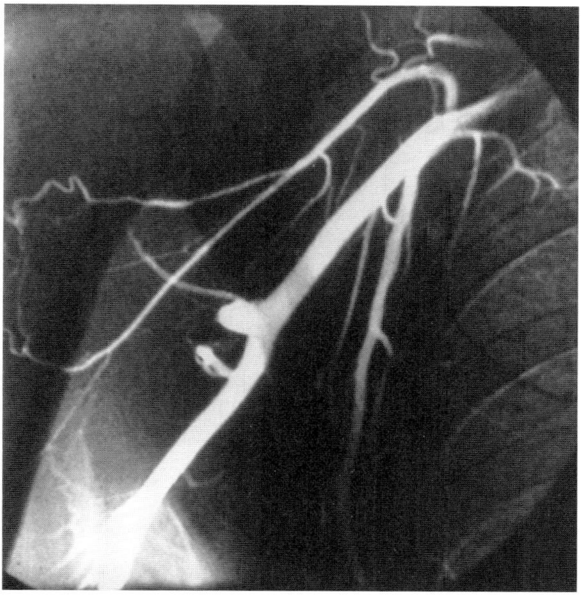

FIGURE 2.—Case 1. Arteriogram shows aneurysm at junction of right axillary artery with circumflex humeral arteries. (Courtesy of Todd GJ, Benvenisty AI, Hershon S: Aneurysms of mid axillary artery in major league baseball pitchers—A report of two cases. *J Vasc Surg* 28?:702-707, 1998.)

► These 2 cases were well-chronicled in the New York Times sports page. Todd's scientific report is very interesting, particularly as a counterpoint to the lay press descriptions. In these examples and other reports, saphenous veins were the grafts of choice. The discussion section of this article describes other shoulder vessel injuries in different types of athletes (eg, posterior circumflex aneurysms in volleyball players). Thank heaven, golfers seem immune to such injuries.

M.J. Pentecost, M.D.

Iliac Arterial Occlusive Disease: Cost-effectiveness Analysis of Stent Placement Versus Percutaneous Transluminal Angioplasty

Bosch JL, for the Dutch Iliac Stent Trial Study Group (Univ of Groningen, The Netherlands)

Radiology 208:641-648, 1998 6–20

Introduction.—Stents are often placed selectively when angioplasty outcomes are suboptimal and are sometimes chosen for primary treatment. The cost-effectiveness of both approaches has not been addressed. The relative benefits and cost-effectiveness of using primary stent placement, percutaneous transluminal angioplasty (PTA), or PTA with selective stent placement to treat lifestyle-limiting claudication caused by iliac arterial stenosis was examined.

Methods.—The cost-effectiveness of treatment was examined in a hypothetical patient cohort with intermittent claudication caused by an iliac arterial stenosis. This hypothetical cohort was followed up over time and a decision and cost-effectiveness analysis was undertaken with the use of a multistate transition (Markov process) model. Alternative treatments, including drug therapy, exercise, or surgery, were not considered. Costs and benefits, expressed as quality-adjusted life years, of the initial procedures and the events during follow-up were calculated. The model combined data from a randomized, controlled trial (the Dutch Iliac Stent Trial) and from published meta-analysis. Complication rates, patency results, and decreases in risk of failure were taken from the meta-analysis. Variables, baseline values, and ranges were examined with sensitivity analysis.

Results.—Mean total costs of primary stent placement, PTA with selective stent placement, and PTA alone were $3,990, $3,033, and $2,343, respectively. The Dutch Iliac Stent Trial showed that PTA with selective stent placement had complication rates, patency results, and quality-of-life outcomes equivalent to those of primary stent placement. The PTA procedure with selective stent placement had higher patency rates, and quality-adjusted life expectancy and had an incremental cost-effectiveness ratio of less than $20,000 per quality-adjusted life year gained, compared with PTA alone.

Conclusion.—The PTA procedure with selective stent placement is a cost-effective strategy, compared with PTA alone, in the treatment of iliac arterial occlusive disease. The gain in effectiveness justifies the additional cost.

► Bosch and colleagues provide a splendid analysis that is important on different levels. First, these economic modeling studies provide powerful tools with which to look at new treatments. Long before such therapies, they can be the subject of controlled trials. That is not to say that such analyses are a substitute for randomized trials, but every day in the real world, practitioners are placed in the predicament of deciding when to use a new device—in this case, primary iliac stenting—and these studies can have a profound effect in the interim. Also, such methods can be invaluable in guiding payment policies before more rigorous analysis is available.

M.J. Pentecost, M.D.

Medical Outcomes Studies in Peripheral Vascular Disease

Murphy TP (Brown Univ, Providence, RI)

JVIR 9:879-889, 1998 6–21

Purpose.—Medical outcomes studies play an increasingly important role in health care research and reimbursement. These studies seek to measure health status from the patients' perspective, including their perceptions of their physical, social, and emotional lives. Current knowledge regarding medical outcomes studies and their use in patients with peripheral vascular disease was reviewed.

Medical Outcomes Studies.—Medical outcomes studies can be broadly classified as utility measurements and health profiles. Utility measures assign a value to patients' perceptions of health status for the purpose of comparing alternative therapies. Simple utility measures are determined using such techniques as rating scales, the standard gamble, the time tradeoff, and, less frequently willingness to pay. Utility measures may be used to calculate quality-adjusted life-years, and cost data can be used to perform cost-benefit or cost-effectiveness analyses. More complex health profile measures use questions addressing the patients' physical, emotional, and social well-being. Some generic health profile questionnaires are the Sickness Impact Profile and the Medical Outcome Study Short-Form 36. The Walking Impairment Questionnaire is an example of a disease-specific health profile. The results are interpreted by comparison with published norms or by comparing pretreatment and posttreatment scores. Unfortunately, health profile measures show poor correlation with utility measures.

Medical Outcomes Studies in Peripheral Vascular Disease.—Several studies have gathered baseline health profiles data on patients with intermittent claudication. These patients report significant deficits in health status, particularly in the areas of physical functioning, bodily pain, social interaction, and emotional health. Some studies have noted sleep problems as well. These reductions in quality of life should be considered in deciding on treatment options for intermittent claudication. Studies of conservative management suggest that exercise therapy can improve physical functioning and bodily pain, although its impact on social, emotional, and role functioning has yet to be demonstrated. Studies have also shown quality-of-life improvements in patients undergoing invasive revascularization. Despite some conflicting results, patients with better baseline functioning, less severe symptoms, and less co-morbidity are more likely to improve. Improvements occur not only in physical functioning and bodily pain but also in vitality, activities, and mental well-being. Cost-effectiveness analyses suggest that a revascularization procedure with a lower patency yield can be cost effective if the risks are lower than with the alternative.

Summary.—Medical outcomes studies have the potential to provide valuable information on the treatment of patients with peripheral vascular disease. The reliance on conservative management for patients with intermittent claudication does not consider the patient's perceptions of health-related quality of life. Unlike exercise therapy, revascularization can improve scores in such areas as vitality and mental well-being. Medical outcomes studies have a potentially important role to play in the evaluation of new percutaneous therapies for patients with peripheral vascular disease.

► History will judge this analysis by Murphy and the corresponding work by Kazmers (Abstract 6–1) (1999) very well. This report is the essence and epitome of outcomes research. That is, using broader, more holistic measures, such as patient preference and quality-of-life, is at least as valid as the typical biological markers such as ankle-brachial index, patency rates, etc. Such analysis can overturn longstanding and widely-held tenets—in this case, the nonoperative or noninterventional management of claudication.

M.J. Pentecost, M.D.

Determinants of Chronic Venous Disease After Acute Deep Venous Thrombosis

Meissner MH, Caps MT, Zierler BK, et al (Univ of Washington, Seattle; Mountain-Whisper-Light Statistical Consulting, Seattle)

J Vasc Surg 28:826-833, 1998 6–22

Background.—The Society for Vascular Surgery/North American Chapter of the International Society for Cardiovascular Surgery standards for reporting of acute and chronic venous disease include a scoring system for thrombotic risk factors, a description of thrombus location and extent, and a definition of diagnostic and treatment standards. These standards were used to assess the relationship between the initial features of acute deep venous thrombosis (DVT) and the natural history and ultimate outcome of the thrombus.

Methods.—Serial clinical and ultrasound examinations were performed in 73 limbs of 68 patients with acute DVT. The extent of the thrombus through 7 venous segments was scored retrospectively, on a scale of 0 to 3, and segmental reflux was scored as present or not present. These grades were used to calculate initial and final thrombus scores, recanalization and recurrent thrombosis rates, and total reflux scores, all of which were assessed as potential predictors of final chronic venous disease (CVD) classification.

Results.—Mean follow-up was 55 months. At the end of follow-up, 27% of limbs were asymptomatic, 18% had pain or prominent superficial veins, 34% had edema, 18% had hyperpigmentation, and 3% were ulcerated. Final CVD classification was correlated with reflux score, but not with initial or final thrombus score or with recanalization or rethrombus rate, on univariate analysis. The only significant predictor of CVD classification on multivariate analysis was tibial thrombosis score. The ability to predict final outcome was greater in a model including follow-up variables such as final reflux score, final popliteal score, and recanalization rate.

Conclusions.—Information on an acute episode of DVT is of limited value in predicting the final severity of CVD. The presenting features of the DVT are less useful in this regard than information on the subsequent natural history of the thrombus. Among the factors affecting the final CVD classification are the extent of reflux, the presence of persistent popliteal obstruction, and the recanalization rate; other factors remain to be identified.

► Before everyone jumps on the bandwagon, it is not altogether obvious that venous thrombolysis will be effective. Sure, clot will be busted aplenty. Veins will be recanalized—you betcha. Patients will tolerate the procedure well—almost certainly. But prevent chronic venous insufficiency?—not so clear. The articles of Browse[1] and Lindhagen[2] suggest that chronic venous insufficiency may be independent of the previous presence or absence of venous thrombosis in the affected extremity. Nonetheless, Meissner and Strandness continue their very productive work in this area. Their thesis is logical: faster clot dissolution leads to less incompetent venous valves, competent valves result in less reflux or retrograde flow, diminished reflux prevents or reduces chronic venous insufficiency—we hope.

M.J. Pentecost, M.D.

References

1. Browse NL, Clemenson G, Thomas ML: Is the postphlebitic leg always postphlebitic? Relation between phlebographic appearances of deep-vein thrombosis and late sequelae. *BMJ* 281:1167-1170, 1980.
2. Lindhagen A, Bergqvist D, Hallbrook T et al: Venous function five to eight years after clinically suspected deep venous thrombosis. *Acta Med Scand* 217:389-395, 1985.

Brachytherapy for Prophylaxis of Restenosis After Long-Segment Femoropopliteal Angioplasty: Pilot Study

Minar E, Pokrajac B, Ahmadi R, et al (Univ Clinic Vienna)
Radiology 208:173-179, 1998 6–23

Introduction.—Restenosis with poor long-term results has been a major limitation of the clinical usefulness of percutaneous transluminal angioplasty. Chronic vessel constriction, or remodeling, and neointima hyperplasia by cell proliferation are the 2 primary phenomena that contribute to restenosis after successful angioplasty. No previous studies have examined postangioplasty irradiation without stent implantation. The feasibility and efficacy of endovascular brachytherapy for prophylaxis of restenosis after angioplasty without stent implantation in patients at high risk of restenosis were evaluated.

Methods.—Percutaneous transluminal angioplasty followed by endovascular irradiation with high–dose-rate afterloading of an iridium-192 rod was performed on 10 patients (6 women, 4 men; mean age, 68 years) who had long-segment restenosis, with a mean length of 16 cm, ranging from 9 to 22 cm.

Results.—In all patients, irradiation was technically feasible without complications. The dilated and irradiated segment remained widely patent in 6 patients at color US. After 12 months, there were corresponding excellent hemodynamic and clinical results (Fig 2a). Recurrence was indicated in the clinical and laboratory findings of 4 patients. Restenosis was

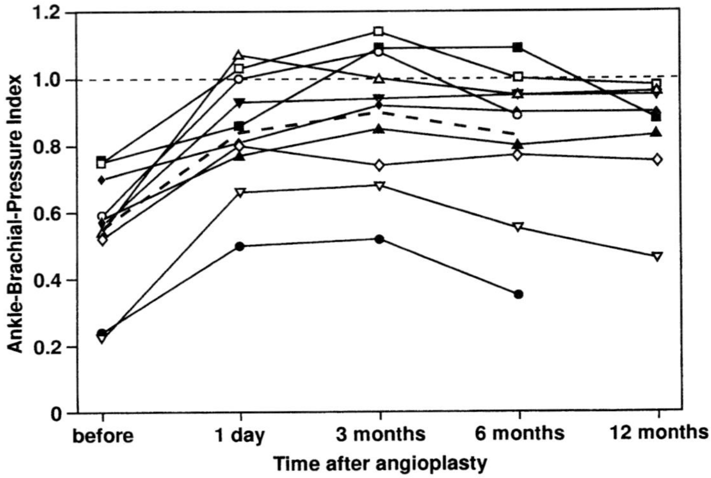

FIGURE 2.—A, Ankle brachial pressure index versus time before and after angioplasty. Mean (*bold dashed line*) and individual values for the 10 patients are graphed. The *dotted line* at an ankle brachial pressure index of 1.0 is indicative of at least 50% stenosis. Values below the *dotted line* are abnormal. *Open circle*, patient 1; *solid circle*, patient 2; *open triangle*, patient 3; *solid triangle*, patient 4; *open square*, patient 5; *solid square*, patient 6; *open inverted triangle*, patient 7; *solid inverted triangle*, patient 8; *open diamond*, patient 9; *solid diamond*, patient 10. (Courtesy of Minar E, Pokrajac B, Ahmadi R, et al: Brachytherapy for prophylaxis of restenosis after long-segment femoropopliteal angioplasty: Pilot study. *Radiology* 208: 173-179, 1998. Radiological Society of North America.)

demonstrated with arteriography, with a diameter reduction of 60%, 70%, 80%, or 90%.

Conclusion.—Concerning the possibility of reduction of restenosis by means of endovascular brachytherapy, the results of this study are promising. The value of this approach should be determined definitively in randomized trials.

► If the results of this study are promising, the authors are real optimists. Twelve patients (not 10) entered this trial and, at the end of 1 year, 6 patients had subjective evidence of therapeutic benefit—maybe. That is a 50% 1-year patency rate. And this patency rate is based on: (1) color-flow US, which is very unreliable in the superficial femoral artery, and (2) patient symptoms (all well and good, but not really dependable). Vascular brachytherapy probably does work in preventing restenosis, especially in small vessels such as the coronaries, but this article adds little to our knowledge of the place of this technique in the peripheral circulation.

M.J. Pentecost, M.D.

Two-Year Follow-up After Catheter-based Radiotherapy to Inhibit Coronary Restenosis

Teirstein PS, Massullo V, Jani S, et al (Scripps Clinic, La Jolla, Calif)

Circulation 99:243-247, 1999 6–24

Background.—Studies have shown that intravascular radiation therapy can prevent restenosis after angioplasty. The longer-term effects of this therapy, however, are not known. Will radiation therapy now increase complications caused by aneurysm formation later? And will the effects of radiation be permanent, or merely delay the redevelopment of restenosis? Patients were studied 2 years after they underwent radiation therapy of restenotic coronary arteries.

Methods.—In this double-blind study, 55 patients with restenosis after coronary angioplasty were randomized to receive either placebo (n = 29) or radiation therapy with ^{192}Ir (dose of 800 to 3,000 cGy; n = 26). In both groups, the study drug was sealed and delivered on a 0.76-mm ribbon into an infusion catheter. Six months later, patients returned for repeat coronary angiography. Between 24 and 33 months after their treatment, patients were contacted so that the authors could evaluate the number of survivors, the incidence of myocardial infarction, and the need for revascularization.

Findings.—Two patients in each group died. The 2 patients receiving placebo died of myocardial infarction. Patient receiving ^{192}Ir died during bypass surgery 23 months after treatment and the other died because of complications of abdominal surgery for diverticulitis at 18 months after treatment. Myocardial infarction occurred in 2 patients in the placebo group and 1 patient in the ^{192}Ir group. Similarly, the revascularization of nontarget lesions did not differ between the placebo and ^{192}Ir groups (20.7% vs 19.2%). There was a great increase in nontarget-lesion revascularizations between years 1 and 2 of follow-up in both the placebo (from 13.8% to 20.7%) and ^{192}Ir (from 3.9% to 19.2%) groups. On the other hand, revascularization of target lesions was significantly less common in the ^{192}Ir group (44.8% vs 15.4%). When the outcomes of death, myocardial infarction, and target-lesion revascularization were combined, patients who received ^{192}Ir were at significantly less risk than those taking placebo (23.1% vs 51.7%). Only 1 of the patients in the ^{192}Ir group required "late" (at 11 months) revascularization of a target lesion.

Conclusions.—At 2 years after treatment of restenotic coronary arteries, patients who received ^{192}Ir required significantly less target-lesion revascularization than those receiving placebo. Thus, the effects of ^{192}Ir in reducing stenosis appear to be permanent. Rates of nontarget-lesion revascularization hovered at 20% in both groups, and increased during the second year of follow-up. During follow-up angiography, none of the patients in the ^{192}Ir group experienced late untoward events. Based on these intermediate results, radiotherapy appears to be effective in treating stenosis.

► Though not an angiographic study, this article is a clinical follow-up of the previously reported trial in which catheter-based ^{132}Ir was used to prevent restenosis after percutaneous transluminal coronary angioplasty.[1] Within the limits of telephone follow-up, the results are encouraging: 15% of lesions that were treated with vascular brachytherapy required further therapy, whereas 45% of areas in the control arm required additional angioplasty or surgery. As an internal control, revascularization of untreated lesions was similar (19% and 21%).

M.J. Pentecost, M.D.

Reference

1. Tierstein PS, Massullo V, Jani S, et al: Catheter-based radiotherapy to inhibit restenosis after coronary stenting. *N Engl J Med* 336:1697-1703, 1997.

Pseudoaneurysm of the Cystic Artery: A Rare Cause of Hemobilia

Kaman L, Kumar S, Behera A, et al (Postgraduate Inst of Med Education and Research, Chandigarh, India)

Am J Gastroenterol 93:1535-1537, 1998 6–25

Background.—Hemobilia may rarely result from erosions of the intrahepatic or extrahepatic bile ducts associated with various conditions. The case of a patient with cystic artery pseudoaneurysm causing hemobilia was reported.

Case Report.—Woman, 32, was evaluated for upper abdominal pain, jaundice, and a 2-week history of low-grade hematemesis and melena. On emergency admission, she had blood pressure of 80/60 mm Hg, a pulse of 110 beats/min, and hepatomegaly, with elevated levels of total bilirubin, aspartate aminotransferase, alanine aminotransferase, and alkaline phosphatase. Immediately after resuscitation, the patient underwent upper gastrointestinal endoscopy, which showed blood in the fundus and blood coming out of the papilla. US showed gallbladder distention with clots and echogenic areas within the lumen. The diagnosis of aneurysm was suggested by the color Doppler finding of persistent pulsatile flow within the echogenic lesion. CT showed only gallbladder thickening with a few stones. Selective hepatic artery angiography was performed and showed a 1-cm aneurysm of the cystic artery. Laparotomy confirmed the diagnosis of cystic artery pseudoaneurysm with acute calculous cholecystitis. The patient recovered after cholecystectomy and cystic artery ligation with proximal control of the hepatic artery.

Discussion.—Cystic artery pseudoaneurysm is a rare cause of hemobilia. Less than 10 such cases have been reported, always in association with gallbladder inflammation. The diagnosis can be made using selective hepatic angiography. Other useful studies include upper gastrointestinal endoscopy and color Doppler US.

► Sure enough, diagnostic angiography is slipping away. The advent of helical CT and MRI have made tremendous inroads into catheter-based interarterial arteriography. Furthermore, radionuclide imaging can allegedly detect minute gastrointestinal hemorrhage (although it has been generally disappointing to me), and the new idea of detecting extravasation into the intestinal lumen on CT or MRI (truly a brilliant idea) promises to cut into our business even more.

So, when a condition comes along, even as a case report, that will probably be diagnosed with conventional angiography, it is encouraging. Such is the case for pseudoaneurysm of the cystic artery causing hemobilia and secondary gastrointestinal hemorrhage. Mention that at surgery grounds and wait for the calls.

M.J. Pentecost, M.D.

Variation in Carotid Endarterectomy Mortality in the Medicare Population: Trial Hospitals, Volume, and Patient Characteristics

Wennberg DE, Lucas FL, Birkmeyer JD, et al (Maine Med Ctr, Portland; Maine Med Assessment Found, Augusta; Dartmouth Med School, Hanover, NH; et al)

JAMA 279:1278-1281, 1998 6–26

Introduction.—According to the 2 largest studies of carotid endarterectomy (CEA), the procedure effectively reduces the risk of stroke and death if performed in centers of excellence, with a low risk of perioperative stroke and death. The 30-day mortality rate at the study centers was very low: 0.6% in the North American Symptomatic Carotid Endarterecomy Trial (NASCET) and 0.1% in the Asymptomatic Carotid Atherosclerosis Study (ACAS). The perioperative mortality among patients undergoing CEA at other hospitals was assessed.

Methods.—The retrospective analysis examined perioperative mortality among 113,300 Medicare patients undergoing CEA over a 2-year period. The procedure was done at 86 NASCET or ACAS hospitals (6,510 patients) and at 2,613 nonfederal institutions (106, 790 patients). The 2 groups were compared for crude and adjusted 30-day mortality rates. The nontrial hospitals were grouped according to CEA volume.

Results.—The perioperative mortality rate was 1.4% at the trial hospitals, significantly higher than in nontrial hospitals. It was 1.7% at high-volume hospitals, 1.9% at average-volume hospitals, and 2.5% at low-volume hospitals. On multivariate analysis, mortality risk was significantly reduced for patients operated on at trial hospitals. It was reduced by 15% compared with high-volume hospitals, 25% compared with average-volume hospitals, and 43% compared with low-volume hospitals.

Conclusion.—This national cohort study suggests that perioperative mortality among Medicare patients undergoing CEA is higher than that reported in the NASCET and ACAS trials. This was shown to be so even at the trial hospitals. The discrepancy between the reported efficacy of CEA in asymptomatic patients and its routine effectiveness is of particular concern.

► The Dartmouth and Maine Medical Assessment Foundation groups have made yet another contribution to our understanding of variation in medical practice. In this case, they examined the mortality from CEA in a Medicare population and compared this with the published trials from the NASCET and ACAS reports. Their conclusion: the mortality rate after carotid endarterectomy is much higher in this group of patients than in the published reports.

This, of course, is the age-old problem of efficacy versus ineffectiveness. That is, an expert develops a new procedure and, by the very nature of concentration in 1 area, performs the surgery, interventional procedure, or whatever better than one who is doing many other things. Yet, standards of practice are developed based on published reports of efficacy (that is, the expert practitioner's publication of results) when, in reality, the real question is effectiveness (that is, how well the procedure is applied to a large population of patients). There is nothing devious about this discrepancy; in fact, it happens every day in medicine. Rather, it is the inevitable consequence of expert versus generalist practice. The real lesson is that we must study effectiveness in addition to efficacy to more completely understand the impact of a new surgery, a new device, or a new drug on our patients.

M.J. Pentecost, M.D.

One-step Needle Aspiration and Lavage for the Treatment of Abdominal and Pelvic Abscesses

Wroblicka JT, Kuligowska E (Boston Med Ctr)

AJR 170:1197-1203, 1998 6–27

Purpose.—Percutaneous catheter drainage under imaging guidance is an effective treatment for abdominal and pelvic abscesses. However, serious complications of this procedure have been reported, with a mortality rate as high as 14% and morbidity as high as 10%. One-step needle aspiration and lavage is a potentially advantageous alternative. This approach was evaluated for use in the treatment of abdominal, retroperitoneal, and pelvic abscesses.

Methods.—The 16-year experience included 82 patients undergoing needle aspiration and lavage of 97 nonenteric, nonpancreatic abdominal and pelvic abscesses. All procedures were performed in a single session using US or CT guidance. Aspiration and saline lavage were performed through an 18-gauge needle, without catheter drainage after the procedure. If the collection was multiloculated, the needle was repositioned for repeat aspiration and lavage during the same session. Management included IV antibiotics for up to 1 week after the procedure. All patients underwent follow-up sonography or CT.

Results.—Needle aspiration and lavage was successful in 90% of abscesses, including 85% of multiloculated abscesses. There were 2 complications: 1 case of transient sepsis and 1 case of hemorrhage requiring transfusion. Fluid reaccumulations were considered treatment failures. Conditions associated with such failures included diffuse peritonitis, occult malignancy, unsuspected enteric communication, and dropped surgical clip.

Conclusion.—For patients with abdominal and pelvic abscesses, 1-step percutaneous needle aspiration and lavage offers a safe and effective alternative to percutaneous catheter drainage. Even if the abscess is multiloculated, needle aspiration and lavage should be considered the initial therapy for patients with focal abscesses larger than 3 cm. If fluid reaccumulates, needle aspiration and lavage should be repeated only if the patient's clinical condition is improving.

▶ One great thing about the minimally invasive or interventional therapies is the inherent way these techniques challenge established medical practices. Draining an abscess with a small catheter was considered heresy when first conceived but now has been proven in thousands of patients.

Now someone wants to just aspirate material and not even leave it in a catheter. Why, this is crazy. Maybe so, but it seems to work also. For sure, the patients, when this technique is used, must be carefully selected and followed. But, nonetheless, one can imagine a group of patients that will be well served with this technique and be spared the time, inconvenience, and morbidity of indwelling catheter drainage.

M.J. Pentecost, M.D.

Difference in Acetylcholine-induced Nitric Oxide Release of Arterial and Venous Grafts in Patients After Coronary Bypass Operations

Nishioka H, Kitamura S, Kameda Y, et al (Nara Med Univ, Japan)

J Thorac Cardiovasc Surg 116:454-459, 1998 6–28

Purpose.—Internal thoracic artery (ITA) grafts offer numerous advantages over venous grafts in coronary artery revascularization. In vitro studies suggest that these 2 grafts differ in terms of nitric oxide (NO) released from endothelial cells. An in vivo study was performed to compare acetylcholine-induced NO release in ITAs versus saphenous veins after coronary artery bypass grafting, as well as the metabolic function of the 2 grafts.

Methods.—The study included 39 patients who had undergone coronary artery bypass grafting a mean of 43 months earlier. Twenty-four ITA grafts were compared with 16 saphenous vein grafts. The mean patient ages were 65 and 68 years, respectively. By selective catheterization, blood was sampled from the distal end of the graft before and after infusion of acetylcholine, 5 μg. Concentrations of NO in these samples were measured as plasma nitrite level by the Griess reaction. After blood sampling, angiography was performed for analysis by cine-densitometry.

Results.—Compared with baseline, plasma nitrite concentration in the arterial grafts rose 34% by 4 minutes after acetylcholine infusion and by 87% at 6 minutes. Corresponding values in the venous grafts were 1% and 8%, respectively. Coronary arteries supplied by arterial grafts dilated 6.3% in response to acetylcholine, whereas those supplied by venous grafts were reduced in diameter by 9.8%.

Conclusion.—This in vivo study demonstrates greater release of NO by ITA grafts than by saphenous vein grafts in coronary artery bypass patients. Thus, ITA grafting may result in transplantation of functional endothelial cells into the coronary circulation. This metabolic effect may protect ITA grafts and the coronary arteries they supply against spasm and atherosclerosis.

► It is hard to believe that it has been little over a decade since endothelium-derived relaxing factor was identified as NO. In that short time, a Nobel prize has been awarded and investigations have defined the omnipresent significance of NO in vascular physiology. Much of the research has been done in vitro. Nishioka and colleagues detail an interesting analysis of acetylcholine-induced NO release in ITA compared with saphenous vein grafts.

M.J. Pentecost, M.D.

Scraping of Aortic Debris by Coronary Guiding Catheters: A Prospective Evaluation of 1,000 Cases

Keeley EC, Grines CL (William Beaumont Hosp, Royal Oak, Mich)

J Am Coll Cardiol 32:1861-1865, 1998 6–29

Background.—The higher complication rate of percutaneous revascularization procedures compared with diagnostic catheterization may be related to the stiff, large-bore guiding catheters used. The authors have observed atheromatous debris exiting the back of guiding catheters during advancement. This study evaluated the incidence and amount of aortic atherosclerotic debris scraped off by guiding catheters during percutaneous interventions.

Methods.—The prospective study included 1,000 consecutive percutaneous procedures. During each intervention, the amount of visible atheromatous material retrieved from the large-lumen guiding catheter was graded on a scale of 1+ to 3+ (Fig 3). The clinical characteristics and in-hospital complications associated with debris were analyzed.

Results.—The Judkins left and multipurpose catheters were most likely to produce visible aortic debris, doing so in 60% or more of procedures. Catheters associated with large debris—grade 2+ or 3+—were the multipurpose catheter (odds ratio, 3.79), the Judkins left catheter (odds ratio, 2.83), and the voda left catheter (odds ratio, 2.73) (Fig 4). The Judkins

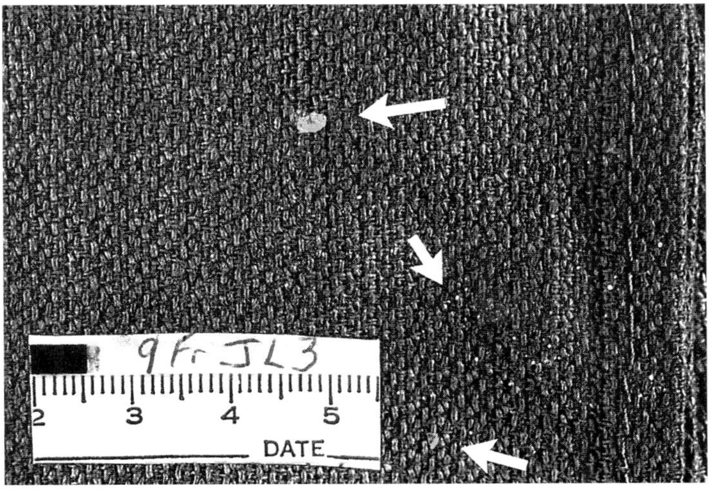

FIGURE 3.—Gross pathologic features of 1+ (*middle arrow*), 2+ (*bottom arrow*) and 3+ (*top arrow*). (Reprinted with permission from the American College of Cardiology courtesy of Keeley EC, Grines CL: Scraping of aortic debris by coronary guiding catheters: A prospective evaluation of 1,000 cases. *J Am Coll Cardiol* 32:1861-1865, 1998.)

right catheter produced debris in only 24% of interventions. Debris production during percutaneous interventions was less likely in patients with previous unstable angina or myocardial infarction. The finding of debris did not carry a higher complication rate.

Conclusion.—In patients undergoing percutaneous revascularization procedures, the coronary guiding catheter scrapes visible debris from the aorta in more than half of cases. Certain catheters are more likely to be associated with debris, especially the Judkins left, multipurpose, and voda left catheters. To ensure that atheromatous debris is not embolized during contrast injection, the operator must allow sufficient "back-bleeding" from the guiding catheter.

▶ For the most part, the complications and hazards of angiography are vastly overstated. No one is more guilty of this than diagnostic radiologists who, in an effort to push their own studies, portray angiography as some sort of medieval torture. That said, Keeley and colleagues, in a very simple and elegant study, point out that half of the patients undergoing percutaneous revascularization have macroscopically visible aortic debris in the lumen of guiding catheters. This article should be required reading for every member of the interventional team that is involved in any way in the handling of catheters.

M.J. Pentecost, M.D.

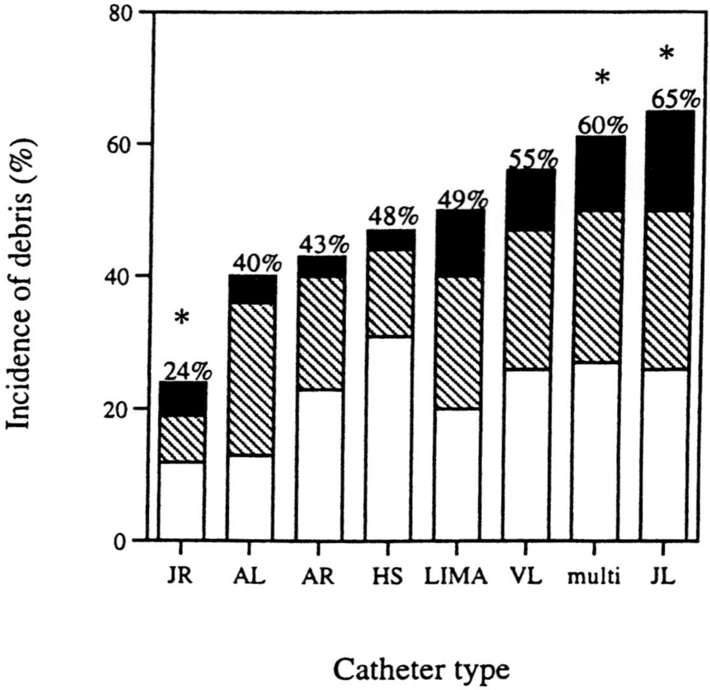

FIGURE 4.—Debris scores expressed as percent of total debris for each catheter type. *Abbreviations*: *AL*, Amplatz left; *AR*, Amplatz right; *HS*, hockey stick; *JL*, Judkins left; *JR*, Judkins right; *LIMA*, left internal mammary artery; *multi*, multipurpose; *VL*, voda left. *Asterisk* indicates *P* value less than 0.05 relative to any catheter; thus, JR catheters scrape less debris, and multi and JL catheters scrape significantly more debris than does the average guiding catheter. Debris score: *open columns*, 1+; *striped columns*, 2+; *solid columns*, 3+. (Reprinted with permission from the American College of Cardiology courtesy of Keeley EC, Grines CL: Scraping of aortic debris by coronary guiding catheters: A prospective evaluation of 1,000 cases. *J Am Coll Cardiol* 32:1861-1865, 1998.)

Acute Traumatic Rupture of the Thoracic Aorta: Delayed Treatment With Endoluminal Covered Stent: A Report of Two Cases

Perreault P, Soula P, Rousseau H, et al (CHU Rangueil, Toulouse, France)
J Vasc Surg 27:538-544, 1998 6–30

Introduction.—In patients with blunt chest trauma, rupture of the thoracic aorta is a life-threatening injury. It is the cause of many deaths after motor vehicle accidents, with many patients dying before attempted surgical repair. The cases of 2 patients with acute rupture of the thoracic aorta who underwent delayed treatment with an endoluminal covered stent were reported.

Patients.—The patients were 2 young men who sustained multiple injuries in motor vehicle accidents. Rupture of the thoracic aorta was detected by CT and angiography. In both cases, the aortic rupture was initially left alone because of the patients' precarious condition, which

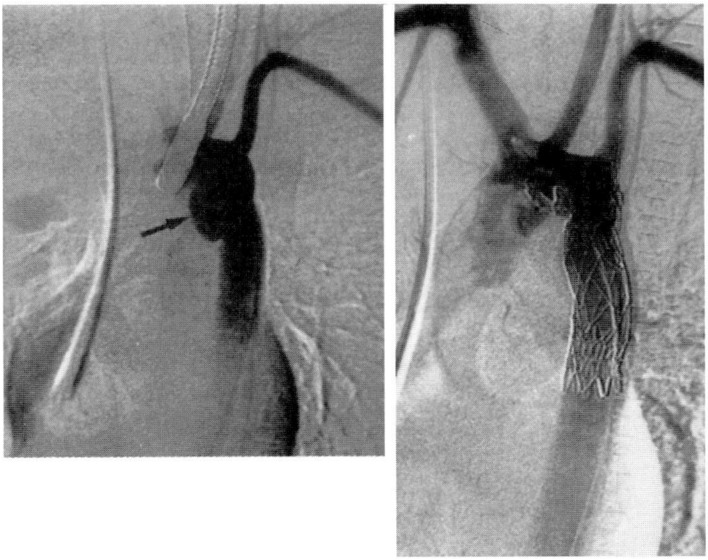

FIGURE 6.—Left anterior thoracic aortography before and after intervention showing complete exclusion of previously communicating isthmic pseudoaneurysm (*arrow*). (Courtesy of Perreault P, Soula P, Rousseau H, et al: Acute traumatic rupture of the thoracic aorta: Delayed treatment with endoluminal covered stent: A report of two cases. *J Vasc Surg* 27:538-544, 1998.)

included head and other injuries. The patients were monitored closely for 1 to 6 months, during which time their neurologic and respiratory condition improved significantly. Both underwent transluminal placement of endovascular covered stents for delayed management of the ruptured aorta. Postoperative imaging studies showed complete involution of pseudoaneurysms associated with the ruptures, with the stents intact and stable (Fig 6).

Discussion.—Delayed endoluminal stent placement for the management of traumatic rupture of the thoracic aorta requires a simple arteriotomy, with no need for thoracotomy or aortic clamping and can be performed in patients with associated head and pulmonary injuries. There are no long-term data on the safety and effectiveness of endovascular grafting. Controlled, prospective trials are needed.

► Perreault and colleagues really push the envelope with stent grafts in the repair of traumatic thoracic aortic pseudoaneurysms. Operative repair of such lesions is virtually 100% effective with minimal morbidity. Further, the 2 patients in this study are teenagers. They are very likely to tolerate the surgery well and, even more important, they could be expected to live with the stent graft for 50 or 60 years. That is a real test of durability for a new device—and a vote of confidence in this new technique.

M.J. Pentecost, M.D.

Cost-effectiveness of Ultrasound-guided Liver Biopsy

Pasha T, Gabriel S, Therneau T, et al (Mayo Clinic, Rochester, Minn)

Hepatology 27:1220-1226, 1998 6–31

Background.—The rate of major complications associated with percutaneous liver biopsy performed without imaging guidance is as high as 4%. However, the efficacy and cost of image-guided liver biopsy remain to be established. The relative cost effectiveness of US-guided liver biopsy was analyzed.

Methods.—The study used decision-tree analysis to compare liver biopsy with and without US guidance. Baseline estimates were drawn from a randomized trial. The clinical outcomes evaluated included minor complications, such as pain requiring analgesics; and major complications requiring hospitalization. Direct medical costs were estimated from the payer's perspective. Cost-effectiveness was determined by comparing the reduction in major complications by the 2 methods. Sensitivity analyses were performed to identify the variables with the greatest effect on cost effectiveness.

Results.—Under baseline assumptions, the average cost from complications per patient was $62 with US guidance versus $129 without, for an incremental cost of $67. Incremental cost per complication prevented with US guidance was $2,731; incremental cost to prevent a major complication was $406. Marginal effectiveness was 1.2 major complications avoided per 100 biopsies. The most important variables on sensitivity analysis were the major complication rate and the incremental cost of US. At a baseline major complication rate of 2%, a favorable cost-effectiveness ratio would result from an additional US cost of $187 or less; a US cost of $127 would equalize the average cost of major complications.

Conclusion.—US guidance during liver biopsy is a cost-effective procedure. Cost effectiveness is sensitive to changes in the major complication rate and the additional cost of US. If the latter cost could be reduced to $67 or less, US-guided liver biopsy would reduce costs as well as complications.

► Pasha and colleagues present another robust example of economic modeling. This is, indeed, a powerful tool when there are substantive underlying clinical and scientific data available. After studying this rigorous and well-designed analysis, one would be skeptical about the need for a prospective study of US-guided versus blinded liver biopsy (at least, if cost effectiveness was the major parameter in question). The results of this model are clear: Seeing what one is doing is better than not seeing what one is doing. And in the long run, it's cheaper too.

M.J. Pentecost, M.D.

Tubal Obstruction After Ligation Reversal Surgery: Results of Catheter Recanalization

Thurmond AS, Brandt KR, Gorrill MJ (Legacy Meridian Park Hosp, Tualatin, Ore; Oregon Health Sciences Univ, Portland; Mayo Clinic, Rochester, Minn)

Radiology 210:747-750, 1999 6–32

Introduction.—For women desiring reversal of sterilization by fallopian ligation, surgery consists of careful resection of the damaged segment of tube and anastomosis. Tubal occlusion is a common cause of nonconception after ligation reversal surgery. The use of fluoroscopically guided tubal catheterization to manage occlusion after ligation reversal surgery was evaluated.

Methods.—The experience included 24 women with tubal obstruction after tubal ligation reversal surgery. Their mean age was 35 years; the mean time since ligation was 22 months. All underwent transcervical fluoroscopically guided catheter recanalization using standard coaxial technique. Selective salpingography was done to confirm recanalization. A total of 38 obstructed tubes were treated.

Results.—Successful recanalization was achieved in 68% of tubes. A total of 8 perforations occurred in the 12 tubes that were not recanalized. Complete patency was achieved in 100% of underfilled tubes, 75% of proximally obstructed tubes, and 53% of tubes obstructed in the middle portion. Follow-up data were available on 13 patients who could conceive only through a recanalized anastomotic tube. Of 6 pregnancies, 2 were successful uterine pregnancies, 2 were early spontaneous abortions, and 2 were tubal pregnancies. Conception occurred at a mean of 2 months after the procedure.

Conclusion.—Fluoroscopically guided catheterization successfully recanalizes 68% of tubal obstructions in women with ligation reversal surgery. Selective salpingography can establish tubal patency in many cases. If conception is to occur, it usually does so soon after the procedure.

► My residents must get very tired of hearing this story about creative thinking. The tale is of a radiology resident at Oregon who has a startlingly simple idea: Recanalize fallopian tubes in infertile women utilizing the same tools used daily in treating vascular disease (Dr. Dotter would be very proud). A decade and hundreds or thousands of children later (including dear friends of mine as parents), the resident, Dr. Thurmond herself, continues this important work. This report describes excellent results with adjunctive percutaneous techniques in the surgically reversed, previously ligated fallopian tube.

M.J. Pentecost, M.D.

Temporary and Retrievable Inferior Vena Cava Filters: Current Status
Millward SF (Univ of Ottawa, Ont, Canada)
JVIR 9:381-387, 1998 6–33

Background.—Although there are no data from large, randomized trials, inferior vena cava (IVC) filters are thought to be effective in preventing recurrent pulmonary embolism. Concerns over the risk of complications and long-term fate of permanent filters have led to the development of temporary and retrievable IVC filters. The author reviewed the current state of temporary and retrievable IVC filters.

Concepts and Indications.—Temporary IVC filters can be attached to a catheter or guidewire, which may project from the insertion site. These filters must be removed after a certain period. Retrievable filters may be left in place indefinitely, but they may also be removed—for example, by snaring a hook on the filter. These new IVC filters vary in their maximum potential implantation time, and there are certain potential problems associated with filter removal. The route of insertion and removal may vary by device and clinical situation. The indications for use of temporary and retrievable IVC filters have not been well established but include prevention of deep venous thrombosis or pulmonary embolism in patients with major trauma, use in thromboembolism patients with a temporary contraindication to anticoagulation, and prophylactic use after PE or deep venous thrombosis. The major contraindication is the need for long-term protection.

Filter Types.—Several different types of temporary filters have been developed. These include the Gunther Temporary Filter, the Protect Infusion Catheter, the Bird's Nest device, a homemade retrievable nitinol filter, and the Tempofilter, among others. Some success has been achieved with all of these devices, including evidence of trapped thrombi; however, various complications also have occurred. Retrievable filters include the Amplatz filter, although this has been withdrawn because of a high rate of IVC occlusion; the Gunther Tulip Filter, and the Irie Filter.

Discussion.—Several different designs of temporary and retrievable IVC filters are being studied, with special attention to their respective indications. The current evidence does not support a recommendation for routine clinical use of these filters. Simple temporary filters with short implantation times are potentially useful in patients undergoing lower extremity venous thrombolysis. However, retrievable filters that could be removed after a relatively longer implantation time appear to have the broadest range of clinical utility.

► The development of a reliable, easy-to-use, temporary or retrievable vena cava filter (some cynics say that's an oxymoron) has been feverishly anticipated—and unexpectedly difficult. The appeal and indications are clear: for brief use in a young patient at risk only for a short time (for example, a trauma victim), as a precaution during venous thrombolysis, etc. Millward provides an excellent review of the current status and technical challenges of the current devices, as well as international experience with their use.

M.J. Pentecost, M.D.

Evaluating Patients With Renal Failure for Renal Artery Stenosis With Gadolinium-enhanced Magnetic Resonance Angiography

Ghantous VE, Eisen TD, Sherman AH, et al (Yale Univ, New Haven, Conn)

Am J Kidney Dis 33:36-42, 1999 6–34

Introduction.—End-stage renal disease is an increasingly common problem, particularly in the elderly population. Major causes include diabetes and high blood pressure; the contribution of renovascular disease is unclear. Several approaches to screening for renovascular disease in the elderly have been evaluated, including MR angiography (MRA). Gd-enhanced MRA was evaluated for use in the detection of renal artery stenosis in elderly patients with progressive renal failure.

Methods.—The prospective study included 40 consecutive older adults with progressive renal failure and suspected atherosclerotic renovascular disease. There were 22 women and 18 men (mean age, 70 years). Sixty-five percent had diabetes, 90% had peripheral vascular disease, 65% had coronary artery disease, and 75% had hypertension. All underwent 3-dimensional volume spoiled grass recall MRA with Gd enhancement. If this study showed significant renal artery stenosis, digital subtraction angiography was performed.

Results.—Both renal arteries were well visualized in 39 of the 40 patients. Of these, 12 had severe renal artery stenosis on MRA. All 12 of these patients had peripheral vascular disease and hypertension. Eleven patients went on to digital subtraction angiography, for a total of 22 renal arteries evaluated by both imaging techniques. Of 12 significant stenoses demonstrated by MRA, 11 were confirmed by angiography and 1 during surgical revascularization. Management consisted of percutaneous transluminal angioplasty in 6 patients, renal artery bypass surgery in 5, and angioplasty followed by stent placement in 1.

Conclusion.—Gd-enhanced MRA can detect renal artery stenosis in elderly patients with compromised renal function. Initial use of this imaging study can reduce the number of patients undergoing intra-arterial digital subtraction angiography, avoiding the associated risks of atheroembolic disease and contrast nephropathy. Larger clinical trials of Gd-enhanced MRA for the detection of renal artery stenosis are needed.

► The number of patients with end stage renal disease continues to grow, and as many as 10% to 20% may have a treatable renovascular cause for their condition. Even in this setting, catheter angiography has never caught on, despite advances such as smaller catheters and digital subtraction angiography. Well, catheters are not going to get any smaller and digital subtraction technology has plateaued, so what are we to do? US, radionuclide studies, CT—none have the appeal of MRA because of operator dependence, lack of reproducibility, or the need for iodinated contrast.

Ghantous and colleagues report their promising experience with Gd-enhanced MRA in the detection of patients with incipient renal failure. The improving technology and experience with renal artery stents provides a legitimate, minimally invasive therapy once renal artery lesions are identified.

M.J. Pentecost, M.D.

Renal Artery Stenosis: Evaluation With Conventional Angiography Versus Gadolinium-enhanced MR Angiography

Gilfeather M, Yoon H-C, Siegelman ES, et al (Univ of Utah, Salt Lake City; Hosp of the Univ of Pennsylvania, Philadelphia)

Radiology 210:367-372, 1999 6–35

Objective.—A small but significant proportion of cases of hypertension are caused by renal artery stenosis, which can also cause renal insufficiency. Both problems can be controlled through repair of renal artery stenosis. For patients at high clinical risk of renal artery stenosis, there is

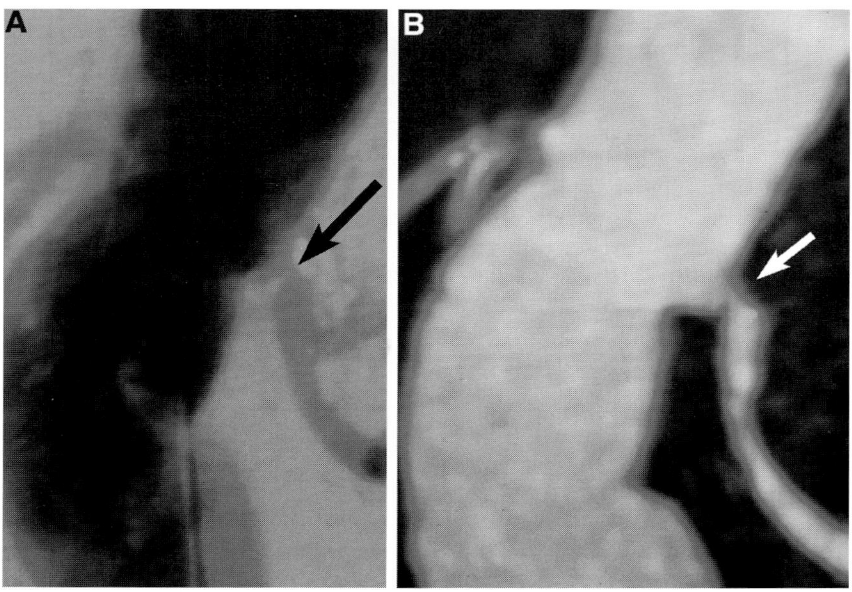

FIGURE 6.—Disagreement between results of MR angiography and conventional angiography. **A**, Conventional angiogram was interpreted by all 3 readers as showing clinically important stenosis (> 80%) of the left renal artery (*arrow*). **B**, MR angiogram (6.3/1.3) was interpreted by all 3 readers as showing less than 50% stenosis of the left renal artery (*arrow*). There was agreement between both sets of readers on the presence of severe right renal artery stenosis. (Courtesy of Gilfeather M, Yoon H-C, Siegelman ES, et al: Renal artery stenosis: Evaluation with conventional angiography versus gadolinium-enhanced MR angiography. *Radiology* 210:367-372, 1999. Radiological Society of North America.)

debate over the optimal test for diagnosis of the condition. Gd-enhanced MR angiography (MRA) was compared with conventional angiography for this purpose, including assessments of intermodality and interreader variability.

Methods.—Ninety-eight consecutive patients underwent both conventional angiography and Gd-enhanced 3-dimensional gradient-echo MRA at a single institution over a 2-year period. Of these, 54 had adequate visualization of the renal arteries by both techniques. The analysis included 31 men and 23 women with an average age of 64 years. Both sets of studies were evaluated by 3 experienced readers without knowledge of each other's findings or the results of the other study. A total of 107 main renal arteries were evaluated.

Results.—The 2 imaging studies had similar interobserver variability for the degree of renal artery stenosis, with a mean standard deviation of 6.9% with MRA versus 7.5% with conventional angiography. Estimates of stenosis among the 3 readers varied by 10% or less in 64% of arteries with MRA and 67% of arteries with conventional angiography. Agreement as to the presence of clinically important disease—defined as 50% or greater maximal stenosis—was 85% with MRA and 92% with conventional angiography. All 3 readers reported clinically significant stenosis in 24 vessels on MRA and 23 on conventional angiography. The 2 interpretations agreed in 18 cases (Fig 6).

Conclusion.—In the evaluation of renal artery stenosis, the interobserver variation with MRA is similar to that of conventional angiography. This supports MRA as a screening study for patients with clinically suspected atherosclerotic renovascular disease. Although conventional angiography has some important advantages, it also carries a higher cost and greater morbidity than does MRA.

► Unlike the earlier article by Ghantous (see Abstract 6–34), in this article, the evidence for detecting renal artery stenosis with MRA is less clear, despite the rosy conclusions of this report. The experience with 54 patients is described. Unfortunately, 98 patients were consecutively screened to identify this group. That means that 44 patients could not be included in the studies because either catheter angiography or MRA was inadequate (the authors do not say which, but my guess is that MRA was the cause in the majority of these). Further, in their blinded analysis of MR angiograms, 3 observers failed to reach agreement on more than one third of the patients. Angiographers were not so good either: About one third of the observers also could not come to an agreement about the degree of stenosis. Even when all 3 observers agreed about MRI, the angiographers concurred only two thirds of the time. All this said, MRA may evolve into a good tool for the detection of renal artery stenosis, but the sobering results from this analysis demonstrate that much work is necessary for this to be a reliable screening tool.

M.J. Pentecost, M.D.

Infrarenal Aortic Stenosis: Long-term Clinical and Hemodynamic Results of Percutaneous Transluminal Angioplasty

Audet P, Therasse E, Oliva VL, et al (Univ of Montreal Med Ctr; Hôpital Saint-Sacrement, Quebec)

Radiology 209:357-363, 1998 6–36

Background.—The traditional treatment for localized stenosis of the infrarenal abdominal aorta and its bifurcation is surgery, either endarterectomy or bypass grafting. Several studies have reported very good results with percutaneous transluminal angioplasty (PTA) of the infrarenal aorta, leading it to be recommended as the procedure of choice for patients with short abdominal aortic stenosis. However, there are few long-term follow-up data. This study reported the 10-year clinical and hemodynamic results of PTA of the infrarenal aorta.

Methods.—The experience included 102 consecutive patients undergoing PTA for symptomatic focal stenosis of the infrarenal aorta. Ninety-two patients had follow-up data available for analysis; they were 75 women and 17 men with a mean age of 52 years. Although the exact lengths of the stenoses were unknown, all could be treated using a 3- to 4-cm balloon catheter. Stenosis was present in the infrarenal abdominal aorta only in 74 patients and in the aortic bifurcation in 18. Study outcome definitions were as follows: technical success, less than 50% residual stenosis or a pressure gradient of less than 10 mm Hg; clinical patency, improvement or resolution of symptoms; and hemodynamic patency, normal Doppler findings in the common femoral arteries, an ankle-brachial ratio of greater than 0.95, or absence of a thigh-brachial pressure gradient.

Results.—The technical success rate was 72%. The 10-year clinical patency rate was 72%, with a hemodynamic patency rate of 46%. Twenty-two patients had had symptomatic recurrence at a mean follow-up of 51 months. Fifteen were the result of aortic restenosis, 11 of which were managed with repeat PTA, sometimes with stent placement. Three patients went on to have aortic surgery. There was no morbidity associated with primary or secondary PTA. On multivariate analysis, dilatation diameter was the only factor significantly associated with symptom improvement survival.

Conclusion.—For patients with focal stenosis of the infrarenal abdominal aorta, PTA offers a safe, minimally invasive treatment. Because of its high success rate and low morbidity, PTA should be considered the treatment of choice. In a relatively young group of patients with infrarenal aortic stenosis, PTA can avoid or delay major vascular interventions.

► On the bright side, this is a very important perspective on the use of PTA in treatment of aortic stenosis. In particular, this is a long-term analysis (> 10 years). On the negative side, this really is a mixture of 2 very different groups of patients. We all recognize a type of aortic stenosis that occurs in young women who are heavy cigarette smokers. Many such patients are included in this analysis because the majority of patients are women, the age ranges down to 30 years, and the mean age is only 52 years. Within this group, there are also a number of elderly patients who doubtless have more diffuse aortoiliac disease that really constitutes a different type of disease. A separate analysis of these 2 groups of patients would have been more informative. Even with this combination, the primary clinical patency at 10 years was 72%, which is quite encouraging.

M.J. Pentecost, M.D.

Concurrent Comparison of Endoluminal Versus Open Repair in the Treatment of Abdominal Aortic Aneurysms: Analysis of 303 Patients by Life Table Method

May J, White GH, Yu W, et al (Univ of Sydney, Australia)
J Vasc Surg 27:213-221, 1998 6–37

Objective.—The long-term outcome after endoluminal repair (ER) of abdominal aortic aneurysm (AAA) is not known and concurrent comparison studies of ER and open repair (OR) have not been done. Results of a concurrent comparison, using a 5-year life table analysis, of ER and OR in consecutive patients with abdominal aortic aneurysms are presented.

Methods.—Primary elective ER (n = 108, 8 female; average age, 70) or conventional OR (n = 195, 44 female; average age, 69) repair of abdominal aortic aneurysm was performed on 303 patients between May 1992 and May 1996. ER patients were monitored with contrast-enhanced CT within the first 10 days, at 6 and 12 months, and annually thereafter. Outcomes were survival and successful repair, which was defined for ER as continuing endograft function without leak or conversion to OR.

Results.—ER was achieved in 95 patients (88%). The remaining 13 were converted to OR. There were 6 perioperative deaths, 3 during initial ER surgeries and 3 in patients converted to OR. There were 10 late deaths. There were 7 perioperative and 6 late endoleaks, and 18 remote/systemic complications. In the OR group, there were 11 perioperative deaths, 10 late deaths, and 38 complications. Perioperative mortality and survival rates were similar in the 2 groups. The incidence of graft failure was significantly higher in the ER group than in the OR group (23% vs. 0.5%, respectively). Kaplan-Meier calculations of graft failure showed a 3-year ER graft success probability of 71%. The ER group had significantly less blood loss than did the OR group.

Conclusion.—Perioperative mortality and survival rates for ER and OR are similar, but failure rates were significantly lower for OR. ER resulted in significantly shorter intensive care stays and less blood loss.

► As the commentators at the conclusion of this article note (an excellent feature of the *Journal of Vascular Surgery* that should be duplicated in the interventional radiology literature), 2 facts are clear. First, the most recent groups of patients in all stent graft studies do better than the earlier enrollees. The equipment is better (namely, smaller) and operator experience grows over time. So all composite data look worse than the most recent results. Second, a randomized trial may already be impractical. If randomized to open procedures, many patients who journeyed to study centers simply opt out of the trial. It is very encouraging, however, that, despite the fact that all stent graft candidates had been turned down for surgery because of the risk, the mortality was the same in the operative and interventional groups.

M.J. Pentecost, M.D.

Results of Treatment of Inferior Vena Cava Syndrome With Expandable Metallic Stents

Fletcher WS, Lakin PC, Pommier RF, et al (Oregon Health Sciences Univ, Portland)

Arch Surg 133:935-938, 1998 6–38

Background.—Obstruction of the intrahepatic inferior vena cava (IVC), or IVC syndrome, often develops in patients with hepatic metastases. Ascites and anasarca make this obstruction debilitating. The diagnosis and treatment of IVC syndrome were reviewed at 1 center.

Methods.—Twenty-eight patients with hepatic metastases who received a diagnosis of IVC syndrome were included in the retrospective review. Treatment consisted of transfemoral placement of Gianturco-Rosch self-expandable Z metallic stents in the intrahepatic IVC. In 1 patient, a Wallstent was used. The stents used were 15 to 25 mm in diameter and 60 to 140 mm long. In all patients, pressure gradients across the IVC were determined before and after stent placement.

Findings.—All patients had a reduction in pressure gradients, followed by a rapid decrease of ascites and anasarca. Median weight loss was 5.9 kg. Mean survival after stent placement was 34 days, with a range from 1 to 99 days. In all patients, stents remained patent until death.

Conclusions.—Transfemoral placement of self-expanding metallic stents into the IVC promptly relieves the increased caval pressure associated with IVC syndrome. Pressure gradients across the constriction decline to normal or near-normal levels, and ascites and edema resolve. With greater awareness of this syndrome, earlier diagnosis, and the use of better systemic agents to control the tumor, improvements in survival can be anticipated.

► Fletcher and colleagues present their experience with efforts to relieve a most difficult problem—malignant inferior vena cava obstruction. Such attempts must always be undertaken against a backdrop of very limited and realistic expectations. Barely half of these patients survived a month and none over a 100 days. Nonetheless, the mean weight loss was over 5 kg, the procedure is simple enough to perform, and the benefits are very substantial in some patients.

M.J. Pentecost, M.D.

Real-Time Measurement of Radiation Exposure to Patients During Diagnostic Coronary Angiography and Percutaneous Interventional Procedures

Cusma JT, Bell MR, Wondrow MA, et al (Mayo Found and Clinic, Rochester, Minn)

J Am Coll Cardiol 33:427-435, 1999 6–39

Introduction.—As part of the increasing complexity of coronary angiographic procedures, coronary artery stenting has become a more frequent procedure. The effects of these changes on radiation exposure to patients and laboratory staff are unclear. This study measured radiation exposure of a large series of patients undergoing diagnostic and interventional cardiac catheterization.

Methods.—Over an 8-week period, the investigators measured radiation exposure to 972 patients undergoing diagnostic coronary angiography and percutaneous interventional procedures. A total of 992 procedures were performed; 706 procedures were diagnostic and 286 were interventional. A real-time exposure measurement system was used for continuous assessment of the radiation exposure rate and total exposure. The effects of various patient and procedure characteristics on exposure were analyzed.

Results.—The median radiation exposure was 41.8 mC/kg overall—34.9 mC/kg for diagnostic procedures and 95.6 mC/kg for interventional procedures. Fluoroscopy exposure time was 4.7 minutes during diagnostic procedures versus 21.0 minutes during interventional procedures. The rate of radiation exposure was significantly greater for patients weighing more than 83 kg than for lighter patients. The difference was 44.9 mC/kg/min for heavier patients versus 27.9 mC/kg/min for lighter patients during cineangiography and 2.3 versus 1.5 mC/kg/min, respectively, during fluoroscopy.

Conclusion.—With modern cardiac catheterization procedures, levels of patient exposure to x-ray radiation have increased. The high frequency of stent placement is associated with significantly increased exposures during both fluoroscopy and cineangiography. Real-time exposure measurement systems, like the one used in this study, will aid in efforts to reduce radiation exposure in the cardiac catheterization laboratory.

► The tumult over radiation skin burns has settled down since the Food and Drug Administration warnings of 1995. Appropriately enough, well-constructed prospective studies such as this work by Cusma and colleagues from the Mayo Clinic can now replace the earlier uncertainty. Inexpensive, reliable thermoluminescent detectors are now readily available.

As those at the head of the table know, most patients who need these procedures—whether a transjugular intrahepatic portosystemic shunt, or a coronary or neurologic intervention—do not have lots of options. That said, real-time monitoring, collimation, tube angulation, and pulsed fluoroscopy (the duties of the entire team) can only be enhanced with understanding of such studies.

M.J. Pentecost, M.D.

Sonography in a Clinical Algorithm for Early Evaluation of 1671 Patients With Blunt Abdominal Trauma

Bode PJ, Edwards MJR, Kruit MC, et al (Leiden Univ Med Ctr, The Netherlands)

AJR 172:905-911, 1999 6–40

Background.—Even with advanced imaging modalities, evaluation of the patient with blunt abdominal trauma is a challenging problem. Many centers use abdominal US in the diagnostic workup of patients with blunt abdominal trauma. This study assessed the efficacy of abdominal US in triage of abdominal trauma patients.

Methods.—The prospective study included 1,671 patients evaluated for blunt abdominal trauma over a 5-year period. According to the researchers' trauma management protocol, abdominal US was performed as the initial imaging study in the trauma room. Emergency laparotomy was performed in all patients seen with US abnormalities plus hemodynamic instability. For hemodynamically stable patients with positive results on US, additional diagnostic tests were performed. Criteria for positive US results were the presence of free fluid or organ injury.

Results.—Ninety patients had positive results on US. Of these, 11 had hemodynamic instability and went on to emergency laparoscopy. In another 6 patients with hemodynamic instability, US ruled out intraperitoneal causes. All patients in need of emergency laparotomy were recognized by means of US; none had inconclusive laparotomy. US had a sensitivity of 88% for intra-abdominal injury, with a specificity of 100% and an accuracy of 99%. There were 12 false negatives (Table 3). Abdominal CT was performed in 132 patients and showed posttraumatic abnormalities in 61%. In 470 patients discharged at 12 hours after admission on the basis of negative US results, the rate of improper discharge was only 0.4%. The revised trauma score or injury severity score had no effect on the efficacy of US.

Conclusion.—Using US as the initial imaging study in patients with blunt abdominal trauma is quick, accurate, and cost effective. It is highly efficient in identifying patients in need of emergency laparotomy and in recognizing relevant injuries. The authors' clinical algorithm for the assessment of suspected blunt abdominal trauma performs well from both a medical and economic point of view.

TABLE 3.—Data for 12 Patients with False Negative US Findings

Patient	Age (yr)	Sex	Delay	Clinical Course	Additional Imaging	Laparotomy	Outcome
1	78	Female	24 hr	Hemodynamic instability in ICU	Some free fluid (RS)	Mesenteric thrombosis, necrotic bowel	Died during laparotomy
2	65	Female	6 hr	Severe neurotrauma, signs of abdominal bleeding	Free fluid, splenic injury (RS)	Bleeding, grade 2 splenic rupture	Splenectomy
3	73	Female	3 days	Signs of peritonitis, hypotension (observed because of cerebral contusion)	Free fluid, free air (RS)	Bowel tear, bleeding splenic rupture	Hemicolectomy, splenectomy
4	24	Male	24 hr	Recurrent hypotension 1 day after initial assessment and discharge	Perihepatic, perisplenic, and paracolic free fluid; free air (RS)	Avulsion of the proximal jejunum, no splenic injury	Surgical repair
5	21	Male	24 hr	Abdominal tenderness	About 1 L of free fluid, suspected splenic injury (RS) Substantial amounts of free fluid, inhomogeneous spleen, suspected bleeding in gastrohepatic ligament (CT)	Small bleeding liver laceration, no splenic abnormalities	Surgical repair of liver laceration
6	21	Male	<1 hr	Multiple lower rib fractures	Grade 1 splenic rupture with subcapsular hematoma, no free fluid (CT)		CT follow-up No complications
7	69	Female	<1 hr	Multiple lower rib fractures	Grade 2 liver laceration, some free abdominal fluid around the liver and in Morison's pouch (CT)		CT follow-up No complications
8	44	Female	<1 hr		Grade 2 liver laceration, no active bleeding, also fracture of L2 vertebra (CT)		CT follow-up No complications

(Continued)

TABLE 3 (cont.)

Patient	Age (yr)	Sex	Delay	Clinical Course	Additional Imaging	Laparotomy	Outcome
9	38	Male	3 days		Inhomogeneous spleen, probably posttraumatic; also suspected liver metastases previously seen on sonography (CT)		CT follow-up No complications
10	17	Male	2 days	Abdominal complaints 2 days after initial assessment	Splenic rupture, substantial amounts of free fluid, no active bleeding (RS, CT)		CT follow-up No complications
11	34	Male	2 days	Blood pressure decrease (not unstable)	Free fluid, perisplenic and perihepatic fluid (RS); liver and splenic hematoma, no bleeding (CT)		CT follow-up No complications
12	1	Female	24 hr		Perihepatic fluid; spleen inhomogeneous, mottled (RS); grade 4 splenic laceration, no active bleeding (CT)		CT follow-up No complications

Abbreviation: RS, Repeated sonography.
(Courtesy of Bode PJ, Edwards MJR, Kruit MC, et al: Sonography in a clinical algorithm for early evaluation of 1671 patients with blunt abdominal trauma. *AJR* 172:905-911, 1999.)

Blunt Abdominal Trauma: The Role of Emergent Sonography and a Review of the Literature

McGahan JP, Richards JR (Univ of California, Sacramento)

AJR 172:897-903, 1999 6–41

Introduction.—There is growing interest among United States physicians in the use of US to evaluate patients with blunt abdominal trauma. Sensitivity and specificity are high, but few studies have examined the effects of US on patient care. Current knowledge regarding US for evaluation of patients with blunt abdominal trauma was reviewed.

Ultrasonography for Blunt Abdominal Trauma.—US evaluation of the patient with blunt abdominal trauma seeks not only to detect free abdominal fluid but also to image all solid parenchymal organs for injury. The usual US appearance of free fluid is a hypoechoic area within the peritoneal cavity or pelvis. Fluid typically accumulates in the upper abdomen, but the location depends on the injury site. US is more sensitive in detecting injuries to the spleen than to other parenchymal organs (Fig 4). Hepatic and renal injuries are more easily missed (Fig 5). Bowel and mesenteric injuries are generally not seen on US. If the procedure does not identify a

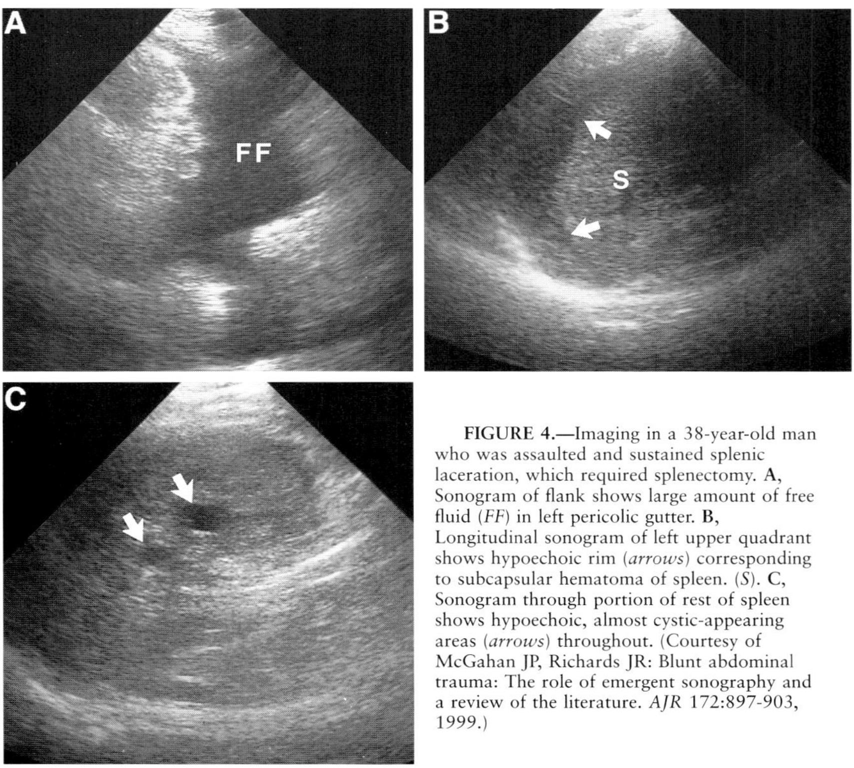

FIGURE 4.—Imaging in a 38-year-old man who was assaulted and sustained splenic laceration, which required splenectomy. **A**, Sonogram of flank shows large amount of free fluid (*FF*) in left pericolic gutter. **B**, Longitudinal sonogram of left upper quadrant shows hypoechoic rim (*arrows*) corresponding to subcapsular hematoma of spleen. (*S*). **C**, Sonogram through portion of rest of spleen shows hypoechoic, almost cystic-appearing areas (*arrows*) throughout. (Courtesy of McGahan JP, Richards JR: Blunt abdominal trauma: The role of emergent sonography and a review of the literature. *AJR* 172:897-903, 1999.)

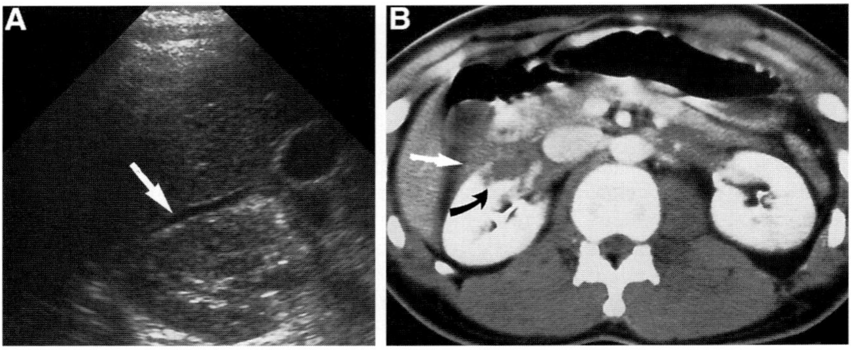

FIGURE 5.—Eleven-year-old boy who was in motor vehicle crash and sustained renal injury, which was treated conservatively. **A**, transverse sonogram of right kidney shows hypoechoic perirenal fluid collection (*arrow*). **B**, corresponding CT scan shows perirenal fluid collection (*curved arrow*) and renal contusion (*curved arrow*) that was not identified on sonogram. (Courtesy of McGahan JP, Richards JR: Blunt abdominal trauma: The role of emergent sonography and a review of the literature. *AJR* 172:897-903, 1999.)

suspected organ injury, contrast-enhanced CT may be useful. US can also identify abnormalities, such as pleural or pericardial effusion, or other nontraumatic causes of abdominal pain.

Studies of Abdominal Ultrasonography.—Although studies of US for blunt abdominal trauma have been performed, design flaws have been common. One of the major problems has been the lack of a gold standard for comparison: Most studies have used clinical improvement as the gold standard; only one used CT for all patients. There are also questions about the ability of US to localize the specific parenchymal organ injured, which has an important impact on the option for nonoperative treatment. US may also overlook vascular injuries, unless color Doppler sonography is performed. No study has examined the therapeutic impact of US on the clinical outcomes of patients with blunt abdominal trauma.

Discussion.—Despite these research limitations, the authors advocate the use of US for evaluation of patients with blunt abdominal trauma. They recommend prompt US performed by an experienced examiner, including images of the right upper quadrant, right and left flank, pelvis, midepigastrum, and heart in patients with chest trauma. Used in combination with physical examination, US can play an important role in determining the need for further examination and treatment.

Sonography as the Primary Screening Technique for Blunt Abdominal Trauma: Experience With 899 Patients

McKenney KL, Nuñez DB Jr, McKenney MG, et al (Univ of Miami, Fla; Ryder Trauma Ctr, Miami, Fla)

AJR 70:979-985, 1998 6–42

Objective.—There is growing interest in the use of US to evaluate patients with blunt abdominal trauma. Since a 1992 study showing US to be sensitive in the detection of hemoperitoneum, trauma surgeons at the authors' institution have come to rely on US as their screening technique of choice. US was evaluated for accuracy as the primary screening technique in patients with blunt abdominal trauma.

Methods.—The study included 899 patients undergoing diagnostic workup for suspected blunt abdominal trauma at a level I trauma center over a 1-year period. Throughout the study period, the initial diagnostic study performed was emergency US. All examinations were performed by a registered sonography technologist under the supervision of an attending radiologist or senior radiology resident. Sonograms showing free fluid or parenchymal injury were considered positive. The results of US were correlated with those of subsequent CT scanning, surgery, or clinical follow-up.

Results.—The results of US were negative in 87% of cases, positive in 11%, and indeterminate in 2%. Ninety-eight percent of the negative results and 94% of the positive results were confirmed by CT, surgery, or clinical follow-up. There were 15 false negative and 6 false positive interpretations (Tables 1 and 2). US screening had a sensitivity of 86%, a specificity of 99%, and accuracy of 98%.

Conclusion.—This study demonstrates the high accuracy of US for routine screening of patients with blunt abdominal trauma. US is well suited to the needs of the trauma patient, although its exact role remains

TABLE 1.—Comparison of 783 Sonograms With Findings Interpreted as Negative

Correlates (Negative Findings)		Noncorrelates (Positive Findings)	
Technique	No. of Patients	Technique	No. of Patients
Observation	557	Observation	1
CT	166	CT	12
Diagnostic peritoneal lavage	39	Diagnostic peritoneal lavage	2
CT and diagnostic peritoneal lavage	6		
Total	768		15

(Courtesy of McKenney KL, Nuñez DB Jr, McKenney MG, et al: Sonography as the primary screening technique for blunt abdominal trauma: Experience with 899 patients. *AJR* 170:979-985, 1998.)

TABLE 2.—Comparison of 101 Sonograms With Findings Interpreted as Positive

Correlates (Positive Findings) Technique	No. of Patients	Noncorrelates (Negative Findings) Technique	No. of Patients
CT	55	CT	6
Diagnostic peritoneal lavage	15	Diagnostic peritoneal lavage	0
Exploratory laparotomy	25	Exploratory laparotomy	0
Total	95		6

(Courtesy of McKenney KL, Nuñez DB Jr, McKenney MG, et al: Sonography as the primary screening technique for blunt abdominal trauma: Experience with 899 Patients. *AJR* 170:979-985, 1998.)

to be defined. It also has the potential for reducing costs in the trauma department.

► The battlefield studies in Vietnam have always been haunting and intriguing to me. Autopsy studies identified fatalities that could have been saved with the simplest of interventions: a tracheostomy for orofacial edema, a chest tube for tension pneumothorax, and so on. Minified portable US equipment could have a huge impact on the assessment of the trauma victim whether battlefield trauma, street trauma, or even iatrogenic injury (for example, hemothorax, hemoperitoneum, or pericardial effusion). McKenney's, Bode's, and McGahan's reports (Abstracts 6–40 through 6–42) validate the accuracy of the procedure in a large sample of patients.

M.J. Pentecost. M.D.

7 Abdomen

Introduction

The chapter on the abdomen in the 1999 YEAR BOOK OF DIAGNOSTIC RADIOLOGY encompasses both the gastrointestinal and genitourinary systems, using all imaging techniques, and also includes covering gynecologic and obstetric US. The US section was edited by Douglas L. Brown, M.D. from the Brigham and Women's Hospital/Harvard Medical School.

This year's abdominal chapter is subdivided into sections to increase clarity. The topics covered in these sections are the gastrointestinal tract, the liver, the biliary tree and pancreas, genitourinary radiology, gynecological US, and obstetrical US. The overall trend for abdominal imaging is the increase in interventional procedures and the continuous application of cross-sectional imaging to areas that, until recently, were reserved for so-called 'conventional studies' (ie, small bowel series, barium enema, and excretory urography).

Finally, we are noticing a resurgence of nuclear medicine applied to abdominal diseases such as the use of colonic scintigraphy for transit time and PET for abdominal malignancies.

Regarding the increased use of interventional radiology, ablation of liver tumors and metastases is becoming a mainstay in abdominal imaging. This certainly represents a new method of offering hope to the sub-set of patients who, until now, had no therapeutic options. We are also including the initial experience of treating benign prostatic hyperplasia with an imaging-guided laser-induced thermotherapy procedure.

In the area of applying cross-sectional imaging to substitute for conventional studies, we have selected articles that present examples of MRI used to study the small bowel (to assess obstruction) and the stomach (to assess motility). Other selections cover further refinements in virtual colonoscopy or CT-colonography that may, in the future, substitute for many barium enema examinations. Another topic covered is the increased application of MR cholangiopancreatography to substitute for endoscopic retrograde cholangiopancreatography.

Furthermore, in areas where cross-sectional imaging has had a role for many years, such as the use of CT in the gastrointestinal tract, we are seeing the expected refinement in clinical applications such as the distinction between diverticulitis and colon cancer.

Finally, we see how the last nails are being placed in the coffin of excretory urography, with further applications of CT and MRI to the complete study of the genitourinary tract.

In a classic area dominated by cross-sectional imaging, such as the study of the liver metastases, we are seeing how arterial portography is being further displaced by the now prevalent helical CT with multi-phasic scanning, and how the use of MRI with liver-specific contrast agent continues to be superior to multi-phasic helical CT.

In US, the trend is to increase the technical capabilities of the modality with the introduction of new sonographic techniques such as tissue harmonic imaging and the use of US contrast agents that hold the promise of increased sensitivity and specificity for liver lesions.

As in prior years, the articles here include selections from both mainstream radiology publications as well as nonradiology journals. We faithfully maintain our commitment to highlight the best articles from the main radiologic journals while finding hidden treasures among journals not routinely reviewed by radiologists.

Finally, we hope that the selections we've made include practical information that can be applied to common clinical situations and will, therefore, be relevant to the daily practice of abdominal imaging.

Pablo R. Ros, M.D., M.P.H.

Gastrointestinal Tract

MR Imaging of the Small Bowel Using the HASTE Sequence
Lee JKT, Marcos HB, Semelka RC (Univ of North Carolina, Chapel Hill)
AJR 170:1457-1463, 1998 7–1

Background.—Because of long imaging times and suboptimal image quality, MR imaging is not often used for assessing small-bowel abnormalities. The normal MR appearance of small bowel on half-Fourier acquisition single-shot turbo spin-echo (HASTE) sequence and the ability of this sequence to demonstrate small-bowel disease were established in the current study.

Methods and Findings.—The HASTE images of 50 patients with no small-bowel disease and of 18 patients with proven small-bowel abnormalities were reviewed. In the first group, no fluid was seen in the jejunum and ileal loops in 8%. Fluid was seen in less than 25% of the small-bowel loops in 40% of the patients, in 25% to 50% of the small-bowel loops in another 40%, and in 50% to 75% of the small-bowel loops in 12%. In 60% of the patients, equal amounts of fluid were seen in the jejunum and ileum. In 32% of the patients, more fluid was seen in the jejunum than in the ileum, whereas the reverse was seen in 8%. The mean diameters of the jejunum and ileum were 2.1 and 1.9 cm, respectively. The mean thickness of the small-bowel wall and valvulae conniventes was 2 mm. In the 18 patients with small-bowel abnormalities, both bowel lumen dilation and

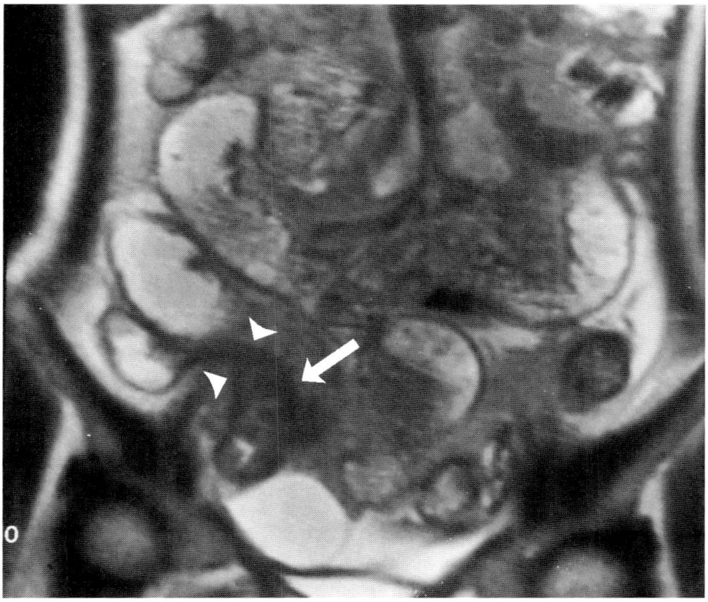

FIGURE 4.—Small-bowel obstruction due to Crohn's disease of distal ileum in 23-year-old woman. Coronal MR image using HASTE sequence reveals numerous fluid-distended jejunal and ileal loops. Note marked narrowing (*arrowheads*) and thickening (*arrow*) of distal ileal loop, representing cause and site of this patient's small-bowel obstruction. (Courtesy of Lee JKT, Marcos HB, Semelka RC: MR imaging of the small bowel using the HASTE sequence. *AJR Am J Roentgenol* 170:1457-1463, 1998.)

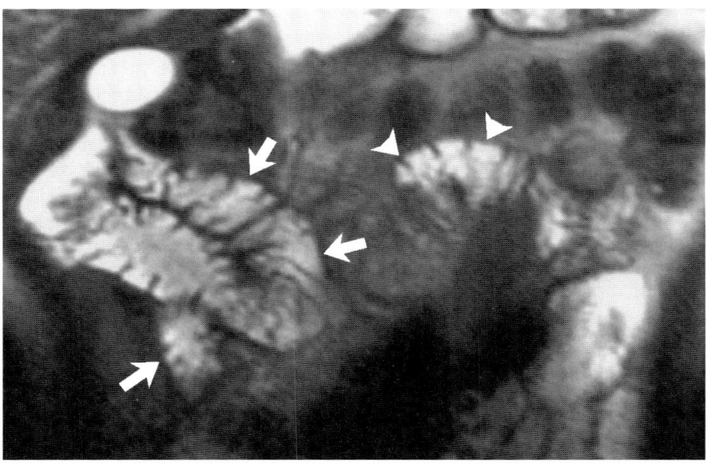

FIGURE 9.—54-year-old man with nontropical sprue. **A**, Coronal MR images obtained with HASTE sequence show several fluid-filled jejunal and ileal loops. Mucosal pattern of ileal loops (*arrows*) in right upper and lower quadrant is similar to that of jejnum (*arrowheads*) in left upper quadrant. (Courtesy of Lee JKT, Marcos HB, Semelka RC: MR imaging of the small bowel using the HASTE sequence. *AJR Am J Roentgenol* 170:1457-1463, 1998.)

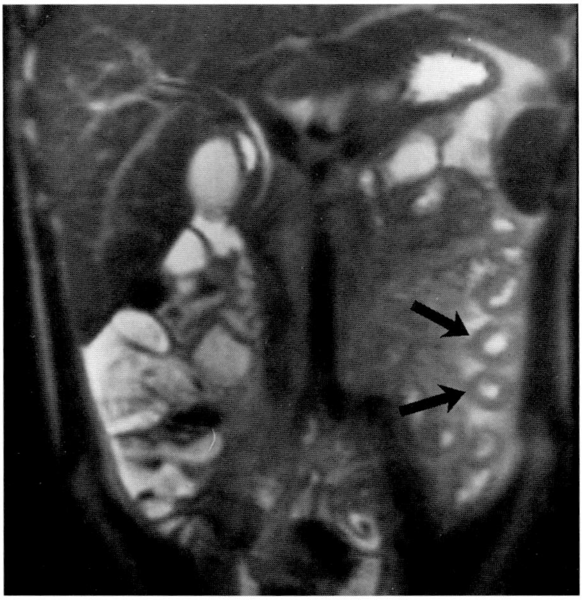

FIGURE 10.—Postchemotherapy jejunitis in 17-year-old boy with acute myelocytic leukemia. Coronal MR image obtained with HASTE sequence shows marked wall thickening of jejunal loops (*arrow*). Signal intensity of jejunal wall is intermediate between intra-abdominal fat and abdominal-wall muscle. (Courtesy of Lee JKT, Marcos HB, Semelka RC: MR imaging of the small bowel using the HASTE sequence. *AJR Am J Roentgenol* 170:1457-1463, 1998.)

increased thickness of the bowel wall and valvulae conniventes were observed (Figs 4, 9, and 10).

Conclusions.—The HASTE sequence can clearly delineate normal small-bowel loops. In addition, MR imaging using the HASTE sequence can demonstrate a variety of small-bowel disorders.

► The final frontier for abdominal MRI has been the gastrointestinal tract and between the different sections of the gastrointestinal tract; the small bowel has been the most difficult to image because of its peristalsis. On the other hand, small-bowel imaging is of primary importance to radiologists because of its inaccessibility to endoscopy.

Researchers at the University of North Carolina have offered us an excellent technique using a HASTE sequence to demonstrate the small bowel. They used the technique for MRI in 50 patients with small-bowel disease and 18 patients with proven bowel abnormalities to assess the ability of HASTE to characterize small-bowel diseases. Detailed findings such as increased thickness of the valvulae conniventes were routinely demonstrated.

It is obvious that the use of MRI will inexorably progress to encompass the small bowel, particularly because its coronal and sagittal capabilities make MR an ideal technique to display it. This article proves how a commonly available sequence affords not only pretty images of the small bowel, but also allows identification of subtle abnormalities and characterization of small-bowel disease.

P.R. Ros, M.D., M.P.H.

Fast MR Imaging and the Detection of Small-Bowel Obstruction

Regan F, Beall DP, Bohlman ME, et al (Johns Hopkins Bayview Med Ctr, Baltimore, Md)
AJR 170:1465-1469, 1998 7–2

Background.—Little information exists on MR imaging of small-bowel obstruction. The accuracy of fast MRI using the half-Fourier acquisition

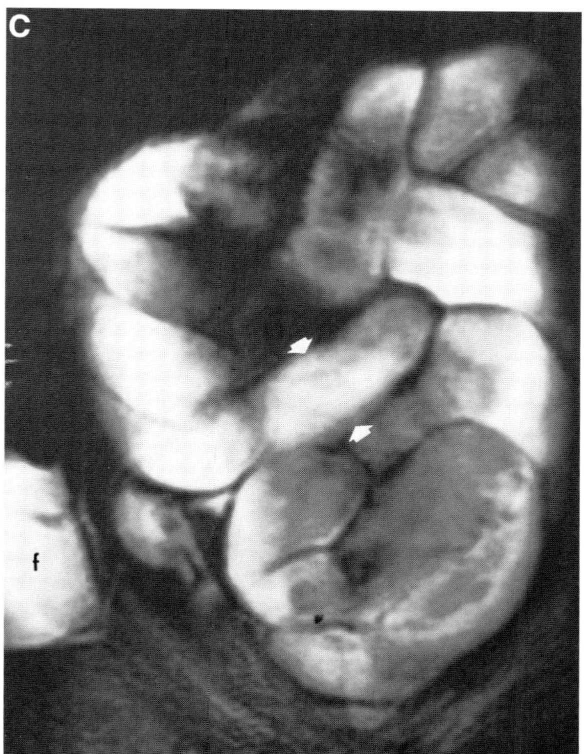

FIGURE 1.—Fifty-year-old man with metastatic bladder cancer and small-bowel obstruction. Patient had undergone cystaprostatectomy with ileal conduit and pelvic radiotherapy. Cause of small-bowel obstruction could not be determined, and patient was managed conservatively but subsequently died of complications of disease. A, radiograph shows dilated loops of bowel and ileostomy in right lower quadrant. B, sagittal HASTE MR image shows dilated small bowel (*closed arrows*) with multiple air-fluid levels. Valvulae conniventes (*open arrows*) can be seen C, Coronal HASTE MR image shows centrally positioned dilated small bowel (*arrows*) and fluid-filled ileostomy (*f*). (Courtesy of Regan F, Beall DP, Bohlman ME, et al: Fast MR imaging and the detection of small-bowel obstruction. *AJR Am J Roentgenol* 170:1465-1469, 1998.)

single-shot turbo spin-echo (HASTE) MR sequence in diagnosing small-bowel obstruction was investigated.

Methods.—Forty-three patients with suspected small-bowel obstruction underwent HASTE MR imaging during 12 months. Images were examined retrospectively for the presence, level, and cause of bowel obstruction. Findings on MR were compared with those of conventional radiography and surgery, when available.

Findings.—Unenhanced or contrast-enhanced radiography or CT showed small-bowel obstruction in 29 patients. Surgical verification was available for 21 patients. In 90% of the 29 patients with small-bowel obstruction, such obstruction was also shown by HASTE MR imaging. In 73%, HASTE MR images showed the correct level of obstruction. In 50%, HASTE MR images demonstrated the cause of obstruction (Fig 1).

Conclusions.—The HASTE MR sequence can provide images within seconds that assess small-bowel obstruction with high accuracy, using intrinsic intestinal fluid as a contrast material. Although this modality probably will not replace radiography and CT in the assessment of small-bowel obstruction, MR imaging may have a future role as technology improves and becomes more available.

▶ The use of cross-sectional imaging in the characterization of small-bowel obstruction has been established within the past few years. The main technique has been CT, but in many cases CT still is far from perfect because of the inherent difficulties of following the small bowel in the axial plane.

Authors from Johns Hopkins Bayview Medical Center used MR with HASTE sequence to determine the accuracy of this technique for the diagnosis of small-bowel obstruction. Forty-three patients with suspected bowel obstruction were evaluated, and MR was successful in 90% of the cases in determining small-bowel obstruction. Furthermore, HASTE MR images showed the correct level of obstruction in 73% of the cases and the cause of obstruction in 50% of the cases.

Again, these researchers prove that MR may be superior to CT in the study of the gastrointestinal tract if the adequate technique is used.

P.R. Ros, M.D., M.P.H.

Occlusive Colon Carcinoma: Virtual Colonoscopy in the Preoperative Evaluation of the Proximal Colon

Fenlon HM, McAneny DB, Nunes DP, et al (Boston Univ)

Radiology 210:423-428, 1999 7–3

Objective.—It is important to evaluate the entire colon before surgery in patients with colorectal cancer. However, this is difficult to achieve in patients with distal occlusive cancers that cannot be traversed endoscopically. Preoperative virtual colonoscopy was evaluated for use in inspecting the proximal colon in patients with distal occlusive carcinoma.

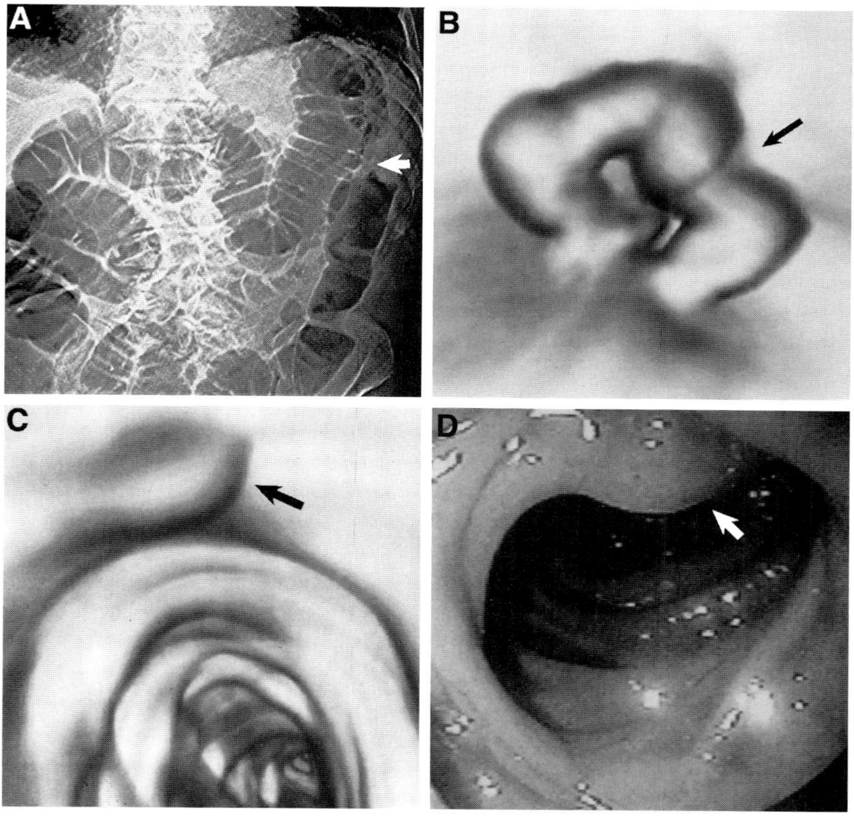

FIGURE 2.—Annular constricting carcinoma of the proximal descending colon with a synchronous proximal colon polyp. A, Anteroposterior scout view image demonstrates a circumferential carcinoma (*arrow*) in the proximal descending colon. Despite the presence of this occlusive cancer, sufficient air was insufflated into the proximal colon to allow adequate evaluation by virtual colonoscopy. B, Virtual colonoscopic image demonstrates the distal margin of the carcinoma (*arrow*) in the descending colon. C, Virtual colonoscopic image demonstrates a 10-mm polyp (*arrow*) in the distal transverse colon. D, Postoperative colonoscopic image shows the same polyp (*arrow*), which was subsequently removed. (Courtesy of Fenlon HM, McAneny DB, Nunes DP, et al: Occlusive colon carcinoma: virtual colonoscopy in the preoperative evaluation of the proximal colon. *Radiology* 210:423-428, 1999, Radiological Society of North America.)

Methods.—The study consisted of 29 patients with distal occlusive colorectal cancers that prohibited visualization of the proximal colon by conventional colonoscopy. Within 3 hours after conventional colonoscopy, each patient underwent virtual colonoscopy using a helical CT scanner. The virtual colonoscopies and axial CT studies were interpreted by 2 experienced GI radiologists who reached a consensus. The findings were compared with those of preoperative colonoscopy, barium enema examination, intraoperative colon palpation, histopathologic examination, and postoperative colonoscopy and barium enema.

Results.—All 29 occlusive carcinomas were successfully identified by virtual colonoscopy. Also depicted were 2 synchronous cancers and 24 polyps in the proximal colon. Both synchronous cancers were confirmed after resection. Postoperative conventional colonoscopy of 12 patients confirmed the presence of 16 polyps seen by virtual colonoscopy and demonstrated 2 small polyps missed by virtual colonoscopy (Fig 2). Two patients underwent postoperative barium studies, which confirmed 2 polyps seen by virtual colonoscopy. The proximal colon was visualized by virtual colonoscopy in 26 of the 29 patients, compared with none by preoperative barium examination.

Conclusions.—In patients with occlusive colon carcinomas, virtual colonoscopy can allow preoperative evaluation of the entire colon. It is superior to preoperative barium studies in visualizing the proximal colon and in identifying synchronous cancers. Preoperative virtual colonoscopy helps to optimize the surgical approach and identify patients who can benefit from early postoperative colonoscopy.

▶ In the current battleground over diagnostic evaluation of the colon, there is one indication where virtual colonoscopy is universally welcomed by gastroenterologists and endoscopists: the preoperative evaluation of the proximal colon in patients with occlusive colon cancer.

Researchers from the Departments of Radiology, Surgical Oncology, and Gastroenterology at Boston University School of Medicine have proven in 29 patients with occlusive colorectal cancer that virtual colonoscopy is the method to use to preoperatively evaluate the proximal colon in patients whose colon cancer cannot be traversed endoscopically. In these 29 patients, virtual colonoscopy confidently demonstrated 2 synchronous cancers as well as 24 polyps, proving that virtual colonoscopy is a useful method to evaluate the entire colon in this subset of patients.

The authors also indicate that virtual colonoscopy is preferable to preoperative enema not only because it visualizes the proximal colon better but also because it is not associated with a risk of colonic obstruction from barium inspissation or potential intraoperative barium contamination of the peritoneum.

P.R. Ros, M.D., M.P.H.

Diverticulitis Versus Colon Cancer: Differentiation With Helical CT Findings

Chintapalli KN, Chopra S, Ghiatas AA, et al (Univ of Texas, San Antonio)
Radiology 210:429-435, 1999 7–4

Background.—Patients with suspected colonic diverticulitis and colon cancer are commonly evaluated using CT. The few reports on this imaging study suggest some overlap between the 2 conditions. This retrospective-prospective study evaluated the CT signs of diverticulitis and colon cancer and the CT differentiation between them.

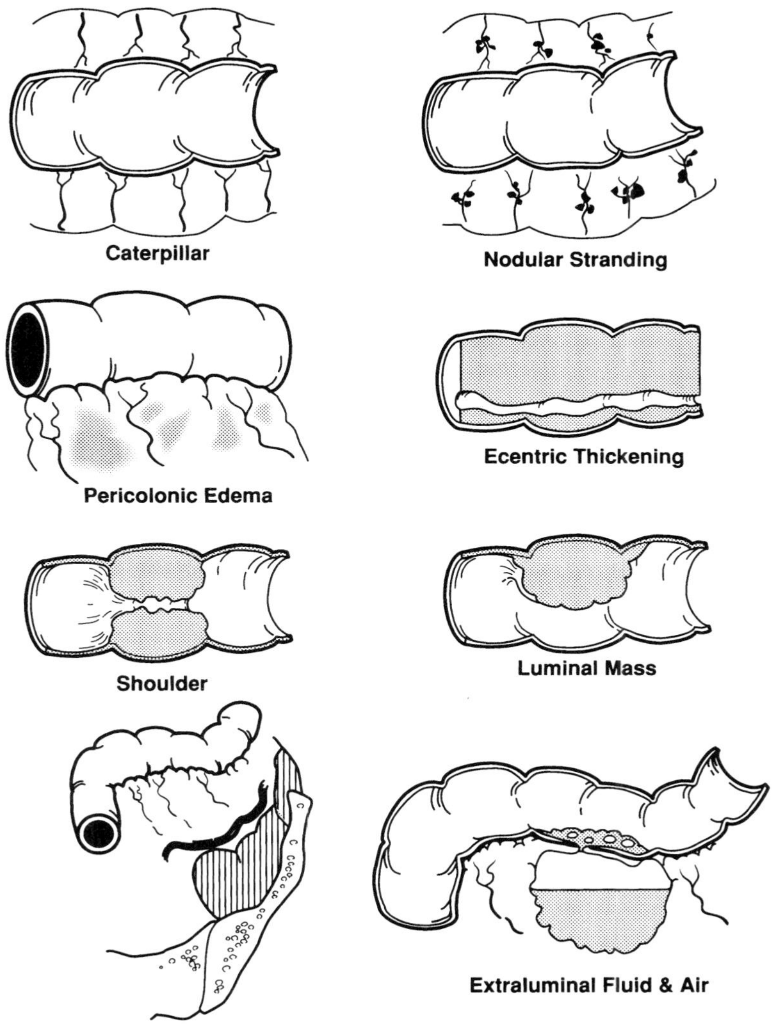

FIGURE 1.—Diagram shows the CT findings (*arrows*) evaluated in the retrospective and prospective parts of this study. Findings that are self-explanatory, such as length of segment and pericolonic lymph nodes, are not included. (Courtesy of Chintapalli KN, Chopra S, Ghiatas AA, et al: Diverticulitis versus colon cancer: differentiation with helical CT findings. *Radiology* 210:429-435, 1999. Radiological Society of North America.)

Methods.—In the retrospective portion of the study, CT scans from 27 patients with confirmed diverticulitis and 31 with colon cancer were reviewed in blinded fashion. The review focused on the presence or absence of CT findings reportedly associated with the 2 conditions (Fig 1). The CT signs associated with diverticulitis and colon cancer were then

TABLE 1.—Prevalence of CT Findings in Colon Cancer and Diverticulitis: Retrospective and Prospective Comparisons

CT Finding	Diverticulitis* Retrospective (n = 27)	Diverticulitis* Prospective (n = 40)	Colon Cancer* Retrospective (n = 31)	Colon Cancer* Prospective (n = 32)	*P* Values Retrospective	*P* Values Prospective
Length of involved segment					<.012	<.0025
<5 cm	1 (4)	2 (5)	8 (25)	10 (32)		
5-10 cm	20 (74)	30 (75)	22 (71)	21 (66)		
>10 cm	6 (22)	8 (20)	1 (3)	1 (3)		
Eccentric wall thickening	NE	10 (25)	NE	16 (50)	NE	<.026
Luminal mass	1 (4)	3 (8)	11 (35)	15 (47)	<.003	<.0002
Shoulder formation	NE	1 (3)	NE	16 (50)	NE	<.0001
Pericolonic inflammation	22 (81)	38 (95)	15 (48)	21 (66)	<.01	<.0005
Pericolonic edema	20 (74)	31 (78)	17 (55)	11 (34)	.10	<.0003
Pericolonic lymph nodes	4 (15)	3 (8)	22 (71)	23 (72)	<.0001	<.0001
Extraluminal fluid or air	7 (26)	12 (30)	1 (3)	2 (6)	<.02	<.011
Fluid in the root of mesentery	NE	20 (50)	NE	3 (9)	NE	<.0002

*Data are the number of cases. Numbers in parentheses are percentages.

Abbreviation: NE, not evaluated in the retrospective study.

(Courtesy of Chintapalli KN, Chopra S, Ghiatas AA, et al: Diverticulitis versus colon cancer: differentiation with helical CT findings. *Radiology* 210:429-435, 1999. Radiological Society of North America.)

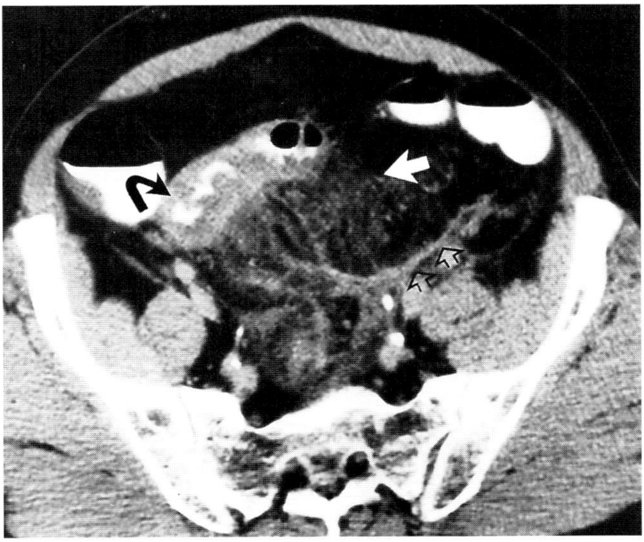

FIGURE 2.—Typical acute sigmoid diverticulitis in a man, 54. CT image of the pelvis shows colonic wall thickening (*curved arrow*), pericolonic inflammation (*white arrow*), and fluid at the root of the sigmoid mesentery (*open arrows*). These findings are characteristic of sigmoid diverticulitis. (Courtesy of Chintapalli KN, Chopra S, Ghiatas AA, et al: Diverticulitis versus colon cancer: differentiation with helical CT findings. *Radiology* 210:429-435, 1999. Radiological Society of North America.)

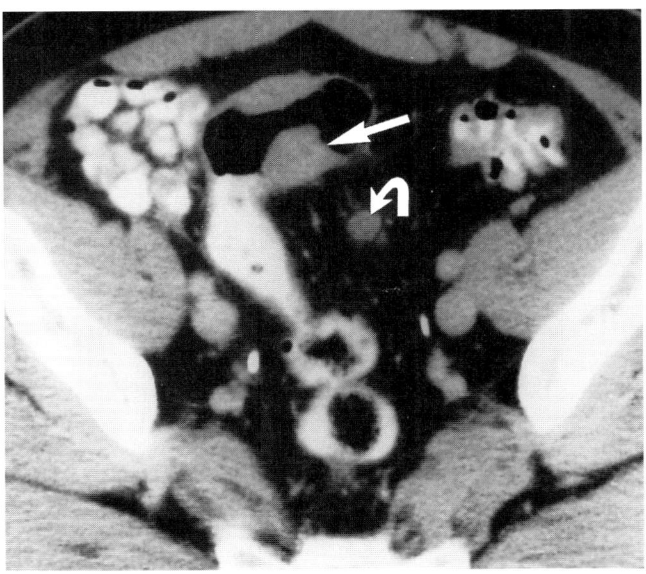

FIGURE 3.—Typical colon cancer in a man, 52. CT image of the pelvis shows a circumferential colonic mass with shoulder formation (*straight arrow*) involving a short segment (<5 cm). A single enlarged lymph node (*curved arrow*) is present in the sigmoid mesocolon. Colon cancer with metastasis to lymph nodes was confirmed at surgery. (Courtesy of Chintapalli KN, Chopra S, Ghiatas AA, et al: Diverticulitis versus colon cancer: differentiation with helical CT findings. *Radiology* 210:429-435, 1999. Radiological Society of North America.)

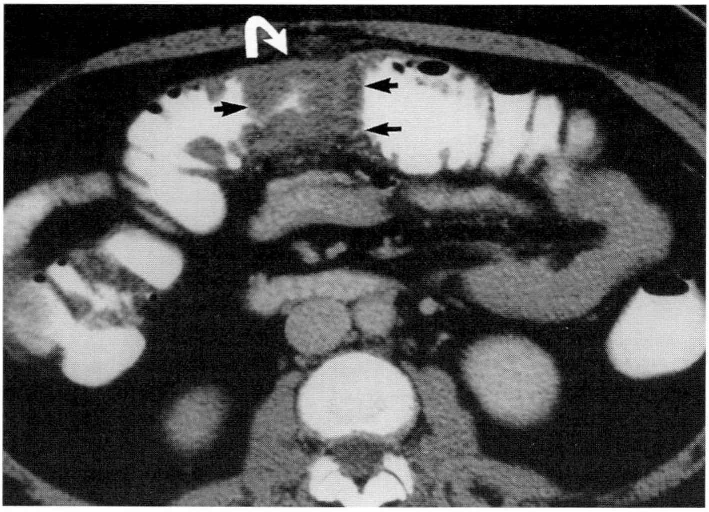

FIGURE 6.—Atypical diverticulitis in a woman, 46 years. CT image of the midabdomen shows a short segment of narrowing with shoulder formation (*black arrows*) of transverse colon and minimal inflammatory changes in adjacent fat (*curved arrow*). The short segment and shoulder formation erroneously suggest cancer. (Courtesy of Chintapalli KN, Chopra S, Ghiatas AA, et al: Diverticulitis versus colon cancer: differentiation with helical CT findings. *Radiology* 210:429-435, 1999. Radiological Society of North America.)

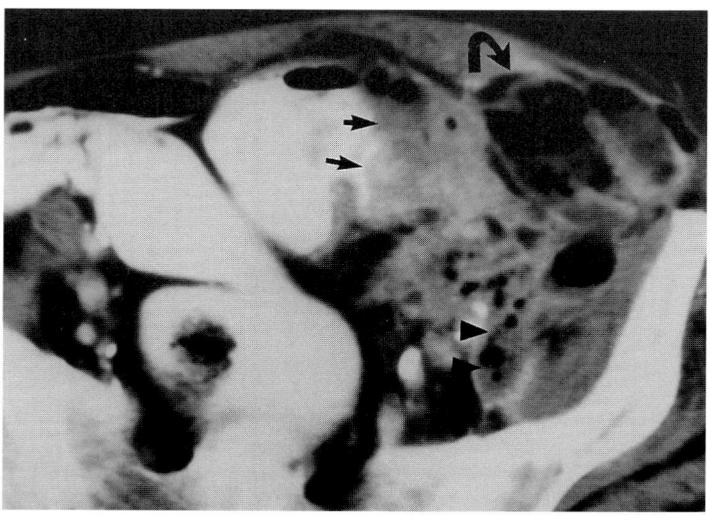

FIGURE 7.—Atypical colon cancer in a man, 64 years. CT image of the pelvis shows focal wall thickening (*black arrows*) and extraluminal fluid and air collection involving the left iliopsoas muscle (*arrowheads*) and extending to the abdominal wall (*curved arrow*). The inflammatory changes and pericolonic abscess suggest diverticulitis and mask the underlying cancer. (Courtesy of Chintapalli KN, Chopra S, Ghiatas AA, et al: Diverticulitis versus colon cancer: differentiation with helical CT findings. *Radiology* 210:429-435, 1999. Radiological Society of North America.)

TABLE 3.—Statistical Analysis of CT Findings for Diverticulitis and Colon Cancer: Prospective Component

CT Finding	Sensitivity (%)	Specificity (%)	PPV* (%)	NPV* (%)	Accuracy (%)
			Diverticulitis		
Inflammation	95	34	64	84	68
Fluid at the root	50	90	87	54	68
Length >10 cm	95	31	63	83	67
Edema	76	66	74	70	67
Extraluminal air or fluid	30	94	86	52	58
Multivariate analysis					
Lymph nodes absent and edema present	70	90	90	71	79
Lymph nodes absent and inflammation and/or edema present	92	78	84	89	86
			Colon Cancer		
Luminal Mass	47	92	83	68	72
Shoulder formation	50	97	94	71	76
Lymph nodes	63	92	87	76	79
Length <5 cm	68	5	37	17	33
Multivariate analysis					
Lymph nodes present with or without edema	90	70	70	90	79
Lymph nodes present with or without edema and no inflammation	78	92	89	84	86

Abbreviations: PPV, positive predictive value; *NPV*, negative predictive value.

(Courtesy of Chintapalli KN, Chopra S, Ghiatas AA, et al: Diverticulitis versus colon cancer: differentiation with helical CT findings. *Radiology* 210:429-435, 1999. Radiological Society of North America.)

used prospectively in the evaluation of 72 new scans. Diagnoses were made from the new scans, including judgments of diagnostic confidence.

Results.—In the retrospective portion of the study, findings significantly associated with diverticulitis were pericolonic inflammation and involvement of a segment larger than 10 cm. Findings associated with colon cancer were pericolonic lymph nodes and a luminal mass (Table 1). The prospective series consisted of 40 cases of diverticulitis and 32 of colon cancer. Both typical (Figs 2 and 3) and atypical (Figs 6 and 7) appearances of each condition were identified. A correct and unequivocal diagnosis was made in 40% of cases of diverticulitis and 66% of cases of colon cancer. On multivariate analysis, pericolonic inflammation and edema markedly improved the diagnostic significance of present or absent lymph nodes (Table 3).

Conclusions.—The study identifies some CT findings significantly associated with diverticulitis and colon cancer. However, there is still substantial overlap between the 2 conditions. Strict diagnostic criteria permit a correct and unequivocal CT diagnosis in about one half of cases.

► With the shift from barium enema to CT in the evaluation of patients with abdominal symptoms of possible gastrointestinal origin, there is a need to better understand the CT appearance of focal colonic diseases.

The 2 most common focal colonic diseases in the United States are diverticulitis and colon cancer. Abdominal imagers from the University of Texas Health Science Center at San Antonio offer a study with retrospective and prospective components to determine the helpfulness of CT signs in differentiating between these 2 conditions. The article includes an excellent diagram showing the different CT findings evaluated in the study (Fig 1).

The authors conclude that the most important finding is the presence of pericolonic lymph nodes, suggesting colon cancer. Of note is the poor yield in the prospective arm of the study, with only 40% correct diagnosis of diverticulitis and 66% correct diagnosis of colon cancer.

Therefore, it seems that the most important lesson to be learned is the considerable overlap in the CT diagnoses of these 2 conditions. In only approximately 50% of the cases can a correct unequivocal diagnosis of diverticulitis or cancer be made by CT. In these cases, the patients may not need further diagnostic evaluation. However, for patients in whom diverticulitis is clinically suspected but radiologically the criteria overlap with those of cancer, follow-up studies must be performed.

P.R. Ros, M.D., M.P.H.

Gastric Emptying and Motility: Assessment With MR Imaging—Preliminary Observations

Kunz P, Crelier GR, Schwizer W, et al (Univ of Zurich, Switzerland; Univ Hosp, Lausanne, Switzerland)

Radiology 207:33-40, 1998 7–5

Background.—The mechanisms of gastric emptying are not clear, and the role of gastric motility in the proximal and distal stomach in liquid meal emptying is still debated. An MR imaging method for the simultaneous assessment of gastric emptying and motility was evaluated.

Methods.—Nine volunteers were assessed after ingesting a liquid meal. The specially designed MR protocol enabled simultaneous assessment of gastric emptying and motility. The former was assessed using a spatial resolution of 1.5 mm, corrected for gastric secretion volume, and the latter using a temporal resolution of 1.2 seconds and a spatial resolution of 3.1 mm. The effect of a prokinetic agent on gastric emptying and motility was determined in 5 volunteers to assess the ability of this protocol to detect small changes in gastric motor activity.

Findings.—Each contraction was visualized individually at MR imaging. Administering the prokinetic agent reduced gastric half-emptying time and increased gastric motility.

Conclusions.—Gastric emptying and gastric motility can be studied simultaneously using MR imaging. In addition, this modality can determine the effect of drugs on gastric motor activity.

► The use of cross-sectional imaging and in particular MRI in the abdomen has been mainly limited to the study of anatomically based derangements, with little or no impact in altered physiology. A group of researchers from the Universities of Zurich and Lausanne in Switzerland present a pioneering use of MRI to assess gastric emptying and motility, still poorly understood physiologic phenomena. This opens an alternative to the established method to evaluate gastric emptying of liquid and solid meals in human subjects with scintigraphic studies. These researchers used 9 volunteers and a liquid meal and imaged the stomach using a specially designed MR imaging protocol. A prokinetic agent on gastric motility also was tested in each volunteer. These authors elegantly demonstrated that it is feasible to study gastric emptying and motility with MR imaging.

P.R. Ros, M.D., M.P.H.

Use of Methylcellulose in Small Bowel Follow-through Examination: Comparison With Conventional Series in Normal Subjects

Ha HK, Park KB, Kim PN, et al (Univ of Ulsan, Seoul, Korea)
Abdom Imaging 23:281-285, 1998 7–6

Background.—Many technique modifications have been made to shorten examination times and improve the quality of small bowel follow-

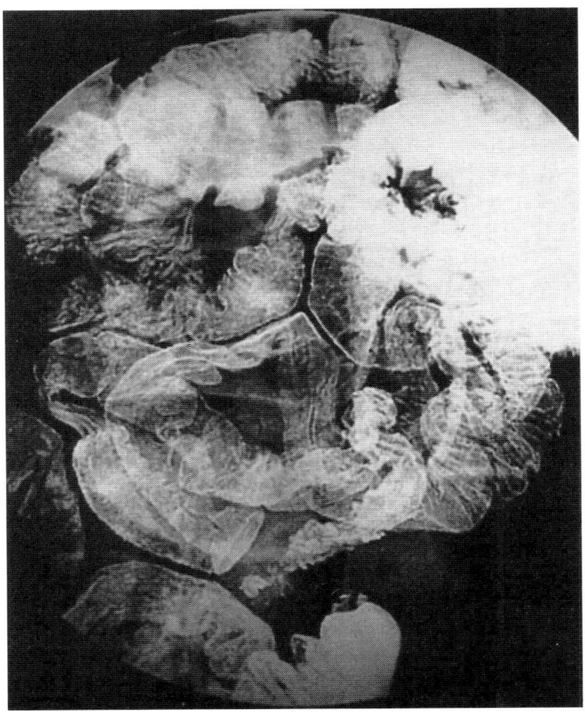

FIGURE 3.—Normal subject who underwent a modified SBFT using oral administration of methylcellulose after taking 100 mL of 120% w/v barium. In spot radiograph with compression, the bowel transradiancy appears excellent. (Courtesy of Ha HK, Park KB, Kim PN, et al: Use of methylcellulose in small bowel follow-through examination: Comparison with conventional series in normal subjects. *Abdom Imaging* 23:281-285, 1998.)

through examination (SBFT). Although the methods proposed have been somewhat effective, none has gained wide acceptance. These authors report on the use of methylcellulose in SBFT examination.

Methods.—Ninety-nine healthy persons underwent modified SBFT with an oral administration of 600 mL of 0.5% methylcellulose after taking 100 mL of 120% or 100, 150, or 200 mL of 70% weight/volume (w/v) barium. Transradiancy and distensibility of the bowel and transit time were compared with those of 39 additional healthy persons undergoing conventional SBFT with 500 mL of 70% w/v barium.

Findings.—Two persons reported diarrhea immediately after the examination. However, none of the other patients had acute symptoms, including abdominal pain and vomiting. Modified SBFT was far better than conventional series in acquiring good bowel transradiancy and rapid transit time. Bowel distention was not significantly better with the modified SBFT. The use of 150 mL of 70% w/v barium resulted in better bowel transradiancy, more rapid transit time, and less flocculation than the other 3 modified methods tested (Fig 3).

Conclusions.—This modified SBFT, which involves the oral administration of a large amount of methylcellulose after ingestion of a small amount of barium suspension, is a simple technique. The current data show that it easily improves the image quality of SBFT by enhancing bowel transradiancy and transit time.

► Debate still exists among gastrointestinal radiologists regarding the ideal small bowel series. Although little doubt remains regarding the superior results with enteroclysis, its detractors point to its invasiveness, increase length of study, and radiation dose as key drawbacks.

A group of authors from Asan Medical Center in Korea have offered what could be an ideal compromise: a modified SBFT examination using large amounts of methylcellulose after ingestion of a small amount of barium (150 mL of 70% w/v barium). They compared 99 normal subjects using this technique with 39 subjects who underwent conventional small barium follow-through with the usual dose of 500 mL of 70% w/v barium. The modified technique had no acute symptoms except for 2 patients who reported diarrhea immediately after the examination. This modified technique was superior in both bowel transradiancy and transit time but did not alter the bowel distention. There was also less occurrence of flocculation.

Again, this may be the ideal compromise to obtain images comparable with those of enteroclysis without some of its drawbacks.

P.R. Ros, M.D., M.P.H.

Segmental Colonic Transit After Oral ^{67}Ga-Citrate in Healthy Subjects and Those With Chronic Idiopathic Constipation

Bartholomeusz D, Chatterton BE, Bellen JC, et al (Royal Adelaide Hosp, Australia)

J Nucl Med 40:277-282, 1999 7–7

Introduction.—Constipation is a relatively common disorder. More commonly found in women, it may be caused by pelvic floor damage, anal sphincter dysfunction, generalized slow bowel transit, abnormal gastrocolic reflex, or irritable bowel syndrome. To assess patients with severe constipation, measurement of the segmental colonic transit is necessary. The tracer of choice has been ^{111}In-diethylenetriamine pentaacetic acid (DTPA), but it is not readily available and is expensive. An inexpensive tracer is ^{67}Ga-citrate. Colonic transit studies were conducted with oral ^{67}Ga-citrate and ^{111}In-diethylenetriamine pentaacetic acid among constipated and nonconstipated women.

Methods.—There were 20 women thought to have slow transit idiopathic constipation and 16 women with normal bowel habits. Eight controls underwent colonic transit studies with ^{111}In-DTPA and the other 8 controls underwent colonic transit studies after ingestion of oral ^{67}Ga-citrate. They were compared with the 20 patients who had slow transit constipation. Serial abdominal imaging was performed up to 96 hours after injection, and computer data were generated from geometric mean images of segmental retention of tracer, mean activity profiles, and a colonic tracer half-clearance time.

Results.—In a comparison between controls and constipated patients, there were no differences in segmental retention of either tracer or in mean activity profiles. There were significantly different results between constipated subjects and controls. For controls, the mean half-clearance time of tracer was 28.8 hours for ^{111}In-DTPA and 29.9 hours for ^{111}In-DTPA. For constipated patients, the time was 75 hours for ^{67}Ga-citrate and 70.8 hours for ^{111}In-DTPA (Fig 6).

Conclusion.—For accurate measurement of segmental colonic transit, oral ^{67}Ga-citrate can be used as a safe alternative to ^{111}In-DTPA.

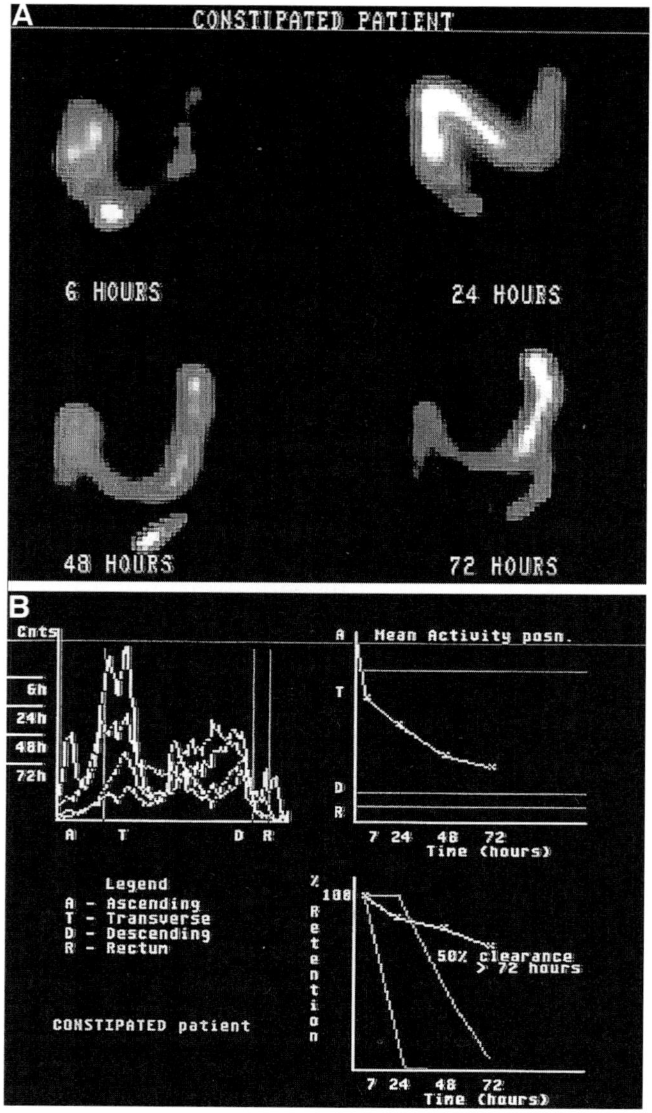

FIGURE 6.—A, ^{67}Ga-citrate colonic transit study in constipated patient. B, Half-clearance time of tracer, mean position of activity, and segmental activity profile. (Reprinted by permission of the Society of Nuclear Medicine from Bartholomeusz D, Chatterton BE, Bellen JC, et al: Segmental colonic transit after oral ^{67}Ga-citrate in healthy subjects and those with chronic idiopathic constipation. *J Nucl Med* 40:277-282, 1999.)

The Utilization of Colon Transit Scintigraphy in the Diagnostic Algorithm for Patients With Chronic Constipation

McLean RG, King DW, Talley NA, et al (Western Nuclear Medicine, Fairfield, NSW, Australia; St George Hosp, Kogarah, NSW, Australia; Miranda, NSW, Australia)

Dig Dis Sci 44:41-47, 1999 7–8

Introduction.—Constipation is a common problem that occurs with differing degrees of severity at various stages of life. Chronic idiopathic constipation is characterized by severe and disabling symptoms that do not respond to dietary treatment and that seem to have no systemic or obstructive cause. Diagnostic procedures are evacuation proctography, anorectal physiology studies, and radionuclide procedures, including colon transit studies. Chronic constipation has multiple causes. Colon transit scintigraphy involves an orally administered tracer that allows repeated imaging over a number of days with no additional radiation dose. A study was undertaken to determine how colon transit scintigraphy was used in clinical decision making by those who are familiar with its application.

Methods.—A questionnaire was sent to 4 referring specialists (1 colorectal surgeon and 3 gastroenterologists), who referred a total of 211 patients for colonic transit scintigraphy during a 4-year period. The specialists were asked to review their records retrospectively.

Results.—After colonic transit scintigraphy, there was a change in frequency and likelihood of diagnosis. In 51% of the patients, the diagnosis was changed. Within this group with a changed diagnosis, 37% were considered to have slow transit constipation, 43% with obstructive defecation, and 64% with functional bowel disease. The diagnostic likelihood was increased in all groups with colonic transit scintigraphy. Of patients in whom with slow transit constipation was diagnosed, 16% of the diagnoses were considered to be "almost certain" before the procedure and 83% were considered to be "almost certain" after the procedure. A number of patients thought to have functional bowel disease were reclassified from primary to slow transit constipation and some to obstructed defecation.

Conclusion.—In the diagnostic workup of patients with chronic constipation, colon transit scintigraphy may play a major role, both altering diagnosis and increasing diagnostic certainty.

► These 2 articles devoted to the imaging diagnosis of constipation, a common problem. In some cases, constipation is determined to be "idiopathic" because, despite conventional investigations and treatments, no obvious dietary systemic or obstructive cause can be found and symptoms continue to be severe and disabling. Assessment and management of chronic idiopathic constipation rely on determination of intestinal transit, usually measured by sequential radiographs after administration of oral markers.

These 2 articles, published respectively in gastroenterology and nuclear medicine journals, report the experience of 2 groups of investigators from Australia. In both cases, either Ga-citrate or In-DTPA was used as a scintigraphic marker. The article from the Royal Adelaide Hospital suggests that Ga-citrate can substitute for In-DTPA because it is inexpensive, available, and can be given orally without absorption by the bowel. The article from St. George Hospital in Kogarah indicates the usefulness of colon transit scintigraphy to manage patients with chronic constipation, with a change of diagnosis in 51% of the cases studied.

P.R. Ros, M.D., M.P.H.

Sclerosing Mesenteritis: Imaging Findings in 17 Patients

Sabaté JM, Torrubia S, Maideu J, et al (Universitat Autònoma de Barcelona)
AJR 172:625-629, 1999 7–9

Introduction.—Sclerosing mesenteritis is a rare, benign, nonspecific process involving mesenteric fat. The disease may represent many pathologic findings, including mesenteric panniculitis and retractile mesenteritis. This rare disorder is difficult to diagnose preoperatively. Radiologic examinations of patients with pathologically proven sclerosing mesenteritis were reviewed to describe the spectrum of imaging features of this rare disorder.

Methods.—There were 17 patients with sclerosing mesenteritis during a 16-year period. Twelve had mesenteric panniculitis, and 5 had retractile mesenteritis. All patients had CT scans. Medical records were reviewed, and surgical procedures were surveyed.

Results.—Bowel involvement was found in 8 patients. CT findings showed retractile mesenteritis in 5 patients and mesenteric panniculitis in 12. Masses ranged from 5 to 25 cm. The presence of the fat ring sign indicated the preservation of the densitometric values of the fat nearest the mesenteric vessels; it was found in 75% of the patients with mesenteric panniculitis and in none with retractile mesenteritis. Tumoral pseudocapsule represented a peripheral band with soft-tissue attenuation and was found in 50% of the patients with mesenteric panniculitis and in none with retractile mesenteritis.

Conclusion.—Important findings for the diagnosis of this disease are the "fat ring" sign and the presence of a tumoral pseudocapsule (Fig 5). Sclerosing mesenteritis is a single disease with 2 radiologically different variants. The diagnosis can be suggested by radiologic features, which can help delineate the extent of the process and help to prescribe or limit surgical procedures.

► Sclerosing mesenteritis (also known as mesenteric panniculitis and retractile mesenteritis), although rare, is an interesting benign process involving the mesenteric fat and often creating confusion because its CT appearance is not well established. Furthermore, as its management is not

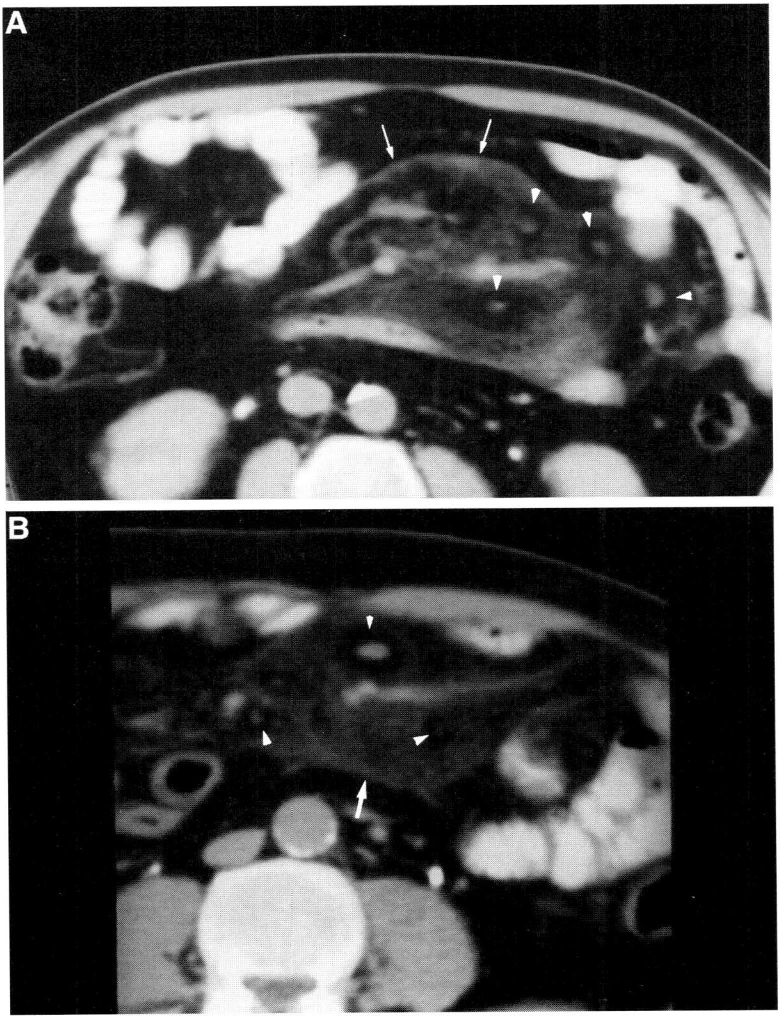

FIGURE 5.—CT scan in 59-year-old man with mesenteric panniculitis shows "fat ring" sign (*arrowheads*) and tumoral pseudocapsule (*arrows*). **B**, CT scan in 64-year-old man with mesenteric panniculitis also reveals fat ring sign (*arrowheads*) and tumoral pseudocapsule (*arrow*). (Courtesy of Sabate JM, Torrubia S, Maideu J, et al: Sclerosing mesenteritis: Imaging findings in 17 patients. *AJR* 172:625-629, 1999.)

primarily surgical, the recognition by radiologists of its imaging appearance is of paramount importance.

Researchers from the Autonomous University of Barcelona in Spain have published one of the largest series of cases of mesenteritis, reporting retrospectively the imaging findings in 17 patients. The authors describe the "fat ring" sign, which may be valuable in suggesting the diagnosis.

P.R. Ros, M.D., M.P.H.

Plain Abdominal Radiography as a Routine Procedure for Acute Abdominal Pain of the Right Lower Quadrant: Prospective Evaluation

Boleslawski E, Panis Y, Benoist S, et al (Hôpital Lariboisière, Paris)

World J Surg 23:262-264, 1999 7–10

Introduction.—The patient with right lower quadrant (RLQ) abdominal pain poses a difficult diagnostic challenge. The white blood cell count and plain abdominal radiographs (PAX) are commonly used to diagnose acute appendicitis, but their accuracy is low. This study prospectively evaluated the use of PAX in the management of acute RLQ abdominal pain.

Methods.—In the study, 104 consecutive patients admitted for evaluation of acute RLQ pain underwent clinical examination, WBC count, and PAX, including both erect and supine abdominal films. Before the PAX results were available, surgeons completed a questionnaire choosing 2 clinical diagnosis and therapeutic option. They then revised those judgments based on the PAX results.

Results.—Seventy-six of the patients underwent surgery for suspected acute appendicitis. The final diagnosis was acute appendicitis in 54 of these cases, for a negative laparotomy rate of 22%. In just 6 cases, PAX altered the clinical diagnosis and proposed management; 1 of these patients went on to have a negative laparotomy. Three of the other 5 patients had laparotomy, 2 for acute appendicitis and 1 for small bowel obstruction. Two patients with urinary calculi were managed conservatively.

Conclusions.—Routine use of PAX does not appear to alter the clinical diagnosis and management for most patients with acute RLQ abdominal pain. Avoiding indiscriminate use of PAX would help reduce health care costs. However, PAX may help in selected patients with suspected small bowel obstruction or ureteral stones.

► Use of plain abdominal radiographs is still the most common radiological examination performed on patients with acute abdominal symptoms presenting to an emergency department. However, with the increasing use of cross-sectional imaging methods, particularly CT for the diagnosis of appendicitis, the yield of plain abdominal radiographs as a routine procedure for right lower quadrant acute abdominal pain is questioned.

Surgeons from a French hospital undertook a prospective evaluation of over 100 patients to try to answer the questions about the procedure. They conclude that the routine use of plain abdominal radiographs altered the clinical diagnosis, and therefore the management, in only 6 patients. Therefore, they suggest that plain abdominal radiographs not be used routinely in patients with acute right lower quadrant pain but be used only in selected cases where small bowel obstruction or urinary symptoms are clinically suspected.

This article deals with the routine use of radiologic procedures without clinical input, but diagnostic imaging evaluation of patients with acute right lower quadrant pain must include adequate clinical input to determine if the findings are suspicious for acute appendicitis, and therefore whether a CT is needed. If gynecologic or pelvic origin is suspected, obtain a pelvic US, if, as the authors suggest, bowel obstruction or urinary origin is suspected, obtain a plain film of the abdomen.

P.R. Ros, M.D., M.P.H.

Transrectal US in Male Infertility: Spectrum of Findings and Role in Patient Care

Kuligowska E, Fenlon HM (Boston Univ)
Radiology 207:173-181, 1998 7–11

Introduction.—Men with demonstrable distal ductal abnormality represent only 1% to 2% of all men who seek medical attention for infertility. It is important to identify these patients so that correctable and uncorrectable causes of infertility can be addressed. The spectrum of findings at transrectal ultrasonographic (US) examination was examined in infertile men with low-volume azoospermia to determine the role of this diagnostic tool in patient care.

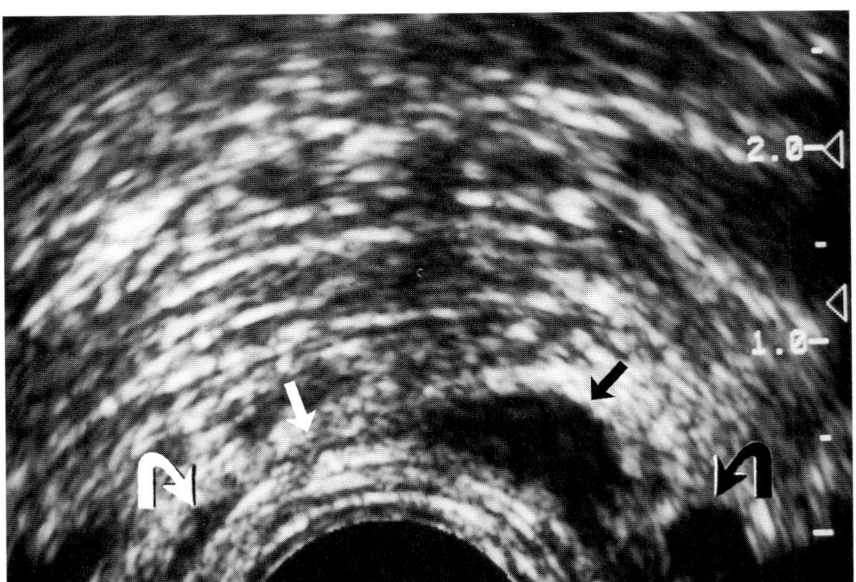

FIGURE 4.—Unilateral absence of the vas deferens as shown at transrectal US. Axial view shows absence of the right vas deferens (*straight white arrow*) and a rudimentary right seminal vesicle (*curved white arrow*). On the left, a normal vas deferens (*straight black arrow*) and a seminal vessicle (*curved black and white arrow*) are seen. (Courtesy of Kuligowska E, Fenlon HM: Transrectal US in male infertility: Spectrum of findings and role in patient care. *Radiology* 207:173-181, 1998. Radiological Society of North America.)

Methods.—Mean patient age was 34 (range, 24-52). All patients were infertile and had documented low ejaculate volumes and azoospermia. Two hundred seventy-six patients underwent transrectal US.

Results.—Seventy (25.4%) of 276 patients had no anatomical abnormalities. Ultrasonographic findings in the remaining patients were congenital bilateral absence of the vas deferens; 94 (34.1%) bilateral occlusion of the vas deferens, seminal vesicles, and ejaculatory ducts by calcification or fibrosis; 43 (15.6%) unilateral absence of the vas deferens, 31 (11.2%) (Fig 4); obstructing cysts of the seminal vesicles, vas deferens, ejaculatory ducts, or prostate, 26 (9.4%) and ductal obstruction secondary to calculi, 12 (4.4%).

Conclusion.—Transrectal US is the ideal method of evaluating the distal ductal system in patients with potentially correctible defects and for eliminating unnecessary investigations and interventions in patients not likely to benefit.

► Little attention has been devoted in the literature to sonographic evaluation of the distal male reproductive tract. Transrectal US, however, is a useful means of evaluating for lesions associated with male infertility. The authors' experience in this area provides useful lessons. Some of the more subtle echotexture abnormalities may be somewhat subjective, but most lesions in the distal male reproductive tract are straightforward. Those who perform such US examinations would be well served by this article.

D.L. Brown, M.D.

Liver

Large-Volume Tissue Ablation With Radio Frequency by Using a Clustered, Internally Cooled Electrode Technique: Laboratory and Clinical Experience in Liver Metastases

Goldberg SN, Solbiati L, Hahn PF, et al (Harvard Med School, Boston; Ospedale Generale, Busto Arsizio, Italy; Radionics Inc, Burlington, Mass)

Radiology 209:371-379, 1998 7–12

Background.—Radiofrequency (RF) ablation under CT or ultrasound guidance has been studied for use in the treatment of metastases in various locations. These studies have all used a single conventional RF electrode, necessitating extended treatment schedules with repeated electrode placement. The use of a cluster of closely spaced electrodes to perform RF ablation was evaluated.

Methods.—A 3-stage experimental study evaluated the use of clustered RF electrodes in ex vivo and in vivo liver and in vivo muscle. The technique used a cluster array of 3 internally cooled RF electrodes spaced 0.5 cm apart. Using optimal RF deposition with a peak mA of 1,400 to 2,150, an RF application of 5 to 60 minutes, and electrode tip lengths of 1.5 to 3 cm, the diameter of coagulation necrosis achieved was compared with that obtained using a single electrode by similar technique. In a clinical study,

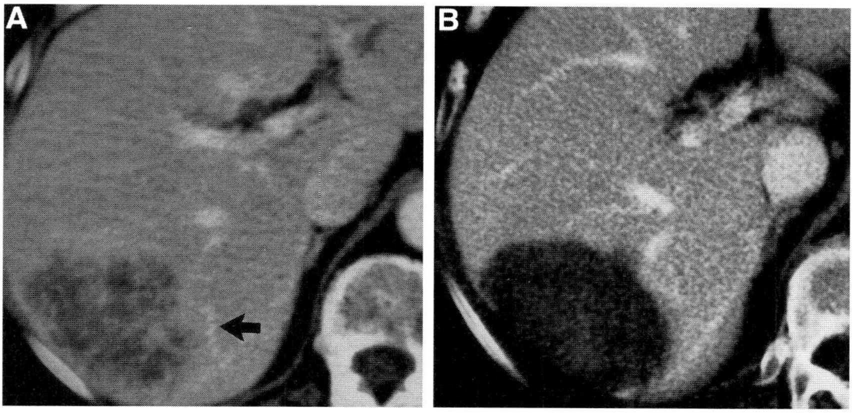

FIGURE 5.—Images in a patient who underwent RF ablation of hepatic colorectal metastases (*M*) with the cluster technique. **A**, contrast-enhanced CT scan reveals a 4.2 × 6.0-cm metastasis. **B**, contrast-enhanced CT scan obtained 2 days after RF ablation (peak current of 1,800 mA for 12 minutes) shows a nonenhancing area of hypoattenuation (which denotes coagulation necrosis) measuring 4.5 × 6.6 cm and enveloping the tumor. (Courtesy of Goldberg SN, Solbiati L, Hahn PF, et al: Large-volume tissue ablation with radio frequency by using a clustered, internally cooled electrode technique: laboratory and clinical experience in liver metastases. *Radiology* 209:371-379, 1998. Radiological Society of North America)

cluster electrode RF ablation was used to treat solitary intrahepatic metastases from colorectal cancer in 10 patients.

Results.—The ex vivo liver studies showed a 4.7-cm area of coagulation necrosis when electrode cluster RF was applied for 15 minutes. The coagulation necrosis area was 6.2 cm with a 30-minute application and 7.0 cm with a 45-minute application. A 12-minute application of electrode cluster RF achieved a 3.1-cm area of coagulation in in vivo liver and a 4.3-cm area in muscle. By comparison, the coagulation area produced by single-electrode RF was 2.9 cm in ex vivo liver, 1.8 cm in in vivo liver, and 4.3 cm in muscle. Patients in the clinical study were treated with a single, 12- to 15-minute application of electrode cluster RF. This treatment produced a 4.5- to 7.0-cm area of coagulation necrosis (Fig 5A and B). One-month follow-up studies showed no evidence of viable tumor in 9 of 10 cases.

Conclusions.—This study demonstrates an electrode cluster RF technique for ablation of intrahepatic metastases. The technique produces a larger area of coagulation necrosis than possible with percutaneous RF ablation using single-electrode techniques. Electrode cluster RF may increase the clinical application of percutaneous tumor ablation therapy.

► Percutaneous ablation of liver metastases is becoming less of an experimental procedure and more of a key component in the practice of abdominal imaging in many centers.

This study was 1 of the largest, combining the experiences at Massachusetts General Hospital and the General Hospital of Busto Arsizio in Italy, and using 68 ex vivo livers as well as 12 in vivo cases. The radiation frequency ablation method used internally cooled electrodes, which allowed a larger diameter of radio-frequency deposition and therefore of coagulation necrosis, as well as using an array of 3 separate electrodes.

The results suggest the effective ablation of the largest hepatic colorectal metastases reported to date, with coagulation necrosis up to 7 cm.

P.R. Ros, M.D., M.P.H.

Hepatic Cavernous Hemangioma: Sonographic Patterns and Speed of Contrast Enhancement on Multiphase Dynamic MR Imaging

Yu J-S, Kim M-J, Kim KW, et al (YongDong Severance Hosp, Seoul, South Korea; Yonsei Univ, Seoul; Yeungnam Univ, Taegu, South Korea)

AJR 171:1021-1025, 1998 7–13

Purpose.—Various sonographic and CT/MRI contrast enhancement patterns of hepatic cavernous hemangioma have been reported. The com-

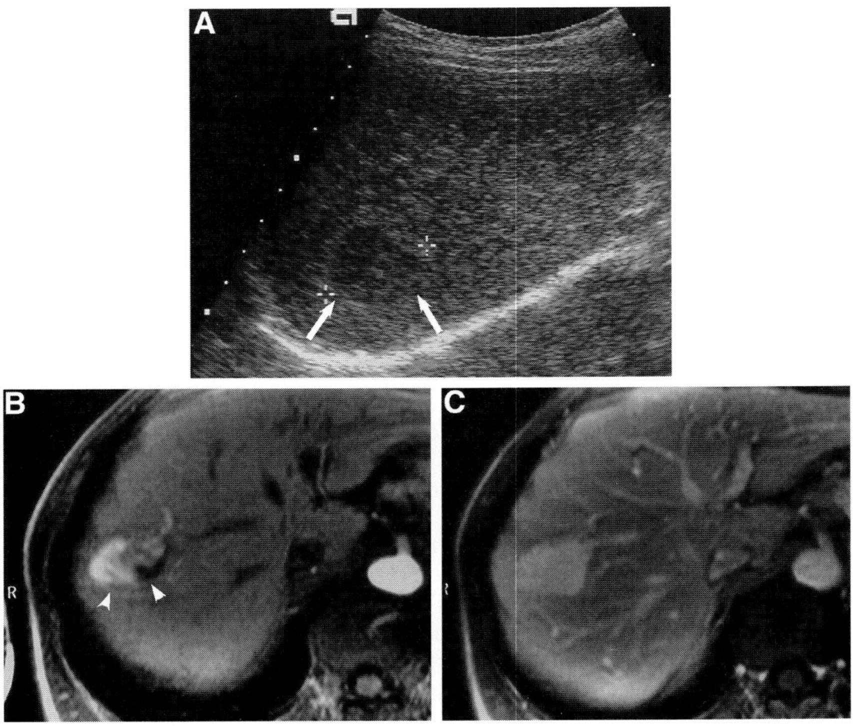

FIGURE 1.—A man, 54, with hypoechoic and rapid-enhancing cavernous hemangioma of the liver. **A**, sonogram shows a 3-cm homogeneously hypoechoic tumor (*arrows*) in right lobe of liver. **B**, contrast-enhanced MR image obtained during first phase (arterial dominant phase), 10 seconds after administration of contrast agent, shows contrast enhancement of more than 50% of tumor (*arrowheads*). **C**, contrast-enhanced MR image obtained during second phase (early nonequilibrium phase), 35 seconds after administration of contrast agent, shows complete contrast enhancement. (Courtesy of Yu J-S, Kim M-J, Kim KW, et al: Hepatic cavernous hemangioma: sonographic patterns and speed of contrast enhancement on multiphase dynamic MR imaging. *AJR* 171:1021-1025, 1998.)

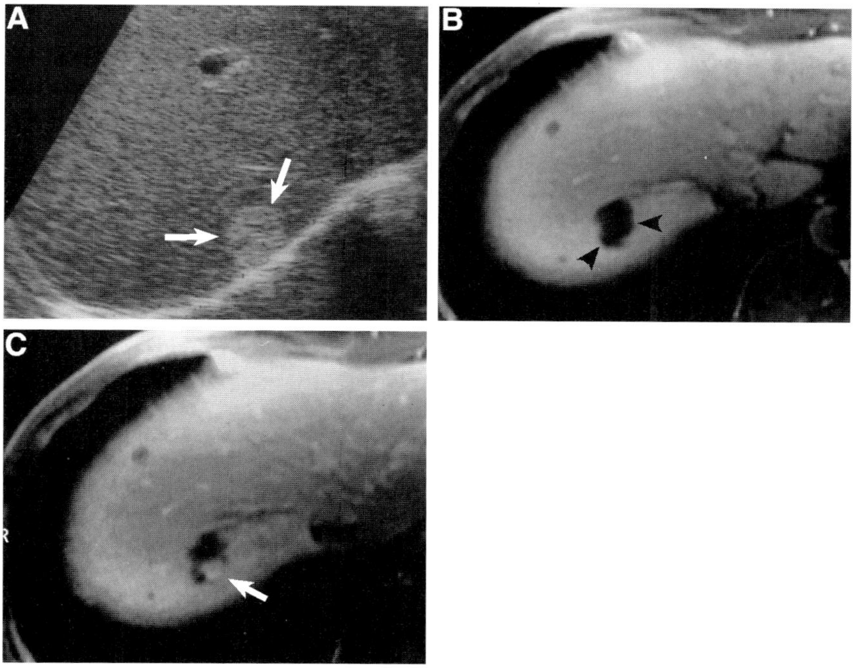

FIGURE 2.—A man, 39, with hyperechoic and slow-enhancing cavernous hemangioma of the liver. **A**, Sonogram shows 2-cm homogeneously hyperechoic tumor (*arrows*) in right lobe of liver. **B**, Contrast-enhanced MR image obtained during third phase (early nonequilibrium phase), 60 seconds after administration of contrast agent, shows no contrast enhancement (*arrowheads*). **C**, Contrast-enhanced MR image obtained 5 minutes after administration of contrast agent (delayed phase) shows globular contrast enhancement at posterior aspect of tumor (*arrowhead*). (Courtesy of Yu J-S, Kim M-J, Kim KW, et al: Hepatic cavernous hemangioma: sonographic patterns and speed of contrast enhancement on multiphase dynamic MR imaging. *AJR* 171:1021-1025, 1998.)

bination of hemodynamic and sonographic data may provide more-reliable diagnostic information. The sonographic pattern of hepatic cavernous hemangioma was correlated with the enhancement pattern on dynamic MRI.

Methods.—The study consisted of 45 patients with 71 hepatic cavernous hemangiomas less than 4 cm in diameter, detected on multiphase IV contrast-enhanced dynamic MRI. The MRI patterns were classified as rapid-, intermediate-, and slow-enhancing, and compared with the findings of sonography. The sonographic patterns were classified as hypoechoic, isoechoic or mixed echoic, or hyperechoic, based on the relative echogenicity between lesions and surrounding liver parenchyma.

Results.—Seventy-five percent of hemangiomas with a rapid-enhancing MRI pattern had a hypoechoic MRI pattern (Fig 1). In addition, 90% of hemangiomas with a slow-enhancing MRI pattern were hyperechoic (Fig 2). All lesions with a hyperechoic sonographic pattern were rapid-enhancing on MRI, while 79% of sonographically hyperechoic lesions were slow-enhancing on MRI. Seventy-two percent of hemangiomas with an intermediate MRI pattern showed an inhomogeneous or mixed echogenic pattern on sonography.

Conclusions.—In patients with hepatic cavernous hemangioma, the pattern of contrast enhancement on multiphase dynamic MRI correlates well with the echo pattern on sonography, and vice versa. The mechanism affecting these patterns is unknown. The findings may simplify the differential diagnosis between cavernous hemangioma and other hepatic diseases.

▶ This study addresses the variability of appearances of hepatic cavernous hemangioma using both contrast-enhanced multiphase dynamic MRI and ultrasound.

Imaging of hemangioma of the liver continues to puzzle abdominal imagers because of its variable appearance by different techniques. Researchers from the YongDong Severance Hospital in South Korea have been astute enough to find a correlation between the sonographic and enhanced MRI patterns in cavernous hemangioma. They conclude that the typical hyperechoic lesion seen with ultrasound also has the classic delayed peripheral, globular (or nodular) contrast enhancement. Interestingly enough, the atypical rapid-enhancing hemangiomas seen on dynamic MRI tend to also have an atypical hypoechoic appearance by ultrasound.

This seems to suggest that the echogenicity, sonography, and speed of contrast enhancement on dynamic MR imaging depend on the internal architecture of hemangiomas in a way not completely understood.

This article helps us better understand these common liver lesions.

P.R. Ros, M.D., M.P.H.

Helical CT Versus CT Arterial Portography in the Detection of Hepatic Metastasis of Colorectal Carcinoma

Valls C, Lopez E, Gumà A, et al (L'Hospitalet de Llobregat, Barcelona)
AJR 170:1341-1347, 1998 7–14

Background.—Preoperative assessment of the number and location of hepatic metastases is essential in patients being considered for curative resection of hepatic metastasis of colorectal cancer. Though CT arterial portography (CTAP) is the current technique of choice for this purpose, its specificity is low. Helical CT is an important advance in imaging of the liver. Helical CT and nonhelical CTAP were compared for detection of hepatic metastases from colorectal cancer.

Methods.—Thirty-five patients with colorectal carcinoma and suspected metastases to the liver underwent helical CT and CTAP before surgery. The imaging findings were compared with the surgical and pathologic results in 26 patients who underwent surgery. The findings of helical CT and CTAP were compared with readings by 3 independent radiologists, with the results analyzed by means of receiver operating characteristic methods.

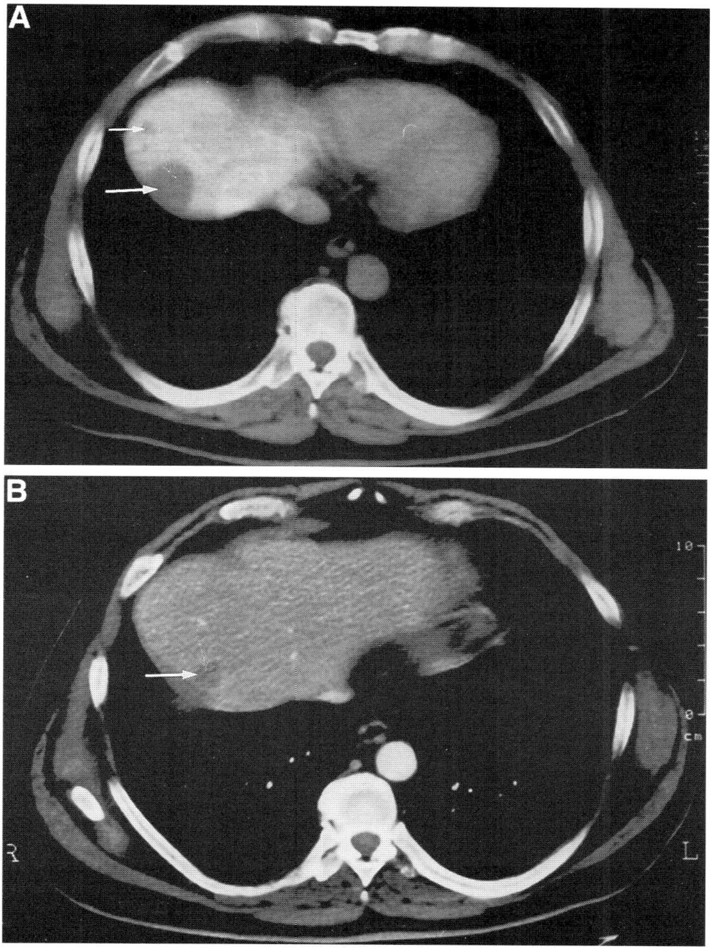

FIGURE 2.—False-positive findings at CT arterial portography in 62-year-old man. **A**, CT arterial portography at dome of liver shows round hypodense lesion in segment VII (*large arrow*) and 2 tiny nodules more anteriorly, in segment VIII (*small arrow*). **B**, Helical CT scan confirms lesions in segment VII (*arrow*). Rest of liver parenchyma is normal. Histologic examination detected only lesion in segment VII. (Courtesy of Valls C, Lopez E, Gumà A, et al: Helical CT versus CT arterial portography in the detection of hepatic metastasis of colorectal carcinoma. *AJR* 170:1341-1347, 1998.)

Results.—A total of 50 metastases were shown with histologic analysis. Sensitivity in the detection of these lesions was 76% with helical CT and 74% with CTAP. Positive predictive values were 90% versus 69%, respectively (Fig 2). According to receiver operating characteristic curve analysis, the area under the curve was significantly greater for helical CT than for CTAP (Fig 4).

Conclusions.—This prospective study finds helical CT to be more effective than nonhelical CTAP in detection of liver metastases from colorectal

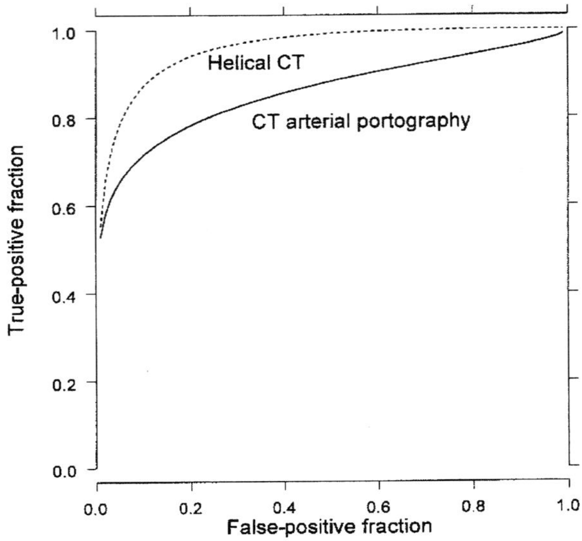

FIGURE 4.—Receiver operating characteristic curve for helical CT and CT arterial portography. Helical CT allowed significantly greater diagnostic accuracy than did CT arterial portography ($P = .001$). (Courtesy of Valls C, Lopez E, Gumà A, et al: Helical CT versus CT arterial portography in the detection of hepatic metastasis of colorectal carcinoma. *AJR* 170:1341-1347, 1998.)

carcinoma. Helical CT also avoids the invasiveness, cost, and inability to detect extrahepatic disease associated with CTAP.

► In the seemingly endless quest to find the most accurate diagnostic imaging method to evaluate the liver for metastases of colorectal cancer, several challenges have occurred to CT arterial portography (CTAP), for years considered the most sensitive of all preoperative imaging methods for liver metastases.

CTAP has been successfully challenged with MRI with the use of tissue-specific contrast agents, particularly the use of ferumoxides, with results indicating the ferumoxides-enhanced MRI was as sensitive as CTAP and, therefore, suggesting the obsolescence of CTAP because of its invasiveness and cost.

With the advent of helical CT scanning that eliminates misregistration artifacts because of breathing, there has been an increase in lesion detection with intravenous administration of contrast when compared with non-helical scanning. This has therefore given rise to the hope that conventional intravenous contrast administration with helical CT could be as sensitive as CTAP.

Researchers from Barcelona, Spain, have recently proved this by comparing prospectively helical CT with CTAP in patients with colorectal cancer with surgical and histologic findings as the gold standard. Their conclusion is that helical CT is superior to CTAP in the detection of hepatic metastases, therefore confirming what was on an anecdotal basis being discussed among abdominal imagers.

P.R. Ros, M.D., M.P.H.

Hepatic Lesion Detection: Comparison of MR Imaging After the Administration of Superparamagnetic Iron Oxide With Dual-Phase CT by Using Alternative-Free Response Receiver Operating Characteristic Analysis

Ward J, Naik KS, Guthrie JA, et al (St James's Univ, Leeds, England)

Radiology 210:459-466, 1999 7–15

Introduction.—Helical CT, using a dual-phase technique with imaging at the arterial and portal venous phases of enhancement, has improved the imaging of hepatic lesions. The liver-specific particulate MRI contrast agent superparamagnetic iron oxide (SPIO) appears to improve accuracy in the depiction of focal liver lesions, compared with unenhanced MRI and contrast-enhanced CT. SPIO-enhanced MRI was compared with dual-phase helical CT for preoperative imaging of hepatic metastases.

Methods.—The study consisted of 52 consecutive patients with known colorectal metastases who were being considered for hepatic resection. All underwent MRI, including fast spin-echo (SE) T2-weighted imaging and T1-weighted gradient-echo (GRE) fast low-angle shot imaging before SPIO enhancement, dual-echo SE imaging, T2-weighted fast low-angle shot imaging, and T1-weighted GRE imaging after SPIO enhancement. They also underwent CT scanning using 8-mm collimation and 1:1 pitch, with imaging starting 20 and 65 to 70 seconds after injection of contrast medium. The results were interpreted in blinded fashion, and the 2 techniques were compared using alternative-free response receiver operating characteristic (ROC) analysis. The CT and MRI findings were correlated with those of surgery, intraoperative US and histopathologic studies in 31 patients, and with imaging and clinical follow-up in 20.

Results.—Overall sensitivity was 80% with MRI vs. 75% with CT. The difference was greater, 81% versus 74%, respectively, for malignant lesions (Fig 2). However, there was no significant difference in the mean areas under the alternative-free response ROC curve: 0.83 with MRI and 0.78 with CT.

Conclusions.—In patients with hepatic metastases from colorectal cancer, SPIO-enhanced MRI is a more sensitive imaging technique than dual-phase CT. Patients who are candidates for segmental hepatic resection should undergo both SPIO-enhanced MRI of the liver and CT of the chest and abdomen, as CT is superior in detecting extrahepatic disease. More research is needed to improve the ability of SPIO-enhanced MRI to detect lesions smaller than 1 cm.

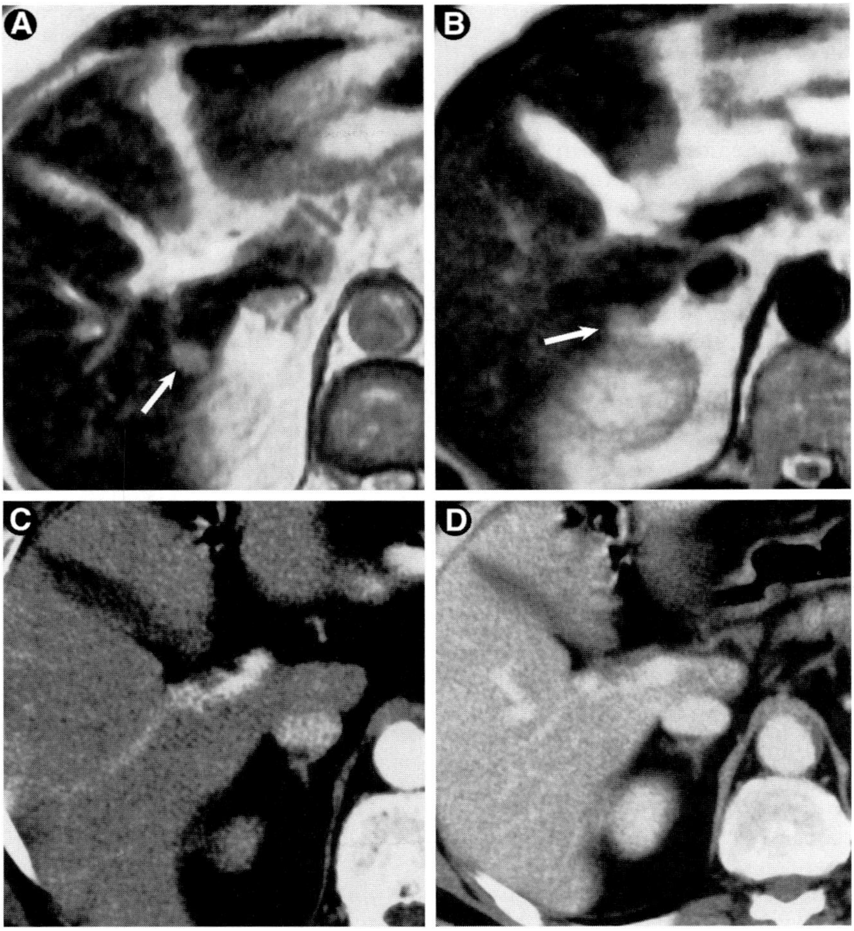

FIGURE 2.—Images obtained in a man, 69. **A**, SPIO-enhanced moderately T2-weighted SE image (2,500/45) shows a highly conspicuous 1.5-cm metastasis (*arrow*). **B**, unenhanced fast SE image (4,000/91) also shows the lesion (*arrow*) but with less conspicuity than in **A**, **C** and **D**, the lesion is not visible on (**C**) the arterial-phase CT image or (**D**) the portal venous-phase CT image. (Courtesy of Ward J, Naik KS, Guthrie JA, et al: Hepatic lesion detection: Comparison of MR imaging after the administration of superparamagnetic iron oxide with dual-phase CT by using alternative-free response receiver operating characteristic analysis. *Radiology* 210:459-466, 1999. Radiological Society of North America.)

► With the advent of advanced techniques to study the liver with helical CT, a common question is whether this technique will suffice in the detection of hepatic lesions.

In the evolution of liver focal lesion detection techniques, intravenous dynamic CT was replaced by CT arterial portography (CTAP), and recently, CTAP has been replaced by MR with contrast-specific contrast-agents (such as superparamagnetic iron oxide).

Dual-phase CT, has now made it necessary to compare these new imaging techniques with the recognized best possible test, MR imaging of the liver after administration of superparamagnetic iron oxide. Researchers from St. James's University Hospital in Leeds, England, have published a sophisticated prospective comparison using ROC analysis. They concluded that MR imaging with ferum oxides was significantly higher than CT regarding mean sensitivity. CT was inferior to MRI with ferum oxide by 5% for all lesions and by 7% for malignant lesions.

This study establishes in an elegant manner that dual-phase CT is not as good as MR with ferum oxides for the detection of liver metastases, and confirms the latter test as the most reliable, particularly in presurgical evaluation before resection for liver metastases.

P.R. Ros, M.D., M.P.H.

Biliary Tree and Pancreas

Use of Magnetic Resonance Cholangiography in the Diagnosis of Choledocholithiasis: Prospective Comparison With a Reference Imaging Method

Zidi SH, Prat F, Le Guen O, et al (Bicêtre Hosp, France)
Gut 44:118-122, 1999 7–16

Introduction.—MR cholangiography (MRC) provides a noninvasive means of biliary tract imaging without contrast medium, sedation, or analgesia. It remains to be demonstrated whether MRC can achieve the accuracy of endoscopic retrograde cholangiography (ERC) or endosonography in diagnosing common bile duct (CBD) stones. MRC was prospectively compared with standard imaging methods for the evaluation of suspected CBD stones.

Methods.—The subjects were 70 consecutive patients with suspected CBD stones. Reasons for referral included cholangitis in 47% of patients and information from US or CT scan in 27%. All patients underwent MRC with 2-dimensional turbo spin echo sequences. In addition, 63 underwent ERC, with or without sphincterotomy, within 12 hours of MRC. Other reference studies included endosonography in 5 patients and

TABLE 3.—Choledocholithiasis Diagnosis in Relation to Stone Size

Size	No of Cases Observed by Reference Method	No of Cases Observed by MRC
≤6 mm	27 (55.1)	9/27 (33.3)
>6 and ≤10 mm	16 (32.7)	15/16 (93.7)
>10 mm	6 (12.2)	4/6 (66.7)
Total	49 (100)	28/49 (57.1)

Values in parentheses are percentage of cases with lithiasis. In patients with stones of various size, the largest one is used for the table.

Abbreviation: MRC, magnetic resonance cholangiography.

(Courtesy of Zidi SH, Prat F, Le Guen O, et al: Use of magnetic resonance cholangiography in the diagnosis of choledocholithiasis: prospective comparison with a reference imaging method. *Gut* 44:118-122, 1999.)

TABLE 4.—Stone Size in the Subgroup of Patients With Small Stones (≤6 mm)

Size (mm)	No of Cases Observed by Reference Method	No of Cases Observed by MRC
1-2	5	1
1-3	6	2
2-4	6	3
4-6	10	3
Total	27	9

Some patients from each size group had two stones or more.
Abbreviation: MRC, magnetic resonance cholangiography.
(Courtesy of Zidi SH, Prat F, Le Guen O, et al: Use of magnetic resonance cholangiography in the diagnosis of choledocholithiasis: prospective comparison with a reference imaging method. *Gut* 44:118-122, 1999.)

intraoperative cholangiography in 2. The MRC findings were evaluated without knowledge of the results of the reference studies.

Results.—Bile duct stones were detected by reference imaging studies in 49 patients, including 44 with CBD stones. Mean stone size was 6 mm, though 55% of patients had stones smaller than this. The sensitivity of MRC in demonstrating bile duct lithiasis was 57%, with a specificity of 100% and positive and negative predictive value of 100% and 50%, respectively. Magnetic resonance cholangiography tended to miss stones smaller than 6 mm (Tables 3 and 4).

Conclusions.—This study does not support the use of MRC for diagnosis of suspected bile duct stones. Small stones are likely to be missed when standard MRC equipment is used. Technical refinements and wider availability will be required before MRC can replace ERC in diagnosing CBD stones.

Magnetic Resonance Cholangiopancreatography Accurately Predicts the Presence or Absence of Choledocholithiasis

Hochwald SN, Dobryansky M, Rofsky NM, et al (New York Univ)
J Gastrointest Surg 2:573-579, 1998 7–17

Introduction.—Appropriate treatment of patients with biliary stones requires accurate imaging studies of the common bile duct (CBD). However, available noninvasive imaging techniques such as US and CT are of limited accuracy. A new noninvasive technique for imaging of the biliary system is MR cholangiopancreatography (MRCP). The use of MRCP in the diagnostic imaging of CBD stones in patients at high risk was evaluated.

Methods.—The retrospective study consisted of 48 patients with biliary stones who were studied with MRCP. In most of them, MRCP was performed because of abnormal liver function tests followed by hyperamylasemia. Nineteen patients had choledocholithiasis, 11 had gallstone pancreatitis, and 18 had uncomplicated cholelithiasis. The presence or absence

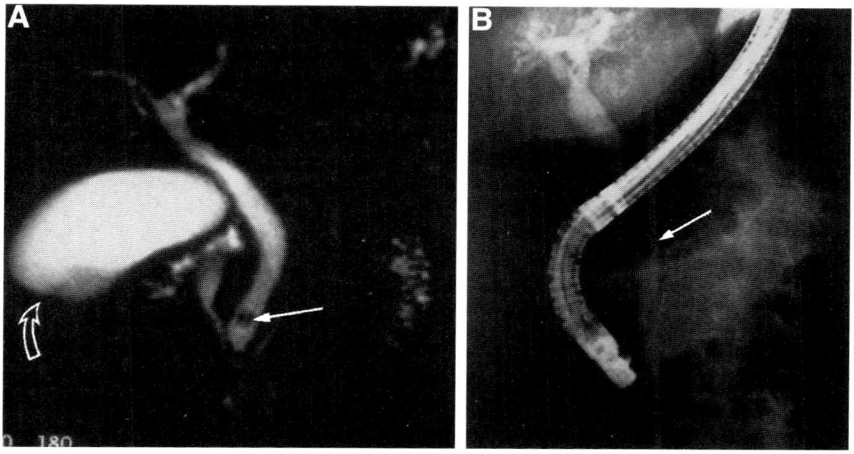

FIGURE 2.—**A**, MRCP study of a patient with a single common bile duct stone. *Open arrow* indicates gallbladder; *closed arrow* indicates stone in common bile duct. **B**, ERCP study of same patient. *Arrow* indicates stone in common bile duct. (Courtesy of Hochwald SN, Dobryansky M, Rofsky NM, et al: Magnetic resonance cholangiopancreatography accurately predicts the presence or absence of choledocholithiasis. *J Gastrointest Surg* 2:573-579, 1998.)

of CBD calculi was evaluated on MRCP. The MRCP findings were correlated with final diagnosis, which was made by endoscopic retrograde cholangiopancreatography in 19 patients, intraoperative cholangiography in 6, CBD exploration in 13, and clinical follow-up in 10.

Findings.—The final diagnosis was CBD stones in 20 patients. Nineteen of them were correctly identified by MRCP (Fig 2); 1 patient with CBD stones associated with gallstone pancreatitis was missed. In addition, MRCP suggested CBD stones in 3 of the remaining 28 patients who proved to have gallstones but no CBD stones. In the remaining 25 patients, including 10 with gallstone pancreatitis, no CBD stones were found on MRCP or at final diagnosis. The sensitivity of MRCP was 95%, with a specificity of 89% and accuracy of 92%.

Conclusions.—Noninvasive MRCP can accurately predict the presence or absence of CBD stones in patients at high risk of choledocholithiasis. The results of MRCP can have a direct impact on patient care by improving the yield of invasive CBD imaging studies and stone extraction procedures. Cost studies of MRCP are needed.

► These 2 articles (Abstracts 7–16 and 7–17) address the use of MRCP in the diagnosis of choledocholithiasis. Both articles were authored by nonradiologists (surgeons at New York University Medical Center and gastroenterologists in France) and radiologists and published in nonradiological journals: the *Journal of Gastrointestinal Surgery* and *Gut*.

The article from New York University was retrospective and included as gold standards, either endoscopic retrograde cholangiopancreatography (ERCP), intraoperative cholangiography, common bile duct surgical exploration, or clinical follow-up. The conclusion in the surgery-focused article is that MRCP is accurate (sensitivity 95%, specificity 89%, and accuracy of 92%) and is the study to recommend in the preoperative evaluation of patients suspected of having choledocholithiasis as the method to influence their therapeutic management.

The article from *Gut* is a prospective study of 70 patients with suspected bile duct stones which used as the gold standard ERC, endosonography, or intraoperative cholangiography. And the conclusion is that MRCP still is not reliable to detect stones smaller than 6 mm. In the subgroup, the sensitivity was only 57%.

These 2 articles provide both sides of the coin of MRCP. Although it is already considered a generally reliable method, when the clinical suspicion of choledocholithiasis is high and MRCP does not reveal a stone, other imaging methods such as ERCP or endoscopic sonography may be used to confirm stones smaller than 6 mm.

P.R. Ros, M.D., M.P.H.

Diagnosis of Pancreatic Carcinoma: Role of FDG PET

Keogan MT, Tyler D, Clark L, et al (Duke Univ, Durham, NC)

AJR 171:1565-1570, 1998 7–18

Purpose.—The imaging technique used in evaluating suspected pancreatic cancer should permit not only accurate diagnosis but also accurate staging. Previous reports have suggested positron emission tomography with ^{18}F-fluorodeoxyglucose (FDG PET) as a useful technique, with higher diagnostic sensitivity and specificity for pancreatic cancer than dynamic contrast-enhanced CT. The ability of FDG PET to detect primary pancreatic cancer and local nodal spread was evaluated.

Methods.—The prospective study consisted of 37 patients with possible pancreatic malignancy, based on the results of CT or ERCP. All underwent FDG PET before biopsy. The PET scan was considered positive if pancreatic FDG activity was greater than background activity, and negative if it was less than or equal to background activity. Standardized uptake ratios of FDG were calculated. The results of FDG PET, interpreted by 2 independent radiologists, were compared with those of CT, ERCP, and biopsy.

Results.—Twenty-four patients showed elevated FDG activity in the pancreas, and 22, or 92% of them were diagnosed as having pancreatic adenocarcinoma (Fig 2). The remaining 2 patients proved to have benign disease, 1 with chronic pancreatitis and 1 with a mucinous cystic tumor. Of 13 patients with low or normal FDG uptake, 10, or 77%, had benign disease. The remaining 3 patients in this group had adenocarcinomas measuring 2 to 4 cm. Mean standardized uptake ratio values were 5.1 for patients with pancreatic cancer versus 1.9 for those with benign disease. The FDG PET studies were 88% sensitive and 83% specific for the diagnosis of pancreatic malignancy.

Conclusions.—This prospective study demonstrates the sensitivity and specificity of FDG PET for diagnosis of pancreatic cancer. The noninvasive

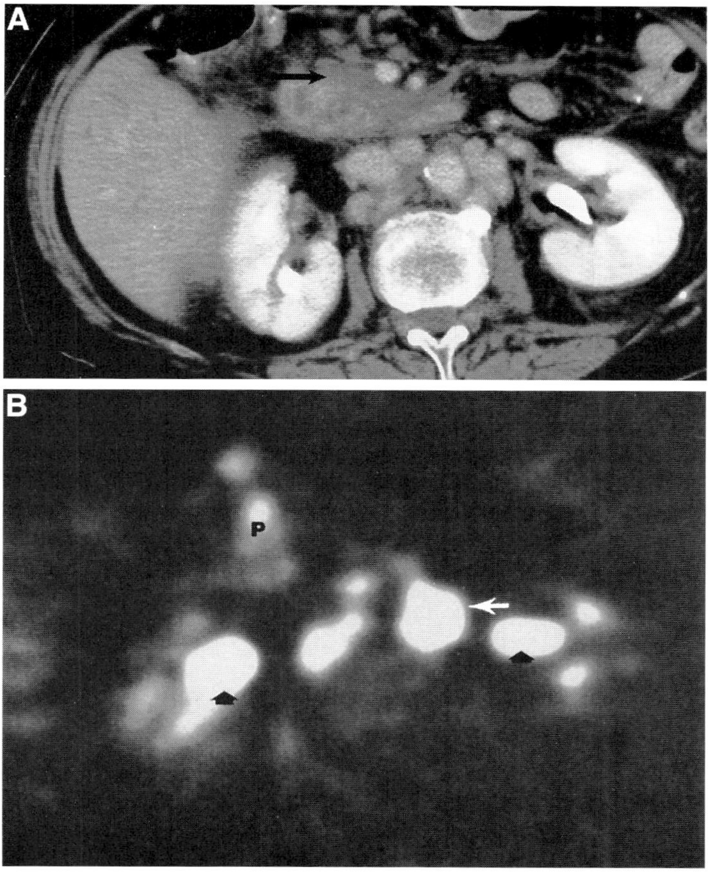

FIGURE 2.—A woman, 75, with adenocarcinoma of the pancreas. **A**, Axial CT scan during portal venous phase shows multiple para-aortic, aorta caval, and retrocaval lymph nodes. Note pancreatic head mass encroaching on superior mesenteric artery (*arrow*). **B**, Axial FDG PET scan at same level as **A** shows semicircular cuff of increased activity (*white arrow*) corresponding to retroperitoneal adenopathy seen on **A**. Note activity in region of pancreatic head mass (*P*) and in both renal collecting systems (*black arrows*). (Courtesy of Keogan MT, Tyler D, Clark L, et al: Diagnosis of pancreatic carcinoma: Role of FDG PET. *AJR* 171:1565-1570, 1998.)

study may be of greatest value in identifying patients with the highest likelihood of pancreatic malignancy, including those with equivocal results on cross-sectional imaging, nonspecific results on ERCP, or indeterminate cytology. A positive FDG-PET result in these groups should prompt an aggressive search for pancreatic cancer.

► In the quest to differentiate benign from malignant (typically ductal adenocarcinoma) pancreatic masses by imaging, researchers from Duke University Medical Center have published their experience using PET with FDG.

The overwhelming majority of cases with malignancy (92%) had increased activity in the pancreas. Only 8% of patients with benign disease had increased activity, including 1 patient with a mucinous cystic tumor who showed no malignancy at laparotomy. The authors conclude that FDG PET is both sensitive and specific to diagnose a pancreatic malignancy in a noninvasive fashion.

This article continues the expanding role of PET outside neuroradiology and its mainstream use in common abdominal malignancies. FDG PET may easily substitute for CT in the evaluation of focal masses in the pancreas when a decision has to be made regarding benign nature (focal chronic pancreatitis vs. malignancy).

P.R. Ros, M.D., M.P.H.

Improved Imaging of Liver Metastases With Stimulated Acoustic Emission in the Late Phase of Enhancement With the US Contrast Agent SH U 508A: Early Experience

Blomley MJK, Albrecht T, Cosgrove DO, et al (Hammersmith Hosp, London; Clinical Development Diagnostics, Schering, Berlin)
Radiology 210:409-416, 1999 7–19

Background.—Accurately detecting and assessing metastatic disease is important in liver imaging. The ability of stimulated acoustic emission

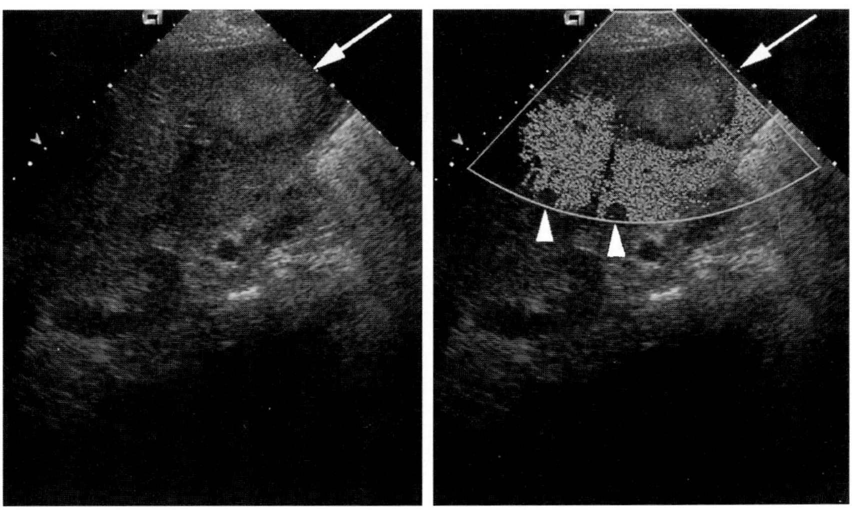

FIGURE 2.—Transverse section through the left lobe of the liver in a 53-year-old male patient with metastatic carcinoid tumor (*arrow*) in (A) gray-scale, and (B) color SAE displays. Note that in B, SAE is confined to the liver parenchyma around the metastasis, increasing its conspicuity. Also note that there are several smaller defects (*arrowheads*) in the SAE inferiorly in B, which may represent further lesions. (Courtesy of Blomley MJK, Albrecht T, Cosgrove DO, et al: Improved imaging of liver metastases with stimulated acoustic emission in the late phase of enhancement with the US contrast agent SH U 508A: Early experience. *Radiology* 210:409-416, 1999. Radiological Society of North America.)

(SAE) in the liver parenchyma in the late phase of enhancement with SH U 508A to increase conspicuity of occult metastases at US was investigated.

Methods.—Eighteen patients known to have hypovascular or hypervascular hepatic metastases were studied. US was performed at least 5 minutes after SH U 508A administration to ensure decay of blood pool enhancement. Sixteen patients had visible metastases. Conspicuity was compared on registered SAE and gray-scale scans by 2 blinded readers and by computerized analysis of relative gray-scale and color Doppler conspicuity scores inside and outside the lesion. Regions suspected of involvement but without definite gray-scale masses in 9 patients were also imaged in this way. Two blinded readers analyzed paired sections for the presence of parenchymal color defects without corresponding gray-scale masses. Nine control images from 3 healthy volunteers were included in this set.

Findings.—In all participants, intense transient parenchymal SAE was noted. Metastases were seen as areas of decreased or absent signal. Conspicuity scores were 80% and 9% for SAE and gray-scale US, respectively. All patients but none of the volunteers had SAE-specific defects. In 3 patients, metastases were seen on SAE but not on gray-scale images (Fig 2).

Conclusions.—SAE with SH U 508A can improve the conspicuity of metastases in patients with liver disease. Defects specific to SAE may demonstrate isoechoic or subtle metastases.

► Most US contrast agents reported thus far remain in the vascular space and provide contrast by increasing backscatter. This study describes a somewhat different approach. This study evaluates what seems to be organ enhancement, not just vascular enhancement. The authors also evaluate a different mechanism of enhancement, SAE. There are other US contrast agents that also work by this mechanism. Several issues remain to be resolved before clinical use of such agents, but this study demonstrates at least the potential of some US contrast agents to improve evaluation of the liver parenchyma.

D.L. Brown, M.D.

Genitourinary Radiology

Unenhanced Helical CT of Ureteral Stones: A Replacement for Excretory Urography in Planning Treatment

Fielding JR, Silverman SG, Samuel S, et al (Brigham and Women's Hosp, Boston; Harvard Med School, Boston)

AJR 171:1051-1053, 1998 7–20

Purpose.—Unenhanced helical CT can detect obstructing ureteral stones and so is widely used in the evaluation of flank pain. Excretory urography is the traditional study used to assess the intervention, and is sometimes ordered to assess the degree of obstruction. The ability of helical CT to replace excretory urography in planning treatment for patients with obstructing ureteral stones was evaluated.

Methods.—The retrospective study included helical CT scans of 100 patients with ureteral stones and a known clinical outcome. The results of excretory urograms performed within 72 hours were reviewed. The helical CT scans were then reviewed for in-plane stone diameter, *z*-axis stone diameter, stone location, periureteral stranding, hydronephrosis, and perinephric fluid. The clinical outcomes were spontaneous stone passage in 71 patients and intervention—including basket retrieval, extracorporeal shock-wave lithotripsy, and/or laser lithotripsy—in 29. Helical CT findings significantly associated with the need for intervention were identified.

Results.—Five patients, all of whom went on to intervention, had excretory urograms. Three of the 5 urograms were ordered to assess stone location, but the studies provided no additional information. Three helical CT findings were correlated with the need for intervention: in-plane diameter, *z*-axis diameter, and stone location. Patients with stones larger than 5 mm in in-plane diameter and those located within the proximal two thirds of the ureter were more likely to require intervention.

Conclusions.—Helical CT appears to be sufficient for treatment planning in patients with obstructing ureteral stones. This study can accurately determine stone size and location, which should be included in the CT report. The information will help assess the severity of obstruction and the likelihood that the stone will pass spontaneously.

► Although CT has been used for several years to detect ureteral stones, no studies have aimed to determine if unenhanced helical CT alone could replace excretory urography for diagnosis and treatment planning of patients with stones.

Researchers from Brigham and Women's Hospital/Harvard Medical School studied 100 patients with ureteral stones. They concluded that helical CT can be used in place of excretory urography to plan treatment of patients with flank pain caused by obstructing ureteral stones.

The potential criticism that CT may not be as accurate as excretory urography in determining exact location and size of stones was dispelled by this study. Both stone size and location can be accurately assessed by CT and should be reported as routinely as it is by excretory urography. Therefore, CT can replace excretory urography to predict the patients who would require endoscopic removal, lithotripsy, or both.

P.R. Ros, M.D., M.P.H.

Gadolinium-enhanced Excretory MR Urography After Low-Dose Diuretic Injection: Comparison With Conventional Excretory Urography

Nolte-Ernsting CCA, Bücker A, Adam GB, et al (Univ of Technology, Aachen, Germany; Univ of Minnesota, Minneapolis)

Radiology 209:147-157, 1998 7–21

Objective.—Although the acquisition of T2-weighted MR urography (MRU) provides "water" images that yield a high signal intensity for

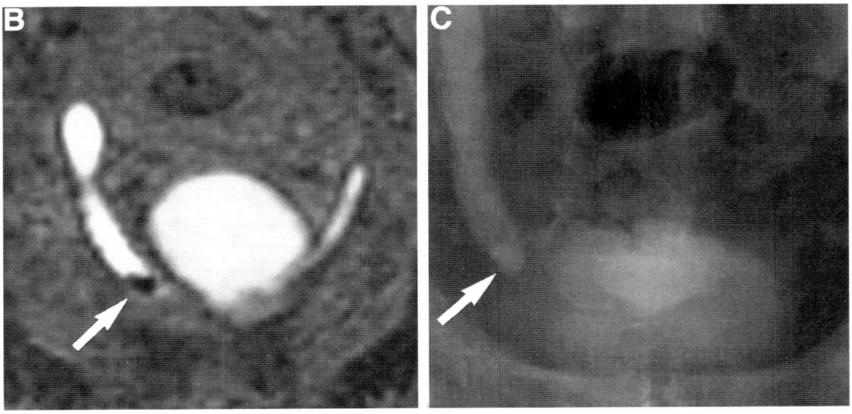

FIGURE 6.—Ureterolithiasis of the ureterovesical junction in a 75-year-old man with ureteral colic. B, Original source image from the 3D MR urography data set (15/4, 70-degree flip angle) shows the calculus (*arrow*) as a sharply delineated filling defect. C, Conventional urogram provides almost equivalent anatomic detail and the additional information that the calculus (*arrow*) is calcified. (Courtesy of Nolte-Emsting CCA, Bücker A, Adam GB, et al: Gadolinium-enhanced excretory MR urography after low-dose diuretic injection: Comparison with conventional excretory urography. *Radiology* 209:147-157, 1998. Radiological Society of North America.)

fluid-filled abdominal and retroperitoneal organs, MRU must be performed with a contrast material to provide morphologic and functional information.

Methods.—Conventional and diuretic-enhanced excretory MRU was performed in 71 patients (27 women), aged 19 to 85 (Figs 6 and 8). Excretory MRU was performed after an IV injection of 5 to 10 mg of furosemide followed by 0.1 mmol of gadopentetate dimeglumine per kilogram of body weight. Results were interpreted by 3 radiologists who were blinded to the clinical outcome.

Results.—Use of the diuretic produced a rapid, uniform distribution of the contrast material, and the furosemide-induced distension was mild. Urograms were obtained within 5 to 20 minutes after injection of contrast material. Ureters were clearly visible, and visibility was not adversely affected by peristalsis or superimposed fluid-filled intestinal loop images. High-resolution kidney images were obtained. Images suggested unilateral renal dysfunction in 11 patients, including poor residual excretory function in 3 of 4 kidneys that appeared on conventional urography to be nonfunctional. Compared with conventional urography, visualization of ureter and bladder function was significantly better with MRU. The procedure was well tolerated, and acquisition time was less than 45 minutes in most patients. The false positive rate ranged from 0 to 15%. MRU does not visualize small caliceal abnormalities as well as conventional urography does, and even fat-suppressed MR images of the pelvicaliceal system are inferior to those obtained with conventional urography.

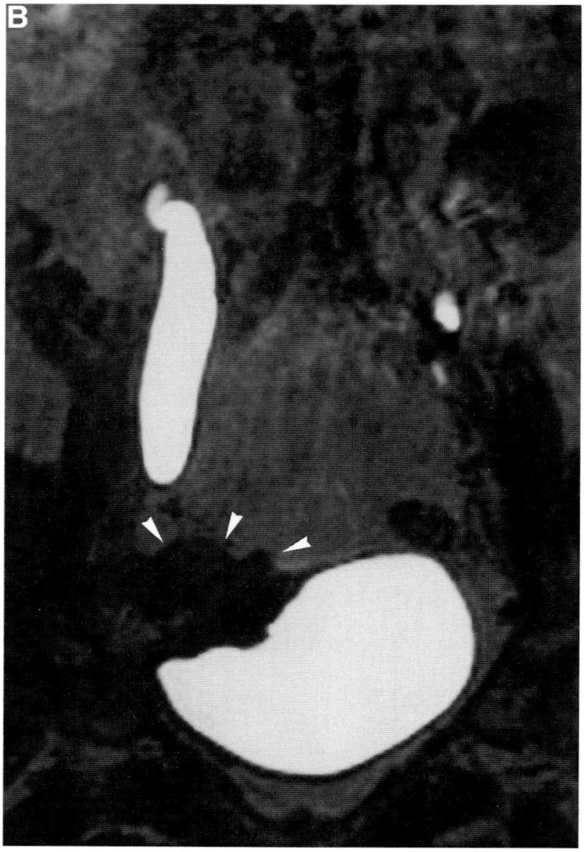

FIGURE 8.—**B**, Single section from the 3D MR urographic sequence (15/4, 70-degree flip angle) enables the best visualization of the retroperitoneal tumor (*arrowheads*). (Courtesy of Nolte-Ernsting CCA, Bücker A, Adam GB, et al: Gadolinium-enhanced excretory MR urology after low-dose diuretic injection: Comparison with conventional excretory urography. *Radiology* 209:147-157, 1998. Radiological Society of North America.)

Conclusion.—Gadolinium-enhanced excretory MR urography is a promising, although expensive, alternative to conventional urography for visualizing the morphology of the urinary tract.

► Although gadolinium-enhanced excretory MR urography is still in its infancy, it is rapidly attracting interest both experimentally and clinically. However, until now there weren't studies between contrast-enhanced MR urography and the radiologic standard of reference, conventional excretory urography. Furthermore, to enhance contrast-enhanced excretory MR urography, the use of a low-dose diuretic injection has been advocated but not carefully studied.

Authors from the Departments of Radiology and Urology at the University of Technology in Aachen, Germany, studied 71 patients with urologic symptoms, performing MR urography after intravenous injection of 5-10 mg of furosemide as well as gadolinium. The injection of diuretic before contrast material led to a rapid, uniform gadolinium distribution inside the collecting system. The MR urograms were subsequently compared with conventional urograms. MR was significantly superior to conventional urography in the assessment of both the ureters and the bladder, although still controversial in the delineation of small caliceal abnormalities.

With this article, MR urography is being established as a new addition to cross-sectional imaging in the evaluation of the urinary tract beyond conventional urography. CT has been established as the method to evaluate urolithiasis, and MR may be the answer for its functional evaluation that urologists seek in the few excretory urograms still performed routinely in our centers.

P.R. Ros, M.D., M.P.H.

Large Degenerated Adrenal Adenomas: Radiologic-Pathologic Correlation

Newhouse JH, Heffess CS, Wagner BJ, et al (Armed Forces Inst of Pathology, Washington, DC)

Radiology 210:385-391, 1999 7–22

Introduction.—Most adrenal adenomas are smaller than 5 cm, are relatively homogeneous, and have rapid and relatively uniform enhancement with rapid washout of iodinated or gadolinium-based contrast material. Intracellular lipid findings are usually associated with rare calcification on imaging. When they have intratumoral hemorrhagic degeneration with avascular and cystic internal regions and fibrosis, they become larger, displaying focal liquefaction, calcification and fibrosis, soft-tissue nodules and, patchy enhancement. The radiologic and pathologic findings of adrenal adenomas were correlated.

Methods.—Thirty large adenomas with cystic regions or areas of heterogeneity were reviewed. Their radiologic and pathologic characteristics were evaluated, as well as the contrast material–enhanced CT or MRI features. To determine whether differentiating characteristics existed, images of 24 adrenocortical carcinomas were also reviewed.

Results.—Most adrenocortical adenomas were found in women who had no symptoms. Calcification was found in 10 adenomas. Pathologic examination showed good correlation between heterogeneity and liquefied regions. Regions of adenomatous tissue with areas of hemorrhage, amorphous degenerated material, calcification, and fibrosis were confirmed by histologic examination. Myelolipomatous foci were found on some tumors. No features could be found that made possible the radiologic differentiation of adenomas from carcinomas, although some clinical and imaging findings differed between the groups.

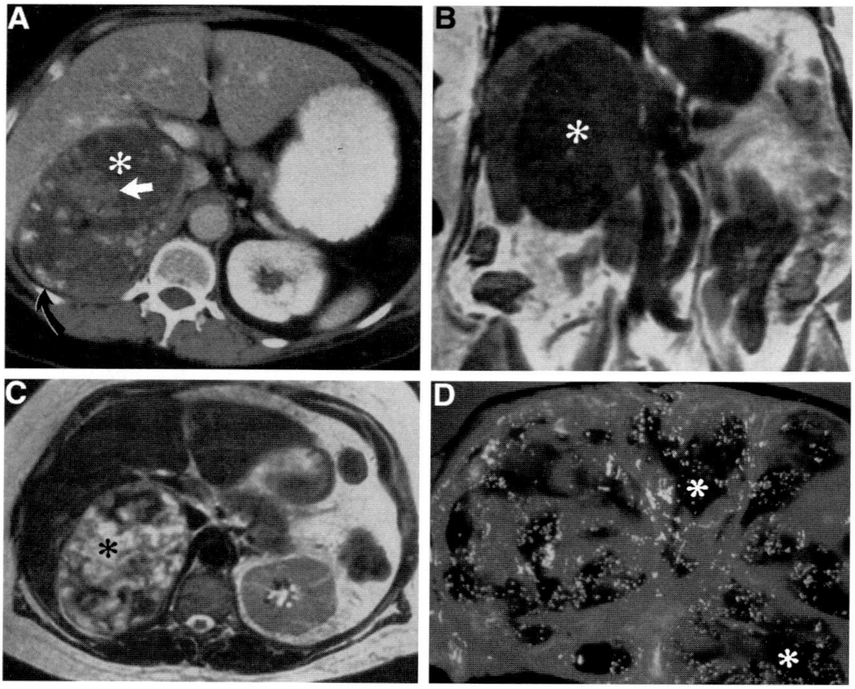

FIGURE 4.—Adrenal adenoma discovered incidentally in a 59-year-old woman many years after a right nephrectomy for multicystic dysplastic kidney. **A**, Contrast-enhanced CT scan shows a low-attenuation mass (*asterisk*) with focal calcifications (*curved arrow*) and enhancement (*straight arrow*). **B**, Coronal T1-weighted MR image shows a low-signal-intensity mass (*asterisk*) with minimal heterogeneity. **C**, T2-weighted transverse MR image shows that the mass (*asterisk*) has marked heterogeneity. **D**, Cut section of gross specimen reveals regions of acute and chronic hemorrhage and necrosis (*asterisk*). (Courtesy of Newhouse JH, Heffess CS, Wagner BJ, et al: Large degenerated adrenal adenomas: Radiologic-pathologic correlation. *Radiology* 210:385-391, 1999. Radiological Society of North America.)

Conclusion.—There is a subgroup of adenomas that are larger, more heterogeneous, and more frequently calcified than those usually found on imaging. Many of the imaging features are caused by central necrosis, hemorrhage, or both (Fig 4). Imaging alone cannot differentiate these lesions from other large adrenal masses, including adrenal carcinoma. For the definitive diagnosis, resection is required.

► Although marked advances have been made in the noninvasive diagnosis of adrenal masses, almost every radiologist has had anecdotal experiences in which the known CT and MRI findings were not as reliable as appears in the literature or prospectively and it has been necessary to determine the management of patients with borderline adrenal masses.

Investigators from the Departments of Radiology and Endocrine Pathology of the Armed Forces Institute of Pathology have summarized their experience in a classic retrospective article correlating the radiologic and pathologic characteristics of 30 large adenomas that had cystic regions or areas of heterogeneity on contrast-enhanced CT or MRI scans.

They conclude that there is a subgroup of adrenal adenomas that are large and heterogeneous, with frequent calcification, and therefore are atypical in imaging appearance. They also conclude that these lesions cannot be differentiated from adrenal carcinoma by imaging.

Therefore, we should not feel bad when, after we have sent these patients for adrenal resections, we receive the pathology report indicating that the original tumor was an adenoma and not a carcinoma.

P.R. Ros, M.D., M.P.H.

Coagulative Interstitial Laser-induced Thermotherapy of Benign Prostatic Hyperplasia: Online Imaging With a T2-Weighted Fast Spin-Echo MR Sequence—Experience in Six Patients

Mueller-Lisse UG, Thoma M, Faber S, et al (Univ of Munich "Ludwig Maximilian," Germany)

Radiology 210:373-379, 1999 7–23

Introduction.—A minimally invasive treatment for benign prostatic hyperplasia is interstitial thermotherapy, predominantly carried out with lasers as the source of thermal energy and also referred to as laser-induced thermotherapy (LITT). It has been suggested that posttherapeutic MRI after LITT of the prostate shows a clear delineation of coagulated tissue from the viable surrounding tissue. To determine whether lesions are permanent and whether their diameters correspond with lesion diameters measured on posttherapeutic T2-weighted fast spin-echo images and contrast-enhanced T1-weighted spin-echo images of the prostate obtained at the end of LITT, a rapid T2-weighted fast spin-echo sequence was applied to the online MRI of LITT in patients with benign prostatic hyperplasia.

Methods.—Six patients with benign prostatic hyperplasia had 12 LITT treatments. They were followed online with repetitive axial T2-weighted fast spin-echo imaging that had a repetition time of 3,700 mseconds, an echo time of 138 mseconds, and an acquisition time of 19 seconds. The investigation included development, time course, correlation with interstitial tissue temperature, and diameters of hypointense lesions around the laser diffusor tip. Comparisons of lesion diameters were conducted on T2-weighted images acquired during LITT, final lesions on T2-weighted images, and unperfused lesions on enhanced T1-weighted spin-echo images obtained at the end of therapy.

Results.—Within 20 to 40 seconds of LITT, hypointense lesions developed. During LITT, the average correlation coefficient between interstitial temperature development and signal intensity developed was 0.92; after LITT, it was 0.90. During LITT, regression slopes were significantly steeper at 0.67% signal intensity change per degree C than after LITT, when it was 0.47% per degree C. For all procedures, lesions remained visible after LITT (Fig 2). Before all treatments, the laser diffusor tip at the active end

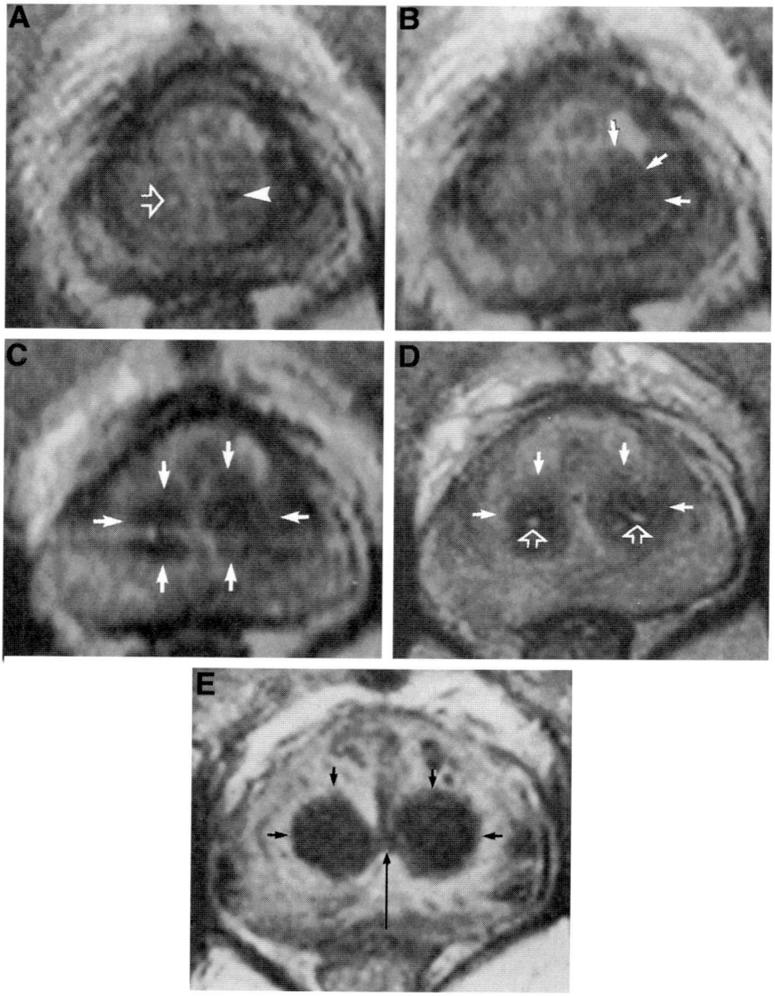

FIGURE 2.—**A**, rapid T2-weighted axial fast spin-echo image (3,700/138) of prostate with benign prostatic hyperplasia before laser-induced thermotherapy. Laser diffusor tip is recognized by a signal void (*arrowhead*). Prior position of laser waveguide in right prostate lobe shows high signal intensity (*open arrow*). **B**, rapid T-2weighted axial fast spin-echo image (3,700/138) of prostate obtained during laser-induced thermotherapy (seventh imaging cycle, 140 seconds of laser irradiation). A hypointense area of round or slightly ovoid shape (*arrows*) spreads from the laser diffusor tip and demarcates from surrounding tissue. **C**, rapid T2-weighted axial fast spin-echo image (3,700/138) obtained immediately after laser-induced thermotherapy (10th imaging cycle, 20 seconds after laser irradiation). *Arrows* demarcate outlines of laser-induced lesions in right and left prostate lobes. **D**, T2-weighted axial fast spin-echo image (4,700/99) obtained at the end of the procedure (similar to level in **C**). Hypointense lesions of laser-induced thermotherapy demarcate from surrounding prostate tissue (*solid arrows*). Prior positions of laser waveguides show high signal intensity (*open arrows*), possibly from interstitial fluid filling the waveguide track. No evidence of periprostatic edema. **E**, Contrast-enhanced axial T1-weighted SE image (714/14) obtained at the end of the procedure shows the same laser-induced lesions (similar to level in **C** and **D**). Tissue necrosis in the hypointense lesions (*short arrows*) is suggested by lack of perfusion. *Long arrow* demarcates prostatic urethra at entry site of laser waveguide tips into prostatic tissue. (Courtesy of Mueller-Lisse UG, Thoma M, Faber S, et al: Coagulative interstitial laser-induced thermotherapy of benign prostatic hyperplasia: Online imaging with a T2-weighted fast spin-echo MR sequence-Experience in six patients. *Radiology* 210:373-379, 1999. Radiological Society of North America.)

of the waveguide was recognized by a signal void. After treatment, a round or slightly ovoid hypointense area was clearly shown. The average maximum diameters of lesions were 1 to 3 mm larger during LITT, than after LITT.

Conclusion.—The development of permanent hypointense prostate lesions was demonstrated on repetitive T2-weighted fast spin-echo MRI during interstitial coagulative LITT of benign prostatic hyperplasia. During LITT, posttherapeutic lesion diameters tend to be overestimated.

► There has been a lot of interest in diagnostic imaging and imaging-guided therapy for prostatic cancer. Conversely, there has been less interest in advanced diagnostic and imaging-guided therapeutic advances for benign prostatic hyperplasia.

Investigators from the Departments of Diagnostic Radiology, Urology and Anaesthesiology at the University of Munich in Germany have published their experience with the use of interstitial LITT to treat benign prostatic hyperplasia and to determine whether MRI is capable of demonstrating the development of permanent changes compared with the benign prostatic hyperplasia findings in pre-LITT MR images.

Although the experience is limited to 6 patients with 12 LITT treatments, it appears that LITT is effective in treating benign prostatic hyperplasia and that MRI is capable of determining the stability of the lesions obtained.

This article confirms the potential use of minimally invasive therapies to solve common problems, such as benign prostatic hyperplasia that until now have relied on more aggressive methods of therapy, such as transurethral prostatic resections.

P.R. Ros, M.D., M.P.H.

Lymph Node Metastases: Safety and Effectiveness of MR Imaging With Ultrasmall Superparamagnetic Iron Oxide Particles—Initial Clinical Experience

Bellin M-F, Roy C, Kinkel K, et al (Hôpital Pitié-Salpêtrière, Paris; CHU, Strasbourg, France; Institut Gustave Roussy, Villejuif, France; et al)
Radiology 207:799-808, 1998 7–24

Objective.—Whereas lymph node staging is an important prognostic factor for patients with urologic and pelvic cancers, there is no general agreement on the best staging method. Studies have shown that ultrasmall paramagnetic iron oxide particles with a long plasma circulation time decrease the MR T2 of normal nodes but not of metastatic nodes. The clinical and biological safety of ultrasmall paramagnetic iron oxide particles (IV infusion of AMI-227 at a dose of 1.7 mg of iron per kilogram of body weight) and the potential of AMI-227 in differentiating benign from metastatic nodes in patients with urologic and pelvic cancers were investigated in a multicenter phase II clinical trial.

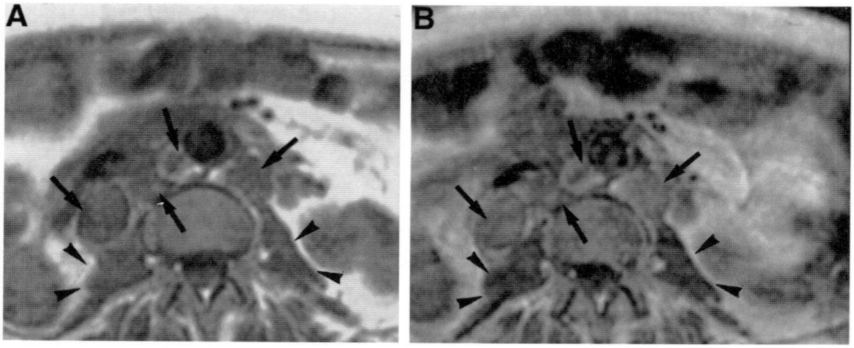

FIGURE 3.—Metastatic retroperitoneal nodes in a patient with transitional cell carcinoma. **A**, Precontrast T1-weighted SE image (400/11) shows multiple bulky retroperitoneal nodes (*arrows*); their SI is comparable to that of the adjacent psoas muscles (*arrowheads*). **B**, Postcontrast T1-weighted image (400/11) shows a homogeneous increase in the SI of these metastatic nodes (*arrows*), which now appear hyperintense relative to the psoas muscles (*arrowheads*). (Courtesy of Bellin M-F, Roy C, Kinkel K, et al: Lymph node metastases: Safety and effectiveness or MR imaging with ultrasmall superparamagnetic iron oxide particles—Initial clinical experience. *Radiology* 207:799-808, 1998. Radiological Society of North America.)

Methods.—The AMI-227 was infused into 30 patients (9 women), aged 29 to 82 years, with suspected metastatic disease. Magnetic resonance imaging studies were performed before and 22 to 26 hours after AMI-227 administration. Sixty nodes were imaged, and 29 of these were analyzed

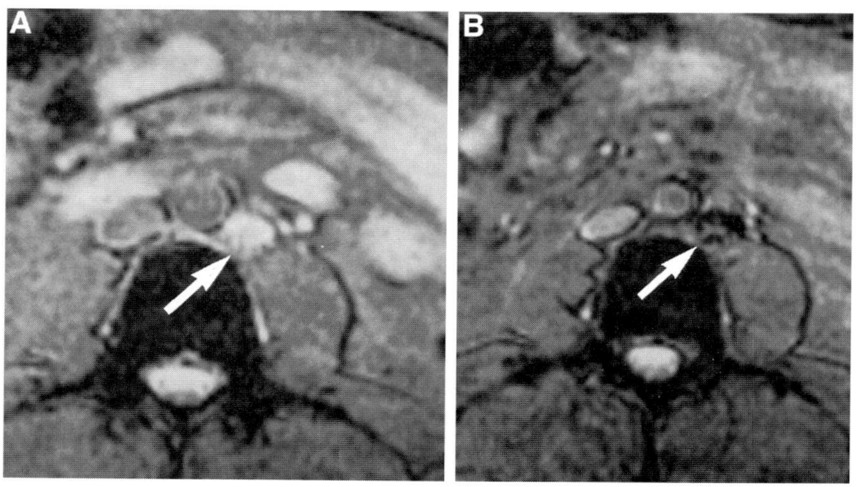

FIGURE 4.—Inflammatory node in a patients with testicular carcinoma. **A**, Precontrast T2*-weighted GRE image (500/18, 15-degree flip angles) shows an 18-mm (diameter) para-aortic node (*arrow*) with high SI. **B**, Postcontrast T2*-weighted GRE images (500/18, 15-degree flip angle) demonstrates partial enhancement, with a peripheral rim of low SI (*arrow*). The node was found to be nonmetastatic at histologic examination. (Courtesy of Bellin M-F, Roy C, Kinkel K, et al: Lymph node metastases: Safety and effectiveness or MR imaging with ultrasmall superparamagnetic iron oxide particles—Initial clinical experience. *Radiology* 207:799-808, 1998. Radiological Society of North America.)

quantitatively to assess AMI-227 uptake. Adverse events were monitored for 3 days after infusion.

Results.—The AMI-227 caused no major adverse reactions. No Perls-staining iron appeared in metastatic nodes or in nonmetastatic areas of metastatic nodes. There was an increase in signal intensity (SI) in 9 of 27 metastatic nodes, but there was no change in SI in 18 metastatic nodes (Fig 3 and Fig 4). Nodal architecture was not characteristic. The sensitivity, specificity, and Youden index were 1005, 77% to 80%, and 0.77 to 0.80, respectively. Whereas the SI of most of the malignant nodes remained unchanged before and after AMI-227 infusion, the decrease in SI of benign nodes after infusion of AMI-227 was more pronounced on GRE images than on SE images.

Conclusion.—AMI-227–enhanced MR images may possibly be used to differentiate between metastatic and nonmetastatic nodes in patients with urologic and pelvic cancers.

► A key pursuit in radiology in general and abdominal radiology in particular has been to characterize benign versus malignant lymph node involvement. The imaging criterion used until now has been size with the innate overlap between benign and malignant etiology.

The advent of ultrasmall superparamagnetic iron oxide particles in 1990 provided a way to assess the internal architecture of lymph nodes experimentally. However, we had to wait until 1998 for the report on the first clinical experience. A group of French investigators studied 30 adults suspected of having lymph node metastases with MRI approximately 24 hours after intravenous infusion of AMI-227, an ultrasmall superparamagnetic iron oxide particle. Sixty lymph nodes were analyzed and MR images were subsequently compared with histopathologic data. None of the 27 metastatic lymph nodes showed a decrease in signal intensity, while a perceptive reduction of signal intensity indicating active AMI-227 update was observed in T2-weighted images on 16 of the 21 benign nodes. The obvious conclusion is that AMI-227 is not only a safe contrast agent but also that it may facilitate a differentiation between metastatic and benign lymph nodes in the abdomen in patients with urologic and pelvic cancers.

P.R. Ros, M.D., M.P.H.

Gynecological Ultrasound

Tissue Harmonic Imaging Sonography: Evaluation of Image Quality Compared With Conventional Sonography

Shapiro RS, Wagreich J, Parsons RB, et al (Mount Sinai Med Ctr, New York)
AJR 171:1203-1206, 1998 7–25

Introduction.—Tissue harmonic imaging (THI) is a new sonographic technique with the potential to provide images of higher quality than those obtained with conventional sonographic techniques. In THI sonography, higher harmonic frequencies produced by propagation of the US beam through tissue are used to create the sonogram. Image quality of THI

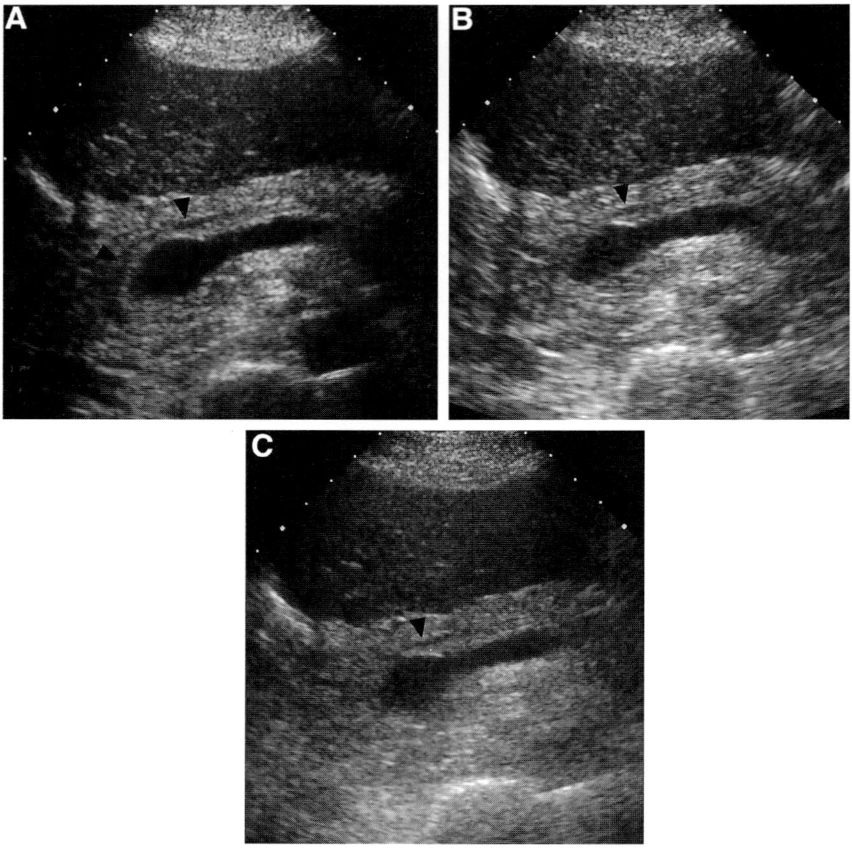

FIGURE 1.—A 73-year-old woman with upper gastrointestinal bleeding and normal pancreas. **A-C**, Sonograms of pancreas using tissue harmonic imaging (THI) (**A**), 2.5-MHz conventional imaging (**B**), and 4.0-MHz conventional imaging (**C**) show that depiction of pancreas duct (*arrowheads*) is best with THI sonography. Echoes within vascular structures are absent in **A**, as opposed to **B** and **C**. (Courtesy of Shapiro RS, Wagreich J, Parsons RB: Tissue harmonic imaging sonography: Evaluation of image quality compared with conventional sonography. *AJR* 171:1203-1206, 1998.)

sonography was prospectively compared with that of conventional sonography in 89 randomly selected patients.

Methods.—Anatomic areas examined were pancreas (60) and other anatomic areas (68, 36 liver, 15 gallbladder or bile ducts, 7 kidney, 3 spleen, 3 uterus, 2 ovaries, 1 transjugular intrahepatic portosystemic shunt, and 1 aorta). All examinations of the same anatomic area were performed in triplicate by means of THI sonography (transmitted frequency, 2.0 MHz, received frequency, 4.0 MHz) and conventional sonography of 2.5 and 4.0 MHz. Images were graded for penetration, detail, and total image quality by graders who were unaware of the sonographic technique used.

Results.—For pancreatic examinations, THI sonography was superior for penetration, detail, and quality in 45, 54, and 50 patients, respectively. For pancreatic examinations, THI sonography was significantly better than both 2.5-MHz and 4.0-MHz conventional sonography for penetration, detail, and total image quality (Fig 1). For the 68 examinations of other anatomic areas, THI was superior for penetration, detail, and total quality image in 42, 57, and 58 patients, respectively. For examinations of other anatomic areas, THI sonography was significantly better than both 2.5-MHz and 4.0-MHz conventional sonography for penetration, detail, and total image quality.

Conclusion.—Images produced by THI sonography were superior to those produced by conventional sonography. Further investigation is needed to determine whether this improvement will produce improved diagnostic accuracy.

► Although much of the initial interest in harmonic imaging US was for US contrast agents, it also is useful without contrast agents. Image quality is generally better than with conventional sonographic imaging and harmonic imaging may be particularly useful for patients in whom optimal images are difficult to obtain with conventional US. The effect on diagnostic accuracy remains to be determined.

D.L. Brown, M.D.

Transvaginal Sonographic Markers of Tubal Inflammatory Disease

Timor-Tritsch IE, Lerner JP, Monteagudo A, et al (Columbia-Presbyterian Med Ctr, New York; New York Univ; Univ of Toronto; et al)

Ultrasound Obstet Gynecol 12:56-66, 1998 7–26

Introduction.—Transvaginal sonography (TVS) permits clear visualization of fallopian tube lesions. There is ongoing confusion over the US diagnosis of pelvic inflammatory disease (PID). The sonographic markers of fallopian tube disease were analyzed, and related to the clinical findings.

Methods.—All gynecologic TVS examinations performed over an 18-month period were reviewed. Of the 77 patients, 15 were referred for evaluation of acute pelvic inflammatory processes, while 62 were referred for various other reasons, including chronic PID. The TVS markers of tubal inflammatory disease evaluated included shape, wall structure, and thickness, extent of ovarian involvement, and presence of fluid.

Results.—Ninety-two percent of patients with acute or chronic tubal inflammation had an incomplete septum of the tubal wall. Among patients with acute tubal disease, 100% had tubal wall thickening and 86% had a "cogwheel" sign wall structure. In contrast, patients with chronic PID were more likely to have a thin tubal wall with a "beads-on-a-string" wall structure. All acute cases and 72% of chronic cases had palpable findings, while 21% and 30%, respectively, had a previous surgical history; these findings were not discriminatory. There were 3 false-positive results: 1

patient with an ovarian cystadenoma, 1 with appendiceal mucocele, and 1 with periovarian fluid.

Conclusions.—TVS is useful in defining the different types and degrees of PID. It allows distinction between the tubo-ovarian complex and tubo-ovarian abscess, with their differing clinical implications. TVS also helps in making the differential diagnosis between chronic tubal disease and ovarian tumor. In addition, it demonstrates hydrosalpinges and infection occurring after tubal ligation or hysterectomy.

► The science of this study can be debated as some of the methods are unclear, however, the article is well illustrated and is a useful teaching aid regarding US and inflammatory disease of the fallopian tubes. The appearance of endosalpingeal folds is well reviewed. It is important to be aware of this appearance so as not to interpret such masses as likely to be malignant. The distinction between tubo-ovarian abscess and tubo-ovarian complex is also discussed. Despite some concerns about methodology, the article provides a useful conceptual framework for the US evaluation of tubal inflammatory disease.

D.L. Brown, M.D.

Sonography of the Female Urethra

Siegel CL, Middleton WD, Teefey SA, et al (Washington Univ, St Louis)
AJR 170:1268-1274, 1998 7–27

Background.—Imaging options for women with symptoms related to the urethra include voiding cystourethrography (VCUG) or direct double-balloon urethrography. Advances in sonographic equipment permit complete sonographic evaluation of the female urethra, including periurethral structures. An experience with sonographic evaluation of women with urethral symptoms is presented.

Methods.—The study included 19 women with urethral symptoms raising suspicion of urethral diverticula. In addition to VCUG, all patients underwent transvaginal, transperineal, and endourethral sonographic examination. The endourethral examination was performed using a 12.5 MHz, 6.2F catheter-based transducer. Both imaging studies were used to seek evidence of diverticula. The sonographic criterion for diverticulum was direct visualization of the neck connecting the periurethral sac with the urethral lumen. Other nonurethral findings were recorded as well.

Results.—A total of 15 urethral diverticula were diagnosed in 14 patients. The sonographic diameter of the diverticula ranged from 2 mm to 5 cm. All but 2 of the diverticula were detected by sonography. Other sonographically detected abnormalities included 2 infected periurethral cysts, a periurethral leiomyoma, a case of diffuse urethritis, and scarring related to a previous diverticulectomy. Eight of the 13 diverticula detected on US encompassed more than half of the circumference of the urethra. In keeping with the study definition, the neck of the diverticulum was visualized sonographically in 13 of 15 cases compared with just 2 of 13 on VCUG.

Conclusions.—US is a useful imaging examination for women with suspected urethral diverticula. US helps to delineate the neck of the diverticulum, which is essential information for surgery. It also demonstrates nonurethral lesions.

► Evaluation of the female urethra is an infrequent but useful application of US. The endoluminal US discussed here is not widely available, but transvaginal and transperineal US are readily available in most locales. We have also found these techniques very useful for evaluating the female urethra, particularly for evaluating urethral diverticula. Awareness of the sonographic appearances discussed in this article will help one use US to evaluate the periurethral area. One must remember however, that with transvaginal assessment the transducer is inserted only slightly into the vagina. With full insertion of the transducer, such as is done with most transvaginal pelvic sonograms, one will not be able to image the urethral region.

D.L. Brown, M.D.

Cystic Teratomas of the Ovary: Diagnostic Value of Sonography

Patel MD, Feldstein VA, Lipson SD, et al (Univ of California, San Francisco)

AJR 171:1061-1065, 1998 7–28

Background.—Patients subsequently found to have cystic teratomas may be commonly referred for MR imaging of the pelvis because of an erroneous preliminary sonographic diagnosis of ovarian cancer. This study determined whether experienced sonologists can make the diagnosis of cystic teratomas of the ovary based only on specific sonographic features.

Methods.—Two sonologists independently reviewed the sonograms of 226 women with a total of 252 adnexal lesions. Each sonologist recorded the sonographic characteristics of each mass using a standardized checklist, then chose a diagnosis from a list of diagnostic possibilities.

Findings.—Seventy-four cystic teratomas were identified. Fifty-five of these masses showed 2 or more associated sonographic features. For each reviewer, the positive predictive value and sensitivity for the diagnosis and identification of cystic teratomas were 98% and 85%, respectively. When an adnexal mass showed 2 or more sonographic features associated with dermoid masses, the positive predictive value was 100%. For individual sonographic features associated with dermatoid masses, the positive predictive value was 80% for a shadowing echodensity, 75% for regionally bright echoes, 50% for hyperechoic lines and dots, and 20% for a fluid-fluid level (Fig 1; Table 1).

Conclusions.—An adnexal lesion that shows 2 or more sonographic features associated with cystic teratomas can be diagnosed confidently as

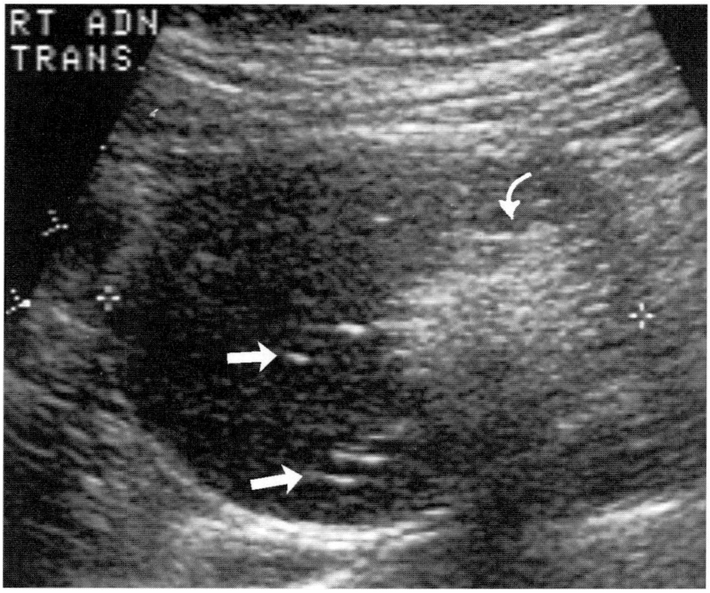

FIGURE 1.—52-year-old woman with cystic teratoma of ovary. Transabdominal sonogram shows regional bright echoes (*curved arrow*) with acoustic shadowing and hyperechoic lines and dots (*straight arrows*). Both reviewers identified all 3 features and made correct diagnosis. (Courtesy of Patel MD, Feldstein VA, Lipson SD, et al: Cystic teratomas of the ovary: Diagnostic value of sonography. *AJR Am J Roentgenol* 171:1061-1065, 1998.)

cystic teratoma. This practice may help reduce unnecessary testing and anxiety.

► Although much has been written about the sonographic findings of cystic teratomas in the ovary, this article attempts to evaluate the various sonographic features that have been described. Because such neoplasms are common, it is important to be aware of all the sonographic findings and how they can best be used to accurately diagnose cystic teratomas. It would be most informative for the reader to review the full article, which is succinct, to understand the various features and their limitations. As the authors state, such knowledge should help decrease patient anxiety and obviate the need for additional imaging tests.

D.L. Brown, M.D.

TABLE 1.—Diagnostic Performance of 2 Reviewers and Sonographic Characteristics Used in Identifying Cystic Teratomas

Reviewer Performance and Sonographic Characteristics	Cystic Teratomas Exhibiting Two or More Features ($n = 55$)	Cystic Teratomas Exhibiting One Feature ($n = 17$)	Nondermoid Masses ($n = 178$)	Sensitivity (%)	Positive Predictive Value (%)	Positive Likelihood Ratio
Reviewer performance						
Reviewer 1 diagnosis of cystic teratoma	52 (95%)	11 (65%)	1	85	98	152
Reviewer 2 diagnosis of cystic teratoma	49 (89%)	14 (82%)	1	85	98	152
Reviewer average	50.5 (92%)	12.5 (74%)	1	85	98	152
Sonographic characteristics						
At least one feature	55 (100%)	17 (100%)	9	97	89	19
At least two features	55 (100%)	0	0	74	100	>132*
Only one feature	0	17 (100%)	9	23	65	5
Shadowing echodensity with no other features	0	12 (71%)	3	16	80	10
Regional bright echoes with no other features	0	3 (18%)	1	4	75	7
Hyperechoic lines and dots with no other features	0	1 (6%)	1	1	50	2
Fluid-fluid level with no other features	0	1 (6%)	4	1	20	1
Cystic with nodular wall	22 (40%)	9 (53%)	30	42	51	3
No features of cyst	24 (44%)	7 (41%)	11	42	74	7

*Exact number lies between 132 and infinity and cannot be determined with more precision.

(Courtesy of Patel MD, Feldstein VA, Lipson SD, et al: Cystic teratomas of the ovary: Diagnostic value of sonography. *AJR Am J Roentgenol* 171:1061-1065, 1998.)

Benign and Malignant Ovarian Masses: Selection of the Most Discriminating Gray-Scale and Doppler Sonographic Features
Brown DL, Doubilet PM, Miller FH, et al (Harvard Med School)
Radiology 208:103-110, 1998 7–29

Background.—The abilities of many gray-scale and Doppler sonographic characteristics to distinguish between benign and ovarian masses have been studied. This study attempted to determine the most discriminating gray-scale and Doppler sonographic features for differentiating between such masses.

Methods and Findings.—The gray-scale and Doppler characteristics of 211 adnexal masses were correlated with final diagnoses. One hundred thirty-eight were benign, and 28 were malignant. All lesions with a markedly hyperechoic solid component or no solid component were benign. Among those with a nonhyperechoic solid component, additional characteristics that significantly discriminated between benign and malignant lesions were location of flow at conventional color Doppler imaging, amount of free intraperitoneal fluid, and the presence and thickness of septations (in decreasing order of importance). A scoring formula based on a logistic regression equation had an area under the receiver operating characteristic curve of 0.98. The cutoff score with the best accuracy had a sensitivity and specificity of 93% each.

Conclusions.—The best predictor of an ovarian mass malignancy is a solid component. These authors developed a multivariate scoring system using 3 gray-scale features and 1 Doppler feature that has a high sensitivity and specificity for predicting malignancy.

► Although this reviewer is somewhat biased in selecting this article, the article tries to integrate the various gray-scale and Doppler sonographic features that have been used to predict malignant and benign ovarian masses. The results show that color Doppler is useful only when there is a nonhyperechoic solid component within the mass. Even if one prefers not to use scoring systems or probability tables, the results provide a practical approach to categorizing ovarian masses.

D.L. Brown, M.D.

Obstetrical Ultrasound

Ultrasonographic Diagnosis of Trisomy 18: Is It Practical in the Early Second Trimester?
Shields LE, Carpenter LA, Smith KM, et al (Univ of Washington, Seattle)
J Ultrasound Med 17:327-331, 1998 7–30

Introduction.—Trisomy 18 is the second most frequent autosomal trisomy and has a prevalence of 1 in 8,000 births. Earlier reports have noted that 80% to 85% of fetuses with trisomy 18 have detectable abnormalities for gestational ages 12 to 40 weeks. Reported is a retrospective review of

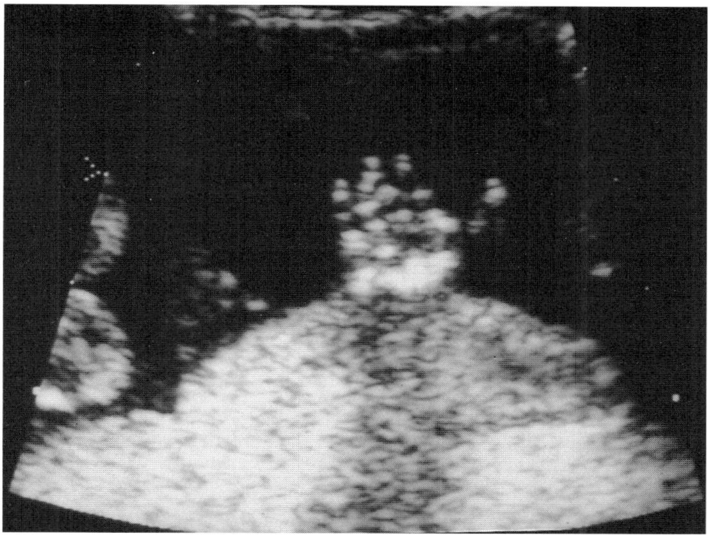

FIGURE 1.—Fetal hand at 16 weeks' gestation shows overlapped third and fourth fingers, which persisted throughout the examination. (Courtesy of Shields LE, Carpenter LA, Smith KM: Ultrasonographic diagnosis of trisomy 18: Is it practical in the early second trimester? *J Ultrasound Med* 17:327-331, 1998.)

experience with the prenatal detection of US abnormalities in fetuses with trisomy 18 early in the second trimester, a time when most pregnant females undergo screening US.

Methods.—The prenatal database was reviewed from January 1987 to June 1996 to identify females referred for prenatal genetic evaluation

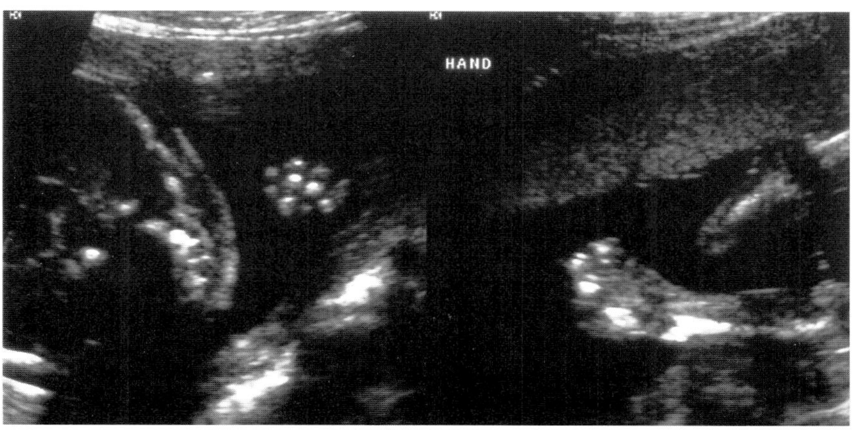

FIGURE 2.—Right and left hands of a fetus with trisomy 18 at 18 weeks' gestation. The image on the left shows a normal fetal hand without overlapping fingers, whereas the image on the left, of the same fetus, demonstrates the hand in a clenched position, which persisted throughout the examination. (Courtesy of Shields LE, Carpenter LA, Smith KM: Ultrasonographic diagnosis of trisomy 18: Is it practical in the early second trimester? *J Ultrasound Med* 17:327-331, 1998.)

between 14 and 22 weeks of gestation who were found to have a fetus with trisomy 18 karoytype. Sonographic reports and films were examined for the presence or absence of fetal anatomic abnormalities.

Results.—Thirty-five fetuses had the trisomy 18 karoytype. Of these, 30 had at least 1 detected abnormality. Mean number of abnormalities per fetus was 3 (range, 0-6); most fetuses had more than 1 abnormality. The most frequently occurring abnormalities were persistent abnormal position of fetal fingers (89%), choroid plexus cysts (43%), abnormally shaped fetal head (strawberry or lemon) (43%), two-vessel umbilical cord (40%), cardiac defects (37%), intrauterine growth restriction (29%), omphalocele (20%), neural tube defects (9%), and cystic hygroma or lymphangiectasia (14%). Abnormalities of amniotic fluid volume and renal defects (12% and 9%, respectively) were not as common.

Conclusion.—Most fetuses with trisomy 18 have sonographically detectable anatomic abnormalities by the early second trimester. The fetal hand seems to be abnormal in many fetuses with trisomy 18 early in the second trimester (Fig 1), and the abnormality may be subtle or unilateral (Fig 2).

► Although the prenatal diagnosis of trisomy 21 has received much attention in the literature, trisomy 18 is also important because it is the second most common autosomal trisomy. The findings in this retrospective study suggest that the majority, but not all, of fetuses with trisomy 18 have some abnormality identifiable by US. The most frequent findings are reviewed. The importance of evaluating the fetal hands is discussed; evaluation of the hands is particularly important in fetuses with choroid plexus cysts.

D.L. Brown, M.D.

Echogenic Peritoneal Fluid As an Isolated Sonographic Finding: Significance in Patients at Risk of Ectopic Pregnancy

Wachsberg RH, Levine CD (Univ Hosp and New Jersey Med School, Newark)

Clin Radiol 53:520-522, 1998 7–31

Introduction.—It is commonly believed that the presence of echogenic fluid in any quantity has a very high positive predictive value for ectopic pregnancy (EP) in patients at risk, regardless of the presence or absence of other abnormal sonographic findings. However, echogenic fluid as an isolated finding is rare.

Methods.—Experience with patients referred because of possible EP and in whom echogenic fluid was the only pertinent positive sonographic finding was reviewed retrospectively. All sonographic reports included the character and quantity of free fluid determined at the time of real-time sonography. Quantity of the fluid was graded as small, moderate, or large. To maximize appreciation of particulate echoes if free fluid was detected, good contact between the probe and the vaginal wall was established and the gain setting was raised to just below the threshold at which artifactual echoes show up in bladder urine. If there was doubt regarding whether apparent echoes were real or artifactual, an attempt was made to cause the echogenic particles to move.

Results.—There was no sonographic evidence of intrauterine pregnancy in 74 patients, among whom EP was verified in 35 (47%). Of these, 29 (39%) had an unremarkable sonogram and 3 (10%) had EP confirmed at laparoscopy. Echogenic fluid was the only extrauterine sonographic abnormality in 13 patients (18%); 1 patient was lost to follow-up. Of the remaining 12 patients, the quantity of echogenic fluid was small in 2 (17%), moderate in 6 (50%), and large in 4 (33%). Of 9 patients who underwent surgery, EP was detected in 7 and there were 2 spontaneous abortions. Eight patients who underwent laparotomy or laparoscopy had confirmed hemoperitoneum. Three additional patients with a moderate quantity of echogenic fluid had passed tissuelike material, were hemodynamically stable, and had low serum β-hCG concentrations. The final diagnosis for these 3 patients was spontaneous abortion. For the series, the final diagnoses were EP in 7 patients (48%) and spontaneous abortion in 5 patients (42%). The prevalence of EP in patients with echogenic fluid as the only sonographic finding was significantly greater than in patients with an unremarkable sonogram. In only 3 of the 8 patients with small or moderate amounts of echogenic fluid was EP diagnosed. This rate was not significantly different from that of patients in whom a large amount of echogenic fluid was detected. Mean serum β-hCG concentrations were similar for both groups. A small to moderate amount of echogenic intraperitoneal fluid as an isolated finding is not highly predictive of EP in patients with a positive pregnancy test and no sonographic evidence of intrauterine pregnancy or adnexal abnormality suggestive of EP. The degree of echogenicity of free pelvic fluid may be diagnostically more significant than the mere presence of intrafluid echoes.

► Although an abnormal amount of intraperitoneal fluid, in the absence of an adnexal mass, is not a frequent sonographic finding in patients with a clinical concern for ectopic pregnancy, it may be problematic when it occurs. Many physicians assume that the echogenic intraperitoneal fluid indicates a high risk of ectopic pregnancy, but there are few studies that have evaluated this as an isolated finding. Hemoperitoneum is likely in the presence of this finding, but ectopic pregnancy is not the only cause of hemoperitoneum. The number of cases in this series is small, but the results suggest caution in using a small to moderate amount of echogenic intraperitoneal fluid, as an isolated finding, to predict ectopic pregnancy.

D.L. Brown, M.D.

Diagnosis of Vasa Previa With Endovaginal Color Doppler and Power Doppler Sonography: Report of Two Cases

Sauerbrei EE, Davies GL (Kingston Gen Hosp, Ont, Canada)
J Ultrasound Med 17:393-398, 1998 7–32

Introduction.—The perinatal mortality rate is high in cases of vasa previa, owing to vessel rupture after spontaneous or iatrogenic rupture of membranes. Diagnosis before onset of labor may prevent fetal morbidity and death. Reported are 2 patients in whom diagnosis was made antepartum with endovaginal color Doppler and power Doppler sonography.

Case 1.—Patient underwent initial dating sonogram at 13 weeks 3 days of gestation. The placenta was reported as anterior and low. There was no vaginal bleeding. The patient underwent transabdominal sonograms without color Doppler sonography at 18, 23, 26, 28, and 31 weeks' gestation. She reported vaginal bleeding before all of these examinations except the one at 28 weeks. Funic

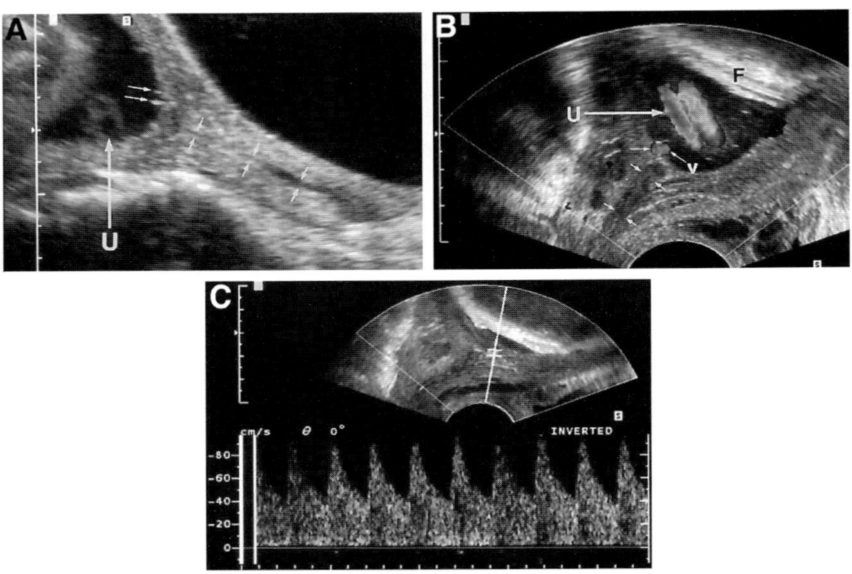

FIGURE 1.—Case 1. **A**, Sagittal transabdominal sonogram, 23 weeks' gestation. The umbilical cord (*U*) was persistently positioned between the fetus and the cervix (ie, funic cord presentation). The significance of the 2 short linear echoes (*short arrows*) was not appreciated at the time of the sonogram. *Shortest arrows* indicate cervical canal. **B**, Sagittal endovaginal sonogram with color Doppler sonography, 36 weeks' gestation. A blood vessel (*V*) is observed at the position of the internal cervical os. *U*, Umbilical cord positioned between the internal cervical os and the fetus (*F*). *Small arrows* indicate position of cervical canal. C, Sagittal endovaginal sonogram with spectral Doppler interrogation, 36 weeks' gestation. The Doppler cursor is placed in the blood vessel at the internal cervical os. The spectral Doppler graph demonstrates fetal arterial blood flow with a rate of 137 beats per minute. The maternal heart rate was 86 beats per minute (the time interval between successive marks at the bottom of the graph is 0.2 second). (Courtesy of Sauerbrei EE, Davies GL: Diagnosis of vasa previa with endovaginal color Doppler and power Doppler sonography: Report of two cases. *J Ultrasound Med* 17:393-398, 1998.)

cord presentation was seen at 23 weeks' gestation. The internal cervical os was clear of placenta; 2 short linear echoes were observed nearby. A transvaginal sonogram performed at 36 weeks' gestation with color Doppler and power Doppler sonography detected vasa previa (Fig 1). Spectral Doppler findings confirmed the arterial fetal cardiac rate. Diagnosis of vasa previa was confirmed during cesarean section. A velamentous cord insertion with blood vessels was observed within the membranes. A male infant was delivered with a weight of 2,355 g and Apgar scores of 9 at 1 minute and 9 at 5 minutes.

Case 2.—Patient was initially seen because of vaginal bleeding at 19 weeks' gestation. A low placenta and possibly marginal placental veins were observed at the internal cervical os on a transabdominal sonogram. Transabdominal sonograms performed at 21 and 23 weeks' gestation indicated marginal placenta previa. A transabdominal sonogram with power and spectral Doppler interrogation performed at 25 weeks' gestation suggested vasa previa. This was confirmed at 28 weeks' gestation by endovaginal color Doppler sonogram. An elective cesarean section was performed at 33 weeks' gestational age. A female infant was delivered with a weight of 1,956 g and Apgar scores of 4 at 1 minute and 6 at 5 minutes. Three or 4 medium sized vessels were seen traversing the membranes. Sections of the placenta had thinned areas with intervillous fibrin deposition, consistent with placenta membranacea.

Conclusion.—Transvaginal color Doppler was significantly more sensitive than transabdominal color Doppler sonography in discerning blood flow in blood vessels near the cervix. It is recommended that transvaginal US be used in patients at high risk of vasa previa.

► This is an illustrative report in which the authors also review the literature for this uncommon, yet potentially lethal, abnormality. It is hoped that increased awareness of the sonographic findings will contribute to improved accuracy in the diagnosis of vasa previa. As the authors discuss, it is important to determine that the vessels in question are umbilical cord (with velanentus insertius) or connecting vessels between placental areas (for succenturiate lobes), so as not to mistake marginal placental vessels or myometrial vessels for vasa previa.

D.L. Brown, M.D.

Using Fetal Nuchal Translucency to Screen for Major Congenital Cardiac Defects at 10-14 Weeks of Gestation: Population Based Cohort Study

Hyett J, Perdu M, Sharland G, et al (Kings College Hosp Med School, London; Guy's Hosp, London)
BMJ 318:81-85, 1999 7–33

Purpose.—Prenatal diagnosis of most major congenital cardiac defects can be made at around 20 weeks' gestation, but it is difficult to identify high-risk pregnancies requiring referral to a specialist center. The current screening approach consists of a 4-chamber view of the heart at 16 to 22 weeks' gestation. US measurement of the fetal nuchal translucency at 10 to 14 weeks' gestation may be a more sensitive approach. This method of screening for major congenital cardiac defects was evaluated in a population-based cohort study.

Methods.—The retrospective analysis included 29,154 singleton pregnancies with a chromosomally normal fetus. All underwent US examination at 10 to 14 weeks' gestation, including measurement of the fetal nuchal transparency thickness. The diagnostic performance of this measurement in screening for major cardiac defects was evaluated.

Results.—Fifty fetuses with major defects of the heart and great arteries were identified, for a prevalence of 1.7/1,000 pregnancies. On US examination, 1,822 pregnancies had fetal nuchal translucency thicknesses above the 95th percentile of normal. Twenty-eight of these fetuses had major congenital cardiac defects. Using the 95th percentile as the cutoff point, measurement of nuchal translucency thickness had a positive predictive value of 1.5% and a negative predictive value of 99.9%.

Conclusions.—US examination at 10 to 14 weeks' gestation identifies increased fetal nuchal translucency thickness in 55% of fetuses with major abnormalities of the heart and great vessels. The good diagnostic performance of this measurement suggests that it may be useful as an indication for specialist fetal echocardiography.

► Increased nuchal translucency of the fetus at 10 to 14 weeks is now well recognized as a useful marker for several chromosomal anomalies. However, there is also a strong association between abnormal nuchal translucency and fetal cardiac anomalies. This study approaches the issue from the standpoint of screening, but its results are useful to emphasize that fetuses with increased nuchal translucency should have follow-up sonographic evaluation of the fetal heart, even if the karyotype is normal.

D.L. Brown, M.D.

The Significance of Choroid Plexus Cysts in an Unselected Population: Results of a Multicenter Study

Chitty LS, Chudleigh P, Wright E, et al (Institute of Child Health, London; St George's Hosp, London; Hammersmith Hosp, London)

Ultrasound Obstet Gynecol 12:391-397, 1998 7–34

Background.—The clinical importance of choroid plexus cysts, commonly detected on routine scans obtained in the second trimester of pregnancy, is unclear. The incidence of choroid plexus cysts in an unselected population was investigated, and the association of cysts with aneuploidy reported.

Methods and Findings.—This prospective, observational, multicenter study included all fetuses found to have choroid plexus cysts with a maximum diameter of 3 mm or greater on scans obtained between 14 and 24 weeks' gestation. Of 101,600 newborns, 658 had choroid plexus cysts. Overall, the incidence of aneuploidy was 2.1%. However, in fetuses with isolated choroid plexus cysts, the incidence of proven aneuploidy was 0.5%. When maternal age was considered, the incidence of aneuploidy associated with isolated choroid plexus cysts was 0.36% among the fetuses of mothers younger than 36 years and 2.4% among the fetuses of older mothers (Table).

Conclusions.—The presence of choroid plexus cysts appears to increase the risk for aneuploidy, primarily trisomy 18. Though the final risk remains small in most fetuses, it increases with maternal age.

► There certainly have been numerous studies addressing this topic. This update is useful because it presents a prospective, multicenter study dealing with an unselected population. It confirms previous reports of a slight increased risk of trisomy 18 with isolated choroid plexus cysts. It adds to

TABLE 6.—Incidence of Aneuploidy for Various Classifications

Sonographic Finding	Maternal Age	Risk Number	Risk %	Risk 95% CI
CPCs	all	14 / 658	2.1 (2.4)	1.2-3.5%
Isolated CPCs	all	3 / 603	0.5 (0.8)	0.1-1.4%
Isolated CPCs	< 36 years	2 / 561	0.36 (0.7)	0.04-1.3%
Isolated CPCs	≥ 36 years	1 / 42	2.4	0.06-12.6%
CPCs and other abnormality	all	11 / 55	20	10-33%
CPCs and other abnormality	< 36 years	8 / 49	16	7-30%
CPCs and other abnormality	≥ 36 years	3 / 6	50	12-88%

Note: Numbers in parentheses represent the risk if the 2 cases (110 and 472) with abnormal findings at birth but no karyotype recorded are assumed to have an abnormal karyotype.

Abbreviation: CPCs, Choroid plexus cysts.

(Courtesy of Chitty LS, Chudleigh P, Wright E, et al: The significance of choroid plexus cysts in an unselected population: Results of a multicenter study. *Ultrasound Obstet Gynecol* 12:391-397, 1998.)

previous evidence that size, unilaterality versus bilaterality, single versus multiple, and spontaneous resolution do not affect the risk for trisomy 18. It also adds to evidence that choroid plexus cysts are not associated with an increased risk of trisomy 21. Because the risk of trisomy 18 increases significantly when other anomalies are seen by sonography, it behooves the sonographer and sonologist to obtain a detailed fetal survey, evaluating especially the heart and extremities.

D.L. Brown, M.D.

8 Neuroradiology

Introduction

In 1999, we saw a continued trend towards broadening the use of advanced imaging techniques such as functional MRI and MR spectroscopy (see Abstract 8–4 on using PET to detect recurrent or residual squamous cell carcinoma of the neck).

The Holy Grail of neuroimaging is pathology specific diagnosis. Early reports that use SPECT and diffusion-weighted MR to distinguish brain abscess and necrotic or cystic brain tumors are encouraging. Blood volume maps, PET, SPECT, and even Xenon CT are being used with greater success to assess tumor grade.

A very hot topic this year is screening for intracranial aneurysm (especially in relatives of patients with so-called "familial intracranial aneurysms") and how unruptured aneurysms should be managed once they are discovered. A recent article (Abstract 8–21) convincingly establishes what I call the Godzilla Principle (ie, size really does matter). Small (ie, less than 10 mm) aneurysms have a very low prospective risk of hemorrhage whereas larger lesions have a much higher change of rupture. We now know what the risk of surgery on unruptured aneurysms is. Early results from neurointerventional techniques are looking pretty good by comparison. The relative long-term outcomes with issues such as regrowth of aneurysms treated conservatively are still pending.

Finally, Jim Smirniotopoulos and I have included a few more traditional articles for your perusal, including a very nice study on nonneoplastic intramedullary lesions that mimic cord tumors and an up-to-the-minute discussion of CT in the early evaluation of acute ischemic stroke. Enjoy!

Anne G. Osborn, M.D.

Head and Neck

ORBIT, NOSE, AND PARANASAL SINUSES

Relative Value of MR Imaging as Compared With CT in the Diagnosis of Inflammatory Paranasal Sinus Disease

Hähnel S, Ertl-Wagner B, Tasman A-J, et al (Univ of Heidelberg, Germany)
Radiology 210:171-176, 1999 8–1

Background.—The technique of choice for paranasal sinuses imaging is CT in the coronal plane, but MRI may have some important advantages over CT. MRI and CT for use in the diagnosis of inflammatory paranasal sinus disease was prospectively compared.

Methods.—The study included 30 patients with suspected paranasal sinus inflammation. All patients underwent imaging of the paranasal sinuses using both coronal CT and coronal T1-weighted, 3-dimensional, gradient-echo MRI. The 2 techniques were compared objectively and subjectively, including anatomic visualization, depiction of inflammatory disease, and artifacts from dental work.

Results.—CT was superior to MRI in visualizing most bone structures of the infundibular complex, whereas MRI was better than CT in visualizing the anatomy of the brain and orbit (Figs 1 and 2). In the areas of diagnostic concern, there were no artifacts from dental work with MRI. The 2 imaging modalities agreed very well as to the type and extent of inflammatory disease, except for mucosal thickening in the maxillary and frontal sinuses, the nasal cavity, and the infundibulum.

Conclusions.—In patients with suspected inflammatory paranasal sinus disease, CT has advantages over MRI in visualization of fine bony details and anatomic variants. As such, CT is the better modality for planning functional endoscopic sinus surgery. However, MRI may be useful in primary diagnosis of certain patient subgroups and in assessing the response to treatment.

► "CT is obviously better than MR in visualizing sinus disease." We hear it; we say it; but where is the real proof? Although only 30 patients were included, this is still the largest prospective comparison of CT and MR in the evaluation of inflammatory sinus disease. As anticipated, CT was the clear winner in planning for functional endoscopic sinus surgery—primarily because of its ability to demonstrate the thin bones of the sinuses and nasal cavity. As we progress along the path of "evidence-based medicine" more and more of our "conventional wisdom" will require validation through scientific study. It is no longer acceptable to practice based on "general knowledge" or opinion.

J.G. Smirniotopoulos, M.D.

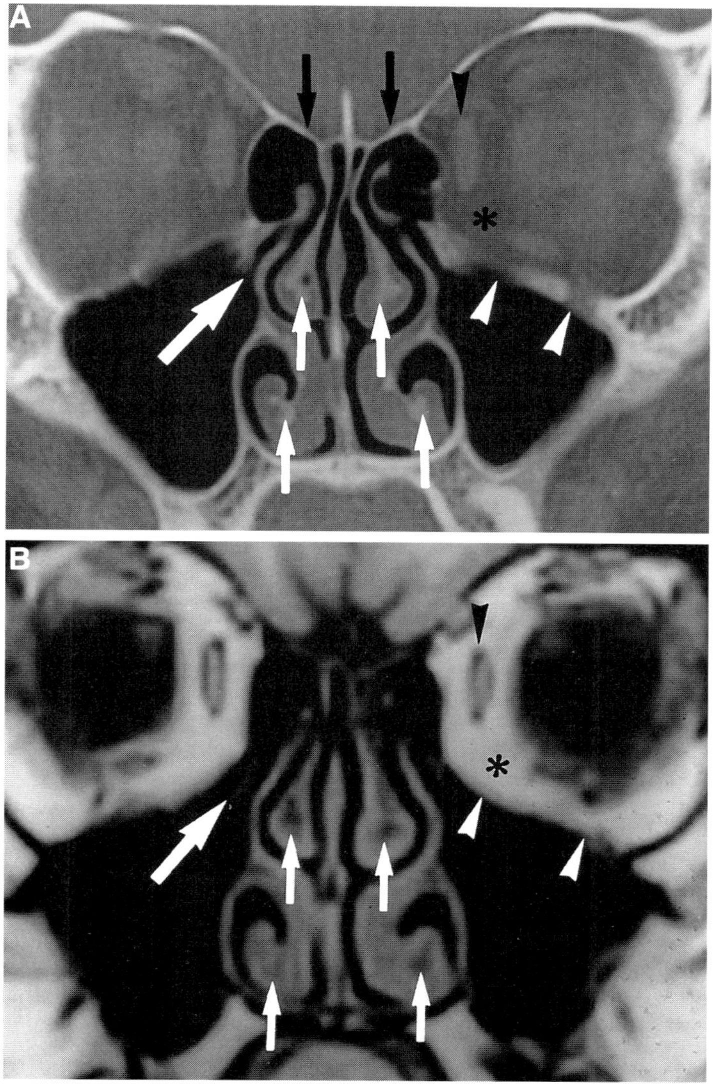

FIGURE 1.—Images obtained in a 36-year-old woman with planned heart valve implantation who was examined for inflammatory paranasal disease. **A**, CT scan depicts the anatomy of the infundibular (*large white arrow*) and parainfundibular complex very well. The bone structures of the inferior and middle conchae (*small white arrows*), the orbital lamina (*small white arrowheads*), the orbital floor (*large white arrowheads*), and the cribriform lamina (*black arrows*) are clearly delineated. Contrast between orbital fat (*) and the medial rectus muscle (*black arrowhead*) is moderate. Inflammatory disease is not present. **B**, MR image (60/12; flip angle, 40 degrees) shows moderately delineated infundibular (*large arrow*) and parainfundibular complex. The bone structures of the inferior and middle conchae (*small arrows*) are visible. The bone structures of the orbital lamina, of the orbital floor, and of the cribriform lamina are not delineated. However, the medial and inferior (*white arrowheads*) borders of the orbit, the border between the frontal lobe and ethmoid cells, and the borders of the maxillary sinuses are clearly seen. Contrast between orbital fat (*) and the medial rectus muscle (*black arrowhead*) is excellent. (Courtesy of Hähnel S, Ertl-Wagner B, Tasman A-J, et al: Relative value of MR imaging as compared with CT in the diagnosis of inflammatory paranasal sinus disease. *Radiology* 210:171-176, 1999.)

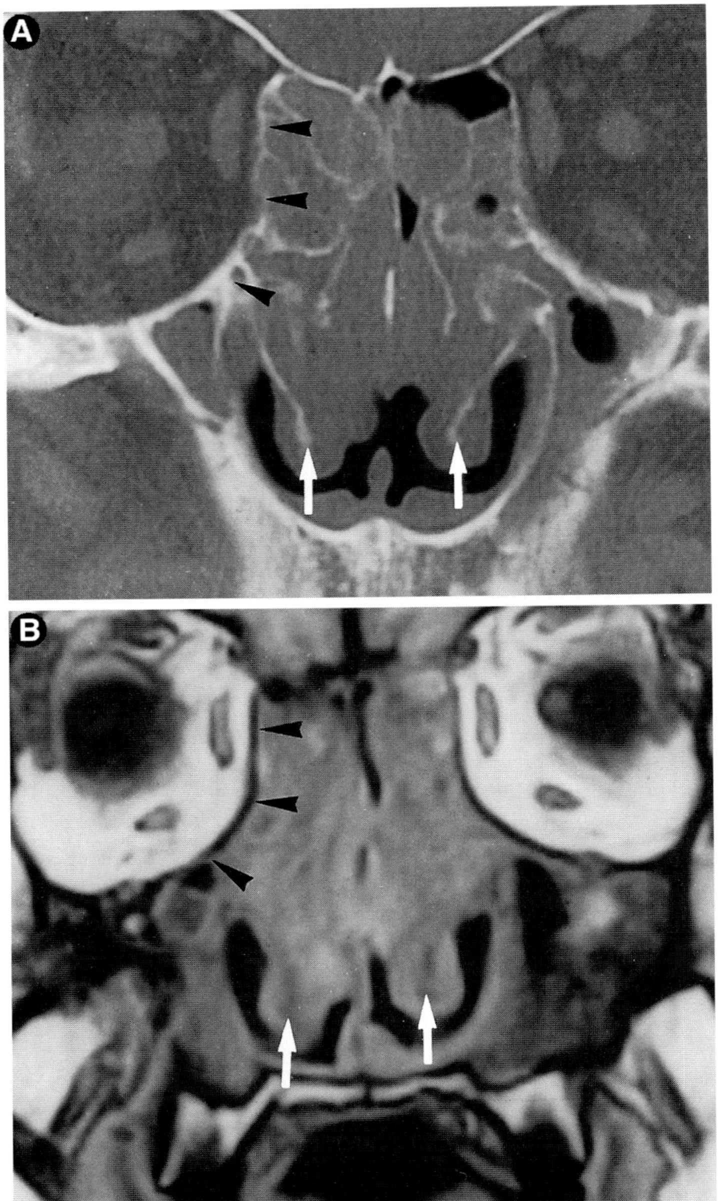

FIGURE 2.—Images obtained in a 49-year-old man suspected of having nasal polyposis. **A**, CT scan shows that despite nearly total opacification of the middle meatus and the ethmoid cell system, the bone structures of the inferior (*white arrows*) and middle conchae, the ethmoid cells, and the orbital lamina (*black arrows*) are excellently delineated. **B**, MR image (60/12; flip angle, 40 degrees) does not depict the fine bone structures of the middle concha and the ethmoid cells. Visualization of the bone structure of the inferior concha (*white arrows*) is indeterminate. The bone structure of the orbital lamina (*black arrows*) is clearly seen as loss of signal intensity, because the adjacent sinuses are filled with material containing water (mucus or mucosa). (Courtesy of Hähnel S, Ertl-Wagner B, Tasman A-J, et al: Relative value of MR imaging as compared with CT in the diagnosis of inflammatory paranasal sinus disease. *Radiology* 210:171-176, 1999.)

Radiology in Focus: Transorbital Penetrating Injury of the Paranasal Sinuses

Wu M-R, Shih C-T, Yeh C-W (Taipei Municipal Jen-Ai Hosp, Taipei, Taiwan; China Med College Hosp, Taichung, Taiwan)

J Laryngol Otol 112:1202-1204, 1998 8–2

Background.—Penetrating injuries of the paranasal sinuses, especially those sustained in traffic accidents, are rare. A patient with a ballpoint pen lodged in the left orbit after a traffic accident was described.

Case Report.—Man, 36, was seen in an emergency department after a pen became lodged in his left eye when the driver of the vehicle braked suddenly at high speed. The patient, a front-seat passenger who was not wearing a seatbelt, was forced forward, and the pen, placed upright on the dashboard, was stabbed into the orbit (Fig 1). About 5 cm of the pen was protruding from the eyelid, near the medial canthus. The patient had bilateral nasal bleeding, but no neurologic deficit was apparent. A skull radio-

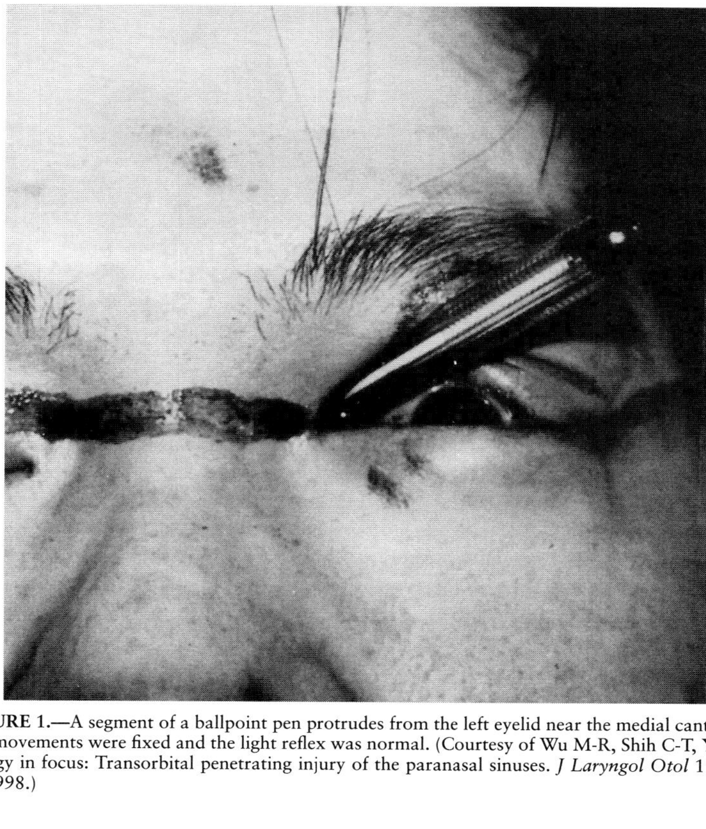

FIGURE 1.—A segment of a ballpoint pen protrudes from the left eyelid near the medial canthus. The left eye movements were fixed and the light reflex was normal. (Courtesy of Wu M-R, Shih C-T, Yeh C-W: Radiology in focus: Transorbital penetrating injury of the paranasal sinuses. *J Laryngol Otol* 112:1202-1204, 1998.)

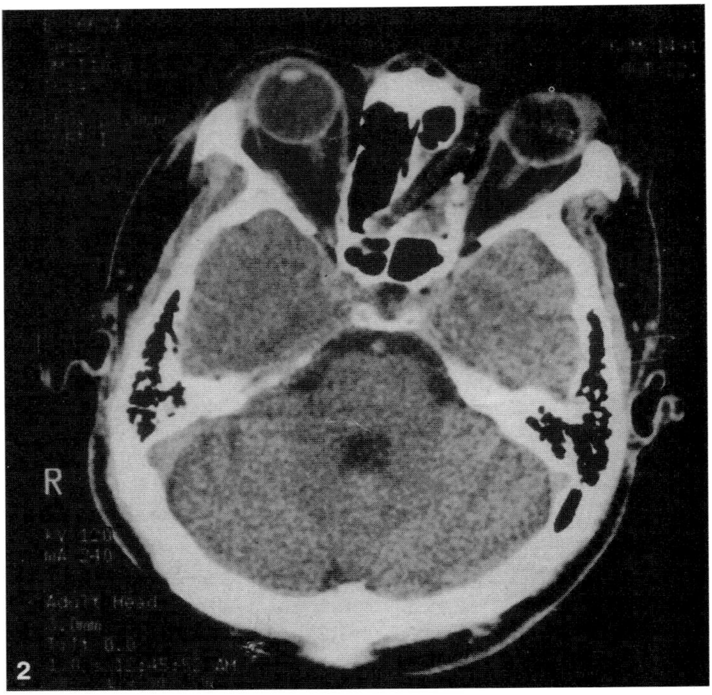

FIGURE 2.—CT scanning reveals the extent of the ballpoint pen penetration. Note the rupture of the left lamina papyracea and the perforation of the nasal septum. The eyeball is intact. The tip of the pen rests on the surface of the right temporal lobe and there is bony dehiscence. (Courtesy of Wu M-R, Shih C-T, Yeh C-W: Radiology in focus: Transorbital penetrating injury of the paranasal sinuses. *J Laryngol Otol* 112:1202-1204, 1998.)

graph showed an oblique longitudinal lucency from the left frontal region to the nasal septum. On CT, a lucent tubular object was seen extending from the medial aspect of the left eye, through the left ethmoid sinus and nasal septum, to the right sphenoid sinus (Fig 2). The dura of the right temporal lobe appeared intact. Endoscopic sinus surgery was performed, and the pen was removed uneventfully through the orbital inlet. After surgery, the patient's condition was good, except for the left upper lacrimal canaliculi rupture. No sequelae occurred in the 1 month of follow-up.

Conclusions.—This case report underscores the need for optimal imaging in transorbital or transnasal penetrating injuries. In this patient, endoscopic surgery was successful.

► I don't usually like to include case reports—but this one was pretty nifty. An unrestrained occupant of a motor vehicle was impaled in the orbit by a ballpoint pen sticking up on the dashboard. This reinforces the need to wear a shoulder harness, and to keep your pens on your desk and not in your car.

Seriously, this case report serves as a reminder about the trauma physiology of the globe and orbit. The eyeball is tough and resilient, and very mobile within the fat-packed orbital cavity. Penetrating injuries to the orbit are very common. However, they are usually not accompanied by damage to the globe or loss of vision. Often, the offending object is inserted and withdrawn with minimal pain at the time of injury. This creates a situation where they may be overlooked by both the patient and the clinician. Perhaps head CT scans should be requested whenever anyone runs with scissors.

J.G. Smirniotopoulos, M.D.

NECK AND SOFT TISSUES

Metastatic Papillary Thyroid Carcinoma Presenting as a Retropharyngeal Mass

DiLeo MD, Baker KB, Deschler DG, et al (Allegheny Univ, Philadelphia)
Am J Otolaryngol 19:404-406, 1998 8–3

Background.—Papillary thyroid carcinoma rarely metastasizes to the retropharyngeal space and presents as an oropharyngeal mass. A patient with metastatic papillary thyroid carcinoma initially presenting as a retropharyngeal mass was reported.

Case Report.—Man, 65, with severe obstructive sleep apnea was referred to an otolaryngologist for consideration of a laser-assisted uvulopalatoplasty. Fullness of the right palate and lateral pharyngeal wall was noted on oral cavity examination, and MRI demonstrated a retropharyngeal space mass. On referral, further MRI showed a bilobed retropharyngeal mass, which had a high-signal and an intermediate-signal lobe on T1-weighted sequences. On T2-fast spin-echo images, both lobes were hyperintense. The intermediate-signal lobe showed minimal enhancement after gadolinium administration (Fig 1). Complete transcervical excision was performed, followed subsequently by total thyroidectomy. The papillary thyroid carcinoma was multifocal and classified as both classic and follicular.

Conclusions.—Thyroid carcinoma only rarely metastasizes to the parapharyngeal and retropharyngeal spaces. Hyperintense lymph nodes on T1-weighted images of the retropharyngeal space suggests the diagnosis of papillary thyroid carcinoma.

► This article contains a very nice review of the anatomy and imaging characteristics of retropharyngeal mass lesions. It also has a very simple take-home message for scanning patients with thyroid carcinoma: You have to scan the neck much higher than you might think! Although most thyroid malignancies spread to the mid- and lower-jugular lymphatics, some may

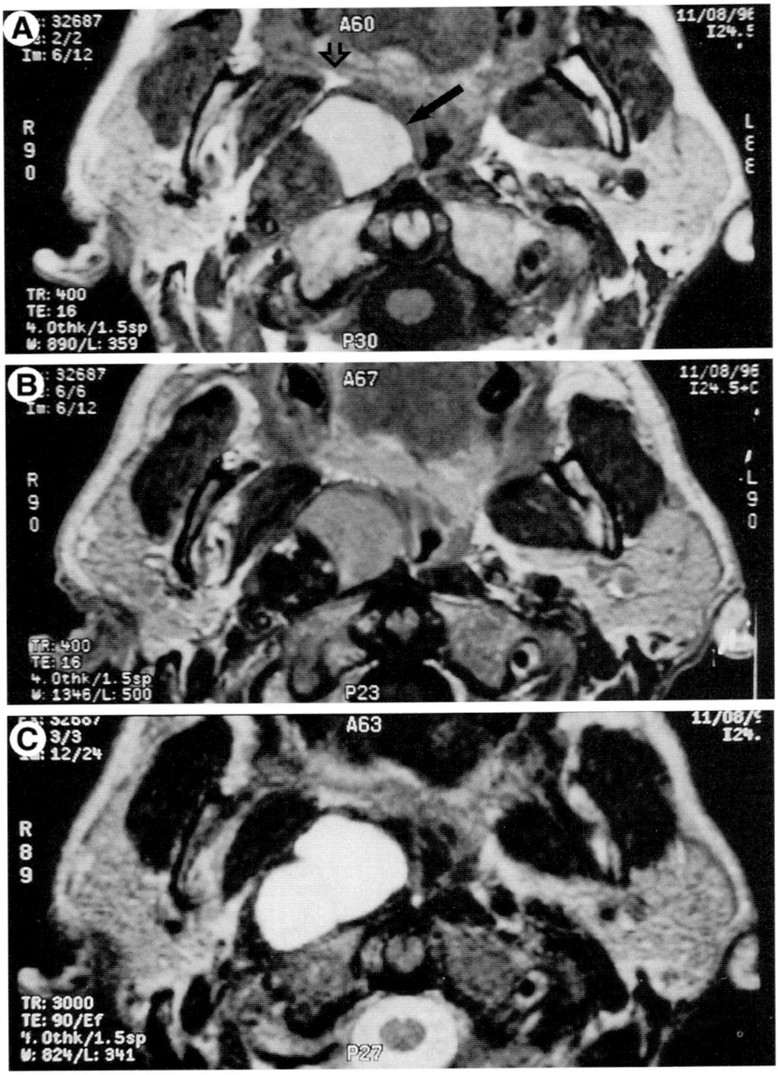

FIGURE 1.—**A**, Axial T1-weighted image (time to repeat[TR]/echo time [TE], 400/12) shows a bilobed mass in the retropharyngeal space. Note the anterior displacement of the parapharyngeal fat (*arrowhead*) and indentation of the longus colli muscle that lies posterior to the mass. One lobe shows high signal (*arrow*). **B**, Axial T1-weighted image (TR/TE, 400/12) after administration of IV gadolinium shows minimal enhancement in the intermediate signal lobe of the mass. **C**, Axial T2–fast-spin echo image (TR/TE, 3000/90) shows both segments of the mass to be hyperintense. MRI of the thyroid (not shown) revealed a heterogeneous gland with multiple small nodules and no focal mass. (Courtesy of DiLeo MD, Baker KB, Deshler DG, et al: Metastatic papillary thyroid carcinoma presenting as a retropharyngeal mass. *Am J Otolarngol* 19:404-406, 1998.)

extend via other channels, involving the retropharyngeal space and superior lymphatic trunks.

So scan from skull base on down, just to be safe. My colleague Ric Harnsberger has seen cases with metastases that were missed just because the radiologists assumed all thyroid tumors drain down. Not necessarily.

A.G. Osborn, M.D.

Clinical Utility of Positron Emission Tomography With ¹⁸F-Fluorodeoxyglucose in Detecting Residual/Recurrent Squamous Cell Carcinoma of the Head and Neck

Fischbein NJ, AAssar OS, Caputo GR, et al (Univ of California, San Francisco)

AJNR 19:1189-1196, 1998 8–4

Introduction.—PET with ^{18}F-fluorodeoxyglucose (FDG-PET) has been evaluated in only small cohorts of patients with squamous cell carcinoma (SCC) of the head and neck. The ability of this technique to distinguish the

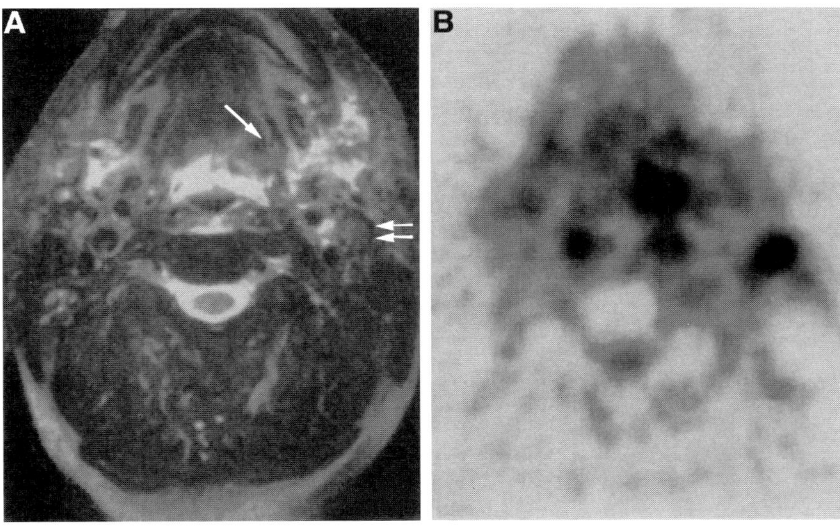

FIGURE 1.—Imaging in a 52-year-old man with a T2N2M0 squamous cell carcinoma of the tongue base, which had been treated with radiation therapy. **A,** follow-up T2-weighted fast spin-echo MR image with fat saturation (4,000/102$_{eff}$/2 [repetition time/echo time/excitations]) shows extensive postradiation change. No definite tumor can be seen at the left base of the tongue (*single arrow*). A left-sided jugulodigastric lymph node (*double arrows*), measuring 11 mm in diameter, is homogeneously low in signal intensity on the T2-weighted image and is significantly decreased in size relative to that on a pretherapy examination (not shown). This study was interpreted as indeterminate for residual disease. **B,** PET scan obtained 1 week after the MR study shows abnormal accumulation of ^{18}F-fluorodeoxyglucose at both the left tongue base and the jugulodigastric lymph node. Mild symmetric activity is also noted in the prevertebral muscles. The patient went on to partial glossectomy, supraglottic laryngectomy, and modified radical neck dissection. The presence of tumor was histologically confirmed at both the primary and the nodal sites. (Courtesy of Fischbein NJ, AAssar OS, Caputo GR, et al: Clinical utility of positron emission tomography with ^{18}F-fluorodeoxyglucose in detecting residual/recurrent squamous cell carcinoma of the head and neck. *AJNR* 19:1189-1196, copyright 1998 by American Society of Neuroradiology.)

presence of tumor at primary and nodal sites was retrospectively assessed in 44 patients with suspicious residual or recurrent SCC of the head and neck.

Methods.—Thirty-five of 44 patients examined over a 2½-year period had sufficient follow-up to be meaningful for analysis. The range of follow-up was 6-33 months. Observers evaluated PET scans visually and with knowledge of the clinical history and correlative anatomical imaging findings. Determination of disease involving primary and nodal sites was evaluated independently. Because patients were referred to resolve a specific clinical problem, the usefulness of PET in addressing these questions reliably was examined.

Results.—The sensitivity and specificity for residual/recurrent disease were 100% and 64%, respectively, for the primary site and 93% and 77%, respectively, for nodal disease. The positive predictive value and negative predictive value of the test result were 65% and 91%, respectively.

Conclusion.—The high sensitivity and negative predictive value of PET scanning in patients with suspicious residual or recurrent SCC of the head and neck indicate an important role for this imagining approach in the care of these patients (Fig 1). The lower figures observed for specificity and positive predictive value reflect the fact that increased FDG uptake may be caused by either tumor or inflammation.

► Detecting tumor in patients treated for head and neck SCC has been a challenge. The distorting effects of surgery and the concealing effects of radiation treatments sometimes make imaging evaluation of these patients difficult. Along comes a somewhat old modality (PET scanning) with a brand-new application. During the past year, several studies have shown that PET is very sensitive and has high predictive value in detecting recurrent/residual tumor, as the authors demonstrate.

Not only that, but PET scans may be useful in patients with a "negative neck" who have oral cavity cancer.[1] They are also useful in predicting survival in patients with head and neck cancers.[2] For an excellent general review of PET in head and neck oncology, see the article by McGuirt and colleagues.[3]

A.G. Osborn, M.D.

References

1. Myers LL, Wax MK: Positron emission tomography in the evaluation of the negative neck in patients with oral cavity cancer. *J Otolaryngol* 27:342-347, 1998.
2. Minn H, Lapela M, Klemi PJ, et al: Prediction of survival with fluorine-18-fluorodeoxyglucose and PET in head and neck cancer. *J Nucl Med* 38:1907-1911, 1997.
3. McGuirt WF, Greven K, Williams D, et al: PET scanning in head and neck oncology: A review. *Head Neck* 20:208-215, 1998.

Spine and Cord

SPINE

Volume Fast Spin-Echo Imaging of the Cervical Spine

Maldjian C, Adam RJ, Akhtar N, et al (Temple Univ, Philadelphia)
Acad Radiol 6:84-88, 1999 8–5

Background.—Routine MRI of the cervical spine currently consists of multiple pulse sequences in sagittal and axial planes. In addition, an axial 3-D gradient-echo (GRE) pulse sequence is used. The standard imaging time is about 30 minutes, which may potentially be shortened by more than half with the use of volume fast spin-echo (SE) imaging. The effectiveness of a T2-weighted 3-D volume fast SE pulse sequence in assessing the cervical spine was investigated.

Methods.—In 18 patients with neck pain, MRI was performed at 1.5 T with 2-D fast SE and axial 3-D GRE protocols and an additional sagittal T2-weighted volume fast SE protocol. Two neuroradiologists examined

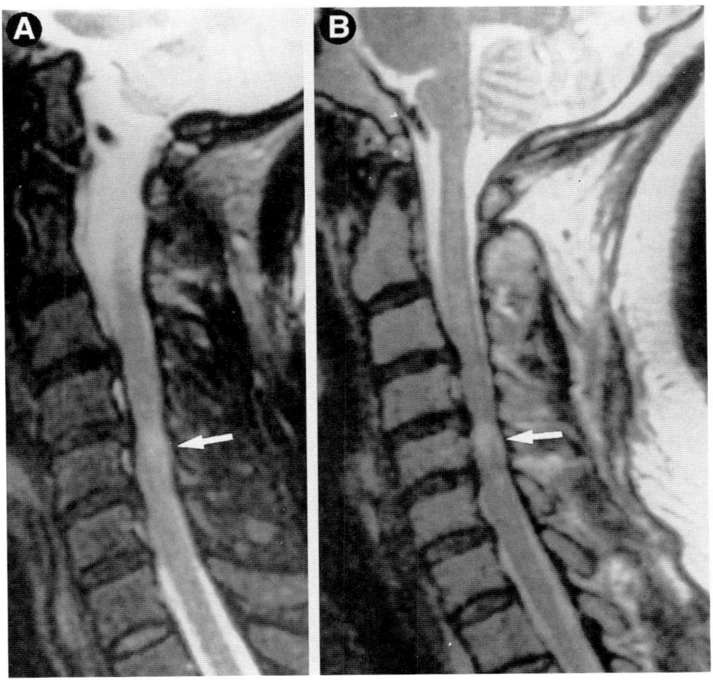

FIGURE 2.—**A**, Sagittal T2-weighted fast SE image shows multilevel disk herniations with a focal area of cord compression and myelomalacia at the C4-C5 level (*arrow*). **B**, Sagittal partition image obtained from a T2-weighted volume acquisition in the same patient shows the area of cord edema (*arrow*) with greater conspicuity. (Courtesy of Maldjian C, Adam RJ, Akhtar N, et al: Volume fast spin-echo imaging of the cervical spine. *Acad Radiol* 6:84-88, 1999.)

the spinal cord and canal, neural foramina, and intervertebral disks, and the results were compared with the standard protocol reports.

Findings.—Two-dimensional fast SE did not differ in assessments of spinal cord disease and disk herniation with volume fast SE imaging. Mild variation in the assessment of the neural foramina was noted. Resolution and contrast were high in partition images, whereas the quality of reconstructed images was consistently lower. However, this did not hinder the detection or grading of disk or spinal abnormalities, which were demonstrated adequately on volume fast SE sagittal images. Neural foramina clearly visualized on axial reconstructions from volume fast SE imaging (Fig 2).

Conclusions.—In the assessment of the spinal cord, canal, disks, and neural foramina, volume fast SE imaging provides information comparable with that provided by routine imaging. The thinner sections and multiplanar reconstruction ability of the former are advantages over 2-D imaging. In addition, its increased tissue contrast with better visualization of the cerval cord, improved signal-to-noise ratio, and reduced susceptibility artifact are advantages over 3-D GRE imaging.

► Faster, better, higher . . . sounds like a motto for the Olympics. It isn't. It's the unrelenting search for new ways to scan more patients in less time. Here's 1 pulse sequence that is worth trying. The authors nicely demonstrate that volume fast SE imaging provides better tissue contrast than do routine sequences. I personally like this technique's excellent visualization of the cervical cord. Some "fast" techniques show the discs and bony anatomy well but sacrifice cord detail. This technique doesn't, as the illustration of spinal stenosis with abnormal cord signal shows (Fig 2). It even shows it better than standard T2-weighted fast SE does.

A.G. Osborn, M.D.

Magnetic Resonance Imaging of Acute Intraosseus Disc Herniation
Seymour R, Williams LA, Rees JI, et al (Univ Hosp of Wales, Cardiff)
Clin Radiol 53:363-368, 1998 8–6

Background.—Schmorl's nodes, which result from intraosseous disc herniation (IODH), are often found incidentally on plain radiographs, CT, and MRI. However, such radiologic features may lead to incorrect suspicion of malignancy or infection. Eight patients with acute IODH were examined to illustrate how this disorder can be diagnosed correctly by MRI.

Methods and Findings.—Six patients underwent isotope bone scintigraphy, which showed focal increased activity at the site of IODH. MRI finding was marrow edema, sometimes localized around the disc herniation and sometimes extensive, extending through the vertebral body into the pedicles. In 3 patients, the diagnosis of IODH may have been possible on plain radiographs, which showed that disc calcification seen on previous radiographs had migrated into an intraosseous location.

Conclusions.—The key to recognizing IODH on MR images is the recognition of the endplate defect and disc herniation. When the diagnosis is unclear, repeating MRI at 2 to 3 months can show the beginning of marrow edema resolution. Percutanoeus biopsy is rarely necessary.

► Schmorl's nodes represent the sequelae of disc herniation through the endplates into the vertebral body. In the "good old days" (when, as they used to say, "men were men and giants roamed the earth"—and women didn't write reviews like this either!) it wasn't too difficult to recognize these lesions. Now we have MRI. Patients with acute onset of back pain are often imaged early in their clinical course. That means we may see worrisome findings in the acute stages of intraosseous disc herniation (IODH) that can mimic more ominous disorders, such as infection or tumor. The edema that surrounds the lesion may involve most of the vertebral body and even extend into the pedicle. Contrast enhancement isn't uncommon either. The key is, as the authors point out, recognizing the end plate defect. In really tough cases we may have to resort to—gasp!—that old-fashioned standby, the plain film.

A.G. Osborn, M.D.

Spinal Cord

Nonneoplastic Intramedullary Spinal Cord Lesions Mimicking Tumors
Lee M, Epstein FJ, Rezai AR, et al (Med College of Georgia, Augusta; Beth Israel Med Ctr, New York; New York Univ)
Neurosurgery 43:788-795, 1998 8–7

Background.—Intramedullary spinal cord tumors are relatively uncommon and not well documented. Nine patients with atypical, nonneoplastic, intramedullary spinal cord lesions were analyzed in a retrospective study.

Methods and Findings.—Of 212 patients undergoing surgery for intramedullary spinal cord lesions between 1989 and 1994, 9 (4%) had nonneoplastic lesions. All 9 had undergone MRI preoperatively. Enhancement with gadolinium ranged from homogenous to none. Marked T2 changes were evident in all lesions. All patients had a lack of significant spinal cord expansion. After surgery, histologic assessment indicated demyelinating lesions in 4 patients, sarcoidosis in 2, amyloid angiopathy in 2, and a mass of nonneoplastic inflammatory cells of unknown origin in 1 (Fig 1).

Conclusions.—Antecedent differentiation of these lesions from neoplastic spinal cord tumors by case history and physical examination was difficult. Absent or minimal spinal cord expansion on preoperative MR images was the most consistent indication of the diagnosis.

► This thought-provoking article is 1 of the largest collections of pathologically proven nonneoplastic intramedullary masses. The authors had long-term follow-up and excellent histopathology in all cases. Most were demy-

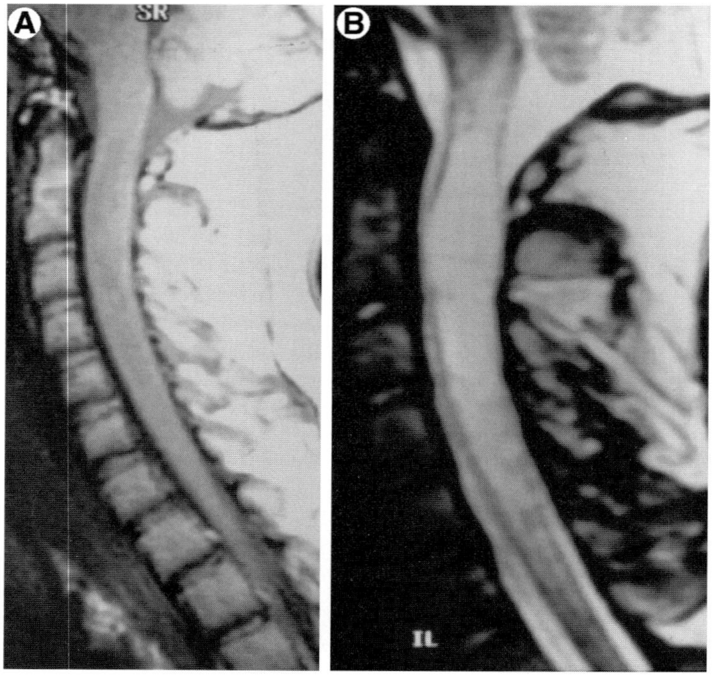

FIGURE 1.—Demyelinating disease of the spinal cord. MR images of patient 1. **A**, Sagittal T1-weighted MR image showing a cervical intramedullary lesion from C2 to C4. Note the minimal spinal cord expansion. **B**, Sagittal T2-weighted MR image. Note the marked T2 changes throughout the cervical spinal cord. The pathologic abnormality proved to be demyelination. (Courtesy of Lee M, Epstein FJ, Rezai AR, et al: Nonneoplastic intramedullary spinal cord lesions mimicking tumors. *Neurosurgery* 43:788-795, 1998.)

elinating disease. The imaging findings of abnormal cord signal and contrast enhancement are always worrisome, of course. A reassuring and helpful finding is the lack of significant cord enlargement, which is usually seen with neoplasms. But this doesn't always happen, as shown in the case illustrated here.

The clinical presentation and course are often helpful as most neoplasms have a longer, more insidious onset than acute demyelinating disease. The neurosurgeons are justifiably loathe to biopsy these lesions. Patience and follow-up imaging are recommended before surgery is contemplated.

A.G. Osborn, M.D.

Skull and Brain

Normal Anatomy

Magnetic Resonance Cisternography for Visualization of Intracisternal Fine Structures

Mamata Y, Muro I, Matsumae M, et al (Tokai Univ, Kanagawa, Japan; Ikegami Gen Hosp, Tokyo)
J Neurosurg 88:670-678, 1998 8–8

Background.—Contrast-enhanced CT and intrathecal gas cisternography have been used to evaluate the subarachnoid cisterns. Now MRI can be used to visualize the cranial nerves and vascular structures in this location. A heavily T2-weighted turbo spin-echo MRI technique was used to assess normal fine structures and pathologic findings in the basal cisterns.

Methods.—Twenty healthy volunteers underwent MR cisternography, with the focus on the parasellar region in 10 participants and the posterior fossa in 10. The ability of the imaging technique to detect the cranial nerves was assessed. Forty-three selected patients were studied as well, including patients with tumors in the juxtasellar regions, cerebellopontine angle lesions, meningiomas, cerebral aneurysms, and facial spasms. Peripheral pulse gating was applied, optimized to reduce artifacts related to CSF flow.

Results.—Peripheral pulse gating with a time delay of 30% of the peripheral pulse gate interval was successful in minimizing the CSF flow artifacts. In all volunteers, the first through third cranial nerves and the seventh through eighth cranial nerve complex were clearly seen. The fifth nerve was visualized in 80% of patients and the sixth nerve in 50%. The fourth and ninth through twelfth nerves were more difficult to see. In the patients, MR cisternography could depict the intracisternal fine anatomy and enhance the contours of juxtacisternal lesions. The T2-weighted turbo spin-echo sequence could depict very small amounts of CSF between lesions and normal structures. Vascular compression of the nerves was demonstrated, in 13 of 13 patients with facial spasm, by axial images and oblique coronal images in a plane parallel to the seventh through eighth nerve complex. In patients with pituitary adenomas, the scans clearly showed the tumor's relationship to the optic nerve and other structures. Cerebral aneurysms and surrounding structures were also clearly seen.

Conclusions.—The use of MR cisternography to visualize the fine structures within the subarachnoid cisterns is described and illustrated. This technique appears to be useful for investigation of patients with neurovascular compression or tumors in this area. Imaging can be performed in a relatively short time. When performed with peripheral pulse gating and a delay time of 30% of the peripheral pulse gate interval, it can aid surgical planning.

► The authors used an inverted gray-scale heavily T2-weighted pulse sequence. Normal volunteers and clinical patients were studied. The course of the cranial nerves was described. The authors demonstrated the advantage of using peripheral pulse gating and found a delay time of 30% of the pulse interval most useful. The authors commented that lesions with a "peritumoral CSF sleeve" were more easily dissected at surgery than those without.

J.G. Smirniotopoulos, M.D.

Microanatomy of the Cerebellopontine Angle and Internal Auditory Canal: Study With New Magnetic Resonance Imaging Technique Using Three-dimensional Fast Spin Echo

Mitsuoka H, Arai H, Tsunoda A, et al (Juntendo Univ, Tokyo; Toshiba Med Engineering Co Ltd, Tokyo)

Neurosurgery 44:561-567, 1999 8–9

Background.—MRI has greatly enhanced the ability to study various abnormal conditions in the cerebellopontine angle (CPA) and internal auditory canal (IAC). A new MR technique using 3-D fast spin echo (FSE) and the minimum intensity projection (Min.IP) method was reported.

Methods and Findings.—Using a 1-mm slice thickness in the axial and parasagittal plane, the authors scanned the CPA and IAC in 10 normal

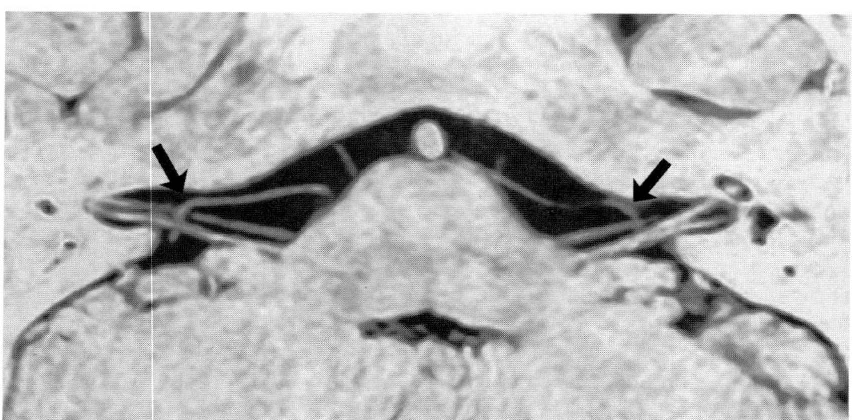

FIGURE 2.—Minimum intensity projection (Min.IP) image generated from 4 contiguous fast spin echo (FSE) images. Because a Min.IP image is similar to an FSE image, the image is displayed in reverse. This image clearly demonstrates that the vessel identified as the antero-inferior cerebellar artery forms a meatal loop, which reaches the porus of the internal auditory canal bilaterally (*arrows*). (Courtesy of Mitsuoka H, Arai H, Tsunoda A, et al: Microanatomy of the cerebellopontine angle and internal auditory canal: Study with new magnetic resonance imaging technique using three-dimensional fast spin echo. *Neurosurgery* 44:561-567, 1999.)

volunteers, 44 patients with acoustic neuromas, and 31 patients with hemifacial spasm. In the normal volunteers, the vestibulocochlear nerve was ovoid near the brain stem, changing to a slightly crescentic configuration as it traveled laterally. In addition, the cochlear and vestibular nerves separated near the central part of the IAC. The superior and inferior vestibular nerves could also be discriminated near the fundus of the IAC. The facial nerve was easy to identify as a discrete nerve at the anterior aspect of the vestibulocochlear nerve. In 44% of 95 CPAs, the meatal loop of the cerebellar artery was medial to the porus, reaching the porus or protruding into the porus in 56%. In a patient with a very small intracanalicular acoustic neuroma, the nerve on which the tumor was located was identified. Cerebrospinal fluid was observed between the tumor and fundus of the IAC in half of the 44 acoustic neuromas. Among patients with hemifacial spasm, the relationship between the responsible artery and facial nerve could be defined clearly (Fig 2).

Conclusions.—Three-dimensional FSE MRI yields ultrahigh-resolution images. These images are extremely useful in defining the surgical anatomy of the CPA and IAC.

► Pulse sequences to evaluate patients who have hemifacial spasm or sensorineural hearing loss and are referred for evaluation of possible vestibulocochlear schwannoma continue to evolve. In 1 of the latest iterations, this group of authors from Juntendo University used 3D-FSE sequences with a minimum intensity projection method to achieve exquisite views of the cerebellopontine angles. Not only does this technique discriminate all 4 nerves in the internal auditory canal, it demonstrated the meatal loup of the cerebellar artery in most all cases. This means the relationship between the compressing artery and facial nerve can be nicely delineated in cases of hemifacial spasm. Even small intracanalicular tumors were identified accurately. This and similar high-resolution techniques will obviate the use (and expense) of contrast in many cases referred to "rule out 'acoustic schwannoma.'"

A.G. Osborn, M.D.

Congenital Abnormalities

Magnetic Resonance Imaging Lesion Analysis in Neurofibromatosis Type 1

DiMario FJ, Ramsby G (Univ of Connecticut, Hartford)
Arch Neurol 55:500-505, 1998 8–10

Background.—Several common brain lesions found on MRI have been associated with neurofibromatosis type 1 (NF-1). The evolution of high-signal brain parenchymal lesions on MR images of patients with NF-1 was investigated.

Methods and Findings.—Thirty patients undergoing a total of 59 MR examinations were studied. Patients were aged from 1 to 53 years. Twenty-two patients were male. Nineteen patients had brain lesions (BL). These lesions were in the hemispheres in all 19 and in the brainstem and cerebellum in 10 each. Of 129 lesions, 87 (67%) were found in the cerebellum and globus pallidus. At initial examination, 97 lesions totalling in size 197 units were identified in the 19 patients with BLs. After a mean of 2.3 years of follow-up, the total number of lesions and their size decreased. In 7 of 13 patients studied serially, the number and size of brainstem lesions increased during follow-up, and hemispheric and cerebellar lesions were more evanescent.

Conclusions.—High-signal T2 lesions on MRI evolve with time in patients with NF-1. The evolution of such lesions is region specific and may be associated with preferential region-specfic effects of the NF-1 gene product.

► A number of brain lesions occur in patients with NF-1. The fact that high-signal intensities in the basal ganglia and white matter occur in these cases is well known. These abnormalities are present in about 45% of NF-1 cases.[2] The few autopsied cases of NF-1 show these lesions are most often myelin vacuolization, not hamartomas or heterotopias as once thought. An earlier article by the same authors showed that these abnormalities are usually transient and most are eventually replaced with more normal myelin during adolescence and childhood.[3]

In this article, the authors observed NF-1 patients with serial scans and found a general decrease in both total number of lesions as well as their size. Most of these lesions were in the cerebellum and globus pallidus. An important observation is that brainstem lesions actually *increased* in number and size, in contrast to the asymptomatic and more evanescent hemispheric and cerebellar abnormalities. The authors suggest that the effect of the NF-1 gene product, neurofibromin, may vary and be region-specific.

Another recent article showed contrast enhancement is useful in baseline MR studies.[1] It maximizes tumor detection and characterization, adds confidence to the diagnosis of benign myelin vacuolization, and is helpful in assessing neoplasm progression on follow-up examinations.

A.G. Osborn, M.D.

References

1. Bonawitz C, Castillo M, Chin CT, et al: Usefulness of contrast material in MR of patients with neurofibromatosis type 1. *Am J Neuroradiol* 19:541-546, 1998
2. DiPaolo DP, Zimmerman RA, Rorke LB, et al: Neurofibromatosis type 1: Pathologic substrate of high-signal-intensity foci in the brain. *Radiology* 195:721-724, 1995
3. DiMario FJ, Ramsby G, Greenstein R, et al: Neurofibromatosis type-1: Magnetic resonance imaging findings. *J Child Neurol* 8:32-39, 1993

Co-localization of TSC1 and TSC2 Gene Products in Tubers of Patients With Tuberous Sclerosis

Johnson MW, Emelin JK, Park S-H, et al (Univ of California, Los Angeles)
Brain Pathol 9:45-54, 1999 8–11

Background.—Researchers have recently reported the cloning of 2 genes containing mutations in the phenotype of tuberous sclerosis (TSC). TSC2 on chromosome 16p13.3 encodes the protein tuberin, which seems to have properties that regulate growth. TSC1 on chromosome 9q34 encodes hamartin, which currently has no specified cellular functions. Antibodies to hamartin and tuberin were developed and characterized. These immunoreagents were used to localize sites of hamartin expression in surgically resected cortical tubers from children with intractable epilepsy associated with TSC. Patterns of hamartin and tuberin expression in these lesions were then compared.

Methods and Findings.—Polyclonal antibodies were raised to synthetic peptides that represent portions of tuberin and hamartin. These antibodies were then used in immunoblots and immunohistochemical studies to localize the proteins in surgically resected neocortical tubers from 4 patients with TSC. Each antibody labeled a single band at the expected molecular weight on Western blots of autopsy brain specimens, K-562 cell, and NT2 lysates. In immunohistochemical studies on paraffin-embedded tissue, antibodies to tuberin and hamartin prominently labeled atypical and dysmorphic neuroglial cells characteristic of TSC tubers. Both tuberin and hamartin antisera labeled some abnormal cells in cortical tuber sections.

Conclusions.—These findings suggest that tuberin and hamartin are expressed robustly in similar populations of neuroglial cells of TSC tubers, even when TSC1 or TSC2 germline mutations are present. Further research is needed to define the roles of these gene products in normal and abnormal cortical development, tuber pathogenesis, and seizure generation.

► We've come a long way in a few short years in our understanding of the genetics that underlie many of the neurocutaneous syndromes. NF-1 and NF-2 were the first disorders to be characterized. Tuberous sclerosis complex (TSC) took a while longer and was more elusive.

TSC is a multisystem disorder with known chromosomal abnormalities. TSC2 is on chromosome 16p13.3 and encodes a protein, tuberin, that appears to have growth-regulating properties. The *TSC1* gene is on chromosome 9q34. It encodes a protein called hamartin. No function for this substance has been defined. The authors demonstrate that antibodies to both tuberin and hamartin are prominent in the atypical, dysmorphic neuroglial cells that comprise the "tubers" found in patients with TSC. What this means for the pathogenesis of tubers is still unknown.

A.G. Osborn, M.D.

Cerebral Ischemia and Infarction

Perfusion CT of the Brain: Diagnostic Approach for Early Detection of Ischemic Stroke

Koenig M, Klotz E, Luka B, et al (Ruhr-Univ Bochum, Germany; Siemens Med Engineering Group, Forchheim, Germany)

Radiology 209:85-93, 1998 8–12

Background.—Detecting parenchymal areas of hypoattenuation and focal brain swelling is crucial for selecting patients who may benefit from fibrinolytic treatment. However, these signs may be difficult to detect in the very early phase of cerebral ischemia. The value of perfusion CT in patients with stroke was compared with that of SPECT.

Methods.—Thirty-two patients with possible stroke underwent perfusion CT within 6 hours of symptom onset. Perfusion CT was obtained at the level of the basal ganglia after iodinated contrast infusion. Based on CT results, cerebral blood volume, cerebral blood flow (CBF), and time to peak contrast material enhancement were determined. A subgroup of 18 patients also underwent cerebral SPECT.

Findings.—Perfusion CT showed areas of reduced CBF in 25 of 28 patients with proven infarct, an 89% sensitivity. The results of CBF maps corresponded well to SPECT findings in 81% of the patients. However, ischemia was outside the scanning level in the remaining 19% and was missed. Perfusion CT demonstrated various changes in CBF, cerebral blood volume, and time to peak enhancement in ischemic territories.

Conclusions.—Perfusion CT enables early detection of cerebral ischemia. In addition, it provides useful information about the extent of perfusion disturbances.

► Some institutions continue to rely on CT assessment in the evaluation of acute stroke. Echo planar MR for diffusion-perfusion imaging is not universally available nor universally applied. This article suggests another CT technique to augment our diagnostic accuracy and treatment planning for therapeutic intervention in patients with acute stroke: CT perfusion imaging. The authors report an 89% sensitivity in identifying areas of reduced CBF on perfusion CT scanning (25 of 28 patients). The authors also demonstrated reasonably good correlation with SPECT scans. This article offers an alternative method of CBF assessment in stroke, a method that can be used in settings where SPECT and diffusion/perfusion MR are not routinely available.

J.G. Smirniotopoulos, M.D.

Diffusion-weighted MR of Acute Cerebral Infarction: Comparison of Data Processing Methods

Chong J, Lu D, Aragao F, et al (Mount Sinai School of Medicine, New York)
AJNR 19:1733-1739, 1998 8–13

Background.—On diffusion-weighted MR images, regions of early cerebral infarction have reduced apparent diffusion coefficient (ADC), reflecting limited diffusion compared with normal brain. In normal brain tissue, diffusion may be relatively more restricted in one direction than in another because of the organization of cellular structures, cell membranes, or pattern of myelination (called *diffusion anisotropy*). The accuracy of simple, orthogonal-axis diffusion-weighted imaging was compared with 3 other sets of postacquisition-processed images in the diagnosis of early cerebral infarction.

Methods.—Twenty-six consecutive adults with signs and symptoms consistent with early cortical or subcortical cerebral infarction and 17 control subjects were assessed. Multisection, single-shot, spin-echo echoplanar diffusion-weighted imaging at 1.5 T was performed to generate a set of 3 orthogonal-axis diffusion-weighted images. In addition, isotropic diffusion-weighted, diffusion trace-weighted, and diffusion trace (mean ADC) images were produced off-line. All 4 sets were interpreted by 2 neuroradiologists.

Findings.—Orthogonal-axis diffusion-weighted images had a mean sensitivity of 98.1%, a specificity of 97.1%, and an accuracy of 97.7%. For isotropic diffusion-weighted images, these values were 88.5%, 100%, and 93%, respectively. For diffusion trace-weight images, the mean sensitivity, specificity, and accuracy were 82.7%, 73.6%, and 79.1%, respectively. These values were 50%, 85.3%, and 64%, respectively, for diffusion trace images.

Conclusions.—Orthogonal-axis diffusion-weighted images are the most sensitive and accurate, with a very high specificity, for diagnosing early cerebral infarction. The current findings are not consistent with the belief that quantitative diffusion maps, which require imaging with multiple diffusion sensitivities or subsequent image processing, are needed for the imaging of stroke.

► This article, like the one by Gonzalez et al[1] concerns the accuracy of diffusion-weighted imaging in the diagnosis of acute stroke. This one addresses the various techniques that can be used. There is an excellent discussion of the important issues involved. The greatest value is in the authors' conclusion that the orthogonal-axis diffusion-weighted image had the greatest accuracy. The authors report that isotropic images and calculation of the mean ADC (apparent diffusion coefficient) or "trace" images are not only unecessary, but may be less accurate than diffusion-weighted images.

J. G. Smirniotopoulos, M.D.

Reference

1. González RG, Schaefer PW, Buonanno FS, et al: Diffusion-weighted MR imaging: Diagnostic accuracy in patients imaged within 6 hours of stroke symptom onset. *Radiology* 210:155-162, 1999.

Studies of Acute Ischemic Stroke With Proton Magnetic Resonance Spectroscopy: Relation Between Time From Onset, Neurological Deficit, Metabolite Abnormalities in the Infarct, Blood Flow, and Clinical Outcome

Wardlaw JM, Marshall I, Wild J, et al (Univ of Edinburgh, Scotland)
Stroke 29:1618-1624, 1998 8–14

Purpose.—Proton MR spectroscopy (MRS) provides useful information on metabolite abnormalities in the brains of patients with stroke, thus indicating neuronal viability. The finding of lactate suggests ischemia, and reduced *N*-acetylaspartate (NAA) suggests a reduction in neuronal viability. The relationship of these MRS variables with infarct size, blood flow, clinical presentation, and outcome were assessed.

Methods.—The study included 50 patients with clinical evidence of a large cortical infarct. Serial proton MRS was performed within 4 days after the stroke, again at 5 to 10 days, and at 11 to 35 days. The studies were performed using a long echo time PRESS single voxel or chemical shift imaging acquisition. Serial transcranial Doppler ultrasonography was performed to estimate blood flow to the infarct. Information on clinical characteristics, demographic variables, and 6-month clinical outcomes was analyzed as well.

Results.—Patients whose initial MRS study showed reduced NAA within the infarct had a more severe clinical stroke syndrome, more extensive infarction, and greater reduction in blood supply to the infarct. They also had higher lactate levels, which were also related to large infarct. Patients with infarct swelling had large infarcts and reduced blood supply to the infarct. However, infarct swelling was unrelated to NAA or lactate levels on MRS. The extent of infarct was the most important predictor of clinical outcome. Outcome was not related to NAA or lactate concentration alone.

Conclusions.—In patients with acute ischemic stroke, a reduction in NAA on MRS is associated with reduced blood flow to the infarct. Reduced blood flow is associated with the size of the infarct, which is the main determinant of clinical outcome. The presence of lactate on MRS is not related to blood flow. The utility of these findings is complicated by the difficulty of performing MRS in clinically ill patients with acute ischemic stroke.

Cerebral Infarction: Time Course of Signal Intensity Changes on Diffusion-weighted MR Images

Burdette JH, Ricci PE, Petitti N, et al (Wake Forest Univ, Winston-Salem, NC)
AJR 171:791-795, 1998 8–15

Purpose.—Diffusion-weighted MRI is a sensitive technique for diagnosis of acute cerebral infarction. However, there are few data on how signal intensity on diffusion-weighted images changes over time. This issue was addressed in a large series of patients with suspected cerebral infarction.

Methods.—During the 6-month study period, 212 patients underwent echoplanar diffusion-weighted MRI because of suspected cerebral infarction. Prototype diffusion acquisition software and a 1.5-T scanner were used to acquire the single-shot spin-echo echoplanar diffusion-weighted imaging sequence. From this series, 85 patients (46 female and 39 male; mean age, 67 years) with clinically definite cerebral infarction were identified. Two neuroradiologists reviewed the conventional and diffusion-weighted MR images, along with the clinical history.

Results.—Thirteen lesions in 12 patients were evaluated within 24 hours; in each case, the diffusion-weighted images showed abnormally increased signal intensity. In 44 patients evaluated between days 1 and 4, 96% of lesions showed abnormally high signal intensity. In contrast, none of 10 infarcts imaged at 15 days or longer showed hyperintensity on diffusion-weighted images. In 10 patients, the infarcts showed hemorrhagic transformation, showing low signal intensity on T2-weighted images or high signal intensity on unenhanced T1-weighted images. The series included 2 false-negative results.

Conclusions.—In patients with acute cerebral infarction, diffusion-weighted MR images show abnormal signal intensity starting within 24 hours and continuing for up to 14 days after the clinical ictus. The overall signal intensity of these images reflects not only changes in the diffusion constant but also in spin density and T2. The presence of blood products may create problems in determining infarct age from diffusion-weighted images (Fig 3).

► Burdette et al reviewed echoplanar diffusion-weighted images (DWI) in 85 patients. They demonstrated a time course for DWI showing that all 13 infarcts imaged in the first 24 hours had abnormal signal, and none of 10 infarcts imaged more than 2 weeks after stroke symptom onset was hyperintense on DWI. They also noted that 2 patients examined within 48 hours after symptom onset had false-negative DWI images. They have downplayed the need for calculated apparent diffusion coefficient images, emphasizing instead that simple visual assessment of DWI is easier, and probably all that is necessary, in acute stroke imaging.

J.G. Smirniotopoulos, M.D.

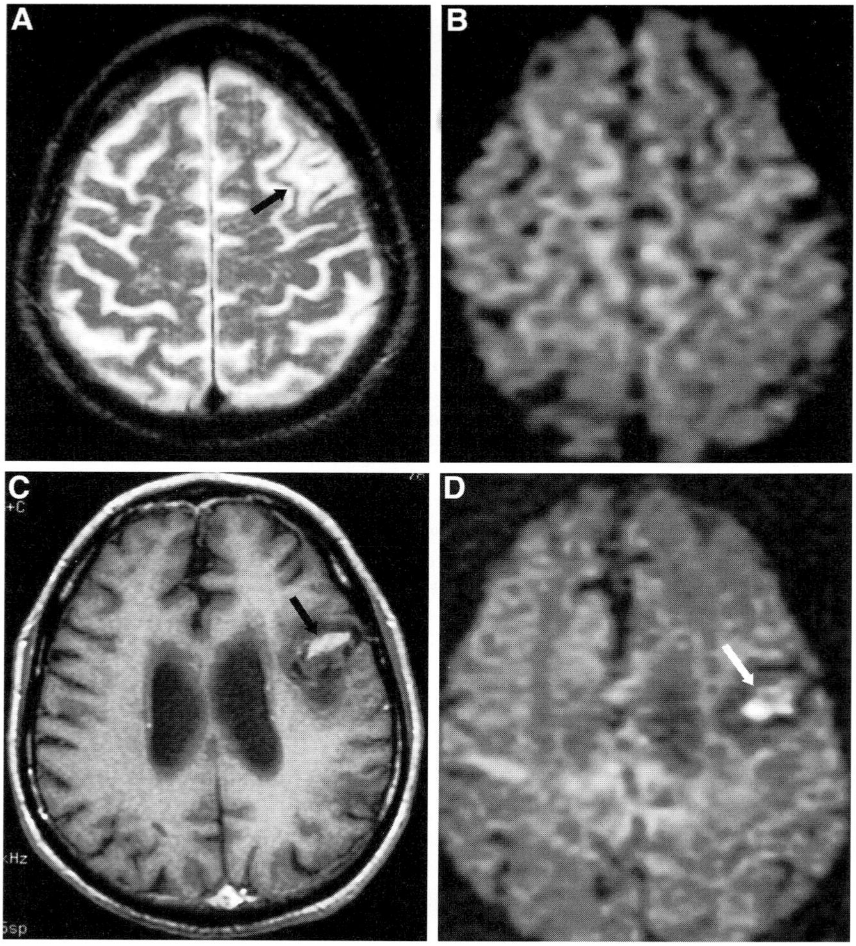

FIGURE 3.—78-year-old man with hemorrhagic transformation of left frontal lobe ischemic infarction resulting in subcortical hematoma. **A**, Axial T2-weighted MR image through high frontal region obtained 13 days after clinical ictus shows abnormally increased signal intensity (*arrow*) in region of infarct. **B**, Axial diffusion-weighted MR image obtained at same time as **A** shows no signal abnormality in same region. **C**, Axial T1-weighted MR image obtained at same time as **A** but located 2 cm inferior to **A** shows subacute hematoma with high-signal-intensity blood products centrally (*arrow*), consistent with methemoglobin formation. **D**, Axial diffusion-weighted MR image obtained at same time as **C** shows focal area of hyperintensity within hematoma (*arrow*) that corresponds to high-signal-intensity area in **C**. (Courtesy of Burdette JH, Ricci PE, Petitti N, et al: Cerebral infarction: Time course of signal intensity changes on diffusion-weighted MR images. *AJR* 171:791-795, 1998.)

Prognostic Value of Proton Magnetic Resonance Spectroscopy in Ischemic Stroke

Federico F, Simone IL, Lucivero V, et al (Univ of Bari, Italy)

Arch Neurol 55:489-494, 1998 8–16

Background.—Single-voxel ^{1}HMR spectroscopy (MRS) is useful in studying neuronal viability and infarct metabolism in patients with acute ischemic stroke. Reduced levels of *N*-acetylaspartate (NAA) is an early finding. Some studies have suggested a further decline in NAA during the subacute phase, possibly reflecting ongoing neuronal loss in the ischemic penumbra. The correlation between variations in MRS measurements of metabolite during the acute and subacute phases and the 6-month outcomes of stroke was studied.

Methods.—The study included 26 patients with recent ischemic stroke in the middle cerebral artery territory. All underwent combined single-voxel proton MRS and MRI, 8 within the first 24 hours after stroke and 18 during the first week. Peak area signals of the metabolites NAA, choline-containing compounds (Cho), and creatine-phosphocreatine (Cr) were compared in the infarcted area vs. the contralateral regions. The MRS findings were evaluated against 6-month clinical outcomes, assessed with the Scandinavian Stroke Scale and the Barthel Index.

Results.—Initial MRS study showed significant reductions in the peak area signals for NAA, Cr, and Cho in the infarcted areas. In 19 patients, MRS revealed a lactate signal. Both NAA and Cr remained significantly reduced at the second examination. The NAA signals were significantly and positively correlated with both outcome measures. Scores on the Scandinavian Stroke Scale were significantly lower for patients in whom lactate was present.

Conclusions.—Performing single-voxel proton MRS as soon as possible after acute stroke provides useful prognostic information. Reduced NAA and the presence of lactate appear to be particularly useful prognostic indications. The findings await confirmation in a larger number of patients studied immediately after stroke.

► This article and the one by Wardlaw et al (Abstract 8–14) examined the potential of MRS to assist in predicting patient outcome in acute cerebral infarction. Federico et al found that most infarcts demonstrated decreased NAA but that elevated lactate correlated with worse outcome measures compared with infarcts without elevated lactate peaks. In their series, the best opportunity for recovery was in those infarcts that had only mild reductions in NAA and no lactate.

In contrast, Wardlaw et al concluded that infarct size and the reduction in the NAA in the infarct were more closely related to an adverse infarct outcome, presumably caused by blood flow changes. In their series the presence of lactate was not as important in predicting outcomes. These studies had different methodologies, but in their area of agreement (reduction in NAA on MRS), they offer yet another tool for predicting the severity of stroke outcome.

Should every patient undergo the additional pulse sequence for MRS? As in the other articles concerning the use of MRS, the ultimate clinical utility of these measures remains to be demonstrated.

J.G. Smirniotopoulos, M.D.

Evaluation of Early Computed Tomographic Findings in Acute Ischemic Stroke

Marks MP, Holmgren EB, Fox AJ, et al (Stanford Univ, Calif; Genentech, South San Francisco, Calif; Univ of Western Ontario, London, Canada, et al)
Stroke 30:389-392, 1999 8–17

Introduction.—CT scanning has demonstrated a possible role as a prognostic and triage test in ischemic stroke with the administration of IV tissue plasminogen activator in the first hours of stroke. Poor outcome has been associated with early infarct signs involving extensive areas of the middle cerebral artery (MCA) territory. In this group, treatment with IV tissue plasminogen activator was found to have no beneficial effect and increased the likelihood of fatal intracranial hemorrhage. It has been difficult to find a means of excluding this group. The reliability of detection with hyperacute CT scans was assessed.

Methods.—Fifty hyperacute CT scans were taken at less than 6 hours after ictus. The scans were evaluated for the degree of MCA territory involvement (less than 33% or more than 33%) and for the presence of a hyperdense MCA territory involvement. Evaluations were made by 3 neuroradiologists. Comparisons of these evaluations were made with baseline stroke scale scores, 30-day infarct volumes, and 24-hour scan results.

Results.—The degree of MCA territory hypodensity was reliably evaluated by readers, with all 3 agreeing in 72% (36 of 50 cases). More than 33% involvement was correctly called with a specificity of 86% to 97% and a sensitivity of 60% to 85% When more than 33% MCA hypodensity was seen, the baseline stroke scale scores were higher. Poorer outcome was correlated with detection of significant hypodensity, or more than 33% The mean 30-day infarct volumes were 27 to 33 cm^3 when more than 33% hypodensity was not detected. When more than 33% hypodensity was detected, the 30-day infarct volumes were 84.3 to 123.1 cm^3.

Conclusion.—A sensitive, prognostic, and reliable indicator of the amount of MCA territory having infarction is the detection of its hypodensity on hyperacute CT scans.

► A simple and succinct take-home message is: MCA territory hypodensity on hyperacute (less than 6 hours after ictus) CT scanning is a sensitive, prognostic, and reliable indicator of the amount of MCA territory undergoing infarction. The implications for treatment are obvious. They have been documented by analysis of the European Cooperative Acute Stroke Study, which showed that patients with hypoattenuation involving less than 33% of the MCA territory benefit from early IV tissue plasminogen activator treatment, whereas those who have involvement of more than 33% do not benefit and, in fact, have increased risk of hemorrhage. Another recent study has shown that hypodensity of greater than 50% is an independent predictor of fatal brain swelling.[1] Still others have shown that early evaluation with triphasic helical CT to detect acute proximal MCA occlusion is useful for assessment of the ischemic zone.[2]

A.G. Osborn, M.D.

References

1. Krieger DW, Demchuk AM, Kasner SE, et al; Early clinical and radiological predictors of fatal brain swelling in ischemic stroke. *Stroke* 30:287-292, 1999.
2. Na DG, Byun HS, Lee KH, et al: Acute occlusion of the middle cerebral artery: Early evaluation with triphasic helical CT—Preliminary results. *Radiology* 207:113-122, 1998.

Cerebral Venous Sinus Thrombosis: Prognostic and Therapeutic Significance of an Early Radiologic Diagnosis

Roncallo E, Turtulici I, Arena E, et al (Universitá degli Studi, Genova, Italy; Ospedale San Martino, Genova, Italy; Centro di Studio per la Neurofisiologia Cerebrale, Genova, Italy)

Rivista di Neuroradiol 11:479-505, 1998 8–18

Introduction.—The etiology, incidence, history, treatment, and outcome of cerebral venous sinus thrombosis are poorly understood. The diagnosis is often suggested by strokelike symptoms with a slow onset. Many predisposing factors and conditions have been associated with cerebral venous sinus thrombosis, including congenital and acquired cardiac diseases, regional infections, and head trauma (Table 3). In terms of course and outcome, cerebral venous sinus thrombosis is unpredictable. Appropriate management that can improve the prognosis of the disease is dependent upon an early diagnosis. The clinical, CT, and MR patterns of cerebral venous sinus thrombosis were described to help establish which patients can be followed conservatively with systemic heparinization and which warrant direct instillation of fibrinolytic agents into the venous sinuses.

Methods.—There were 11 patients with cerebral venous sinus thrombosis who had clinical, CT/CT angiography, and MRI/MR angiography findings reviewed. The patients ranged in age from 24 years to 69 years; they were divided into 2 groups. One group had morphological patterns with vascular signs, such as spontaneous sinusal hyperdensity, spontaneous all-sequences hyperintensity, venous engorgement, empty delta sign, lack of sinusal contrast-enhancement, delayed sinusal transit-time, and lack of flow-related signal (Table 2). The other group had morphological patterns with parenchyma signs, such as mass effect and cortical sulcal

TABLE 3.—Aetiologies of Non-infective Cerebral Venous Sinus Thrombosis

A)	Local Aetiologies	B)	General Aetiologies
1)	*Cranial trauma*	*1)*	*Surgical*
•	Open or closed	•	All interventions with or without inferior limb thrombosis
•	With or without fracture		
2)	*Arterial thrombosis*	*2)*	*Pregnancy and Post-partum*
3)	*Intracranial tumours*	*3)*	*Autoimmune diseases*
•	Meningioma	•	Crohn disease and ulcerous colitis
•	Lymphoma		
•	Astrocytoma	•	Behcet disease
•	Paraganglioma	•	Lupus erythematosus
		•	Horton's disease
		•	Wegener's granulomatosis
4)	*Intracranial malformations*	*4)*	*Hemopathies*
		•	Polyglobulia
•	Porencephalic cavities	•	Paroxysmal nocturnal hemoglobinuria
•	Arachnoid cysts		
		•	Thrombocythemia
		•	Leukemia and Lymphoma
5)	*Vascular malformations*	*5)*	*Coagulation diseases*
•	Dural AVM	•	Antithrombin III deficit
		•	C and S protein deficit
		•	DIC and Thrombopenia
		•	Cryoglobulinemia
6)	*Venous catheterization*	*6)*	*Drugs*
		•	Oral contraceptive
		•	Androgens
		•	Chemotherapy
		7)	*Others*
		•	Cardiopathies
		•	Dehydration
		•	Nephrotic syndrome
		•	Cirrhosis
		8)	*Visceral cancers*
	Idiopathic 20%-25%		

(Courtesy of Roncallo E, Turtulici I, Arena E, et al: Cerebral venous sinus thrombosis: Prognostic and therapeutic significance of an early radiologic diagnosis (*original in Italian*). *Rivista di Neuroradiologia* 11:479-505, 1998.)

effacement, white matter edema, venous ischemia, hemorrhagic infarct, breakdown of the blood-brain barrier, and hydrocephalus.

Results.—It was found that cerebral venous angioarchitecture and underlying pathophysiologic mechanism of venous thrombosis are related to the clinical and radiologic pictures. Vessels related to parenchymal lesions develop progressively and damage slowly, thus their clinical symptoms reverse more frequently.

Conclusion.—A good prognosis is possible with a prompt CT- MRI diagnosis. On MRI, the thrombus in the early stage has an isointense signal on T1-weighted images and a hypointensity on T2-weighted images, reflecting the presence of oxyhemoglobin and deoxyhemoglobin within the clot (Fig 9). When the patient does not improve clinically and radiologi-

TABLE 2.—Radiological Data

Pt n°	Occlusion Site	CT-Direct Signs	MR-Direct Signs	Mass Effect	Edema	Venous Stasis	Ischemia*	Haemorrhage
1	SSS	Cord sign, Delta Sign	T1-hyperintensity	Yes	Yes	Yes	Yes	No
2	SSS, cortical veins	No	No	Yes	Yes	Yes	Yes	No
3	SSS	Cord sign	T1-hyperintensity	No	No	Yes	No	No
4	TS, SSS, SS	Cord sign, Delta sign	T1-hyperintensity	Yes	Yes	Yes	Yes	No
5	SSS, TS	Delta sign	Delta sign	Yes	Yes	Yes	Yes	No
6	TS	Cord sign	Delta sign	Yes	Yes	Yes	Yes	No
7	TS	Cord sign	No	No	No	No	No	No
8	TS bilateral, SSS, SS	Cord sign, Delta sign	No flow enhancement	No	No	No	No	No
9	LS	Cord sign	No flow enhancement	Yes	No	Yes	No	No
10	SS, SSS	Cord sign	T1 hyperintensity	Yes	Yes	Yes	No	No
11	LS, JB	Cord sign	No flow enhancement	Yes	Yes	Yes	Yes	No

*Ischemia also includes hemorrhagic infarcts.

(Courtesy of Roncallo E, Turtulici I, Arena E, et al: Cerebral venous sinus thrombosis: Prognostic and therapeutic significance of an early radiologic diagnosis (*original in Italian*). *Rivista di Neuroradiologia* 11:479-505, 1998.)

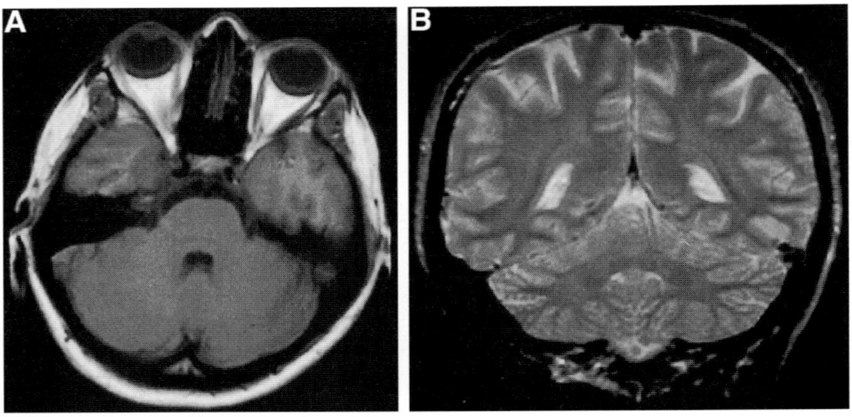

FIGURE 9.—Signal intensity of the thrombus within the superior sagittal sinus in the acute stage. **A**, axial T1-weighted MRI image: isointensity. **B**, coronal T2-weighted MR image: hypointensity (false flow-void). (Courtesy of Roncallo E, Turtulici I, Arena E, et al: Cerebral venous sinus thrombosis: Prognostic and therapeutic significance of an early radiologic diagnosis. *Rivista di Neuroradio* 11:479-505, 1998.)

cally within the first 2 weeks after heparinization, treatment using selective sinusal instillation of urokinase is considered.

► This article presents a very nice overview of the patterns of cerebral venous sinus thrombosis that we observe on imaging studies, showing how they are based on the venous angioarchitecture as well as the underlying pathologic mechanism. Another nice article on this subject is a pictorial essay on dural sinus thrombosis.[1]

The authors also argue that selective sinusal instillation of urokinase should be considered only when the patient does not improve clinically and radiologically within the first 2 weeks after heparinization. This contrasts with an aggressive, early approach in symptomatic patients recently advocated elsewhere.[2]

A.G. Osborn, M.D.

References

1. Provenzale JM, Joseph GJ, Barboriak DP: Dural sinus thrombosis: Findings on CT and MR imaging and diagnostic pitfalls. *AJR* 170:777-783, 1998.
2. Phillips MF, Bagley LJ, Sinson GP, et al: Endovascular thrombolysis for symptomatic cerebral venous thrombosis. *J Neurosurg* 90:65-71, 1999.

Vascular Malformations

The Prospective Natural History of Cerebral Venous Malformations
McLaughlin MR, Kondziolka D, Flickinger JC, et al (Univ of Pittsburgh Med Ctr, Pa)
Neurosurgery 43:195-201, 1998 8–19

Background.—Venous malformations, or developmental venous anomalies, are congenital vascular malformations in the brain believed to be anomalies of venous drainage. These anomalies are the most common intracranial vascular malformations observed on brain imaging and at autopsy. Some authorities have suggested that some venous malformations have an aggressive course, with a high rate of hemorrhage and morbidity. However, others have reported a benign natural history that makes treatment unnecessary. The current prospective clinical and MRI study was performed to determine the natural history of venous malformations.

Methods and Findings.—Eighty patients with venous malformations were referred to one center for evaluation between 1986 and 1996. All patients were managed by observation. Twenty-two patients had neurologic signs or symptoms thought to be associated with malformations, including headaches in 9, seizures in 4, sensory symptoms in 3, motor deficits in 3, trigeminal neuralgia in 2, and an extrapyramidal disorder in 1. Twenty-three patients had headaches thought to be unrelated to brain malformations. The retrospective bleeding rate (projected back to birth) was 0.61%. Sixteen patients had had previous brain hemorrhage in the area of the venous malformations, including 2 patients with subsequent hemorrhage. During follow-up, 2 patients had hemorrhage (0.68% per year), but only 1 patient, who had not previously bled, had a symptomatic bleed (0.34% per year). One of these patients remained free of symptoms, and the other experienced worsening of facial paresthesias. None of the patients died of venous malformations.

Conclusions.—The hemorrhage rate in a patient with venous malformations is comparable to that in a patient with cavernous malformations without previous symptomatic hemorrhage. Hemorrhage in patients with venous malformations may be associated with an underlying, as yet undocumented, cavernous malformation. Because the risk of new neurologic events is low, conservative management is indicated.

► This article reviews the "natural history" of 80 patients with venous malformations, collected between 1986 and 1996. Venous malformations were diagnosed either by "classic" MRI findings of a radiating crown of tubular flow-voids or angiographic confirmation.

The article confirms the benign course of these malformations, with a projected rate of complication that warrants "watchful waiting" rather than operative interventions. Using previously published risk models, the annual rate of bleeding was calculated to be approximately 0.68% per year. Of particular note was the association of cavernous angiomas with the venous malformations. The authors have reiterated earlier assertions that bleeding in venous malformations is usually the result of an (occult) cavernous hemangioma—and not from the venous malformation itself.

J.G. Smirniotopoulos, M.D.

Cavernous Malformations of the Brainstem: Experience With 100 Patients

Porter RW, Detwiler PW, Spetzler RF, et al (Barrow Neurological Inst, Phoenix, Ariz; Mercy Healthcare Arizona, Phoenix; Univ of California San Francisco; et al)

J Neurosurg 90:50-58, 1999 8–20

Introduction.—Autopsy or surgery were the only means of diagnosing cavernous malformations of the brain stem before the era of MRI. Only small surgical series have been reported in the literature; thus, their natural history remains poorly understood. To clarify and define the natural history of this entity, the cases of 100 patients with cavernous malformations of the brain stem were reviewed.

Methods.—The 100 patients comprised 38 males and 62 females with a mean age of 37 years and with 103 cavernous malformations of the brainstem during a 13-year period. During the retrospective review, evaluations were conducted of clinical histories, radiographs, pathology records, and operative reports.

Results.—There were 39 patients with lesions in the pons; 15 in the medulla; 16 in the midbrain; 15 in the pontomesencephalic junction; 10 in the pontomedullary junction; 2 in the midbrain–hypothalamus/thalamus region; and 5 at more than 2 brain stem levels. The annual hemorrhage rate was about 5% per lesion per year. In 86 of the 100 patients, standard skull base approaches were used to resect lesions. A venous anomaly was found in association with the cavernous malformation of the brain stem in all 86 patients (Fig 2). In 87% of the surgical patients, the follow-up found them to be the same or better; 105 were worse and 4% died. Ten of the surgically treated patients (12%) had incidences of permanent or severe morbidity. After a mean follow-up of 35 months, the average postoperative Glasgow Outcome Scale score for the surgically treated patients was 4.5. One patient had had previous resection of 1 of her lesions in the right temporal lobe, and 2 years later, she had a de novo pontine lesion in the brain stem (Fig 1)

Conclusion.—Compared with cavernous malformations in other locations, the natural history of cavernous malformations of the brain stem is worse. Skull base approaches can be used to resect these cavernous malformations. In patients with symptomatic hemorrhage who harbor lesions that approach the pial surface, these approaches should be considered. Cavernous malformations of the brain stem are associated with venous anomalies and they must be preserved.

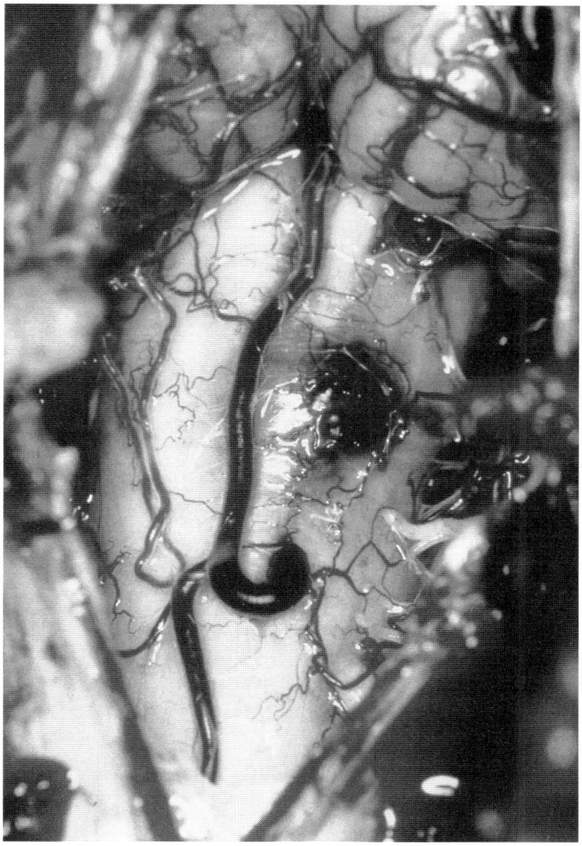

FIGURE 2.—Intraoperative photograph depicting a venous malformation associated with a cavernous malformation located on the dorsal medulla. (Courtesy of Porter RW, Detwiler PW, Spetzler RF, et al: Cavernous malformations of the brainstem: Experience with 100 patients. *J Neurosurg* 90: 50-58, 1999.)

► Cavernous malformations ("angiomas") of the brain represent a challenging management problem. They occur in approximately 0.5% to 1% of the population. Because of their propensity to hemorrhage repeatedly, estimating the risk of bleed vs. the risk of surgery is important. The authors show that the natural history of cavernous angiomas in the brain stem is worse than that of those in other locations. Perhaps their most important observation is that venous anomalies are "always" associated with cavernous angiomas and, because they drain normal brain, must be preserved during surgery.

The authors' findings are supported by another recent article[1] demonstrating that patients with cavernous malformations also often have venous malformations and that these patients are more likely to be female, have associated symptomatic hemorrhage, have posterior fossa lesions, and suffer from repeated symptomatic hemorrhage. They are also less likely to

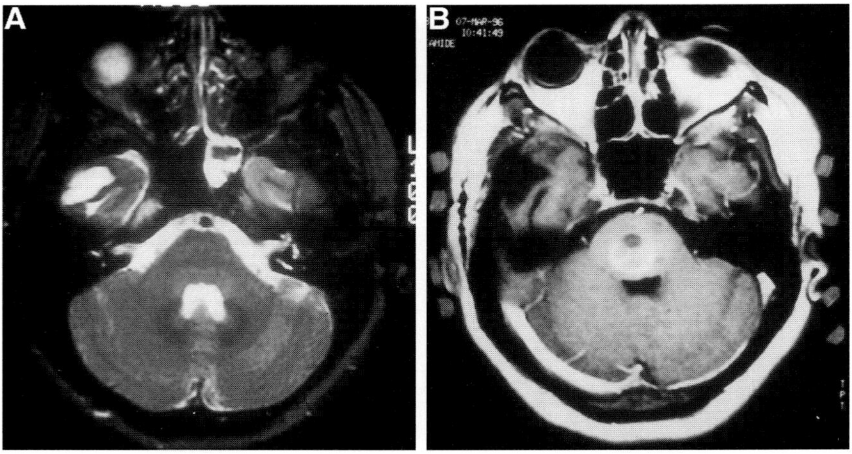

FIGURE 1.—Axial T_2-weighted (*left*) and T_1-weighted (*right*) MR images showing a familial de novo cavernous malformations of the brainstem that developed in the center of the pons. The images were taken 2 years apart in the same patient. (Courtesy of Porter RW, Detwiler PW, Spetzler RF, et al: Cavernous malformations of the brainstem: Experience with 100 patients. *J Neurosurg* 90: 50-58, 1999.)

present with seizures or to have familial histories.[1] For further information and a nice review on cavernous malformations, see the article by Bellon and Seeger.[2]

A.G. Osborn, M.D.

References

1. Abdulrauf SI, Kaynar MY, Awad IA: A comparison of the clinical profile of cavernous malformations with and without associated venous malformations. *Neurosurgery* 44: 41-47, 1999.
2. Bellon RJ, Seeger JF: Cavernous angiomas. *Int J Neuroradiol* 3:343-355, 1997.

Aneurysms and Intracranial Hemorrhage

Should We Screen for Familial Intracranial Aneurysm?

Crawley F, Clifton A, Brown MM (St George's Hosp Med School, London; Atkinson Morley's Hosp, London; Inst of Neurology, London)
Stroke 30:312-316, 1999 8–21

Introduction.—Half of patients with subarachnoid hemorrhage from a ruptured intracranial aneurysm die. Surgery is associated with a low risk of stroke or death. Whether screening individuals with a family history of intracranial aneurysm would help reduce morbidity and mortality of this disease was investigated. An analysis of the usefulness and cost effectiveness of screening healthy individuals for cerebral aneurysm using theoretical models was conducted.

Methods.—There were 3 models used. One model involved MR angiography followed by digital subtraction angiography if MR angiography

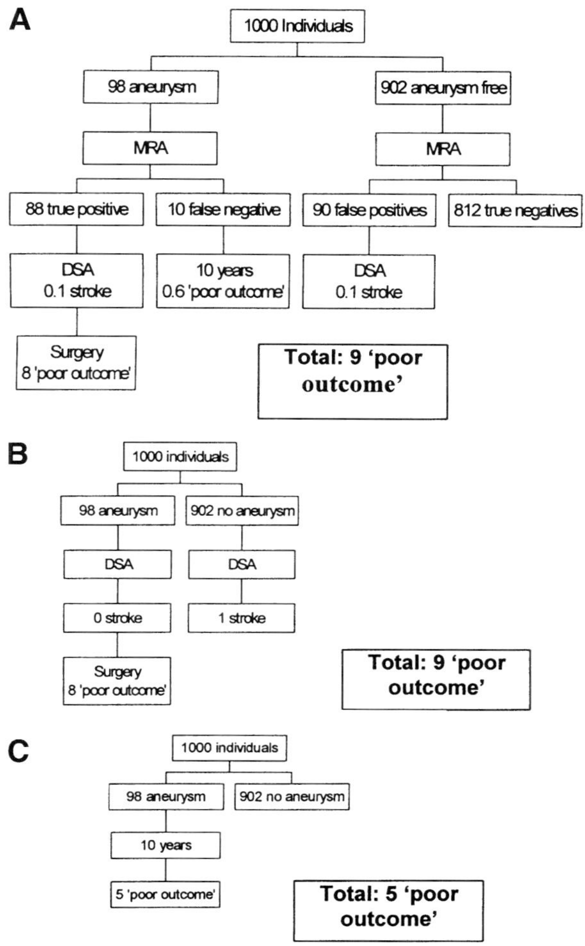

FIGURE 1.—A, Model 1: outcome of screening 1,000 individuals on 1 occasion with MR angiography followed by digital subtraction angiography and by surgery if aneurysm was detected (mean risk of prevalence and risk of rupture of aneurysm). B, Model 2: outcome over subsequent 10 years of screening 1,000 individuals on 1 occasion with digital subtraction angiography, followed by surgery if aneurysm was detected (mean risk of prevalence and risk of rupture of aneurysm). C, Model 3: outcome over 10 years of not screening 1,000 individuals using mean estimate of prevalence and risk of rupture of aneurysm in the calculations. (Courtesy of Crawley F, Clifton A, Brown MM: Should we screen for familial intracranial aneurysm? *Stroke* 30: 312-316, 1999. Reproduced with permission of *Stroke*. Copyright 1999, American Heart Association.)

results were positive. Another model was screening by digital subtraction angiography alone. A third model involved no screening. Every 10 years, screening was repeated and detected aneurysms were surgically treated. In the population screened, the prevalence of aneurysm was assumed to be 9.8%. The annual rupture rate of asymptomatic aneurysm was assumed to be 0.8%. The chance of poor outcome from rupture was assumed to be

75%. The sensitivity and specificity of MR angiography was assumed to be 90% for both, and the risk of digital subtraction angiography was assumed to be 0.1%. The risk of surgery was assumed to be 5.1%.

Results.—Over 30 years, a poor outcome occurred in 14 and 18 individuals, respectively, after screening 1,000 individuals on 3 occasions with MR angiography and digital subtraction angiography or with digital subtraction angiography alone followed by surgery (Fig 1). Poor outcome occurred in 15 individuals over the same period in the group with no screening.

Conclusion.—For individuals with a history of 2 or more affected first-degree relatives with ruptured intracranial aneurysm, screening is not an effective way of reducing morbidity and mortality from ruptured intracranial aneurysm, unless the expected incidence of asymptomatic aneurysm is considerably more than 10%.

▶ Talk about a hot topic! As the noninvasive screening for intracranial aneurysms has improved, the issues raised have also become more pressing. What should be done if an aneurysm is, indeed, found? Now that the entity of familial intracranial aneurysms is firmly established (and may represent up to 27% of cases), we know that the prevalence of aneurysms, in such cases, is very high.[1]

A recent article from the International Study of Unruptured Intracranial Aneurysms Investigators found a strong effect of what I call the Godzilla principle (size really does matter).[2] In fact, it may be about the only thing that really matters in assessing the risk of aneurysm rupture. Aneurysms less than 10 mm in diameter have a very low risk of hemorrhage. The risk of morbidity and mortality related to surgery in this group seems greater than the 7.5-year rupture risk. Combined with the excellent recent reports on endovascular treatment of aneurysms, these data are making the neurosurgeons a bit nervous.

A.G. Osborn, M.D.

References

1. Kojima M, Nagasawa Sh, Lee Y-E, et al: Asymptomatic familial cerebral aneurysms. *Neurosurgery* 43:776-781, 1998.
2. The International Study of unruptured Intracranial Aneurysms Investigators: Unruptured intracranial aneurysms: Risk of rupture and risks of surgical intervention. *N Engl J Med* 339:1725-1733, 1998.

Worst Headache and Subarachnoid Hemorrhage: Prospective, Modern Computed Tomography and Spinal Fluid Analysis

Morgenstern LB, Luna-Gonzales H, Huber JC Jr, et al (Univ of Texas, Houston)

Ann Emerg Med 32:297-304, 1998 8–22

Background.—Although lumbar puncture (LP) may be the best assessment for subarachnoid hemorrhage (SAH), this procedure causes discomfort and is time consuming and costly. The ability of modern head CT to exclude SAH was investigated.

Methods and Findings.—One hundred seven patients seen at 1 center during a 16-month period were enrolled in the study. All reported having "the worst headache of their lives." CT confirmed SAH in 17% of the patients. Among those with negative CT imaging results, only 2 (2.5%) were found on CSF analysis to have SAH. The most sensitive test was CSF spectrophotometric detection. Three patients with fewer than 6 red blood cells in tube 1 had positive spectrophotometric findings. However, tube 4 was negative on spectrophotometric analysis for all 3 patients, suggesting a high false-positive rate.

Conclusions.—Patients reporting the "worst headache of their lives" should undergo noncontrast head CT. If the CT result is negative, patients should undergo LP with spectrophotometric analysis of the CSF. LP should be recommended because of the potentially devastating consequences of undiagnosed SAH.

► Here is another article confirming the accuracy—and potential false-negative rate—for head CT in patients with "the worst headache of my life." This study is important because it was prospective and because of the use of "modern" CT equipment (GE 9800 Hi-Lite Advantage) and contemporary scanning protocol (5-mm sections through the posterior fossa and 10-mm thick above). During the study period, more than 38,000 patients were prospectively screened for headache; and if results were positive, then for "worst headache of my life." Although all 107 patients had CT, only 79 underwent LP (10 refused). Roughly half the patients were scanned during the first 24 hours after onset of headache. Eighteen patients had positive CT scans. Of the 79 with negative CT who had an LP, 2 were positive. This works out to a CT false-negative rate of 2.5%. Of note, neither of those 2 CT negative/LP positive patients had an angiographically detectable aneurysm "after an exhaustive search." It's important to remember that the relative sensitivity of LP and CT behave differently over time: CT may become negative after 48 hours and LP may not become positive until after 12 hours. The overall conclusion of this article is that, even with contemporary or "modern" scanners, an LP is still required in the face of a negative CT, when the patient presents with a history of "worst headache of my life"—especially when the headache has an abrupt onset.

J.G. Smirniotopoulos, M.D.

Value of Repeat Angiography in Patients With Spontaneous Subcortical Hemorrhage

Hino A, Fujimoto M, Yamaki T, et al (Saiseikai Shigaken Hosp, Shiga, Japan)
Stroke 29:2517-2521, 1998 8–23

Introduction.—Some patients with spontaneous subcortical hemorrhage do not show a source of bleeding clinically or neuroradiologically. The etiology of such a hemorrhage is usually classified as unknown. It may be angiographically occult vascular malformations or true arteriovenous malformations. In some instances, a repeat angiogram will reveal a vascular malformation. The usefulness of follow-up angiography in a patient who had an angiogram that did not show a vascular malformation has not been demonstrated. Whether repeat angiography was justified in identifying occult vascular lesions was determined.

Methods.—There were 137 patients with subcortical hemorrhage studied during a 10-year period. Repeat angiography was recommended if the patient was younger than 65 years and the first angiogram or MR image did not show a source of bleeding. A review was conducted of all angiographic and MRI studies. An examination was conducted to determine the relationship between the identified bleeding source and clinical variables such as patient age, sex, history of hypertension, and the size and location of the hematoma.

Results.—Angiography on admission was performed on 107 patients (78%). Immediate surgery for hematoma without angiography was performed on 10 patients (7%). Neither angiography nor surgery was performed on 20 patients (15%). In 55 patients (40%), an etiology for the hemorrhage was found. In young patients without preexisting hyperten-

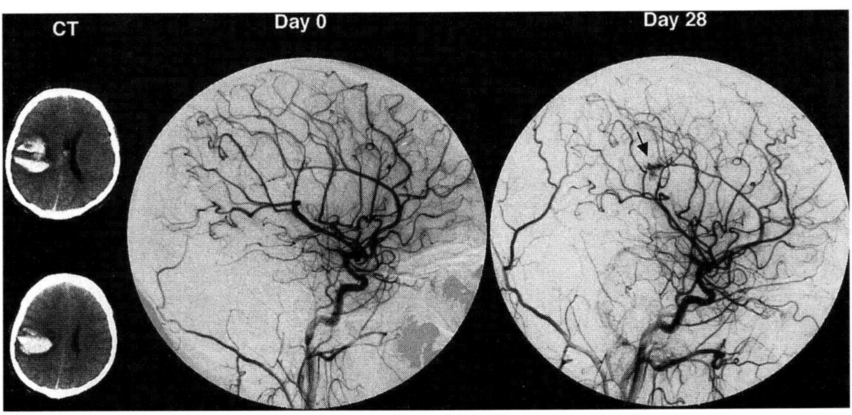

FIGURE.—A case of subcortical hematoma caused by a small arteriovenous malformation that was occult on the initial angiogram was identified on repeat study. Right carotid arteriogram on the day of admission showed no vascular abnormality, but a repeat study 28 days later revealed a small arteriovenous malformation (*arrow*) in the right parietal lobe. (Courtesy of Hino A, Fujimoto M, Yamaki T, et al:Value of repeat angiography in patients with spontaneous subcortical hemorrhage. *Stroke* 29: 2517-2521, 1998. Reproduced with permission of *Stroke*. Copyright 1998, American Heart Association.)

sion, vascular malformations were common. In 22 patients, a second angiogram was obtained, and 4 arteriovenous malformations were shown (Figure). Rebleeding at the site of the initial hemorrhage was not seen after a mean follow-up of 68 months.

Conclusion.—Vascular malformations may not be demonstrated by angiography performed acutely after hemorrhage. For patients who do not have a specific cause for hemorrhage, consideration should be given to repeat angiography.

► It is always a difficult problem, isn't it? A normotensive patient comes to the hospital with sudden onset of a focal neurologic deficit and CT scanning shows a subcortical hematoma. In elderly patients, primary brain tumor or metastasis is always a concern. In those who have dementia, amyloid angiopathy is common.

In younger patients in whom there is no evidence for hypertension, drug abuse, or other predisposing factors, an underlying vascular malformation is always an issue. MR in these cases may show only a focal hematoma, and angiography performed acutely after hemorrhage may not demonstrate abnormal vessels. Sometimes that is because a cavernous malformation, or perhaps a brain tumor, is the underlying cause. In others, an arteriovenous malformation may be present but angiographically "occult." The authors suggest that once the mass effect and edema are resolved, repeat angiography may be warranted. I would suggest another possibility: repeat the MR scan and add MR angiography.

A.G. Osborn, M.D.

DEMYELINATING DISEASE

Serial Whole-Brain Magnetization Transfer Imaging in Patients With Relapsing-Remitting Multiple Sclerosis at Baseline and During Treatment With Interferon Beta-1b

Richert ND, Ostuni JL, Bash CN, et al (NIH, Bethesda, Md; Children's Natl Med Ctr, Washington, DC)

AJNR 19:1705-1713, 1998 8–24

Background.—MRI, the most sensitive and specific technique for imaging multiple sclerosis (MS) disease activity and estimating total disease burden, has been used as a primary or secondary outcome measure in new treatment trials. In most such trials, only conventional MR sequences, with or without contrast material, have been used. Magnetization transfer (MT) was performed monthly to determine whether occult disease fluctuates with macroscopic lesions in the natural history of MS and whether therapeutic agents affect occult disease.

Methods.—Eight patients with relapsing-remitting MS and 4 control participants were studied. Serial whole-brain MT ratios (MTRs) were plotted as normalized histograms. MTR parameters were compared with contrast-enhancing lesions and bulk white matter lesion load noted with standard MR sequences.

Findings.—The MS Patients had a mean histographic peak of 0.25 and a histographic mean of 0.21, which were both significantly lower than corresponding values (0.27 and 0.23) in the control group. In an analysis of histograms by quartiles based on histographic area, voxels with low MTRs in quartile 1 increased during the baseline period, corresponding to bulk matter lesions load. Interferon beta-1b decreased enhancing lesions by 91% and mean bulk white matter lesion load by 15%. However, it did not affect MTR.

Conclusions.—In patients with relapsing-remitting MS, occult disease in normal-appearing white matter, as measured by MTR, parallels the pattern of enhancing lesions and bulk white matter lesion load during the baseline period. Interferon beta-1b does not affect MTR, which suggests that disease may be ongoing even in normal-appearing white matter.

▶ Several authors have demonstrated that MTR may be abnormal in regions of demyelination that are "normal" on routine MR pulse sequences. Richert et al. have demonstrated that the MTR peak is both lower (shorter) and shifted to the left in patients with MS, as compared to matched controls. During treatment there was a dissociation of lesion burden, as measured by contrast enhancement, compared to whole-brain MTR. MTR, and whole-brain MTR, are thought to reflect changes in the cellular microenvironment that are directly related to the process of demyelination. Only 8 patients were involved in this study, and therefore it must be viewed as preliminary. However, if this whole-brain MTR can provide a more sensitive assessment of lesion burden in MS, it may add a parameter that can be used in measuring the effects of various treatment protocols. To quote the authors:

"With the variety of MR pulse sequences available, future MS treatment trials could be designed such that the outcome measure of MR imaging would specifically evaluate the mechanism of action of the drug being tested." I think that this deserves future exploration.

J.G. Smirniotopoulos, M.D.

Sensitivity of Enhanced MR in Multiple Sclerosis: Effects of Contrast Dose and Magnetization Transfer Contrast

Bastianello S, Gasperini C, Paolillo A, et al (Univ "La Sapienza," Rome; Univ of Milan, Italy; Natl Inst for Cancer Research, Genoa, Italy; et al)

AJNR 19:1863-1867, 1998 8–25

Background.—Several new strategies for improving the sensitivity of contrast-enhanced MR imaging in quantifying multiple sclerosis (MS) activity have been reported. The sensitivity of T1-weighted images after injection of a triple dose of contrast material and application of a magnetization transfer (MT) pulse and the sensitivity of the conventional approach were compared in detecting enhancing lesions.

Methods.—Thirteen patients with relapsing-remitting MS underwent monthly MR imaging for 3 months. The MR examinations were done on

2 occasions, using single- and triple-dose contrast material. On each occasion, T1- and T2-weighted spin-echo images were acquired, with and without the MT pulse, before and after contrast administration. Two interpreters assessed all images in a blinded fashion, scoring them in random order and consensually, and counting both the number of new lesions and the total number of lesions.

Findings.—Compared with single-dose non-MT sequences, triple-dose sequences demonstrated 86% more enhancing lesions and 54% more new enhancing lesions. Single-dose MT images showed 33% more enhancing lesions and 18% more new enhancing lesions than the single-dose non-MT images. Triple-dose non-MT images showed 29% more lesions than did single-dose MT images. Combining a triple dose of contrast material and MT did not significantly improve the detection of enhancing lesions, compared with a triple dose of contrast without MT.

Conclusions.—A triple dose of contrast material maximizes the sensitivity of enhanced MR imaging. Larger, longer longitudinal studies are needed to determine the impact the additional lesions have on disease evolution.

▶ This is another in this short series of articles investigating more sensitive assessments of MS lesions. These authors explored 2 different contrast regimens (single- and triple-dose) both with and without MT imaging. Adding MT to a standard-dose contrast study increased overall sensitivity 33% (18% increase in finding new lesions). Using triple, the contrast dose increased sensitivity 86%, with 54% more new lesions found.

J.G. Smirniotopoulos, M.D.

The Effect of Section Thickness on MR Lesion Detection and Quantification in Multiple Sclerosis

Molyneux PD, Tubridy N, Parker GJM, et al (Inst of Neurology, Queen Square, London; Natl Hosp for Neurology and Neurosurgery, Queen Square, London)

AJNR 19:1715-1720, 1998 8–26

Background.—Because serial quantification of brain lesion volume in multiple sclerosis (MS) can be used to determine disease evolution, several investigators have used it as an outcome measure in MS treatment trials; however, a marked proportion of white matter disease is undetectable on standard two-dimensional conventional spin-echo (CSE) sequences with 5-mm thick sections. This undetected lesion load may be important in functional terms. The effect of section thickness on MR detection of brain lesion volume and measurement precision in patients with MS was investigated.

Methods.—Eight patients with MS underwent MR imaging at 1.5 T. With a 3D fast fluid-attenuated inversion-recovery (fast-FLAIR) sequence, contiguous axial brain images were obtained at section thicknesses of 5, 3,

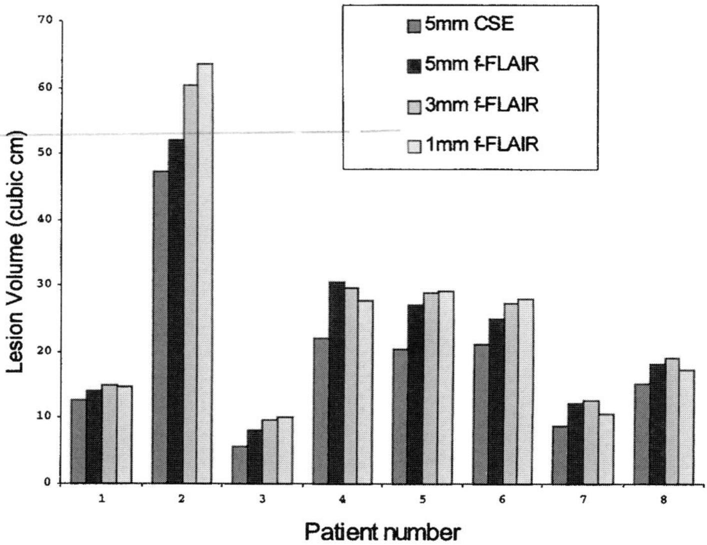

FIGURE 2.—The effect of sequence/section thickness on total lesion volume. For each patient, the mean volume of the 2 measurements (scan and rescan) is shown for each section thickness of the fast-FLAIR sequence to reduce the impact of random measurement error. (Courtesy of Molyneux PD, Tubridy N, Parker GJM, et al: The effect of section thickness on MR lesion detection and quantification in multiple sclerosis. *AJNR* 19:1715-1720, 1998, copyright by American Society of Neuroradiology.)

and 1 mm. Two sets of images were obtained at each section thickness in 2 sessions. Lesion volumes were measured at each section thickness with a semiautomated local thresholding method.

Findings.—The progressive reduction in section thickness resulted in identification of smaller lesions, resulting in an 8% increase in lesion volume on MR images with the decline from 5 to 3 mm. Changes from 3 mm to 1 mm, however, did not result in an increase in total lesion volume depicted, despite a further increase in lesion detection, indicating that the relationship between section thickness and lesion volume on MR images is not linear. Reducing section thickness improved scan-rescan reproducibility, but analysis time increased (Figs 2 and 3).

Conclusions.—The acquisition of very thin sections increases the sensitivity and precision of MS lesion measurement. Serial studies that evaluate lesion changes over time are required to determine the impact of this increase on sample size requirements for MS treatment trials.

▶ The article by Molyneux et al scientifically evaluates and proves the almost obvious and intuitive notion that thinner sections detect more lesions in MS. The added yield may be worth the time and effort, but should be weighed in the context of the other scan protocols. In addition, while this may have great applicability in the research environment, the clinical need for such finely tuned information can still be discussed.

J.G. Smirniotopoulos, M.D.

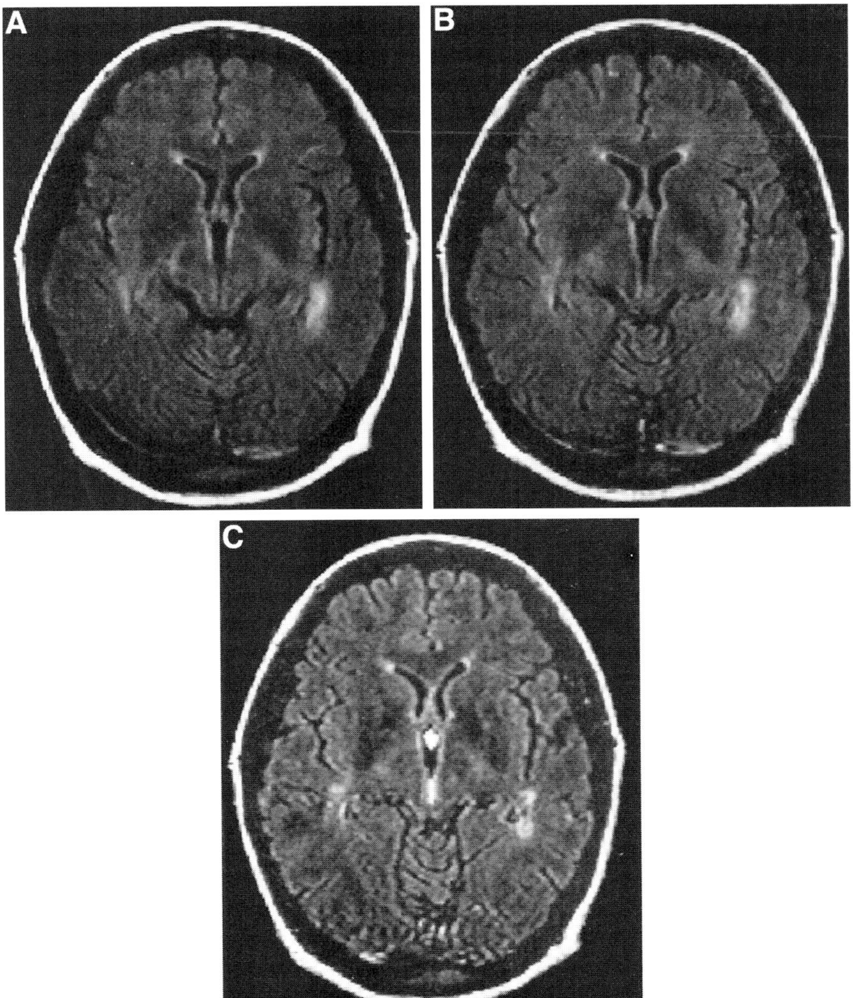

FIGURE 3.—A-C, 3D fast-FLAIR images (TR/TE, 4,600/140; inversion time, 1,740; echo train length, 24) of a patient at section thicknesses of 5 mm (**A**), 3 mm (**B**), and 1 mm (**C**). The signal to noise ratio can be seen to deteriorate as section thickness is reduced. However, despite this, there is an increase in resolution of periventricular lesions with decreasing section thickness. Lesions that look confluent at 5 mm appear as smaller, discrete areas of high signal at 1 mm. (Courtesy of Molyneux PD, Tubridy N, Parker GJM, et al: The effect of section thickness on MR lesion detection and quantification in multiple sclerosis. *AJNR* 19:1715-1720, 1998, copyright by American Society of Neuroradiology.)

MR Outcome Parameters in Multiple Sclerosis: Comparison of Surface-based Thresholding Segmentation and Magnetization Transfer Ratio Histographic Analysis in Relation to Disability: A Preliminary Note

van Waesberghe JHTM, van Buchem MA, Filippi M, et al ("Vrije Universiteit," Amsterdam; Leiden Univ, The Netherlands; Univ of Milan, Italy)

AJNR 19:1857-1862, 1998 8–27

Background.—MRI is now widely used to monitor the progression of multiple sclerosis (MS). The association between disability status and various existing and new MR parameters in patients with MS was investigated.

Methods.—Forty-one patients underwent T2-weighted and T1-weighted MR imaging and gradient-echo imaging with and without magnetization transfer (MT) contrast. Surface-based thresholding segmentation methods were used to obtain T2 and T1 lesion load, the T1 to T2 ratio, and several MT ratio lesion load parameters. Histographic analysis of MT ratio included measures of absolute peak height (aHp), relative peak height (rHp), MT ratio of the peak (MTRp), and mean MT ratio (MTRm). In addition, MTR_{25}, MTR_{50}, and MTR_{75}, related to the integrals of the histogram at 25%, 50%, and 75%, respectively, of the total area under the curve were determined.

Findings.—Surface-based thresholding segmentation methods yielded relatively low correlations with Expanded Disability Status Scale (EDSS) scores. The T1 lesion load and T1 to T2 ratios showed the best correlation. Among MTR histographic parameters, EDSS was most strongly associated with rHp; with the other parameters, this correlation was weak. Comparable associations occurred with disease duration but not patient age.

Conclusions.—Among the MR parameters studied, the best correlations with disability were found for several MTR histographic parameters. The use of these MR parameters may be better than the T2 lesion load for monitoring disease progression in patients with MS. Longitudinal studies are warranted.

► In cases where the clinical responses reflect gross (or grosser) pathology, newer means of assessing treatment efficacy must be sought. MS is such a disease. These authors have chosen to test MTR as a measure of lesion load in MS patients. They used a semiautomated system with good results. But before we all switch to this method, more patients must be studied. In addition, researchers in many institutions are pursuing other techniques. Which will prevail as the best remains to be determined.

J.G. Smirniotopoulos, M.D.

Miscellaneous White Matter and Metabolic Disorders

Usefulness of CT and MR Imaging in the Diagnosis of Acute Wernicke's Encephalopathy

Antunez E, Estruch R, Cardenal C, et al (Univ of Barcelona)
AJR 171:1131-1137, 1998 8–28

Background.—Wernicke's encephalopathy, seen primarily in chronic alcoholics, is a neurologic disease caused by thiamine deficiency. The sensitivity and specificity of CT and MRI in the diagnosis of this condition were reported.

Methods.—Fifteen patients with acute Wernicke's encephalopathy (group 1), 15 symptom-free alcoholics (group 2), and 15 non-drinking control subjects (group 3) were studied. Clinical and laboratory studies were done in addition to CT and MR imaging of the brain.

Findings.—Low-density abnormalities in the paraventricular regions of the thalamus were present on the CT scans of 13% of the group 1 patients and none of the group 2 patients. On MR images, the T2 signal of paraventricular regions of the thalamus was increased in 46% of group 1 and in 6% of group 2. The T2 signal of periaqueductal regions of the midbrain was increased in 40% of group 1 and in 6% of group 2 patients. Groups 1 and 2 did not differ significantly in the prevalence of mammillary body shrinkage. The sensitivity and specificity of MRI in demostrating evidence of disease were 53% and 93%, respectively (Figs 1 and 3; Table 2).

Conclusions.—MRI is useful for confirming the diagnosis of acute Wernicke's encephalopathy, although the absence of MR abnormalities does not exclude it. CT was not useful in diagnosing this disorder.

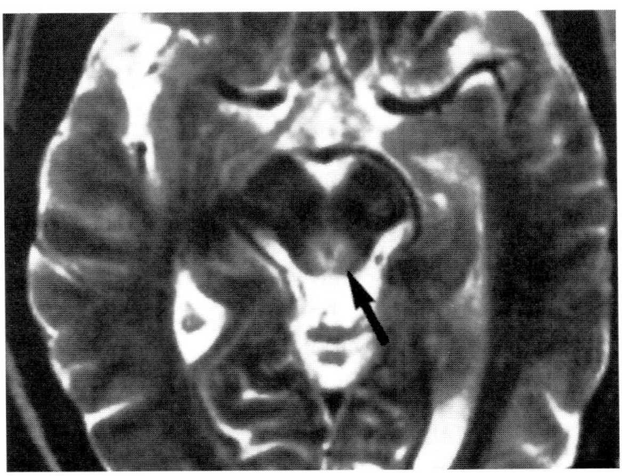

FIGURE 1.—Wernicke's encephalopathy in a 52-year-old man. **A**, Unenhanced T1-weighted spin-echo MR image reveals atrophic mamillary bodies (*arrow*) and atrophy pf posterior fossa structures (vermis and encephalic stem). (Courtesy of Antunez E, Estruch R, Cardenal C, et al: Usefulness of CT and MR imaging in the diagnosis of acute Wernicke's encephalopathy. *AJR* 171:1131-1137, 1998.)

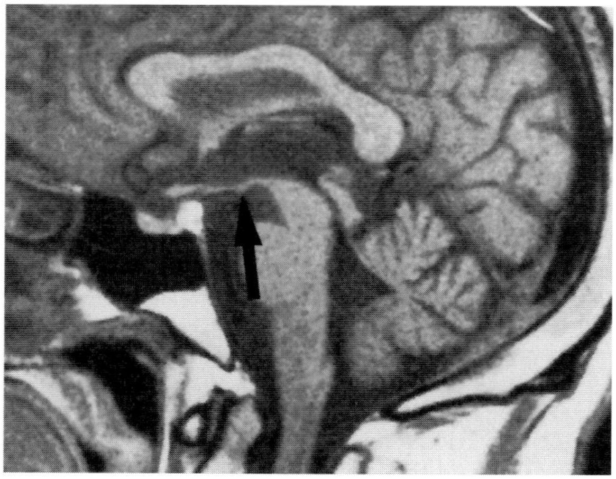

FIGURE 3.—Wernicke's encephalopathy in a 38-year-old man. Unenhanced T1-weighted fast spin-echo MR image obtained at parasagittal level, adjacent to midline, reveals marked atrophy of mamillary bodies (*arrows*). (Courtesy of Antunez E, Estruch R, Cardenal C, et al: Usefulness of CT and MR imaging in the diagnosis of acute Wernicke's encephalopathy. *AJR* 171:1131-1137, 1998.)

► The authors compared three groups of subjects: 15 patients with acute Wernicke encephalopathy (AWE), 15 symptom-free alcoholics, and 15 normal controls. The authors concluded that CT had little value. The suggestive findings on MRI included paraventricular (thalamic) hyperintensity on T2

TABLE 2.—Analysis of CT and MRI Findings

Imaging Finding	Patients with WE (n = 15)	Asymptomatic Alcoholics (n = 15)	Control Subjects (n = 15)
CT			
Low density of PR	2 (13)	0 (0)	0 (0)
Cortical shrinkage	13 (86)*,†	8 (53)‡	1 (6)
Frontal lobe shrinkage	8 (56)†	7 (46)‡	0 (0)
Cerebellar shrinkage	9 (60)*,‡	3 (20)	1 (6)
Vermis shrinkage	8 (53)*,‡	2 (12)	0 (0)
MR imaging			
Mamillary body shrinkage	6 (40)‡	4 (27)§	0 (0)
Increased T2 signal of PR	7 (46)‡,‖	1 (6)	0 (0)
Increased T2 signal of PAR	6 (40)*,‡	1 (6)	0 (0)
Cortical shrinkage	14 (93)†	13 (86)†	1 (6)
Frontal shrinkage	14 (93)†	13 (86)†	1 (6)
Cerebellar shrinkage	15 (100)†,¶	5 (33)§	0 (0)
Vermis shrinkage	15 (100)†,¶	5 (33)§	0 (0)

*$P<.05$ compared with symptom-free alcoholics.
†$P<.001$ compared with control subjects.
‡$P<.01$ compared with control subjects.
§$P<.05$ compared with control subjects.
‖$P<.01$ compared with symptom-free alcoholics.
¶$P<.001$ compared with symptom-free alcoholics.
Abbreviations: WE, Wernicke's encephalopathy; *PR*, paraventricular regions of the thalamus and hypothalamus; *PAR*, periaqueductal regions of the midbrain.
(Courtesy of Antunez E, Estruch R, Cardenal C, et al: Usefulness of CT and MR imaging in the diagnosis of acute Wernicke's encephalopathy. *AJR* 171:1131-1137, 1998.)

images (7 of the 15 with AWE, 1 of the 15 symptom-free alcoholics) and 6 of the 15 with AWE had hyperintensity in the mesencephalic paraventricular (periaqueductal) regions. Surprisingly, 4 of the 15 symptom-free alcoholics had mamillary body atrophy, not significantly different from the six with AWE. The most important conclusion, however, was that overall sensitivity was only 53%, meaning that a normal MR image cannot exclude acute Wernicke encephalopathy.

J.G. Smirniotopoulos, M.D.

Marchiafava-Bignami Disease: Reversibility of Neuroimaging Abnormality

Gass A, Birtsch C, Oster M, et al (Universität Heidelberg, Mannheim, Germany)

J Comput Assist Tomogr 22:503-504, 1998 8–29

Background.—Marchiafava-Bignami disease (MBD) is a rare but often fatal disease, first described about 100 years ago in Northern Italian men who drank excessive amounts of red wine. The disorder is characterized by isolated demyelination and axonal loss in the central layer of the corpus callosum (CC). Often, nonspecific, severe clinical deficits that can be associated with interhemispheric disconnection are present. A patient with resolution of the characteristic CT and MR abnormalities accompanied by marked clinical improvement was described.

> *Case Report.*—Man, 34, was malnourished, with chronic alcoholism, severe generalized extrapyradmidal rigid syndrome, Gegenhalten ("ratchet" resistance), and severe dyspraxia. Cranial CT and MRI showed isolated lesions in the genu and splenium of the CC, characteristic of MBD (Fig 1). Thiamine treatment produced slow, steady resolution of clinical signs and symptoms. Serial CT and MR studies showed pronounced reversal of the CC abnormalities.

Conclusions.—In addition to clinical improvement with good functional outcomes, thiamine replacement therapy and normal nutrition can reverse CT and MR abnormalities. Cranial imaging provide confirmatory information on the characteristic pathologic features of lesions in the callosal fibers for diagnosing MBD.

► Although I don't usually include case reports, I thought that this one was interesting, and relates to the article about high-altitude cerebral edema. The classic lesions of Marchiafava-Bignami disease are destructive (demyelination) in the deep white matter, and involvement of the splenium of the corpus callosum is most suggestive. This patient survived, and the white-matter low-attenuation changes resolved on CT with thiamine therapy.

J.G. Smirniotopoulos, M.D.

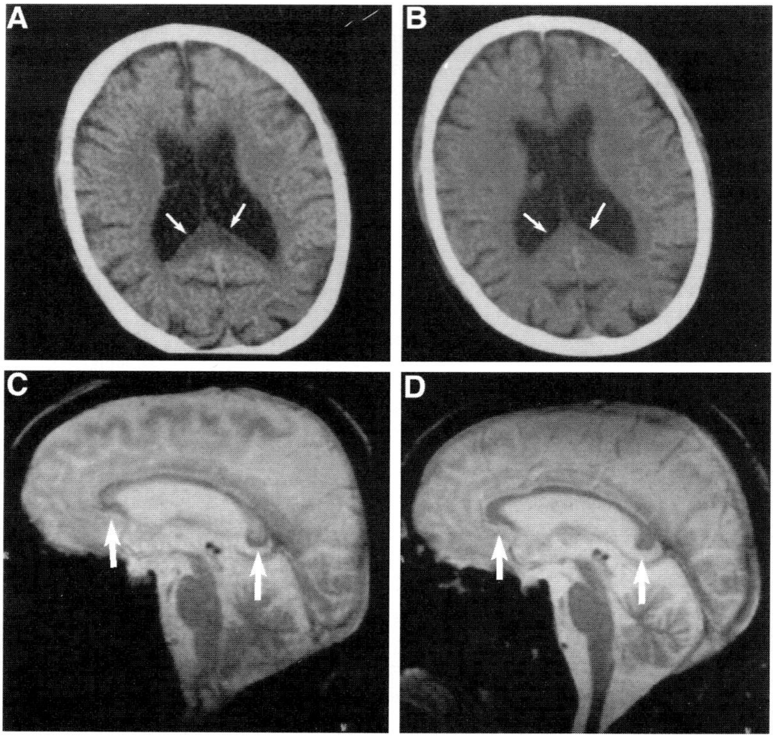

FIGURE 1.—CT and MRI on admission and at follow-up. A, cranial CT on admission shows hypodense splenium (*arrows*) of the corpus callosum and slightly enlarged ventricles and subarachnoid CSF spaces. B, follow-up CT after 7 weeks shows unequivocal improvement of the initially hypodense changes (*arrows*) in the corpus callosum that are isodense to normal-appearing white matter. C, midsagittal T2*-weighted image on the day after admission shows hyperintense lesions (*arrows*) in the genu and splenium of the corpus callosum. D, follow-up MR image after 7 months shows normal signal (*arrows*) in the genu and splenium of the corpus callosum on the T2*-weighted image. There are no obvious atrophic changes in the corpus callosum. (Courtesy of Gass A, Birtsch C, Oster M, et al: Marchiafavia-Bignami disease: Reversibility of neuroimaging abnormality. *J Comput Assist Tomogr* 22:503-504, 1998.)

Serial MRI of Extrapontine Myelinolysis of the Basal Ganglia: A Case Report

Waragai M, Satoh T (Funabashi Chuo Hosp, Tokyo)
J Neurol Sci 161:173-175, 1998 8–30

Background.—The basal ganglia are vulnerable in extrapontine myelinolysis (EPM). Previous studies have shown lesions of T1 and T2 prolongation on MRI. A patient with EPM of the basal ganglia but without central pontine myelinolysis (CPM), who had changes on MR, was examined.

Case Report.—Man, 21, was hospitalized with an adrenergic crisis following a cold. At age 16, this patient had had pineal gland germinoma, and underwent radiation therapy. After treatment, panhypopituitarism developed, which was treated with levothyroxine sodium, hydrocortisone, and desmopressin acetate. On this admission, he had confusion, generalized convulsions, and was hyponatremic (serum sodium 105.3mEq/l) At the current admission, initial brain CT and MRI yielded normal findings. Physiologic saline solution was administered intravenously, (6300 ml/3 days) and his condition gradually improved. However, 16 days after admission, dysarthria, swallowing difficulties, and weakness in one hand were noted. Two more days later, bradykinesia and limb rigidity developed, along with akinetic mutism. Brain CT at that time demonstrated low density regions in the striatum bilaterally. The lesions appeared as bilateral symmetric areas of high signal intensity on T2-weighted images and low or normal signal intensity on T1-weighted images of the basal and caudate nuclei. Amantadine hydrochloride, IV hydrocortisone, and physiotherapy produced gradual improvement of symptoms. Follow-up T1-weighted MRI 2 weeks later showed symmetric areas of abnormal high signal intensity of both basal ganglia, with low signal intensity along the rim of the lesion.

Conclusions.—In this patient, the MRI findings may have reflected microchemorrhagic lesions resulting from vascular endothelial injury associated with EPM. This is consistent with the theory that vascular endothelial injury caused by rapid osmotic change and subsequent demyelination are involved in the pathogenesis of EPM.

► This article serves to remind all of us about one of the more unusual causes of leukoencephalopathy. Osmotic myelinolysis (OM) was formerly called central pontine myelinolysis. This disease was originally linked to rapid correction of hyponatremia with hypertonic (>0.9%) saline. However, our current understanding of this "entity" is that the white matter lesions may occur in many locations outside of the pons, hence the title "extrapontine" myelinolysis. This syndrome was originally associated with rapid "correction" of hyponatremia with hypertonic saline solutions—often in the context of chronic (not acute) hyponatremia, alcoholism, and nutritional problems (vitamin deficiency). But the lesions of osmotic demyelination may also occur even when hyponatremia is corrected using normal saline, and are not limited to cases where hypertonic saline has been used. Cyclosporine therapy can also produce "central pontine myelinolysis." It has also been postulated that an associated hypokalemia is present in the majority of patients who develop OM.[1] [Potassium levels were not reported in this case.] I was particularly intrigued with the resolution images in this patient, which showed the development of signal hyperintensity in the lenticular nuclei bilaterally. The authors postulate hemorrhage. I wonder if this hyperintensity may be caused by microcalcifications—especially since survivable OM is usually not associated with hemorrhage. Last, a clinical note: Osmotic demyelination is uncommon when the rate of correction of the hyponatremia is less than 12 mmol/L per day of therapy.[2]

J.G. Smirniotopoulos, M.D.

References

1. Lohr JW: Osmotic demyelination syndrome following correction of hyponatremia: Association with hypokalemia. *Am J Med* 1994;96:408-413.
2. Sterns RH, Riggs JE, Schochet SSJ: Osmotic demyelination syndrome following correction of hyponatremia. *N Engl J Med* 1986;314:1535-1542.

High-Altitude Cerebral Edema Evaluated With Magnetic Resonance Imaging: Clinical Correlation and Pathophysiology

Hackett PH, Yarnell PR, Hill R, et al (Univ of Alaska, Anchorage; Univ of Washington, Seattle; Univ of Colorado, Denver)

JAMA 280:1920-1925, 1998 8–31

Background.—Understanding the pathophysiology of high-altitude cerebral edema (HACE) may have implications for preventing and treating this disorder as well as the more common acute mountain sickness. The clinical imaging correlate for HACE and whether the edema is mainly vasogenic or cytotoxic were investigated.

Methods.—Nine consecutive men with HACE, aged 18 to 35, were studied. Eight men also had pulmonary edema. All were assessed after evacuation from high-altitude locations. Five were mountain climbers, and 4 were skiers. A control group consisted of 3 men with high-altitude pulmonary edema only and 3 who had been completely well at a high altitude, matched for age and altitude exposure. Four of the male patients were followed up with imaging after complete clinical recovery.

Findings.—Seven patients with HACE had hyperintense T2 signal in white matter areas, especially in the splenium of the corpus callosum, without abnormalities in gray matter. The control group had no such abnormalities. All 9 patients recovered completely. In the 4 patients followed up with MRI, the signal abnormalities were completely resolved.

Conclusions.—HACE is characterized by reversible white matter edema on MR images, with a predilection for the splenium of the corpus callosum. These data suggest that the predominant mechanism is vasogenic edema. Thus the blood-brain barrier may play a role in the pathophysiology of HACE.

► The authors reviewed 9 cases of HACE studied with modern neuroimaging (MRI). This is the largest such series yet reported. Seven patients showed abnormal increased T2 signal intensity in the white matter, especially in the splenium of the corpus callosum. Clinically, all the patients recovered, and in the 4 with follow-up MRI, the signal changes also resolved.

Although the authors proposed a mechanism of vasogenic (rather than cytotoxic) edema, none of the lesions enhanced. The authors speculated that the "unique vessels" of the splenium, specifically the short penetrating arterioles, are responsible for the localization of the lesions in this particular region of the deep white matter. They suggest that the primary injury in HACE is a loss of integrity of the blood-brain barrier, with the formation of vasogenic edema rather than cytotoxic edema. A similar mechanism has been suggested for the reversible changes seen in hypertensive encephalopathy, ecclampsia, etc.

J.G. Smirniotopoulos, M.D.

Central Nervous System Lesions in Liver Transplant Recipients: Prospective Assessment of Indications for Biopsy and Implications for Management

Bonham CA, Dominguez EA, Fukui MB, et al (Univ of Pittsburgh, Pa; Univ of Nebraska, Omaha; Princess Alexandra Hosp, Brisbane, Australia; et al)
Transplantation 66:1596-1604, 1998 8–32

Objective.—As many as 8% of liver transplant recipients experience serious neurologic complications, such as CNS lesions of diverse causes. It is difficult to diagnose CNS lesions in this group of patients; the presence of coagulopathy may make brain biopsy infeasible. The ability of clinical or radiologic characteristics to predict the cause of CNS lesions in liver transplant recipients was examined.

Methods.—The observational cohort study included 1,730 consecutive liver transplant recipients at 4 transplant centers. Neuroimaging studies, performed at the discretion of the transplant teams, depicted CNS lesions in 60 patients. Clinical and radiologic findings were analyzed for their ability to predict the likely cause of the CNS lesions, and thus to target patients for invasive diagnostic procedures.

Results.—Of the patients with CNS lesions, 52% had vascular events, 18% had infections, 12% had immunosuppressive associated leukoencephalopathy, 8% had central pontine myelinosis, and 3% had malignancies. Forty-three percent of CNS lesions occurred within the first month after transplantation, most commonly caused by central pontine myelinolysis, subdural hematoma, acute infarcts, and *Aspergillus*-related brain abscesses (Fig 2). Of 11 brain abscesses, all were fungal, and 8 of the affected patients had pulmonary infection with the same fungal pathogen. Ischemic or infectious CNS lesions were the most frequent reason for patients who are receiving dialysis, whereas patients who had received more than 1 transplant were more likely to have vascular events. One-fourth of the CNS lesions developed more than 1 year after transplantation. All of these delayed lesions were small vessel ischemic lesions, malignancies, or fungal abscesses caused by pathogens other than *Aspergillus*.

Conclusions.—For liver transplant recipients with CNS lesions, a presumptive diagnosis is usually possible on the basis of clinical and neuroim-

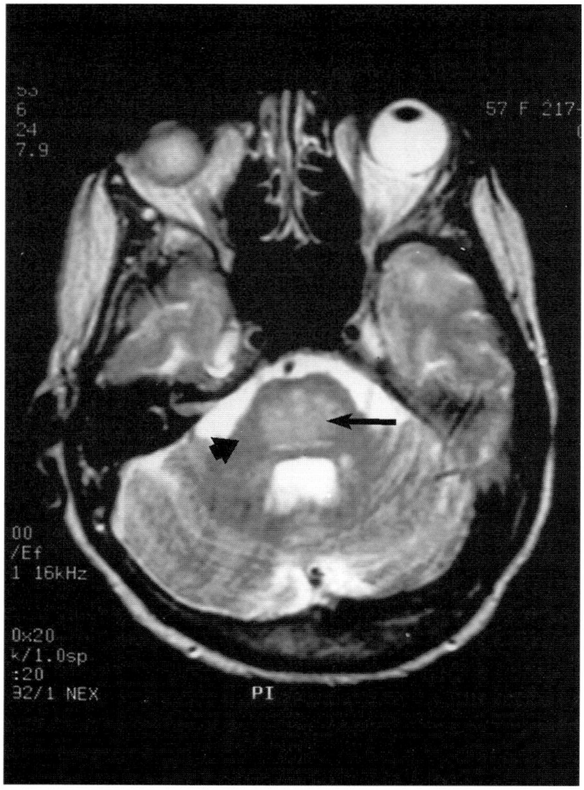

FIGURE 2.—Axial T2-weighted MR image of the brain at the level of the pons (middle cerebellar peduncle) in a patient with central pontine myelinolysis. There is increased signal density in the central pons (*arrow*) compared with the normal signal intensity of the adjacent cerebellar peduncle (*arrowheads*). (Courtesy of Bonham CA, Dominguez EA, Fukui MB, et al: Central nervous system lesions in liver transplant recipients: prospective assessment of indications for biopsy and implications for management. *Transplantation* 66:1596-1604, 1998.)

aging characteristics; the findings will aid in the prompt recognition and treatment of brain abscesses. Brain biopsy is not indicated in patients with suspected brain abscess who have a documented pulmonary fungal infection. For late-developing CNS lesions, vascular causes are the most frequent.

► The metabolic and hemodynamic changes associated with chronic liver disease can produce serious damage to the brain. These consequences, in association with the stress of transplant surgery and immunosuppressive therapy, can take a heavy toll on the CNS. This prospective study found that approximately 3% of liver transplant recipients had CNS lesions. Approximately half (52%) of these were vascular events. Infections, immunosuppressive leukoencephalopathy, central pontine myelinolysis were frequent, but less common than ischemic or hemorrhagic sequelae.

J.G. Smirniotopoulos, M.D.

Proton MR Spectroscopic Measurement of Neurometabolites in Hepatic Encephalopathy During Oral Lactulose Therapy

Haseler LJ, Sibbitt WL Jr, Mojtahedzadeh HN, et al (Univ of New Mexico, Albuquerque; Regional Federal Med Ctr, Albuquerque, New Mexico)

AJNR 19:1681-1686, 1998 8–33

Purpose.—MRI and MR spectroscopy have come into increasing use for monitoring response to drug therapy. Patients with hepatic encephalopathy (HE) may develop abnormal cerebral metabolites; however, the response to treatment of HE is still primarily assessed using arbitrary clinical scales. The use of MR spectroscopy for monitoring neurometabolic changes in response to lactulose therapy in patients with HE was studied.

Methods.—The study included 23 patients with HE, grades I to III; and 10 healthy control subjects. All subjects underwent proton MR spectroscopy, with TR/TE 2,000/26. The investigators calculated metabolic ratios for *myo*-inositol (mI)/creatine (Cre), choline (Cho)/Cre, (glutamine + glutamate) (Glx)/Cre, *N*-acetylaspartate (NAA)/Cre, and (Cho + mI)/Glx. In 8 patients with HE, MR spectroscopic findings were compared before and after oral lactulose therapy, 60 mL 3 times daily.

Results.—Compared with control subjects, patients with HE had a 43% reduction in mI/Cre, a 64% reduction in (Cho + mI)/Glx, and a 5% reduction in Cho/Cre. There was a relative 75% increase in Glx/Cre, but no difference in NAA/Cre. With lactulose treatment, I/Cre increased by 29%, (Cho + mI)/Glx by 37%, and Cho/Cre by 7%, and Glx/Cre decreased by 15%. These changes were accompanied by a 42% reduction in HE grade. There was no change in NAA/Cre.

Conclusions.—In patients with HE, treatment with lactulose is associated with improvement in brain metabolite levels, as measured with MR spectroscopy. The most sensitive indicators of therapeutic effect appear to be mI/Cre and (Cho + mI)/Glx. The findings support the use of MR spectroscopy to monitor the effects of drug therapy in patients with HE in research settings.

► This second article on the brain and liver physiology focuses on MR spectroscopy (MRS) and the changes associated with HE and its treatment with lactulose. The true physiology of HE is not yet completely elucidated. HE was shown to cause a reduction in mL/Cre and Cho/Cre ratios while increasing Glx/Cre. Oral lactulose is thought to act by reducing the toxic nitrogen load. Proposed mechanisms include reduced gut transit time (diarrhea), alteration in intestinal flora, and other speculations. Successful therapy with lactulose reversed most of the MRS abnormalities, except the NAA/Cre ratio. Now direct changes in brain metabolism, as reflected in MRS, can be measured directly. This could open the door to more accurate monitoring of treatment efficacy, and may also allow new and subtler therapeutic regimens to be tested.

J.G. Smirniotopoulos, M.D.

Acquired Hepatocerebral Degeneration: MR and Pathologic Findings

Lee J, Lacomis D, Comu S, et al (Univ of Pittsburgh, Pa; Children's Hosp of Pittsburgh, Pa)
AJNR 19:485-487, 1998 8–34

Background.—Patients with repeated episodes of hepatic encephalopathy rarely develop the progressive, irreversible syndrome called acquired hepatocerebral degeneration (AHD). The neurologic signs include those of hepatic encephalopathy, with the addition of abnormal movements, dysarthria, rigidity, intention tremor, ataxia, and intellectual impairment. The pathologic changes observed in AHD do not always correlate with the clinical course. The MRI findings in a patient with AHD were presented.

> *Case.*—Man, 65, was diagnosed as having alcoholic cirrhosis with ascites and liver failure. His neurologic status had been normal until 2 months earlier, when he developed the first of several episodes of hepatic encephalopathy. At the same time, movement and speech abnormalities developed, including limb tremors, chorea of the tongue, ataxia, and dysarthria. These abnormalities were unassociated with the encephalopathy. MRI showed punctate areas of mildly increased signal on T2-weighted images of the putamen and globus pallidus bilaterally. The basal ganglia showed no T1 signal abnormalities. Postmortem examination of the brain revealed histologic spongiform, myelinolytic white matter changes in several areas.

Discussion.—Some unusual deep cerebellar white matter changes are noted on the MR images of patients with AHD. The findings suggest that AHD may be associated with white matter changes in the middle cerebellar peduncles. The cause of these nonspecific changes is unknown; they may reflect a spectrum of radiologic and pathologic changes in patients with advanced liver disease and extrapontine myelinolysis.

► This patient exhibited bilateral white matter (leukoencephalopathic) lesions in the brachium pontis bilaterally, in relation to hepatic failure. This certainly qualifies as "extrapontine myelinolysis," but the etiology, especially with regard to "osmotic myelinolysis," is uncertain—especially since the serum sodium and potassium concentrations were not provided. However, once again we see a symmetric bilateral pattern very suggestive of a systemic disease, probably toxic-metabolic.

J.G. Smirniotopoulos, M.D.

SEIZURE EVALUATION

Acute Postictal Cerebral Imaging

Silverstein AM, Alexander JA (Crawford Long Hosp, Atlanta, Ga)

AJNR 19:1485-1488, 1998 8–35

Background.—Postictal imaging is done to investigate causes of seizure, such as space-occupying lesions or other structural processes. However, there may be abnormalities that reflect physiologic or pathologic changes caused by seizure activity. Brain imaging findings in patients immediately postictal with altered mental status or weakness were discussed.

Methods.—Ten patients underwent CT or MRI within 12 hours of ictus. Four of the 9 CT studies and the 1 MR study included contrast material administration. The patients were reexamined 1 day to 11 months later.

Findings.—Findings on CT included focal gyral swelling, effacement of adjacent cortical sulci, reduced gyral attenuation by CT, and mild-to-moderate gyral enhancement after contrast material injection. Findings on MRI included gyral swelling, increased signal intensity on T2-weighted images, and enhancement after contrast agent injection. Abnormalities were found in the frontal, parietal, temporal, and occipital lobes in 9, 4, 2, and 1 patient, respectively. Follow-up assessment demonstrated complete or subtotal resolution of these abnormalities (Fig 3).

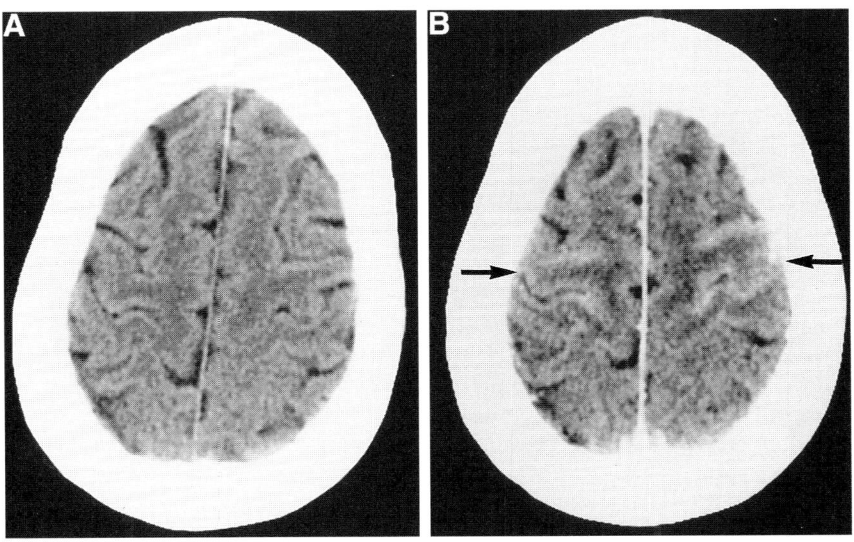

FIGURE 3.—58-year-old woman with profound acute postictal lethargy and bilateral weakness. **A**, axial noncontrast CT scan shows subtle decreased attenuation of superior frontal and precentral gyri bilaterally. **B**, axial contrast-enhanced CT scan obtained at same time reveals symmetric gyriform enhancement of the pre- and postcentral gyri and superior frontal gyri (*arrows*). (Courtesy of Silverstein AM, Alexander JA: Acute postictal cerebral imaging. *AJNR American Journal of Neuroradiology* 19:1485-1488, 1998. Copyright by American Society of Neuroradiology.)

Conclusions.—Gyral swelling and enhancement have many causes, such as infarction and neoplasm. However, if these conditions are reversible and correspond to clinical findings, then the differential diagnosis is limited to postictal change, reversible ischemia, complicated migraine, or resolved inflammation or infection.

► Increasingly, patients are being imaged during or immediately after having had a first-time seizure. One of the difficulties encountered in evaluating scans in these patients is that some disorders such as tumors, encephalitis, and stroke may present initially with a seizure. Seizures, especially if prolonged, may also cause transient blood-brain barrier disruption with subsequent edema and abnormal enhancement. These changes are usually reversible and follow-up scans show resolution of gyral swelling and enhancement. The authors suggest that tumor or infarction are less likely if the cerebral swelling is bilateral, overlaps arterial distribution, and spares the basal ganglia and other deep structures.

I show a particularly striking example of post-ictal gyral swelling and enhancement in my textbook,[1] if you're interested in seeing how dramatic some cases can be.

A.G. Osborn, M.D.

Reference

1. Osborn A: *Diagnostic Neuroradiology*. St Louis, Mosby, 1994, p 384.

Epileptology of the First-Seizure Presentation: A Clinical, Electroencephalographic, and Magnetic Resonance Imaging Study of 300 Consecutive Patients

King MA, Newton MR, Jackson GD, et al (Univ of Melbourne, Australia; Austin and Repatriation Med Centre, Victoria, Australia; Latrobe Univ, Victoria, Australia)

Lancet 352:1007-1011, 1998 8–36

Background.—The prognosis and treatment of a first seizure require the identification of a specific epilepsy syndrome. The value of EEG, MRI, and standard clinical methods in prompt diagnosis of specific epilepsy syndromes was investigated.

Methods.—Three hundred consecutive patients with unexplained seizures were included in the study. Performance of EEG within 24 hours of the seizure was attempted. When the EEG was negative, a sleep-deprived EEG was performed. MRI was performed on an elective basis in 277 patients.

Findings.—Generalized or partial epilepsy syndrome was diagnosed clinically in 47% of the patients. Subsequent analyses showed that these diagnoses were correct in all but 3 patients. Adding the EEG data increased the diagnosis of an epilepsy syndrome to 77% of the patients. An EEG obtained within 24 hours was more useful for the diagnosis of epileptiform abnormalities than an EEG performed after 24 hours. Neuroimaging demonstrated 38 epileptogenic lesions, including 17 tumors. Patients with EEG-confirmed generalized epilepsy had no lesions. The final diagnoses were generalized epilepsy in 23% of the patients, partial epilepsy in 58%, and unclassified seizures in 19%.

Conclusions.—Most first-seizure patients can be diagnosed as having an epilepsy syndrome. Ideally, EEG should be performed within 24 hours of the seizure. A sleep-deprived EEG should be performed if necessary. MRI provides relevant data for diagnosis and should be performed in all patients except those with idiopathic generalized epilepsy and children with benign rolandic epilepsy.

► A new onset of seizures is a very common cause of referral for neuroimaging. In addition, the use of MRI has created a virtual revolution in our understanding of the organic causes (tumors and dysplasias) and consequences (mesial temporal sclerosis) of seizures. This article from Australia records the outcome of the prospective evaluation of 300 consective patients with new onset of seizures. The patient population served included approximately 500,000 persons. More than 90% of these patients (277) had neuroimaging. Only 1 of 50 patients with "generalized epilepsy" had an abnormal scan—an occipital lobe tumor. In contrast, 17% of the 154 patients with partial epilepsy had lesions, including 17 tumors; 7 cortical dysplasias, 4 hippocampal sclerosis, and 2 cavernous hemangiomas (1 of these also had ipsilateral hippocampal sclerosis). Of great importance in planning the screening examinations for this group of patients was the documented insensitivity of CT as compared with MRI. Fewer than half (12 of 28) of the lesions found on MRI were noted on CT. This is of even greater importance when one considers that the missed lesions are, in general, surgically curable.

J.G. Smirniotopoulos, M.D.

Relevance of Temporal Lobe White Matter Changes in Hippocampal Sclerosis: Magnetic Resonance Imaging and Histology

Meiners LC, Witkamp TD, De Kort GAP (Univ Hosp Utrecht, The Netherlands)

Invest Radiol 34:38-45, 1999 8–37

Background.—Hippocampal sclerosis (HS) consists of diffuse pyramidal cell loss and concurrent gliosis in hippocampal subsectors CA1, CA3, and CA4. The relevance of temporal lobe white-matter changes on MRI in patients with HS was investigated.

Methods.—Eighty patients with HS and 30 age-matched control subjects without epilepsy were studied. Hippocampal signal intensity and size of atrophy of the collateral white matter in the parahippocampal gyrus (ACWMp) and temporal lobe gray/white-matter demarcation loss

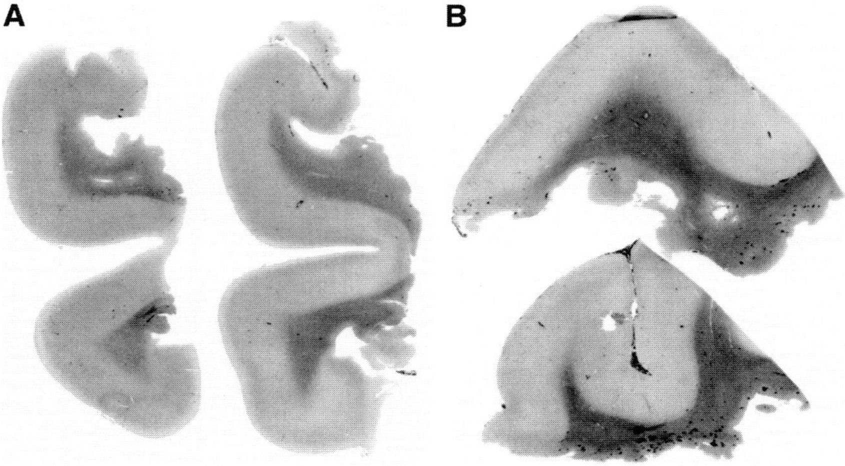

FIGURE 4.—Histologic specimens of temporal lobe stained using Weil's method for myelin sheaths. **A**, a specimen from a patient with temporal lobe gray/white-matter demarcation loss on MRI. **B**, a specimen from a patient without this feature. The white matter stain is lighter in specimen **A** than in specimen **B**. The images have not been manipulated separately in the postprocessing stage. (Courtesy of Meiners LC, Witkamp TD, de Kort GAP: Relevance of temporal lobe white matter changes in hippocampal sclerosis: Magnetic resonance imaging and histology. *Invest Radiol* 34:38-45, 1999.)

(GWDL) on 4- to 5-mm coronal T2-weighted spin-echo MR images were assessed retrospectively. In addition, neocortical temporal lobe specimens were assessed histologically.

Findings.—In the patient group, 68% had ACWMp and 65% had GWDL on MR images. Both findings had an infinite positive likelihood ratio. Seventy-eight percent of the patients had concomitant hippocampal signal increase and smaller size. Twenty-three percent had no or limited hippocampal abnormalities on MR images. When ACWMp and GWDL were used as additional diagnostic parameters, 13 of these 18 patients could be more definitively diagnosed as having HS. No significant morphologic differences were noted between GWDL-positive and negative specimens. The white matter of the GWDL-positive group had a significantly lower average myelin stain than the GWDL-negative group (Fig 4).

Conclusions.—The finding of ACWMp and GWDL can improve the visual diagnosis of HS, especially in patients with no or limited hippocampal abnormalities. These findings suggest that myelin loss may be the underlying cause of GWDL associated with HS.

► Hippocampal (mesial temporal) sclerosis accounts for almost half of the cases operated on for temporal lobe epilepsy (TLE). The pathologic substrate of diffuse pyramidal cell loss with gliosis in the CA1, CA3, and CA4 areas of Ammon's horn is classically seen as hippocampal volume loss with increased signal intensity on T2-weighted scans. But, as we are all too well aware, not all cases are classic. What are we to make of the white-matter signal alterations that are sometimes seen in patients with TLE? Some authors have suggested that seizures may themselves induce benign premature myelination.[1]

These authors show that white-matter atrophy with abnormal signal intensity and loss of gray/white discrimination are often due to myelin loss. The presence of these abnormalities also improves the visual diagnosis of hippocampal sclerosis, especially in patients with minimal or no abnormalities in the hippocampus. A word of caution: if abnormal signal intensity and gray/white effacement occurs without atrophy, watch out for tumor. Look for the subtle mass effect that is often the harbinger of temporal lobe tumors. Many of these are low-grade astrocytomas that don't enhance.

In addition to the usual high-resolution scans, I personally find fluid-attenuated inversion recovery (FLAIR) scans are very helpful in evaluating patients with epilepsy.

A.G. Osborn, M.D.

Reference

1. Duprez T, Ghariani S, Grandin C, et al: Focal seizure-induced premature myelination: Speculation from serial MRI. *Neuroradiology* 40:580-582, 1998.

Neurocysticercosis in Persons With Epilepsy in Medellín, Columbia

Palacio LG, and the Neuroepidemiological Research Group of Antioquia (Instituto Neurológico de Antioquia, Medellín, Colombia; Universidad Peruana Cayetano Heredia, Lima, Peru; Universidad de Antioquia, Medellín, Colombia; et al)

Epilepsia 39:1334-1339, 1998 8–38

Introduction.—Neurocysticercosis (NCC), caused by the tapeworm *Taenia solium*, is a major cause of epilepsy in developing countries. The unpredictable clinical presentation of this condition contributes to the difficulty of diagnosis. CT and enzyme-linked immunoelectrotransfer blot assay (EITB) were used to examine the prevalence of NCC among Colombian patients with epilepsy.

Methods.—The prospective study included 643 adult patients (mean age, 33 years) with epilepsy seen at the institute over a 6-month period. Cerebral CT was performed in 546 patients, and serum EITB in 376 of these. CT findings considered positive for NCC were living or degenerating cysticercosis lesions or the presence of calcifications consistent with NCC.

Findings.—Fourteen percent of patients were found to have NCC at CT. Approximately 10% were found to have *T. solium* antibodies at EITB, including 17.5% of those with epilepsy onset after age 30 years and 19% of those from outside the urban area of Medellín. Eighty-eight percent of patients with mixed cysts and calcifications and 64% of those with live cysts had positive EITB test results. In contrast, the results of EITB were positive in only 3% of patients without CT evidence of NCC.

Conclusions.—This study documents NCC as an important preventable cause of epilepsy in Colombia. Despite some discordance, many patients with epilepsy show radiologic or serologic evidence of *T. solium* infection. The possibility of NCC must be considered in patients with epilepsy who are living in or migrating from developing countries.

► When I was a fellow, I was taught that the most common causes of seizures outside the United States were infections: cysticercosis in Latin America and tuberculosis in Southeast Asia. Over the years, many articles have been written that prove, to 1 degree or another, the validity of that simple statement. Frankly, I was surprised at the low percentage of seizures (about 14%) that were attributed to cysticercosis in this study from Colombia. I think we should ponder how ingenious these parasitic diseases actually are. They have very complex life cycles, require 2 different species as host, and usually require either blood or fecal contamination. How did they ever devise such clever lives?

J.G. Smirniotopoulos, M.D.

PRIMARY BRAIN TUMORS AND NONNEOPLASTIC CYSTS

The Significance of Lack of MR Contrast Enhancement of Supratentorial Brain Tumors in Adults: Histopathological Evaluation of a Series

Ginsberg LE, Fuller GN, Hashmi M, et al (Univ of Texas, Houston)
Surg Neurol 49:436-440, 1998 8–39

Introduction.—In the initial evaluation of brain tumor patients, MRI plays a critical role A highly informative feature of preoperative neuroimaging is the assessment of tumor contrast enhancement. Little is known, however, about nonenhancing brain tumors in adults. A correlative histopathologic evaluation was conducted on a series of nonenhancing supratentorial brain tumors in adults.

Methods.—A retrospective review was conducted of 40 patients whose preoperative MRI studies showed a nonenhancing supratentorial brain neoplasm. A board-certified neuropathologist reviewed biopsy material from all patients.

Results.—There were 24 (60%) low-grade gliomas according to histopathologic examination. There were 4 (10%) low-grade astrocytomas, 10 (25%) low-grade gliomas (not further classified), 9 (20%) low-grade oligodendrogliomas, and 2 (5%) low-grade mixed oligoastrocytomas. There were 16 (40%) nonenhancing lesions that were anaplastic gliomas (Fig 2). There were 12 (30%) anaplastic astrocytomas, 1 (2.5%) anaplastic mixed oligoastrocytomas, 1 (2.5%) anaplastic oligodendrogliomas, and 2 (5%) anaplastic infiltrating gliomas of indeterminate subtype.

Conclusion.—Low-grade malignancy is not equated with nonenhancement of supratentorial brain neoplasms in adults. When biopsy and treatment are being planned in patients with nonenhancing brain tumors, this factor should be taken into account. Such lesions may require more aggressive or surgical therapy, particularly lesions in the nondominant hemisphere or in nonmotor areas.

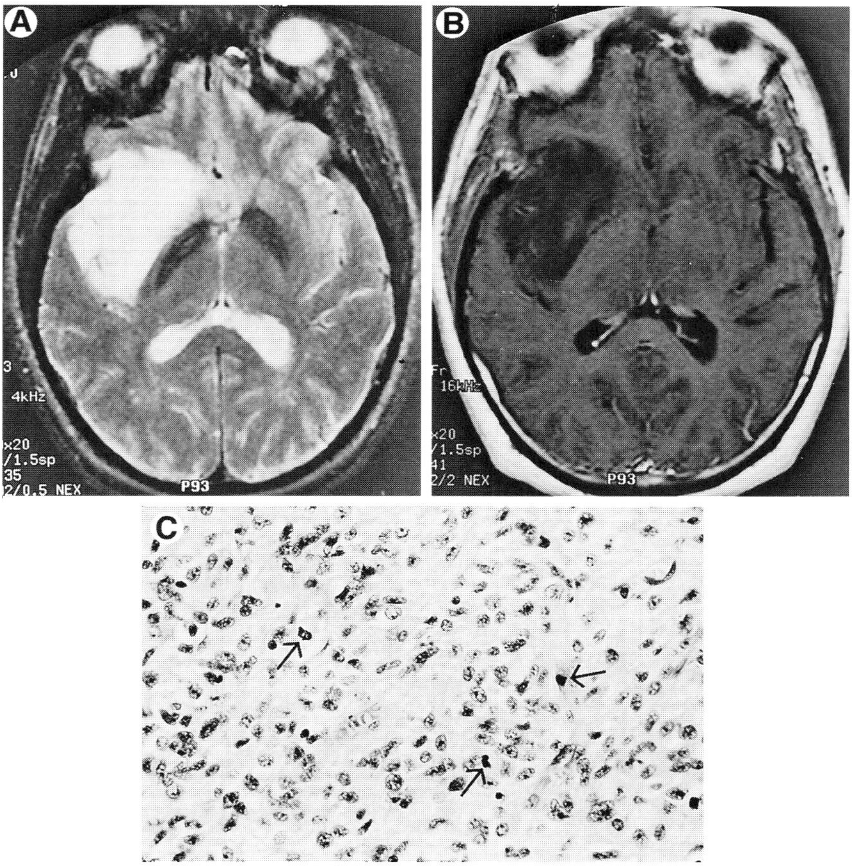

FIGURE 2.—Right insular anaplastic astrocytoma in a 26-year-old woman. **A**, Axial T2-weighted (3,000/100) MRI shows a large hyperintense mass centered in the right insular cortex. **B**, Axial T1-weighted (600/8) postcontrast MRI shows no tumor enhancement. **C**, Tissue section shows a densely cellular astrocytic neoplasm composed of pleomorphic cells with fibrillar cytoplasmic processes. Note the presence of numerous mitotic figures (*arrows*). No microvascular proliferation or necrosis is present, (hematoxylin-eosin; original magnification × 100). (Reprinted by permission of the publisher from Ginsberg LE, Fuller GN, Hashmi M, et al: The significance of lack of MR contrast enhancement of supratentorial brain tumors in adults: Histopathological evaluation of a series. *Surg Neurol* 49: 436-440, copyright 1998 by Elsevier Science Inc.)

► This nice article demonstrates a truism that isn't true, that is, that lack of contrast enhancement on MR scans in patients with brain tumors correlates with low-grade tumor. In fact, most anaplastic astrocytomas *do not* enhance; if they do, one must suspect that foci of grade IV tumor (glioblastoma) are present.[1] The pathologic hallmarks of glioblastoma are vascular proliferation and necrosis. In this series, 30% of nonenhancing lesions were anaplastic astrocytomas (World Health Organization grade III astrocytoma). New techniques such as dynamic contrast-enhanced MR imaging look promising in the preoperative evaluation of tumors and in predicting histologic tumor grade.[2,3]

A.G. Osborn, M.D.

References

1. Rutherford GS, Hewlett RH, Truter R: Contrast enhanced imaging is critical to glioma nosology and grading. *Intl J Neuroradiol* 1:28-38, 1995.
2. Daldrup H, Shames DM, Wendland M, et al: Correlation of dynamic contrast-enhanced MR imaging with histologic tumor grade: Comparison of macromolecular and small-molecular contrast media. *AJR* 171:941-949, 1998.
3. Wong ET, Jackson EF, Hess KR, et al: Correlation between dynamic MRI and outcome in patients with malignant gliomas. *Neurology* 50:777-781, 1998.

Classification of Biopsy-confirmed Brain Tumors Using Single-Voxel MR Spectroscopy

Meyerand ME, Pipas JM, Mamourian A, et al (Dartmouth-Hitchcock Med Ctr, Hanover, NH)

AJNR 20:117-123, 1999 8–40

Introduction.—Tumor types most likely have unique metabolic fingerprints because of differences in the cell type and growth characteristics of tumors. A classification scheme of tumor types that is relative to the treatment program and that can be correlated with biopsy results was created. This is a noninvasive alternative to intracranial biopsy. By using a combination of single-voxel spectroscopy, biopsy confirmation, and tumor classification, brain tumors were differentiated.

Methods.—Using the point-resolved spectroscopic pulse sequence as part of the Probe spectroscopy package on a G.E. 1.5-T Signa scanner, single-voxel spectra were acquired. There were 27 patients with biopsy-confirmed brain tumors. There were 13 with glioblastoma multiforme, 6 with anaplastic astrocytoma, and 8 with low-grade astrocytoma. The histologic subtype of the tumor was used to divide the patients into groups for different treatment protocols.

Results.—For each metabolite (choline, creatine, *N*-acetylaspartate, lactate), metabolic peak areas were normalized to the area of the unsuppressed water peak and to the area of the creatine peak. Statistically significant differences among the tumor groups were shown for all the area ratios (Fig 1). All 3 tumor groups were distinguished by the lactate-water ratio. Low-grade astrocytomas were distinguished from the 2 high-grade groups by the choline-water ratio. The high-grade tumors could be separated from the low-grade by both the choline and lactate ratios.

Conclusion.—To classify astrocytoma according to histopathologic grade, specific relative metabolic peak area ratios acquired from regions of contrast-enhancing brain tumor can be used.

► The "Holy Grail" of neuroimaging (or, at least, 1 of the prized goals) is more pathologically specific lesion diagnosis. Every time we think we've

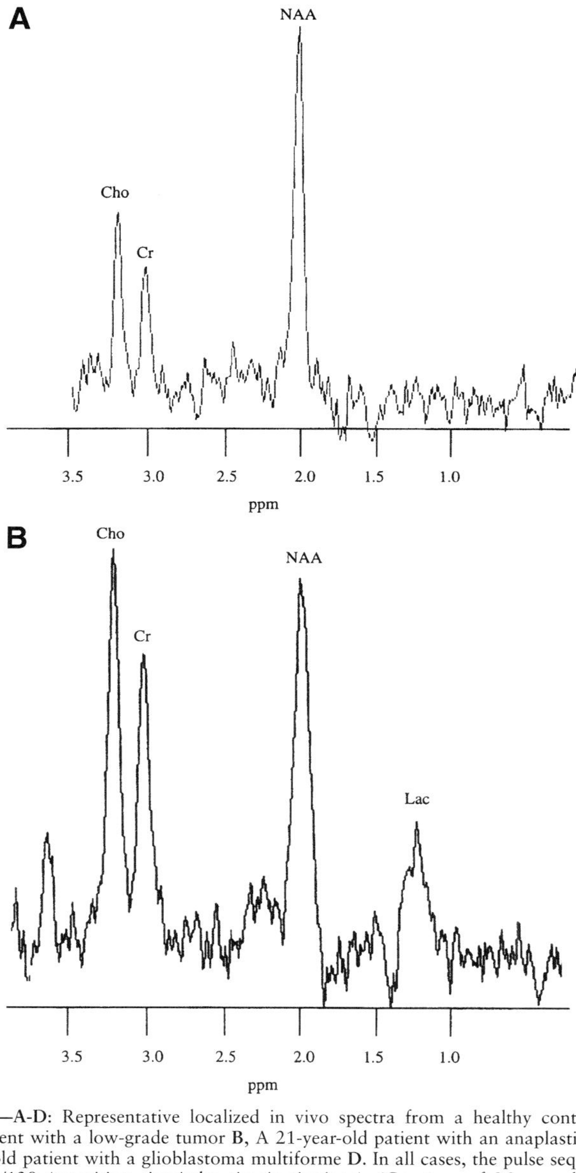

FIGURE 1.—A-D: Representative localized in vivo spectra from a healthy control subject **A**, A 36-year-old patient with a low-grade tumor **B**, A 21-year-old patient with an anaplastic astrocytoma **C**, And a 57-year-old patient with a glioblastoma multiforme **D**. In all cases, the pulse sequence parameters were 2,000/272/128 (repetition time/echo time/excitations). (Courtesy of Meyerand ME, Pipas JM, Mamourian A, et al: Classification of biopsy-confirmed brain tumors using single-voxel MR spectroscopy. *AJNR* 20: 117-123, 1999. Copyright by American Society of Neuroradiology.)

(*Continued*)

FIGURE 2 (cont.)

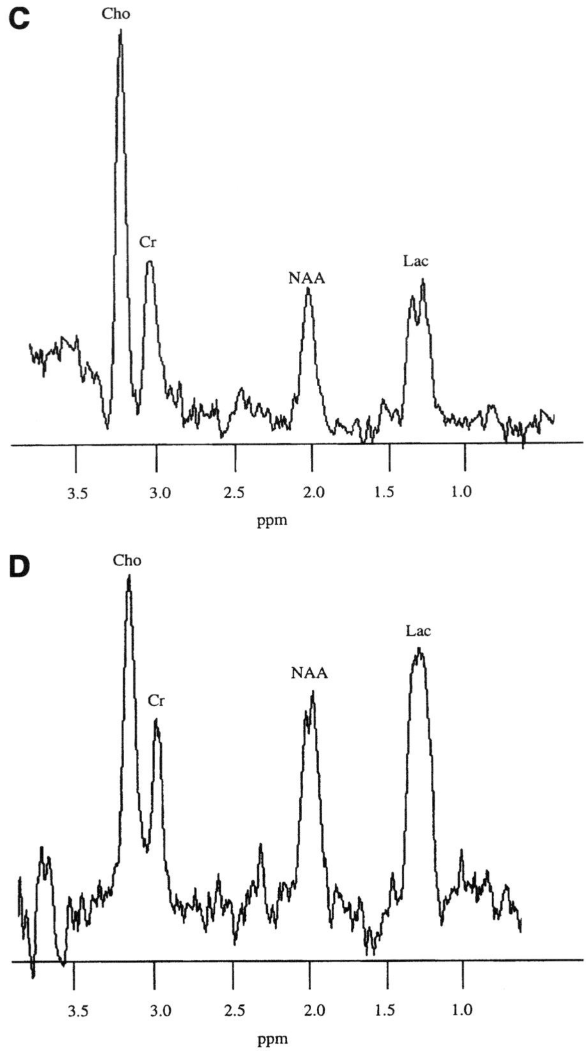

found it, the prize seems elusive. Remember the early days of CT? We were so excited. How much better it seemed than angiography and pneumoencephalography! It was, in lesion detection. It wasn't, in terms of specificity. I still remember that during the early days of CT, Hillier ("Bud") Baker, the much-respected neuroradiologist from the Mayo Clinic, threw up his hands during a heated discussion at a meeting of the American Society of Neuroradiology and exclaimed, "Anything can look like anything else!" Then along came MR and its vastly improved sensitivity for lesion detection in the CNS. Again we hoped for more histologic specificity. Again we were disappointed.

Are we now on the verge of discovering the Grail, at long last? MR spectroscopy and other techniques such as SPECT imaging look promising.[1,2] There are encouraging reports of using diffusion-weighted MR to help distinguish brain abscess and necrotic or cystic brain tumor.[3] The jury is still out but, as always, we are hopeful. Tune in next year—maybe "promising" will turn into "prognostic."

A.G. Osborn, M.D.

References

1. Chang LL, Chang I-W, Louis DN, et al: Correlation of high-resolution magic angle spinning proton magnetic resonance spectroscopy with histopathology of intact human brain tumor specimens. *Cancer Res* 58:1825-1832, 1998.
2. Reiche W, Schaefer A, Schmidt S, et al: ^{18}FDG-SPECT imaging of brain tumours. *Rivista Neuroradiol* 11:149-160, 1998.
3. Kim YJ, Chang K-H, Song IC, et al: Brain abscess and necrotic or cystic brain tumor: Discrimination with signal intensity on diffusion-weighted MR imaging. *AJR* 171:1487-1490, 1998.

Correlation of MR Imaging–Determined Cerebral Blood Volume Maps With Histologic and Angiographic Determination of Vascularity of Gliomas

Sugahara T, Korogi Y, Kochi M, et al (Kumamoto Univ, Japan)

AJR 171:1479-1486, 1998 8–41

Introduction.—Previous studies have shown that the vascularity of gliomas demonstrated by spin-echo echoplanar MRI is well correlated with their histologic vascularity. However, brain cancers are often associated with larger neovascular structures, including feeding arteries and draining veins. Gradient-echo echnoplanar MRI can be used to create hemodynamic maps representing not only total blood volume but also relative cerebral blood volume (rCBV). Gradient-echo echoplanar imaging was used to create rCBV maps of gliomas.

Methods.—The prospective study included 30 consecutive patients with intraaxial gliomas. The tumors were histologically confirmed as glioblastoma, anaplastic glioma with or without enhancement, or low-grade glioma. In each patient rCBV maps were generated using lipid-suppressed gradient-echo echoplanar imaging before, during, and after injections of contrast agent. Angiographic vascularity was calculated as well using a point system: 1 point each for tumor vessels, tumor stain, and early draining veins. For each tumor, maximum rCBV ratio was compared with the histologic and angiographic vascularity. The maximum rCBV ratio for each type of glioma was determined as well.

Results.—Enhanced areas were found in all glioblastomas studied, in some of the anaplastic gliomas, and in none of the low-grade gliomas. Angiographic vascularity was 1 or greater in 10 of 12 glioblastomas and

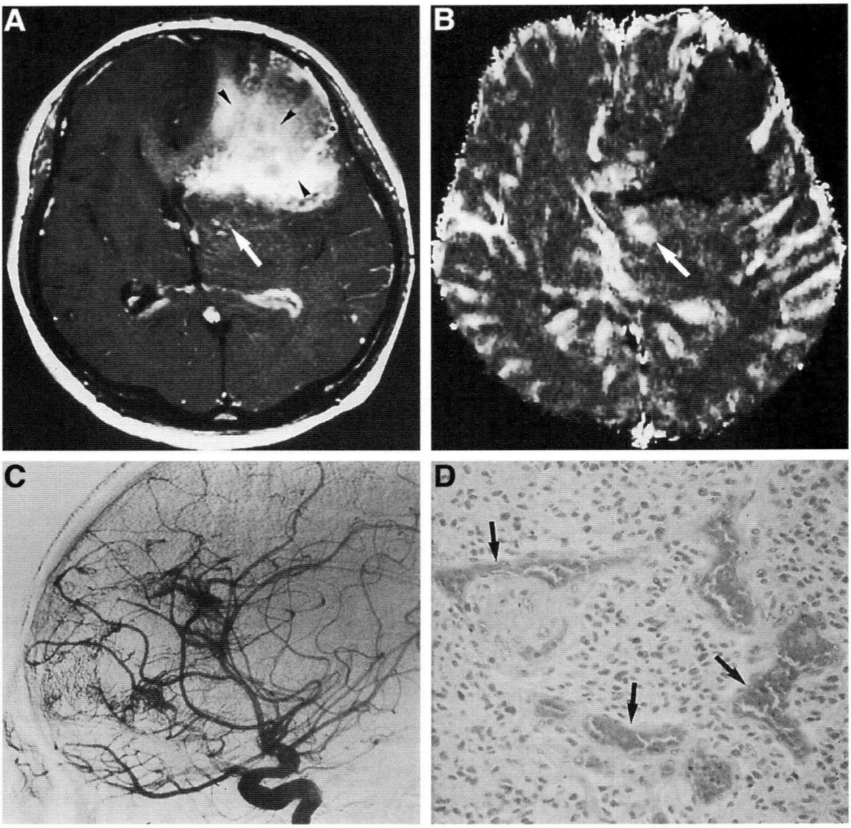

FIGURE 5.—37-year-old man with glioblastoma in left frontal lobe extending to corpus callosum and striate nuclei. **A**, Contrast-enhanced T1-weighted image. Minimal enhancement was observed within tumor (*arrow*). Hyperintense areas indicated tumoral hemorrhage (*arrowheads*). **B**, Relative cerebral blood volume (rCBV) map. Hypervascular areas (*arrow*), which are not consistent with enhanced areas, were clearly shown. Maximum rCBV ratio was 8.65. **C**, Conventional angiogram. Multiple tumor vessels and marked tumor stains were observed, and angiographic vascularity was rated as 3. **D**, Histologic specimen. Multiple tumor vessels with heterogeneity of vessel diameter and endothelial proliferation were observed (*arrows*); histologic vascularity was 3 (hematoxylin-eosin, × 120). (Courtesy of Sugahara T, Korogi Y, Kochi M, et al: Correlation of MR imaging–determined cerebral blood volume maps with histologic and angiographic determination of vascularity of gliomas. *AJR* 171:1479-1486, 1998.)

5 of 14 anaplastic gliomas (Fig 5). All other tumors had an angiographic vascularity score of 0, reflecting no abnormal angiographic vasculature. The areas of high vascularity shown on rCBV maps did not always agree with the enhanced areas on contrast-enhanced T1-weighted images. Glioblastomas had a significantly higher maximum rCBV ratio than anaplastic gliomas without enhancement and low-grade gliomas (Fig 7).

Conclusions.—Gradient-echo echoplanar MRI is useful in depicting the tumor angiogenesis of gliomas. The maximum rCBV ratios provided by this technique are well correlated with both angiographic and histologic

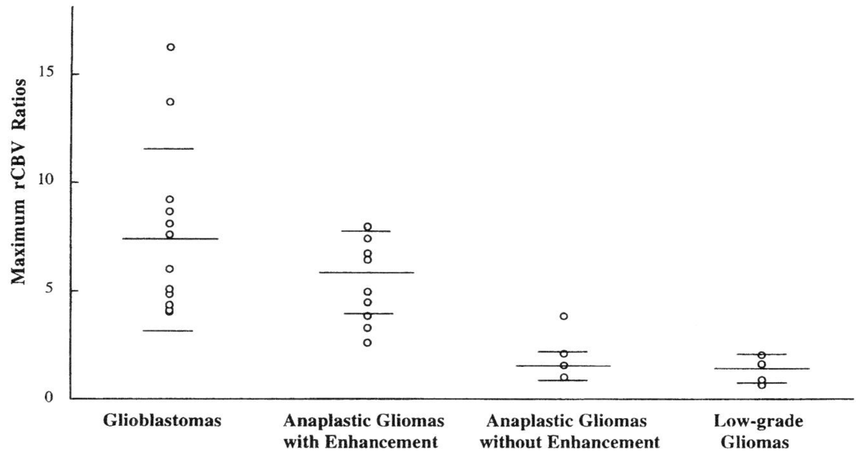

FIGURE 7.—Graph shows relationship between maximum relative cerebral blood volume (rCBV) ratios and gliomas. Maximum rCBV ratios of glioblastomas were significantly higher than those of anaplastic gliomas without enhancement ($P = 0.002$) and low-grade gliomas ($P < 0.001$). Maximum rCBV ratios of glioblastomas (mean = 7.32 ± 4.39) were higher than those of anaplastic gliomas with enhancement (mean = 5.84 ± 1.82), although difference did not reach statistical significance ($P = 0.04$). Maximum rCBV ratios of anaplastic gliomas with enhancement were higher than those of anaplastic gliomas without enhancement (mean = 1.53 ± 0.75) and low-grade gliomas (mean = 1.26 ± 0.55), but not significantly so ($P = 0.08$ and 0.03, respectively). No significant difference was found between anaplastic gliomas without enhancement and low-grade gliomas in this regard ($P = 0.68$). (Courtesy of Sugahara T, Korogi Y, Kochi M, et al: Correlation of MR imaging–determined cerebral blood volume maps with histologic and angiographic determination of vascularity of gliomas. *AJR* 171:1479-1486, 1998.)

assessments of vascularity. Low-grade gliomas show low vascularity with all 3 techniques.

► These authors studied 30 patients with histologically verified (by resection in 27 and biopsy in 3) gliomas. They included a mixture of astrocytomas, oligodendrogliomas, and oligoastrocytomas, which they lumped together into the categories of glioblastoma (GBM), anaplastic glioma with enhancement (AG+), anaplastic glioma without enhancement (AG−), and astrocytoma or "low-grade astrocytoma" (LGA). The 12 GBMs included 11 GBMs and 1 gliosarcoma. The 14 anaplastic gliomas included 11 anaplastic astrocytomas, 1 anaplastic oligodendroglioma, and 2 anaplastic oligoastrocytomas. There were only 4 LGAs.

All patients had contrast-enhanced images with "lipid-suppressed gradient-echo" protocols. This technique requires about half the contrast dose to create perfusion images. All 12 of the GBMs enhanced, and none of the LGAs enhanced. Among the 14 anaplastic gliomas, 10 were AG+ and 4 were AG−. The enhancing regions did not always correlate with the blood flow (rCBV) maps. Angiographic neovascularity was not present in 2 GBMs, 5 AA+ lesions, all 4 AA− lesions, and all 4 LGAs, again illustrating that contrast enhancement may be uncoupled from both angiographic neovascularity and blood flow maps. There was good general correlation between angiographic vascularity and the rCBV maps. However, there also were cases that had high rCBV that did not correlate with the angiograms, suggesting that microvasculature (e.g., increased and/or dilated capillaries) contributed to increased blood flow, along with large arteries and veins.

The authors also state: "In fact, low-grade gliomas have neither histologically high vascularity nor angiographically abnormal vessels...." Therefore, any assessment that reveals increased vascularity, whether by rCBV mapping or angiography, should suggest a higher grade glioma.

J.G. Smirniotopoulos, M.D.

Haemodynamic Evaluation of Cerebral Gliomas Using XeCT
Nakagawa T, Tanaka R, Takeuchi S, et al (Niigata Univ, Japan)
Acta Neurochir (Wien) 140:223-234, 1998 8–42

Background.—Although the use of stable Xe-enhanced CT (XeCT) for measurement of cerebral blood flow is widespread, few reports on its use for measuring blood flow in patients with brain tumors have been published. In the current study, regional blood flow was characterized in untreated cerebral gliomas (CG) with the use of XeCT.

Methods and Findings.—Thirty-eight patients with untreated CG underwent XeCT, and the findings were compared with those obtained by CT, MRI, and histopathologic analysis. Individual mean blood flow values in 29 high-grade gliomas (HGGs) and in 9 low-grade gliomas (LGGs) were intermediate between averaged blood flow values for cortex and white matter in the non-tumor-bearing hemisphere. Mean blood flow values for cyst and central necrosis were very low. Blood flow in 27/29 HGGs was relatively high in ring-enhancement lesions on CT and MRI but was low, even in viable tumor centers demonstrating no contrast enhancement. Blood flow in the remaining 2 HGGs was low in the center and relatively high in the periphery, even with homogeneous enhancement. The averaged blood flow value of the cortex outside surrounding edema in 5 HGGs was greater than that of cortex in the non-tumor-bearing hemisphere. The blood flow distribution in 3 small LGGs was homogeneously low. It was heterogeneous in 6 large lesions, including regions with both moderately high and low blood flow.

Conclusions.—In this study, averaged blood flow value in central necrosis or cyst was very low, as was that in surrounding edema. High blood flow regions in HGGs were most consistent with regions of ring enhancement seen on CT and MRI. Blood flow distribution was homogeneously low in small LGGs and heterogenous in large LGGs.

► This article used stable Xe-CT to evaluate cerebral blood flow (CBF) in a series of 38 patients with untreated cerebral gliomas. The spatial resolution was approximately 0.5 × 0.5 × 10 mm. The authors confirmed these findings: (1) small low-grade tumors had homogeneously low CBF; (2) larger low-grade tumors had heterogeneous CBF, with some tumor areas higher than normal; (3) as expected, "cysts" and necrotic regions had low CBF; (4)

CBF was high in the ring of ring-enhancing high-grade gliomas but low in the central nonenhancing areas, even when they contained viable but nonenhancing tumor; (5) CBF in normal cortex overlying the tumor was increased (compared with the opposite normal side); (6) CBF in the contralateral hemisphere was lower than in normal controls, presumably because of increased intracranial pressure. This article confirms the belief that high-grade gliomas are intrinsically more vascular and better perfused than low-grade gliomas.

J.G. Smirniotopoulos, M.D.

Assessment of Malignancy of Glioma by Positron Emission Tomography With ^{18}F-Fluorodeoxyglucose and Single Photon Emission Computed Tomography With Thallium-201 Chloride

Tamura M, Shibasaki T, Zama A, et al (Gunma Univ, Maebashi, Japan)
Neuroradiology 40:210-215, 1998 8–43

Background.—Histologic diagnosis is universally accepted for assessment of the malignancy of astrocytic tumors. However, the proliferative potential measured by bromodeoxyuridine (BrdU) labeling index (LI) reflects proliferative potential more accurately than the histologic diagnosis. Correlations between the histologic diagnosis, BrdU LI, and several imaging modalities were investigated.

Methods.—Forty-three patients with various grades of glioma were studied. The histologic diagnosis and the proliferative potential measured by BrdU LI were correlated with preoperative CT and contrast-enhanced MRI, ^{18}F-fluorodeoxyglucose PET, and ^{201}Tl SPECT.

Findings.—^{201}Tl SPECT was slightly more sensitive to tumors with a BrdU LI of 5% or greater than ^{18}F-FDG PET. ^{18}F-FDG PET was better than ^{201}Tl SPECT for identifying tumors with a BrdU LI of less than 1%. Tumor accumulation of ^{201}Tl differed slightly from contrast enhancement on CT or MRI, producing false positive results in some low-grade gliomas.

Conclusions.—In this series, high-grade gliomas typically had a BrdU LI of 5% or more, obvious contrast enhancement on CT or MRI, glucose hypermetabolism on PET, and high thallium uptake on SPECT. Low-grade glioma, astrocytoma, and oligoastrocytoma had a BrdU LI of less than 1%, no enhancement on CT or MRI, hypometabolism of glucose, and no thallium uptake.

► Our knowledge of the biology and imaging of gliomas continues to evolve, even though our treatment success seems to falter. Recent articles have shown a lack of specificity in the MRI characteristics used for grading gliomas. Therefore, we continue to seek other methods for assessing and predicting tumor grade. This article compares BrdU labeling with MR/CT evaluation, and both ^{18}FDG with ^{201}Tl-SPECT. High-grade tumors typically show hypermetabolism (^{18}FDG uptake), an increased BrdU labeling of tissue specimens, contrast enhancement on CT/MRI, and high uptake of thallium.

However, as has also been found earlier, some low-grade lesions (in particular, pilocytic astrocytomas) may also show both enhancement and thallium uptake.

The authors have demonstrated that thallium-SPECT could be useful in the assessment of gliomas. Since SPECT scanning is much more widely available than PET, this should stimulate renewed interest and the accumlation of more data from a larger series of patients.

J.G. Smirniotopoulos, M.D.

Benign Cerebellar Astrocytomas in Children

Pencalet P, Maixner W, Sainte-Rose C, et al (Hôpital Necker-Enfants Malades, Paris)

J Neurosurg 90:265-273, 1999 8–44

Introduction.—Five-year survival rates for children with astrocytomas of the cerebellum are 90% to 100%. Complete tumor excision is closely linked to survival rates. A more significant factor may be the presence of brain stem involvement; however, this has not been identified as a sole independent negative prognostic factor. To clarify the interplay between the degree of resection and brain stem involvement, patients were reviewed.

Methods.—A total of 168 cases of children who were surgically treated for a cerebellar astrocytoma during a 40-year period were retrospectively reviewed. The patients had a mean age of 6.9 years and a mean follow-up of 7.7 years. The review included an examination of their clinical files, a review of the histologic characteristics of their tumors, and an assessment of their outcomes.

Results.—In 76.2% of patients, tumors were strictly located in the cerebellum, and in 23.8%, they involved the brain stem. In 88.7% of patients, complete surgical excision was possible. The mortality rate was 4.2% and the tumor recurrence rate was 9.5%. No neurologic sequelae occurred in 58% of patients. Negative factors included a long preoperative duration of symptoms, brain stem involvement, incomplete tumor excision, and severe ventricular dilation.

Conclusion.—A significant negative prognostic factor was the presence of brain stem involvement, which should be treated as a distinct nosologic entity. The risk of tumor recurrence is significantly affected by the extent of surgical excision.

► Wasn't it the Mad Hatter in *Alice in Wonderland* who said, "Words mean what I mean them to mean"? Or something like that. So what does "benign" mean? If it is merely a tumor with low histologic grade, that is one thing. If it includes outcome, that is quite another matter. This article nicely demonstrates that the same grade of tumor may have such a different outcome when it involves 1 specific area (in this case, the brain stem) vs. another (the cerebellum) that it ought to be treated as a distinct nosologic entity. It is worth noting that the rare primary cerebellar glioblastoma may look very similar to what the authors refer to as the "transitional" solid, low-grade astrocytoma.[1]

A.G. Osborn, M.D.

References

1. Kulkarni AV, Becker LE, Jay V, et al: Primary cerebellar glioblastoma multiforme in children. *J Neurosurg* 90:546-550, 1999.

Tumor-related Venous Obstruction and Development of Peritumoral Brain Edema in Meningiomas

Bitzer M, Topka H, Morgalla M, et al (Univ of Tübingen, Germany)
Neurosurgery 42:730-737, 1998 8–45

Introduction.—Peritumoral brain edema (PTBE) is a common finding in patients with meningioma. Among the many pathophysiologic explanations considered is a tumor-related venous obstruction. The contribution of venous stasis to PTBE in patients with meningioma was studied.

Methods.—The 10-year retrospective study included angiograms of 134 patients with 136 intracranial meningiomas. The venous-phase angiograms were reviewed and graded for tumor-related alterations of venous drainage involving the cortical veins, sylvian veins, bridging veins, deep and transmedullary veins, and dural sinuses. Preoperative CT scans were used to assess total tumor volume; tumor/PTBE volume ratio, expressed as the edema index (EI); and location of the edema.

Results.—The incidence of PTBE was 62.5% overall, 20.7% for small meningiomas ($<10cm^3$) vs. 92.3% for large meningiomas ($\geq 100cm^3$). However, the incidence of PTBE and the mean EI were not significantly affected by the presence of unselected signs of obstructed venous drainage. The incidence of edema was not increased for meningiomas involving the cortical veins, bridging veins, or dural sinuses. However, mean EI was significantly increased for lesions associated with venous changes in the sylvian veins, 4.9 versus 2.7 in size-matched controls (Fig 2); or with dysplastic transmedullary veins, 3.3 versus 1.7.

Conclusions.—For most patients with meningiomas, tumor-related venous obstruction does not appear to be a significant factor in the development of PTBE. Alterations in venous drainage may contribute to preexisting PTBE in some patients with meningiomas involving the sylvian veins or dysplastic transmedullary veins. The larger the meningioma, the greater the incidence of PTBE.

► Meningiomas are the most common nonglial primary tumors of the CNS, and they are the most common primary extraaxial lesion. One of the most common questions about these extraaxial masses is why and how extraaxial meningiomas produce intraaxial brain edema. The edema is almost universally of the "vasogenic" type, spreading through the white matter. But why?

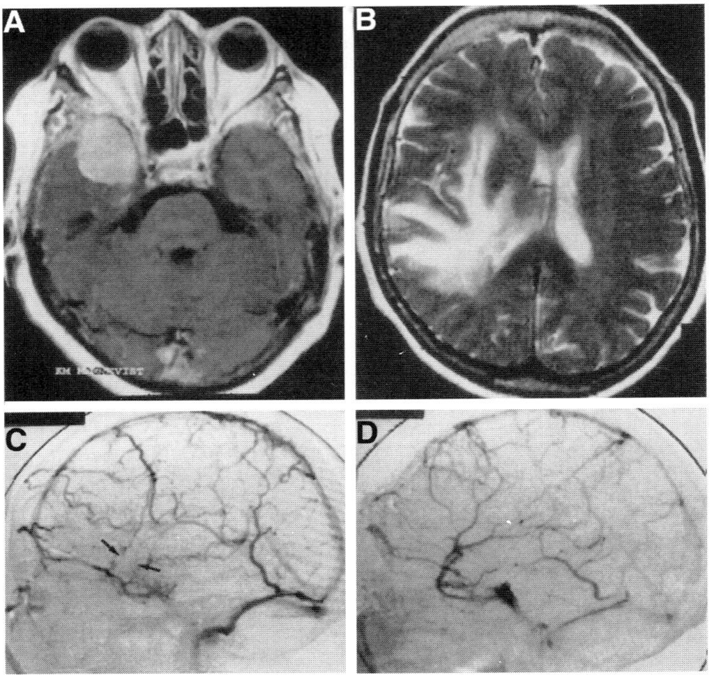

FIGURE 2.—**A**, Contrast-enhanced, T1-weighted, axial MR imaging scan from a patient with a right temporobasal sphenoid wing meningioma. **B**, T2-weighted MR imaging scan, revealing striking brain edema adjacent to the sylvian fissure. **C**, Right internal carotid artery angiogram (lateral view, venous phase), showing abrupt cut-off of the sylvian veins at the tumor border (*arrows*). There was typical prolonged vascular staining of the meningioma. **D**, Contralateral left internal carotid artery angiogram (lateral view, venous phase), demonstrating normal sylvian veins. (Courtesy of Bitzer M, Topka H, Morgalla M, et al: Tumor-related venous obstruction and development of peritumoral brain edema in meningiomas. *Neurosurgery* 42:730-737, 1998.)

Many suggest that meningiomas with edema are more histologically aggressive. Nothing could be farther from the truth. Witness this article by Bitzer et al., who reviewed the angiographic characteristics of 136 meningiomas in 134 patients. With the exception of those tumors that affected the sylvian veins, there was no correlation between edema in the brain and any compromise in venous drainage. This confirms earlier reports that focused on sinus obstruction as one specific type of venous interference. In general, most meningiomas have associated intraaxial edema, probably related to the intimacy of the brain-tumor interface more than any other parameter.

J.G. Smirniotopoulos, M.D.

Preoperative Identification of Meningiomas That Are Highly Likely to Recur

Nakasu S, Nakasu Y, Nakajima M, et al (Shiga Univ, Ohtsu, Japan)
J Neurosurg 90:455-462, 1999 8–46

Introduction.—Recurrence of meningiomas occur even after seemingly complete removal and can occur in up to 15% of benign meningiomas within 10 years after their total removal. Before surgery, it is important to identify high-risk groups for recurrence. Preoperative clinicoradiologic features of recurrent meningiomas were compared with those of nonrecurrent ones to find high-risk factors for recurrence. A strategy for treating meningiomas was devised by investigating their recurrence patterns with use of imaging studies.

Methods.—One hundred one patients who had macroscopically complete removal of meningiomas were observed for 5 years or until recurrence of the tumor. Assessments were made of preoperative radiologic findings and clinical characteristics.

Results.—During the follow-up period, 15 meningiomas recurred, which extended to a maximum duration of 18 years. Significant predictive factors of recurrence were tumor size and shape, relation to the major sinuses, calcification, bone changes, and characteristics of the tumor-brain interface. Gender and patient age were not significant. It was found that

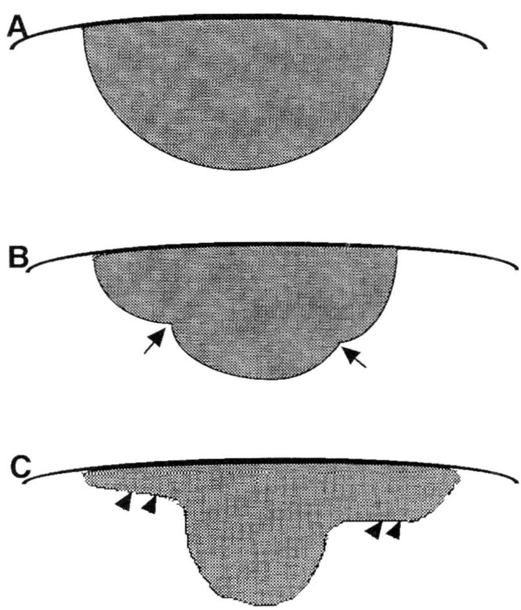

FIGURE 1.—Schematic drawings showing the shapes of meningiomas. A, Round. B, Lobulated tumor showing distinct notch (*arrows*). C, Mushrooming tumor extending a pileus (*arrowheads*) over the brain surface from the globoid mass. (Courtesy of Nakasu S, Nakasu Y, Nakajima M, et al: Preoperative identification of meningiomas that are highly likely to recur. *J Neurosurg* 90:455-462, 1999.)

lobulated and mushrooming meningiomas were more likely to recur than round tumors (Fig 1). After a Simpson Grade II or III removal, local recurrences were predominant. After a Simpson Grade I removal, recurrences most frequently occurred at the edge of the dural resection.

Conclusion.—A more aggressive treatment with a wider dural excision should be used for meningiomas with mushrooming or lobulated shapes. Round tumors do not usually need such aggressive treatment; however, in younger patients, it may be beneficial.

► Although it is difficult to determine the histologic subtype of meningioma on the basis of imaging findings alone, it is important to alert the neurosurgeons to those tumors that may be atypical or anaplastic. The recurrence rate for these more aggressive meningiomas is much higher than for their garden-variety, "vanilla" typical counterpart. So-called mushrooming or lobulated meningiomas recur more often than globose (round) meningiomas. If "size matters" is a motto for cerebral aneurysms, here is one where "shape matters."

A.G. Osborn, M.D.

Pathogenesis of Intracranial Germ Cell Tumors Reconsidered

Sano K (Univ of Tokyo)

J Neurosurg 90:258-264, 1999 8–47

Introduction.—The germ cell theory is that germ cells give rise to germinomas and to tumors composed of totipotential cells that cause embryonal carcinomas. From these, endodermal sinus tumors are created, as well as choriocarcinomas, and teratomas. Germ cell tumors include germinoma, mature and immature teratoma, malignant teratoma or teratoma with malignant transformation, embryonal carcinoma, yolk sac tumor, choriocarcinomas, and mixed germ cell tumors. The classification maintains that these tumors originate from germ cells. The pathogenesis of intracranial germ cell tumors was determined.

Methods.—There were 153 patients with intracranial germ cell tumors; of these, 62.7% had tumors with monotypic histologic patterns and 37.3% had mixed tumors. Six patients died after admission, and the rest had surgery followed by radiotherapy and/or chemotherapy.

Results.—Within 1 year, all patients with a choriocarcinoma had died. There were poor outcomes in patients with a yolk sac tumor (endodermal sinus tumor) or an embryonal carcinoma. Both the 5- and 10-year survival rates were 93% for patients with a mature teratoma. Patients with an immature teratoma had 5-year and 1-year survival rates of 86% each, whereas the 3-year survival rate was 50% for patients with a teratoma with malignant transformation. The 5-year survival rate was 96% for patients with a germinoma and the 10-year survival rate was 93%. Germinoma, the most undifferentiated tumor, was the most benign; choriocarcinoma and yolk sac tumor, the most differentiated tumors, were the most malignant.

Conclusion.—Other than germinomas, germ cell tumors may not originate from 1 single type of cell (primordial germ cell). At the time of primitive streak formation, the embryonic cells of various stages of embryogenesis may be misplaced in the bilaminar embryonic disk, becoming involved in the stream of lateral mesoderm and carried to the neural plate area to become incorrectly enfolded into the brain at the time of neural tube formation. One hypothesis is that tumors composed of cells resembling the cells that appear in the earlier stage of embryogenesis (ontogenesis) are more malignant than those composed of cells resembling the cells that appear in the later stages of embryogenesis.

► This article is a wonderful discussion of the embryogenesis, ontogenesis, and pathogenesis of intracranial germ cell tumors. The bottom line is that they may not be as simple as supposed. There are reasons to agree with Dr. Sano that tumors resembling cells that appear in the earlier stages of embryogenesis are more malignant than those composed of cells that appear later. From an imaging point of view, I do not think that we can tell germinomas from embryonal carcinomas and other more malignant tumors. Practically speaking, the recommended approach is biopsy as necessary to establish the diagnosis that will, in turn, determine treatment.[1] The treatment differs; teratomas, yolk sac tumors, and embryonal carcinomas may do better with adjuvant therapy.[2,3]

An interesting sidelight comes from the therapy literature; a recent report shows that tumor response to radiation therapy correlates negatively with the presence of a cystic region in germinomas.[4] This may be more important than trying to guess the histopathology from the imaging studies.

A.G. Osborn, M.D.

References

1. Sawamura Y, de Tribolet N, Ishii N, et al: Management of primary intracranial germinomas: Diagnostic surgery or radical resection? *J Neurosurg* 87:262-266, 1997.
2. Sawamura Y, Kato T, Ikeda J, et al: Teratomas of the central nervous system: Treatment considerations based on 34 cases. *J Neurosurg* 89:728-737, 1998.
3. Ushio Y, Kochi M, Kuratsu J-I, et al: Preliminary observations for a new treatment in children with primary intracranial yolk sac tumor or embryonal carcinoma. *J Neurosurg* 90:133-137, 1999.
4. Moon WK, Chang KH, Han MH, et al: Intracranial germinomas: Correlation of imaging findings with tumor response to radiation therapy. *AJR* 172:713-716, 1998.

Correlation Between Appearance on Magnetic Resonance Imaging and Tumor Histology

Sartoretti-Schefer S, Aguzzi A, Wichmann W, et al (Univ Hosp of Zürich, Switzerland)

Int J Neuroradiol 4:357-365, 1998 8–48

Introduction.—Gangliogliomas are mixed neurogliogenic and rare intracranial tumors that occur most frequently in children and young adults. Patients with ganglioglioma often have a history of epileptic seizures, especially complex partial seizures. To discern different histologic and MRI subtypes and to correlate the specific histologic features with those observed neuroradiologically, histopathologic specimens were analyzed and compared with preoperative MRI findings from patients who underwent surgery for ganglioglioma.

Methods.—There were 23 patients with histologically proven cerebral ganglioglioma. Histologic findings seen on specimens stained with hematoxylin and eosin were correlated with 1.5 T multiplanar spin echo T2-

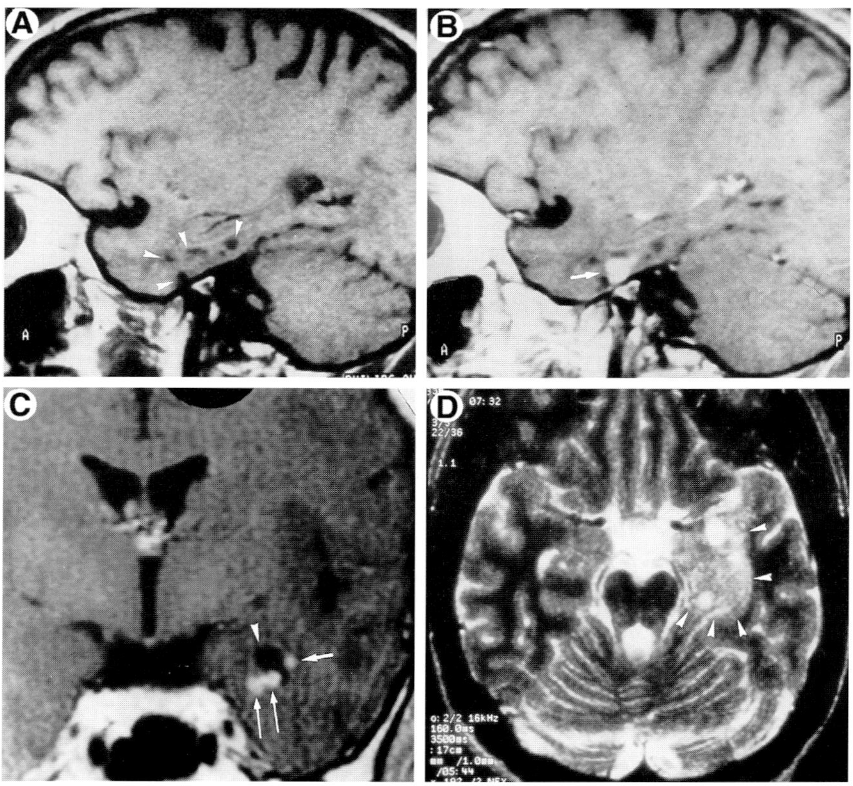

(*Continued*)

FIGURE 1 (cont.)

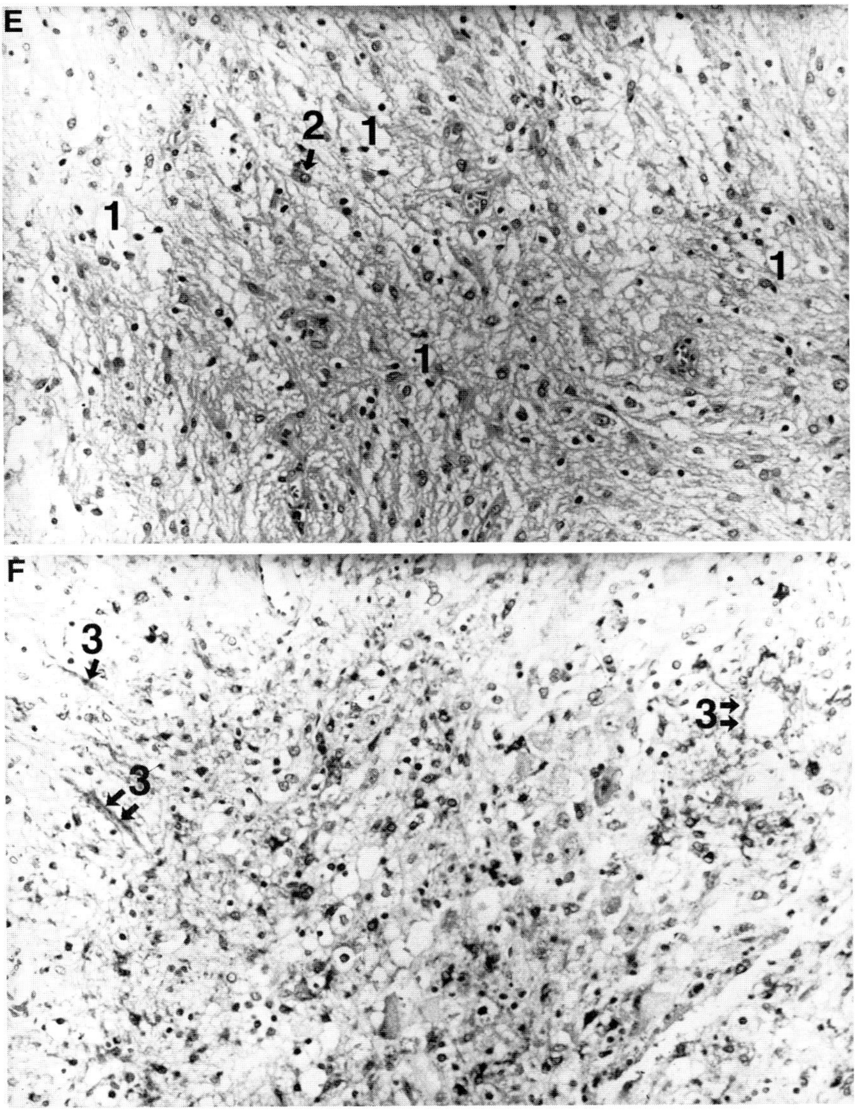

FIGURE 1.—Pilocytic ganglioglioma with a classic MRI appearance. Precontrast sagittal T1-weighted image (**A**), postcontrast sagittal (**B**), and coronal (**C**) T1-weighted images, and transverse T2-weighted MRI (**D**). Multiple, very small nonenhancing cystic areas and a few punctate contrast-enhancing nodules are seen on the T1-weighted images. The tumor borders cannot be delineated. On T2-weighted images, the tumor is well demarcated and appears larger than on the T1-weighted images. Hematoxylin and eosin stain of the tumor specimen (**E**) shows microcystic degeneration (*1*), a population of piloid astrocytes and partly binucleated ganglion cells (*white arrow, 2*) within the tumor matrix. Broad astrocytic fibers (*white arrow, 3*) are seen on the glial fibrillary acidic protein stain (**F**). This histologic pattern is called the pilocytic type. (Courtesy of Sartoretti-Schefer S, Aguzzi A, Wichmann W, et al: Correlation between appearance on magnetic resonance imaging and tumor histology. *Int J Neuroradiol* 4:357-365, 1998.)

weighted MRI, silver-impregnation techniques, and immunohistochemical examinations.

Results.—The histologic features showed 4 subtypes of ganglioglioma: the fibrillar, the pilocytic, the mixed fibrillary and focally pilocytic, and the anaplastic. Four different patterns could be differentiated on MRI. A small tumor with a few small cysts and punctate contrast-enhancing nodular areas was the most classic tumor type (Fig 1). This type was most often found in the mediobasal temporal lobe. The other 3 MRI patterns resembled a pilocytic astrocytoma, a low-grade astrocytoma, or a nonspecific, probably malignant tumor type. The type of glial cell participating in the neoplasia correlated with the differing MRI features of these gangliogliomas. The proportions of neurons and glial cells within the tumors were not correlated with the MRI features.

Conclusion.—Based on the differences in the nature of their glial cell population, gangliogliomas can be classified into several subtypes. The pilocytic histologic variant of ganglioglioma was the most common, or classic, MRI appearance. The fibrillary histologic variant of ganglioglioma correlated with the astrocytic MRI appearance.

► This article is a nice radiologic-pathologic correlation showing that imaging sometimes can predict histology. There are at least 2 subtypes of ganglioglioma based on the type of glial cell that they contain. The most common MR appearance in the authors' series, a solid lesion that contains small cysts and lacks definable margins, correlates with what they term the "pilocytic" histologic variant.

Other variants include a solid mass with a large well-defined cyst (the "piloid" type) and an astrocytic type that has a more solid appearance. The distinction is important because the biologic behavior of these tumors depends on the nature of its astrocytic component.[1] There is some evidence that FDG-PET and ^{201}Tl-SPECT may be helpful in the preoperative grading of these interesting tumors.[2]

A.G. Osborn, M.D.

References

1. Quinn B: Diagnosis of ganglioglioma. *J Neurosurg* 88: 935-937, 1998.
2. Kincaid PK, El-Saden SM, Park S-H, et al: Cerebral gangliogliomas: Preoperative grading using FDG-PET and ^{201}Tl-SPECT. *Am J Neuroradiol* 19: 801-806, 1998.

Cystic Lesions Accompanying Extra-axial Tumours

Lohle PNM, Wurzer HAL, Seelen PJ, et al (St Elisabeth Hosp, Tilburg, The Netherlands; Med Centre Haaglanden, The Hague, The Netherlands; Univ of Groningen, The Netherlands)

Neuroradiology 41:13-17, 1999 8–49

Introduction.—Little is known about the pathogenesis of cysts accompanying extra-axial tumors. One theory is that these cysts are formed because of disruption of the blood-brain barrier with exudation of plasma proteins into the brain parenchyma, resulting in accumulation of fluid and, eventually, in the formation of a cyst. Nine peritumoral cysts accompanying 8 extra-axial tumors were analyzed, and protein concentrations were measured.

Methods.—There were 8 patients with 9 peritumoral cysts who had their cyst fluid, CSF, and blood plasma analyzed. Four patients had meningiomas, 2 had intracranial schwannomas, and 2 had spinal intradural schwannomas.

Results.—Insight into the state of the semipermeability of the blood-brain barrier and blood-CSF barrier was provided by measuring concentrations of various proteins. Disruption of the blood-brain barrier and edema formation caused peritumoral cysts accompanying intra-axial brain

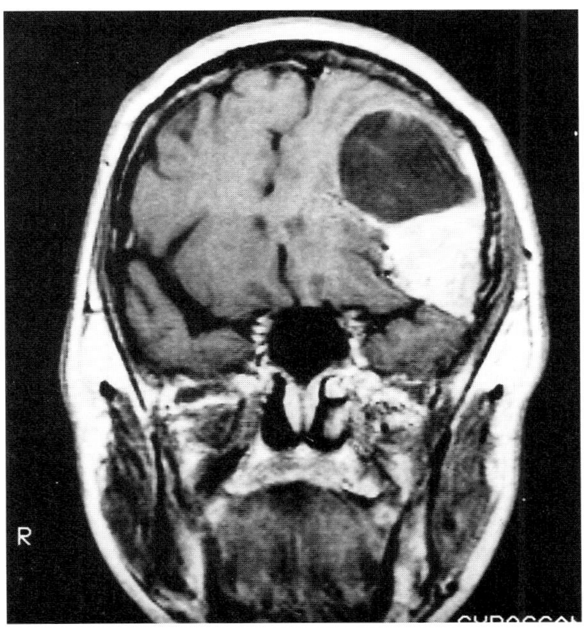

FIGURE 2.—Coronal T1-weighted image after gadolinium administration, with a cystic meningiotheliomatous meningioma. Contrast enhancement of the tumor associated without cyst wall enhancement. (Courtesy of Lohle PNM, Wurzer HAL, Seelen PJ, et al: Cystic lesions accompanying extra-axial tumors. *Neuroradiology* 41: 13-17, copyright 1999, Springer-Verlag.)

tumors. This was evidenced by the lack of contrast enhancement in brain tissue surrounding the meningiomas on CT or MRI (Fig 2). Extra-axial tumors are separate from nervous tissue by arachnoid and pia mater, whereas intra-axial tumors are embedded within nervous tissue. A local barrier disruption and passage across the arachnoid, pia mater, and cortical/medullary layer into the CNS parenchyma was suggested by high concentrations of proteins in the cyst fluid, approaching blood plasma levels.

Conclusion.—Tumor cysts have very high concentrations of protein, with 90% of the total protein in the cyst being formed by plasma proteins. The majority of the proteins in cyst fluid in extra-axial, intradural schwannomas and meningiomas are plasma proteins. The pathogenesis of extra-axial intradural tumor cysts may be formed by leakage of plasma proteins out of the tumor vessels into the nervous tissue.

► The authors point out that 10% of intracranial tumors have cysts. True, but most cysts are inside the mass itself. A classic example is necrotic high grade astrocytomas (usually glioblastoma multiforme). Other tumors such as hemangioblastoma and pleomorphic xanthoastrocytoma may have a neoplastic nodule and a nonneoplastic cyst wall. In the cerebellopontine angle, schwannomas are associated with cysts in nearly 20% of cases. Their pathogenesis is controversial, but the authors make a strong case that tumor vessels leak plasma proteins into nervous tissue. Fluid-fluid levels within cystic neurogenic neoplasms also occur. In these cases, blood breakdown byproducts are often found in the cyst.[1] Determining whether a cystic lesion is neoplastic or nonneoplastic may be difficult. Early evidence is that single-voxel proton MR spectroscopy is helpful in distinguishing inflammatory and neoplastic cysts from arachnoid and porencephalic cysts.[2]

A.G. Osborn, M.D.

References

1. Patankar T, Prasad S, Pardiwala D, et al: Fluid-fluid levels in benign neurogenic tumors. *Rivista Neuroradiol* 11:893-896, 1998.
2. Chang K-H, Song IC, Kim SH, et al: In vivo single-voxel proton MR spectroscopy in intracranial cystic masses. *Am J Neuroradiol* 19:401-405, 1998.

METASTASES

Metastatic Brain Tumors With Dural Extension

Rumana CS, Hess KR, Shi WM, et al (Baylor College of Medicine, Houston; Univ of Texas, Houston)

J Neurosurg 89:552-558, 1998 8–50

Introduction.—Each year, there are about 100,000 new metastatic brain tumors, with most tumors occurring subcortically at the gray-white matter junction. Less commonly seen is metastatic lesions based on or abutting the dura. Patients with metastatic tumors with dural extension may have

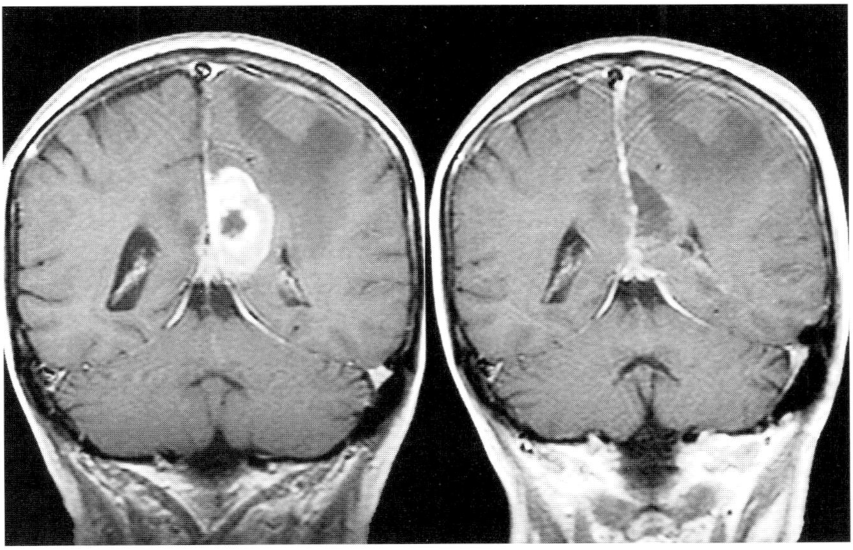

FIGURE 1.—Representative gadolinium-enhanced T1-weighted magnetic resonance MRI imaging performed in a patient with a metastatic brain tumor showing dural extension to the falx. *Left*: preoperative coronal image showing tumor attached to the falx. *Right*: coronal MR image obtained after tumor resection. The falx was not resected. (Courtesy of Ruman CS, Hess KR, Shi WM, et al: Metastatic brain tumors with dural extension. *J Neurosurg* 89:552-558, 1998.)

poorer outcome as a result of their incidence of recurrent disease and leptomeningeal disease compared with patients with subcortical lesions; however, this has not been previously studied. Patients with solitary metastatic tumors with dural extension treated surgically were compared with patients with the disease with no dural involvement to evaluate the clinical behavior and outcome.

Methods.—There were 22 patients with dural extension (median age of 58 years) and who had a median preoperative Karnofsky Performance Scale score of 90 (range 70 to 100) (Fig 1). Most patients had breast cancer, adenocarcinoma and squamous cell carcinoma of the lung, and renal cell carcinoma. Gross-total resection of the tumor was performed, and 86% of patients had radiation therapy. They were compared with 26 patients who did not have dural extension.

Results.—Eleven months was the median patient survival time, with a median time to recurrent intracranial disease of 19 months. In 41% of patients with dural extension, recurrent disease occurred. Three patients (14%) had leptomeningeal disease. Dural resection did not affect the frequency and time course of the development of recurrent disease or survival. In patients without dural extension, the median survival was 1 month, and the median time to recurrence was not reached. One patient (4%) had leptomeningeal disease.

Conclusion.—Patients with metastatic brain tumors with dural extension may be more likely to have recurrences develop along the dura and leptomeningeal disease. In these patients, the overall survival time is no different from those with intraparenchymal lesions.

► The so-called dural tail sign is not pathognomonic for meningioma. We've long known that occasionally nonmeningiomatous tumors such as schwannoma and glioblastoma multiforme may cause reactive dural hyperplasia. So can tumor mimics such as tumefactive tuberculosis, sarcoid, and idiopathic hypertrophic pachymeningitis. Now, we can add parenchymal brain metastases to the list of lesions that may involve the dura. From the outcome point of view, with brain metastases it doesn't matter. It's still a dismal diagnosis. When the disease is subtle, high-dose imaging may be helpful.[1]

A.G. Osborn, M.D.

Reference

1. Kallmes DF, Gray L, Glass JP: High-dose gadolinium-enhanced MRI for diagnosis of meningeal metastases. *Neuroradiol* 40: 23-26, 1998.

The Status of Stereotactic Radiosurgery for Cerebral Metastases in 1998

Mehta MP, Boyd TS, Sinha P (Univ of Wisconsin, Madison)
J Radiosurg 1:17-30, 1998 8–51

Background.—The number of radiosurgery facilities worldwide has greatly increased in the last 10 years. Brain metastases, the most common intracranial neoplasm, are often treated radiosurgically. The major issues of such treatment for brain metastases are discussed.

Discussion.—Twenty independent English-language articles were reviewed. In these studies, more than 1,250 patients with more than 2,100 lesions underwent γ-knife or linear accelerator-based radiosurgery. Composite data showed a mean local control rate of 82%, with a median survival of 9.6 months. These values are comparable to those cited in recent surgical reports. Radiosurgery is associated with a low morbidity, the most serious risks being necrosis (in 4%) and cranial nerve damage (in 1%). Volume of lesions and previous radiation may help to predict late damage. The most important prognostic factors for survival appear to be controlled extracranial disease, Karnofsky performance score, and the presence of 3 or fewer lesions.

Though the impact of dose has not been clearly defined, there seems to be a dose-response relationship, especially for doses of 18 Gy and higher. Whole-brain radiotherapy may enhance local control, but data about survival improvement are unconvincing. In some series, whole-brain radiotherapy is associated with an increased risk of late complications, with an average incidence of less than 5%. Chronic steroid dependence and increased intracranial edema do not seem to be common problems.

► This article is from the inaugural issue of a new journal, *The Journal of Radiosurgery*. I thought I would include it, because it summarizes an important and common problem, the treatment of metastatic disease. The authors reviewed the literature published in English from 1987 to 1997, encompassing more than 2,100 lesions in more than 1,250 patients. Patients with fewer lesions (1 or 2) did better than those with 3 or more. In addition, higher Karnofsky scores and controlled disease outside the CNS correlated with a better prognosis. Even though the "local control" rate achieved was greater than 80%, the median survival of patients with cerebral metastases was just under 10 months.

J.G. Smirniotopoulos, M.D.

Clinical Practice and Miscellaneous Techniques

Magnetoencephalographic Mapping of the Language-Specific Cortex

Papanicolaou AC, Simos PG, Breier JI, et al (Univ of Texas, Houston)
J Neurosurg 90:85-93, 1999 8–52

Introduction.—A completely noninvasive method of functional brain imaging, magnetoencephalography, is complementary to other imaging methods such as functional MRI or PET scanning. For mapping the primary sensory cortex, as well as the association cortex activated in the context of cognitive tasks, this technique has emerged as the method of choice. Whether magnetoencephalographic mapping could be useful in identifying the language-specific cortex was investigated. The reliability and validity of estimates of hemispheric dominance were established, as well as the locus and extent of the language-specific cortex.

Methods.—In patients who had the Wada procedure or language mapping through intraoperative cortical stimulation, magnetoencephalographic data were collected and the reliability, validity, and topographic accuracy of the data were assessed. Results were also compared with those of healthy volunteers. Six experiments were conducted on groups ranging from 4 to 16 individuals.

Results.—Simple language tasks can reliably activate receptive language-specific areas, and this can be readily recorded in short magnetoencephalographic sessions. Reliability was demonstrated because results remained stable and were independent of whether visual or auditory stimuli were used to activate the brain. The results of this technique concurred with the Wada procedure in assessing hemispheric dominance for language and with the results of cortical stimulation in identifying the precise topography of receptive language regions within the dominant hemisphere, which further demonstrated this technique's validity.

Conclusion.—By correctly identifying the language-dominant hemisphere and specific language-related regions within this hemisphere, the magnetoencephalographic mapping technique has been shown to be effective; however, it should be further refined. Many patients who harbor tumors or have epilepsy would benefit from further development of the technique, which could become a valuable adjunct for routine presurgical planning.

► Magnetoencephalography has become an important adjunct to presurgical planning in patients who have neoplasms or intractable epilepsy. Magnetoencephalography mapping is very useful for the neurosurgeons but difficult to do in the average radiology practice. It takes a lot of technical support and designing of the protocols, for evaluating these patients is not easy. These kinds of "niche imaging" procedures are 1 reason that some large institutions are establishing full epilepsy centers. The prevalence of epilepsy, estimated at 11% of the population, means there is a significant patient group out there which needs expert clinical and imaging evaluation.

A.G. Osborn, M.D.

Focal Brain Lesions: Effect of Single-Voxel Proton MR Spectroscopic Findings on Treatment Decisions

Adamson AJ, Rand SD, Prost RW, et al (Med College of Wisconsin, Milwaukee)

Radiology 209:73-78, 1998 8–53

Background.—Single-voxel, image-guided proton MR spectroscopy can measure the amplitudes of various chemicals in brain lesions, including choline, creatine, glutamine, glutamate, *N*-acetylaspartate (NAA), and lactic acid. This information is useful in distinguishing between radiation necrosis and recurrent brain tumors. In this way, MR spectroscopy can avert brain biopsy in some cases, thus reducing morbidity and costs. The impact of single-voxel proton MR spectroscopy on the treatment of patients with suspected brain tumors was studied.

Methods.—The 7-month study included 78 patients undergoing MR spectroscopic evaluation of focal brain lesions suspicious for brain tumor. A neuroradiologist interpreted the MR spectra with the use of clinical, laboratory, and other imaging findings. Spectra showing a choline/NAA ratio of greater than 1 were considered positive for brain tumor. The finding of lactic acid or lipid in the presence of an elevated choline concentration suggested relatively high-grade neoplasia. If lactic acid was elevated but choline was not, infarct was suspected rather than tumor. All spectra were obtained at 0.5 T using a head coil for deep lesions or a surface coil for superficial lesions.

Results.—In 49 patients, MR spectroscopy suggested a neoplasm. In 8 of these patients (16%), MR spectroscopy had a positive influence on treatment in that they received irradiation or chemotherapy without biopsy. In 2 of the patients with positive findings (4%), MR spectroscopy had a potentially negative effect on treatment in that surgery or biopsy showed a nonneoplastic process. Twenty-nine patients had negative results on MR spectroscopy. In this group, MR spectroscopy had a positive influence on treatment in 15 patients (52%), who received medical treatment or were followed up for interval changes.

Conclusions.—This preliminary study suggests that MR spectroscopy may have a beneficial effect on the management of patients with suspected brain tumors. The study is limited by the fact that biopsy was not routinely performed to confirm the MR spectroscopic diagnosis. Prospective studies are needed to assess the true impact of MR spectroscopy in clinical practice.

► This was a retrospective review of 78 cases where MR spectroscopy (MRS) had been performed. In many institutions MRS is readily available and commonly used to augment conventional MR. However, the availability and common use of MRS vary widely. Many radiologists are misinformed, considering MRS to be an experimental or a least a highly specialized procedure requiring the support of a physicist on-site. The article by Adamson et al attempts to demonstrate that MRS may have a more common role in the differential diagnosis of focal brain lesions. The authors state, and I heartily agree, that MRS has great potential in distinguishing neoplastic from non-neoplastic masses. This distinction may alter the patient's treatment path significantly by obviating the need for a biopsy. Clearly, more work needs to be done, and outcome studies would be most helpful in validating the potential for improved patient care. But even without "proof," I think that MRS has moved "out of the lab" and should be used more often in narrowing the differential diagnosis for focal brain lesions.

J.G. Smirniotopoulos, M.D.

Computed Imaging-assisted Stereotactic Brain Biopsy: A Risk Analysis of 225 Consecutive Cases

Sawin PD, Hitchon PW, Follett KA, et al (Univ of Iowa Hosps and Clinics, Iowa City)

Surg Neurol 49:640-649, 1998 8–54

Background.—Image-guided stereotaxy is a relatively safe and accurate method of sampling tissue from small or deep-seated intraparenchymal lesions. Although complications of this procedure are infrequent, devastating neurologic sequelae can occur as a result of hemorrhage or direct trauma. Factors associated with an increased risk of morbidity from stereotactic brain biopsy were investigated.

Methods.—Data on 225 consecutive computer-assisted stereotactic brain biopsy procedures were analyzed. The patients ranged in age from 3 to 84 years, and the male-to-female ratio was about 2:1. Nearly half had pre-existing medical conditions. Sixty-one percent of the biopsied lesions were lobar, and the remaining were deeply seated in the thalamus, basal ganglia, pineal gland, hypothalamus, cerebellum, and brainstem. Glial tumors accounted for 44.4% of the biopsied lesions. Metastases occurred in 12.9%, and lymphoma in 11.6%.

Findings.—Twelve patients had procedural complications—8 from hemorrhage and 4 from direct trauma. Morbidity was major in 8 patients (3.6%). These patients had hemiparesis, aphasia, or obtundation. Another 3 patients (1.3%) had transient, mild neurologic deficits. One patient died during the procedure, for an operative mortality of 0.4%. Factors associated with an increased risk of morbidity were the preoperative use of antiplatelet agents, chronic use of corticosteroids, deep-seated lesions, malignant gliomas, and a higher number of attempted biopsies. Morbidity was not increased by sex, age, pre-existing illness, extracranial cancer, cardiac disease, hypertension, diabetes, HIV status, or the instrument used to obtain the specimen.

Conclusions.—Although complications associated with stereotactic brain biopsy are infrequent, they can be disastrous. Such morbidity may be minimized by modification of risk factors.

► It is important for us in radiology to keep up with the issues that face our surgical colleagues. We commonly, and occasionally very glibly, suggest or help plan stereotactic biopsies. It is also important for us to know the diagnostic yield, pathologic results, and complications of these procedures. This article was a retrospective review of 225 stereotactic biopsies from the "modern era" of 1983-1996. There was 1 fatality (from massive bleeding), 1 infection, and a nondiagnostic procedure in 10 patients (4.4%). The "morbidity group" included 12 patients, 5.3% of the study population. Most of these patients had lesions that were deep (eg, thalamus, brain stem) and often underwent multiple biopsy attempts (up to 44 in1 case). The other risk factors for complications of stereotactic biopsy included high-grade tumors (anaplastic astrocytoma and glioblastoma multiforme), preoperative medication with antiplatelet agents (including aspirin), and chronic steroid use.

J.G. Smirniotopoulos, M.D.

Diagnosis of Brain Death Using Two-Phase Spiral CT

Dupas B, Gayet-Delacroix M, Villers D, et al (Centre Hospitalier Universitaire de Nantes, France)

AJNR 19:641-647, 1998 8–55

Background.—Although clinical criteria alone are sufficient to establish brain death in some countries, additional procedures are needed in other countries. The usefulness of spiral CT in the diagnosis of brain death was investigated prospectively.

Methods.—Spiral CT was performed in 14 brain-dead and 11 healthy individuals by means of a 2-phase protocol. A nonionic iodinized contrast medium was injected intravenously, and 20 seconds later the CT table was drawn through the gantry at a rate of 10 mm/second while scanning was in progress. The second scanning phase was begun automatically at a mean 54 seconds later, using the same parameters. For each image in both phases, opacification or absence of opacification of carotid, vertebral, and basilar arteries and intracerebral veins was determined. Electroencephalopathy, angiography, or both verified the diagnosis of brain death.

Findings.—In the brain-dead individuals, the pericallosal and terminal arteries of the cortex did not opacify during the 2 phases of spiral CT. However, the superficial temporal arteries were always visible. The internal cerebral veins, the great cerebral vein, and the straight sinus did not opacify. The superior ophthalmic veins were visible on both sides on 13 occasions. The specificity was 100% for nonvascular opacification criteria on the right and left sides for each vessel type.

Conclusions.—Conventional angiography, which demonstrates the cessation of cerebral flow and establishes the diagnosis of brain death, is costly and time-consuming. The current 2-phase spiral CT protocol is an easy to apply, accurate method for demonstrating the absence of intracerebral blood flow in brain death.

► The diagnosis of brain death is usually not a pleasant enterprise for anyone involved. Traditional imaging methods for confirming brain death have relied on the cessation of cerebral blood flow. In addition to clinical examination and monitoring, angiography and nuclear medicine blood flow techniques are generally accepted as confirmatory tests for brain death. Recent reports have suggested that transcranial doppler and MRI or MR angiography may also be useful in the diagnosis of brain death. However, finding the ideal test to accurately confirm the clinical suspicion or diagnosis of brain death has received little attention from the newer CT imaging techniques.

This study is a prospective evaluation of the use of spiral CT in 14 patients. For comparison purposes, there were 11 healthy (not brain-dead) control subjects. The technique for demonstrating the absence of cerebral blood flow involved a two-phase multislice (spiral CT) imaging protocol—a bolus injection with imaging timed to illustrate first arterial and then venous opacification.

This protocol demonstrates the potential for spiral CT to replace angiography in the diagnosis of brain death. The appropriate role of this test, as compared with isotope scanning, is as yet unresolved. In legal jurisdictions where nuclear medicine tests are accepted in the diagnosis of brain death, there is the added advantage of using a portable gamma camera at the patient's bedside. However, in locales where angiography is still necessary, spiral CT may serve an important role. Further validation of this method with a larger series of cases, as well as acceptance by the appropriate legal and ethical organizations, will be needed before spiral CT can become a "standard" in the diagnosis of brain death.

J.G. Smirniotopoulos, M.D.

Outwitting the Blood-Brain Barrier for Therapeutic Purposes: Osmotic Opening and Other Means

Kroll RA, Neuwelt EA (Oregon Health Sciences Univ, Portland)
Neurosurgery 42:1083-1100, 1998 8–56

Background.—The presence of an intact blood-brain barrier (BBB) at the proliferating edge of a tumor has been proposed as a major factor in the failure of chemotherapy for CNS neoplasia. Recent advances in the delivery of therapeutic agents across the BBB for the treatment of intracerebral tumors and other neurologic diseases were discussed (Fig 2).

Discussion.—The osmotic BBB disruption procedure has been found to be a clinically useful technique. Such disruption seems to cause endothelial cell shrinkage, associated with the hypertonic environment, which opens the endothelial tight junctions constituting the BBB (Fig 3). Preclinical animal studies, which have played a fundamental role in advancing the understanding of the BBB and delivery of agents to the brain, will continue to have an integral function in efforts to improve the diagnosis and treatment of many neurologic disorders. Methods that modify the BBB or blood-tumor barrier to increase delivery of therapeutic agents have been tested clinically, with very favorable results in patients with brain tumors (Fig 6).

Conclusions.—Methods for "outwitting" the BBB are increasing in the treatment of patients with malignant CNS tumors. Such methods may also be useful for improving the delivery of diagnostic and therapeutic agents to infectious, genetic, and degenerative disorders of the CNS.

► This article provides a concise review of the basic principles of the BBB. The authors also discuss the means and the methods that can be used to disrupt the BBB for the therapeutic delivery of drugs into the brain.

J.G. Smirniotopoulos, M.D.

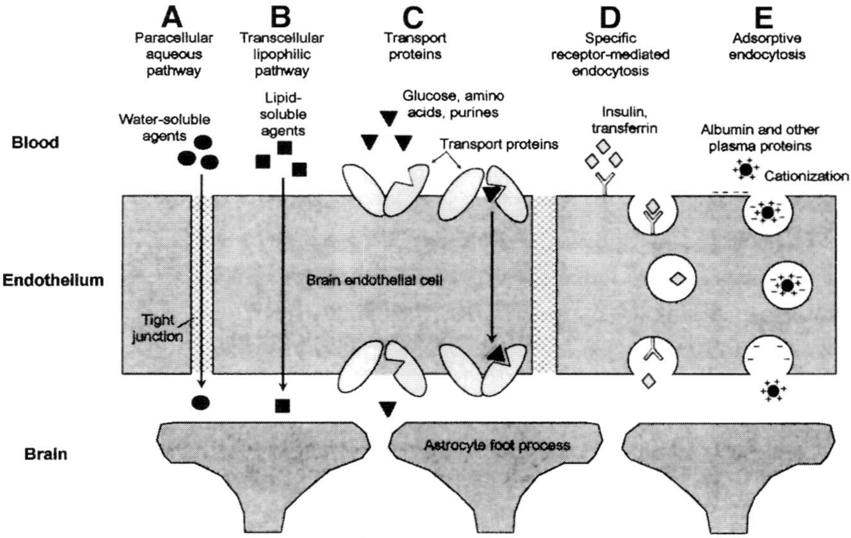

FIGURE 2.—Routes across the BBB. (Adapted from Aboot NJ, Romero IA: Transporting therapeutics across the blood-brain barrier. *Mol Med Today* 2:106-113, 1996. Courtesy of Kroll RA, Neuwelt EA: Outwitting the blood-brain barrier for therapeutic purposes: Osmotic opening and other means. *Neurosurgery* 42:1083-1100, 1998.)

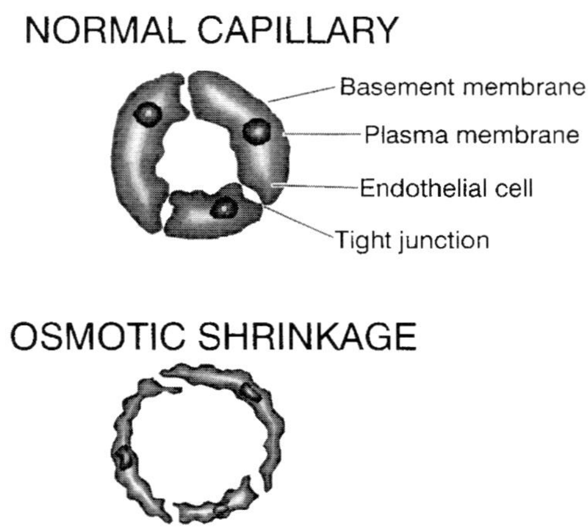

FIGURE 3.—Osmotic opening of the BBB. Osmotic disruption of the BBB seems to cause endothelial cell shrinkage, associated with the hypertonic environment, opening the endothelial tight junctions that constitute the anatomical basis of the barrier. (Adapted from Rapoport SI: *Blood-Brain Barrier in Physiology and Medicine*, New York, Raven Press, 1976. Courtesy of Kroll RA, Neuwelt EA: Outwitting the blood-brain barrier for therapeutic purposes: Osmotic opening and other means. *Neurosurgery* 42:1083-1100, 1998.)

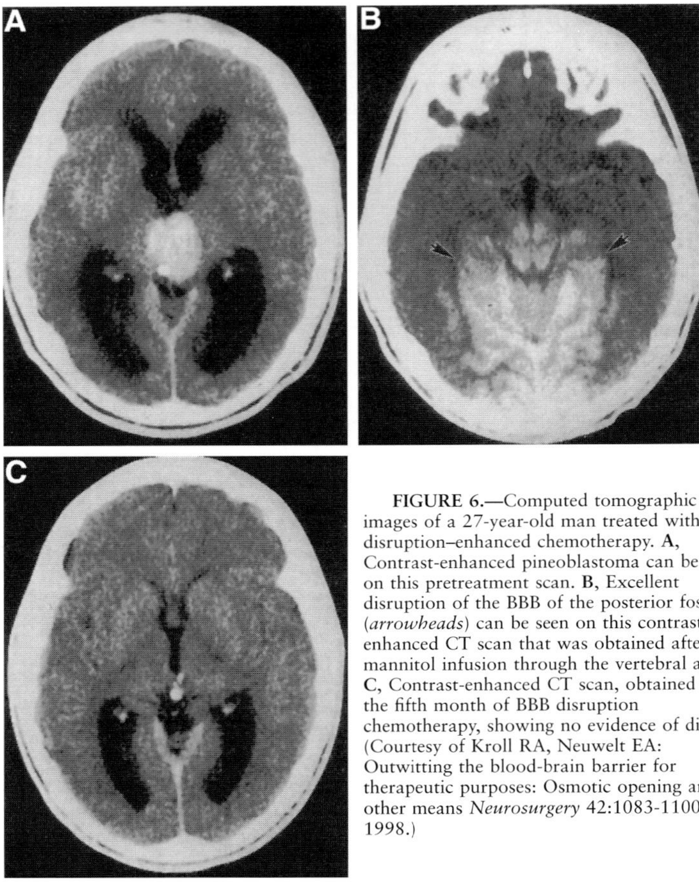

FIGURE 6.—Computed tomographic images of a 27-year-old man treated with BBB disruption–enhanced chemotherapy. **A**, Contrast-enhanced pineoblastoma can be seen on this pretreatment scan. **B**, Excellent disruption of the BBB of the posterior fossa (*arrowheads*) can be seen on this contrast-enhanced CT scan that was obtained after mannitol infusion through the vertebral artery. **C**, Contrast-enhanced CT scan, obtained after the fifth month of BBB disruption chemotherapy, showing no evidence of disease. (Courtesy of Kroll RA, Neuwelt EA: Outwitting the blood-brain barrier for therapeutic purposes: Osmotic opening and other means *Neurosurgery* 42:1083-1100, 1998.)

A Comparison of Two or Three Radiographic Views in the Diagnosis of Skull Fractures

McGlinchey I, Fleet MF, Eatock FC, et al (Western Infirmary, Glasgow, Scotland)

Clin Radiol 53:215-217, 1998 8–57

Background.—Many investigators have addressed the problem of appropriate patient selection for skull radiography, but few have studied which radiographic series of films should be obtained. The adequacy of a 2-view skull series compared with a 3-view skull series for diagnosing skull fracture in patients with a reliable history of the trauma site was reported.

Methods and Findings.—The radiographs of 50 patients diagnosed as having skull fractures were mixed with 200 normal skull series and independently reviewed by 3 interpreters. The films were tailored to the site of trauma: Taone's view G-occipital injury; occipitofrontal for frontal injury; and the appropriate lateral view. Diagnostic confidence levels were 94.4% and 94.6% for the 2-film and 3-film series, respectively. Of 150 skull fracture series viewed as 2 films, 58% were diagnosed correctly, with a confidence level of 92.7%. When viewed as 3 films, 61.3% were diagnosed correctly, with a confidence level of 93%. In an analysis of false-positive and false-negative results, the 2-film and 3-film series did not differ.

Conclusions.—A 2-view skull series did not hinder diagnostic accuracy or the confidence of interpretation, compared with a 3-view series, in patients with an accurate clinical history of head trauma. Thus, a 2-view skull series can be safely adopted in the routine evaluation of head injury in such patients.

► We often forget about the issues of radiation exposure when most of our work is controlled by technology such as CT for examination of the head. However, we all must be proactive in working to limit patient exposure to ionizing radiation, especially when the exposure has limited value or efficacy. Using a blinded comparison, these authors were able to show that for most patients only 2 views (1 lateral and 1 frontal) are necessary for a screening skull series. Most of us would recommend a screening CT, rather than a skull series, when an ER patient needs a neuroradiologic evaluation. Still, this study is significant in that it provides some objective statistical validity for those who wish to limit X ray exposure in the context of a "skull series."

J.G. Smirniotopoulos, M.D.

Analysis of Missed Cases of Abusive Head Trauma

Jenny C, Hymel KP Lt Col, Ritzen A, et al (Brown Univ, Providence, RI; Lifespan Med Computing, Providence, RI; Natl Naval Med Ctr, Bethesda, Md; et al)

JAMA 281:621-626, 1999 8–58

Background.—Abusive head trauma (AHT) is a form of child abuse that is both dangerous and difficult to diagnose in young children. The current study determined how often AHT was missed at 1 center and the factors associated with the unrecognized diagnosis.

Methods.—All cases of head trauma seen between 1990 and 1995 at an academic children's hospital were reviewed. The chart review disclosed 173 children younger than 3 years with head injuries caused by abuse.

Findings.—Physicians did not recognize AHT in 31.2% of the abused children. Among this group, mean time to correct diagnosis was 7 days, with a range of 0-189 days. The diagnosis was more likely to be missed in very young white children from intact families and in children without respiratory compromise or seizures. In 7 children with unrecognized AHT, misinterpretation of radiologic studies contributed to the delay in diagnosis. Twenty-eight percent of the children were injured again after the missed diagnosis. Complications associated with the missed diagnosis occurred in 40.7%. Four of the 5 deaths among the children with unrecognized AHT might have been prevented had abuse been recognized earlier.

Conclusions.—Diagnosing AHT in very young children can be difficult in the absence of a history of abuse. Clinicians must consider this diagnosis in infants and young children with nonspecific clinical signs.

▶ The authors studied cases of AHT in children under 3 years of age, ultimately including 173 patients. Psychosocial bias on the part of health care providers was a significant source of error; when the patient came from an intact (2-parent) white family, child abuse was likely to be underdiagnosed. Similarly, when the signs and symptoms were mild (the patient did not have seizures or respiratory problems), AHT was also likely to be overlooked. The authors pointed out that in the youngest children (younger than 6 months) neurologic development does not yet provide good objective criteria for evaluation of the neurologic status.

The authors made several recommendations for improvement in clinical practice:

1. There should be a thorough inspection of the head and face for bruises.
2. Always consider AHT in young children with nonspecific symptoms (irritability, vomiting, etc.)
3. Watch the supernatant from a lumbar puncture for signs of xanthochromia to rule out a traumatic spinal tap
4. "Pediatrically trained radiologists should be consulted . . ."

Dilated retinal examination and routine CT scans probably may not be needed in every child. However, both are probably underutilized, partially accounting for missed cases of child abuse.

J.G. Smirniotopoulos, M.D.

Cerebrospinal Fluid Fistula: Detection With MR Cisternography

El Gammal T, Sobol W, Wadlington VR, et al (Univ of Alabama, Birmingham)

AJNR 19:627-631, 1998 8–59

Background.—MR cisternography has been used recently to diagnose a variety of intracranial lesions, including CSF fistulas. The role of MR cisternography in the assessment of patients with possible CSF rhinorrhea was reported.

Methods.—Magnetic resonance cisternography was performed in 37 patients over a period of 3 years. A heavily T2-weighted fast spin-echo study with fat suppression and video reversal of the images was used. Subsequently, 24 patients underwent exploratory surgery for fistula.

Findings.—Findings on MR cisternography were significantly correlated with surgical findings. The sensitivity, specificity, and accuracy of MR cisternography were 87%, 57%, and 78%, respectively (Figs 3, 4, and 9).

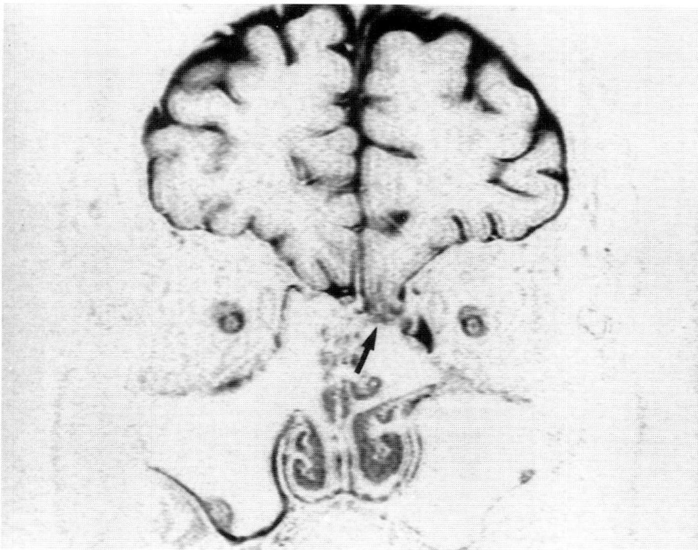

FIGURE 3.—Positive MR cisternography in a patient with brain herniation (*arrow*) into the left anterior ethmoidal sinus after endoscopic surgery. The brain herniation was confirmed at surgery. (This case was not included in the statistical evaluation.) (Courtesy of El Gammal T, Sobol W, Wadlington VR, et al: Cerebrospinal fluid fistula: Detection with MR cisternography. *AJNR* 19:627-631, 1998, copyright by American Society of Neuroradiology.)

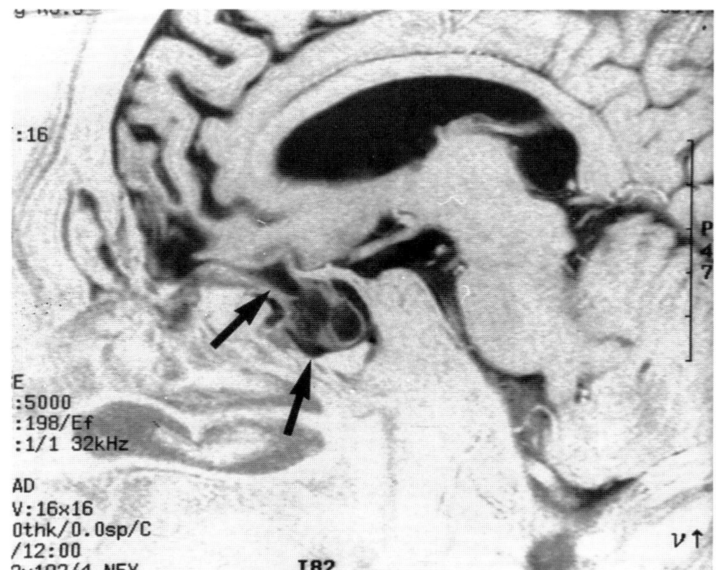

FIGURE 4.—Positive MR cisternography in a patient with posttraumatic herniation of contused brain into the sphenoidal sinus (*arrows*). The patient also had another fistula into the anterior ethmoidal sinus. (Courtesy of El Gammal T, Sobol W, Wadlington VR, et al: Cerebrospinal fluid fistula: Detection with MR cisternography. *AJNR* 19:627-631, 1998, copyright by American Society of Neuroradiology.)

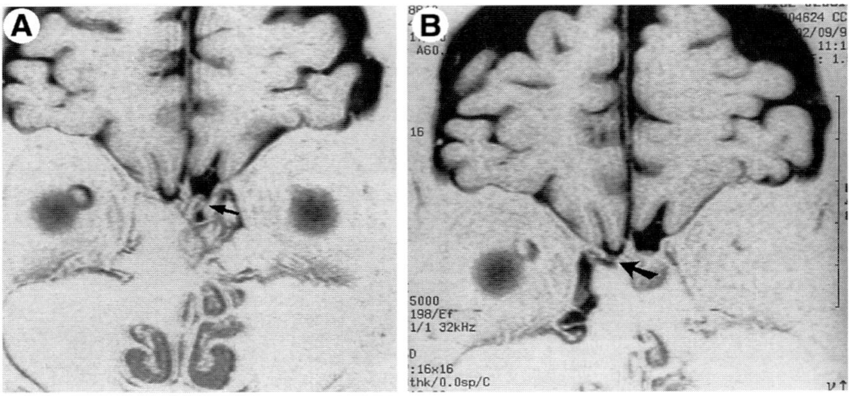

FIGURE 9.—Postendoscopic sinus surgery fistula. **A**, narrow left anterior ethmoidal fistulous tract. No bone defect was seen on coronal CT scan (not shown). The fistula was confirmed and repaired at endoscopic surgery. **B**, a relatively wide right ethmoidal fistula (*arrow*) is seen on coronal MR cisternogram. The fistula and rhinorrhea occurred in the same patient as in **A** 11 months after successful endoscopic closure of the left ethmoidal fistula. The right-sided fistula was confirmed and repaired at endoscopic surgery. (Courtesy of El Gammal T, Sobol W, Wadlington VR, et al: Cerebrospinal fluid fistula: Detection with MR cisternography. *AJNR* 19:627-631, 1998, copyright by American Society of Neuroradiology.)

Conclusions.—MR cisternography is an accurate imaging modality for the diagnosis of suspected CSF rhinorrhea. The authors recommend the use of plain thin-section coronal CT scans followed by MR cisternography in such patients.

► MR cisternography offers considerable advantages over previous techniques, including the obvious distinction of being a noninvasive and noncontrast examination. The authors report here the results of 45 studies in 37 patients. The protocol used is fairly generic and can be applied on many commonly used clinical scanners. The total examination time was reported as 48 minutes, which is certainly tolerable when this type of information is needed. The authors recommend, however, that thin-section CT should be performed routinely before MR cisternography to allow the exam to be focused in areas of visible bone defects.

J.G. Smirniotopoulos, M.D.

Subject Index

A

B

C

D

F

G

M

N

O

P

Q

R

S

T

U

V

W

X

Author Index

A

B

C

D

Y

Z